pursuit:365

365 Inspiring Stories, in 365 Words, by 365 Canadian Women

Shelly Lynn Hughes

Editor: Andreia McLean

Creative Director & Typeset: Justin Lloyd

Book Cover Design: Nicole O'Keefe

First Printing, March 2021

Published by Ho'ola Publishing

hoolapublishing.com

pursuit365.ca

Foreword

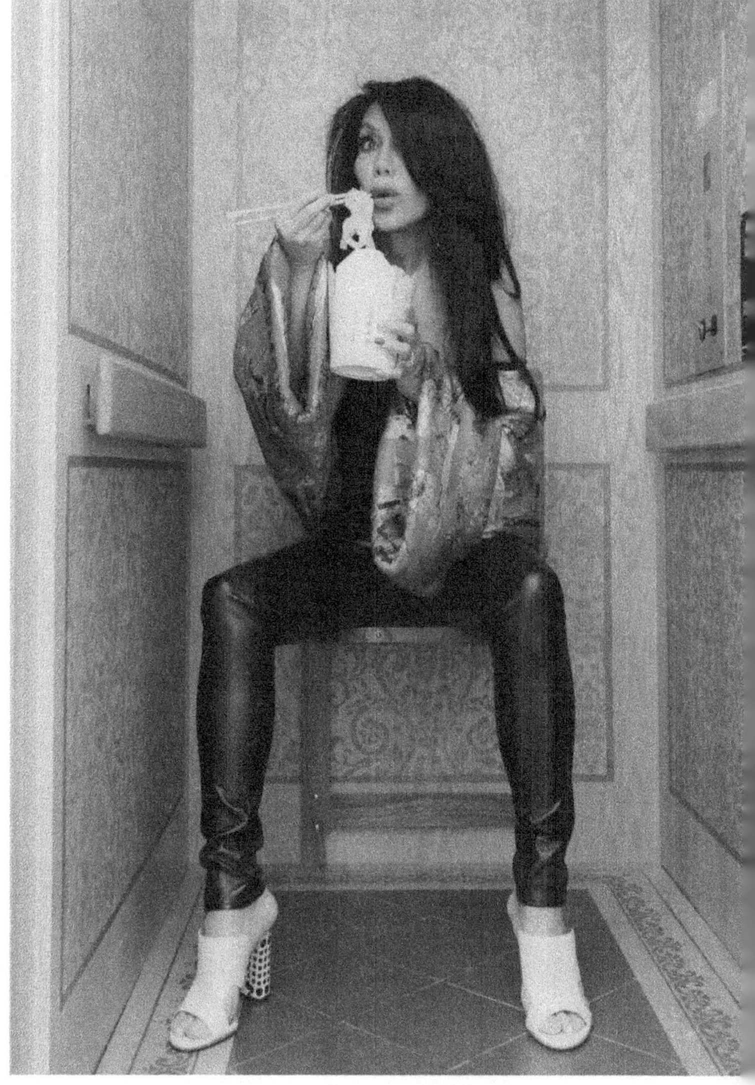

My mother, in her infinite wisdom, had sat me down one day and told me the story about the end of her marriage. I had always had her on a pedestal, had thought she was strong, and everything had come easy... until then. Apparently, she had taken her diamond encrusted wedding ring off, thrown it at her husband (my father), and walked out. Five children, years of being physically beaten and belittled, she had (in a moment which likely seemed like a surprise to him) tossed the symbol of their unity and never looked back.

That moment, that moment she told me, it did not describe the pain she endured, it did not equate to years of abuse or the mere fact that she just may have married the wrong person... it did not tell of the courage it took for her to tell me the story or the pain that was behind what led to that action ... but it did tell me, succinctly, that she had survived, that she was human and she had done and could find hope, even at the most difficult of times. It is her story, and no one could tell it better than the author.

There are 365 stories captured in these pages ... stories that took courage to write, to peel back sometimes painful layers. What we learn from stories is that we are not alone, that someone else had to overcome something similar (or sometimes worse) – these stories tell us that others share our fears, our challenges and that we are human....and through this we can, like others, find hope...even in the most difficult times.

At the end of the day, when I set off on my own life, I was stronger. I did not blame my mother for the pain she had endured, I looked at her as someone I loved and someone that was not brought into the world for me to put on judgement day... her sharing her story made me see the other side of her and realize there is always "a story"... we just have to listen. These 365 stories are for you, they are a gift presented from the heart. Open your gift and you will open your mind.

Dr. Ann Kaplan, DBA, MSc, MBA, ICD.D
President & CEO of iFinance Canada Inc.

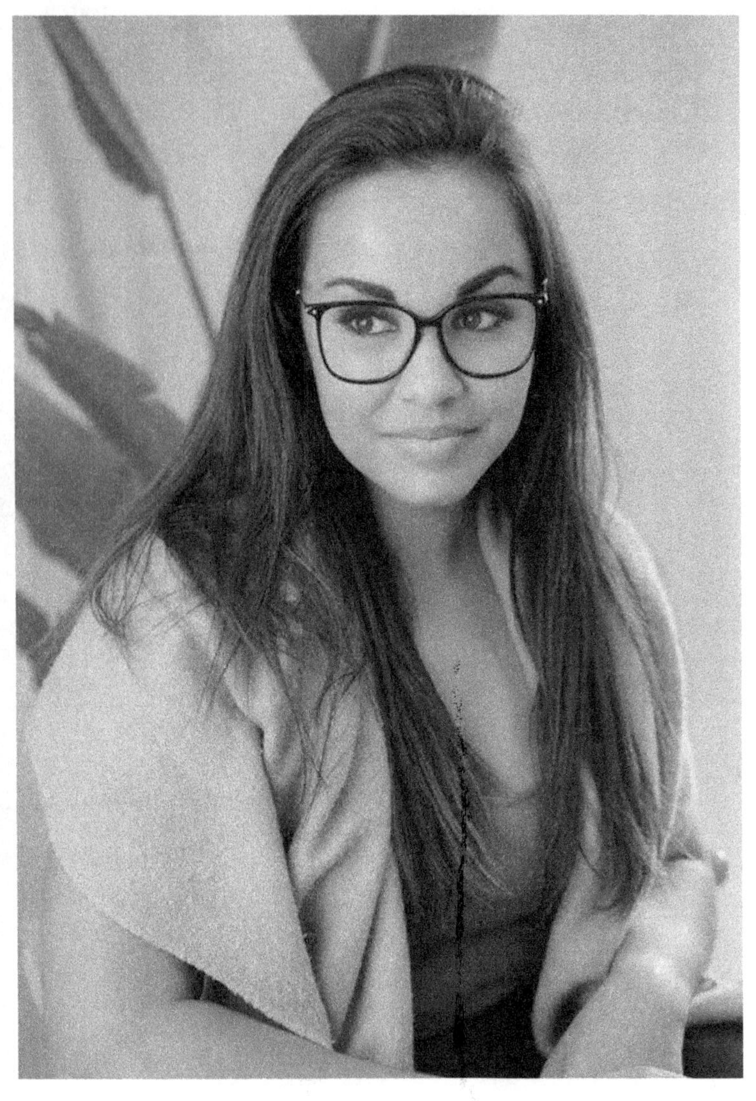

Andreia McLean sees potential, homes in on it, and works tirelessly to amplify it. Specializing in communicating and connecting, taking on the role of editor for the pursuit:365 book came naturally. Andreia (Dre) is the founder of Events by Dre. She works predominantly with women-owned businesses, elevating their interactions with in-person events, digital experiences, and communications-based projects.

Editor

Andreia McLean

When Shelly came to me with this concept, my first reaction was, "yes!" My second reaction was, "wait... how fast do we want to execute this?" But Shelly is a person of action, and with full trust in her, the team she put together, and the idea that in the midst of 2020, I could be part of a team working to elevate and inspire people, I was in.

There is a tremendous responsibility with the nature of this project as an editor. I was the first to read these incredible stories of heartache, loss, and triumph. The pursuit of fulfillment, success, and happiness is such a broad topic, and yet, I found so many patterns emerge throughout editing these amazing stories. It seems that true happiness and fulfillment require adversity, that people will always matter infinitely more than titles or money, and that through time, we can heal even the most inconceivable emotional wounds if we find the courage to push through.

It is my hope that when you pick this book up, you feel inspired, moved, motivated, and feel connected to these women's stories. Going through these stories while editing, I cried real human tears, laughed, got angry, and felt second-hand pride. It has been an amazing experience connecting with each of these women and I can't wait for these stories to be read. There is a piece of each of us to be found in every story in this collection.

Shelly Lynn Hughes is always on the go, finding new ways to elevate the people around her and showcase amazing stories. Through her businesses, Project Her and Fresh Magazine, Shelly is always looking to connect great people in a way that makes their lives richer.

Publisher

Shelly Lynn Hughes

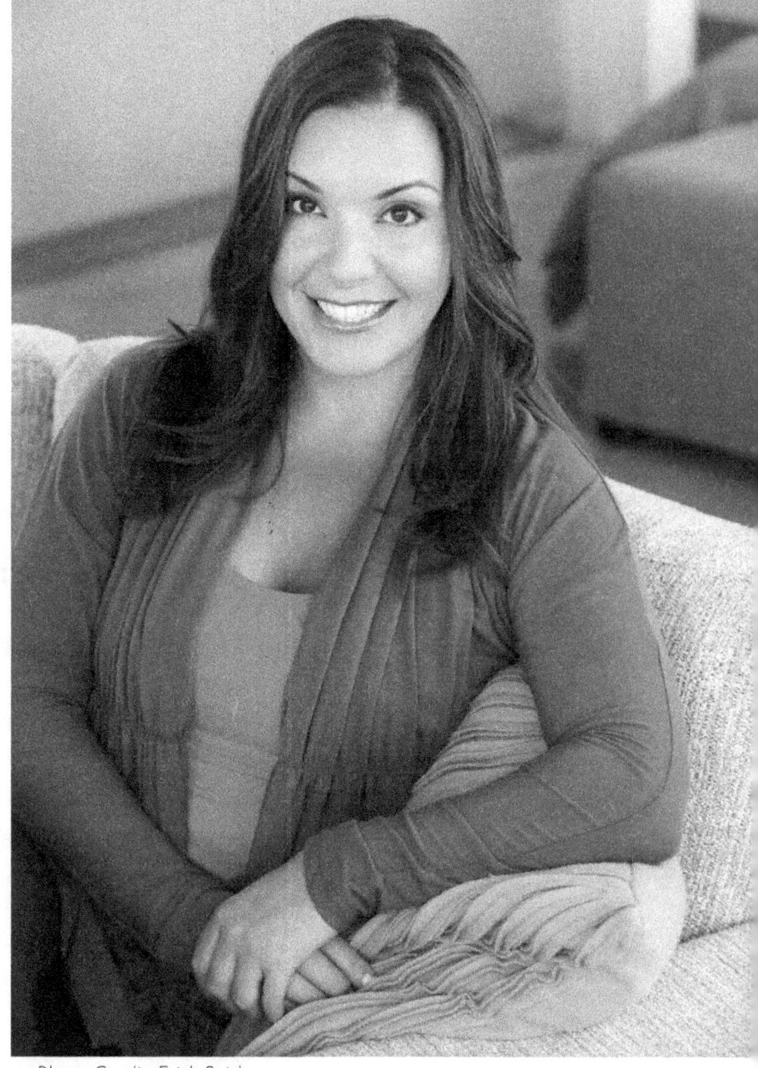

Photo Credit: Erich Saide

There are so many stories to tell. Women are the backbone of society and with this book, I sought out to find Canadian women to tell their own stories through the lens of what is most important to them. We filled this book with an incredible and diverse group of women, all connected through a network of referrals, and with the collaborative intent to elevate one another.

I love when women feel like they're not alone. A lot of the time we go through life thinking we're by ourselves and everyone else's lives are perfect. When we hear other people's stories, it emboldens and empowers us to know that things will always get better. We're allowed to feel, and we're not alone.

This project was created with the intention of connecting women together – to connect us all. I want to bring people hope by highlighting 365 talented, kind, interesting, and valuable women, and put forth the concept that we can accomplish so much when we collaborate.

I hope you enjoy the journeys encompassed in this book as much as we have!

Dedicated to my daughters Ainslee and Tasha, my mother Suzette, my grandmother Elspeth. And to every little girl and woman, never doubt you are valuable, powerful, and beautiful inside and out.

Tosca Reno is a New York Times bestselling author, founder of Eat Clean® Revolution, Gemini Award winner, motivational speaker, lightworker, and a voice for women.

Tosca Reno

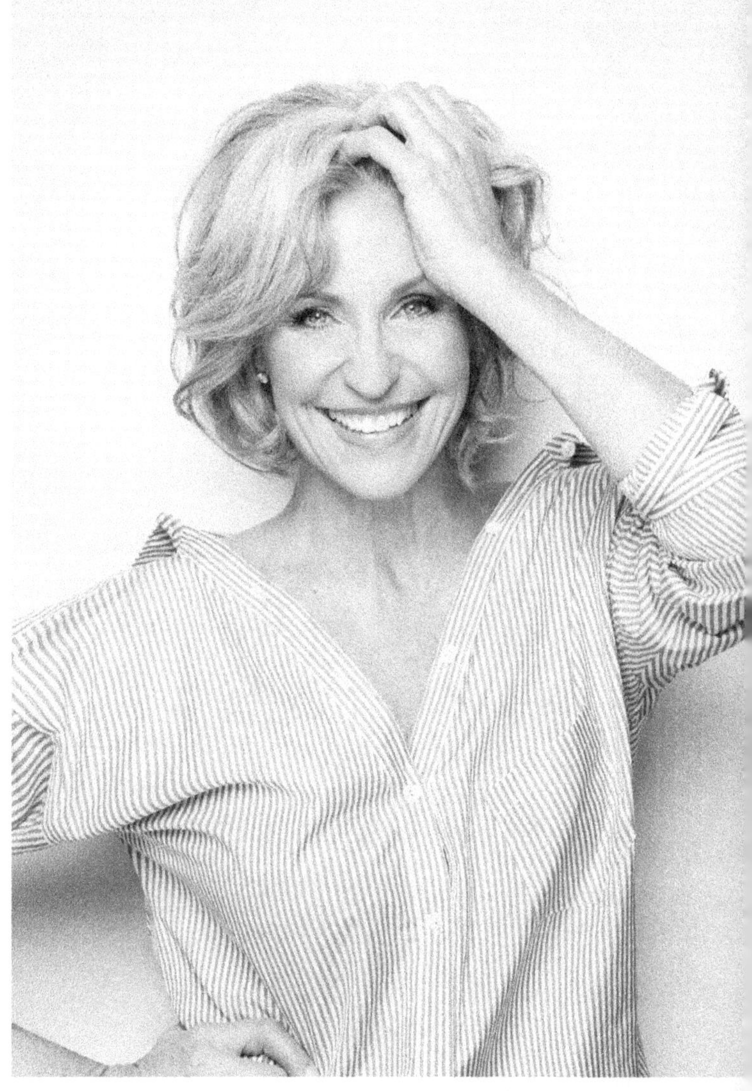

This is me showing up as me. Not someone else's idea of what they think I should be. I had a good ride; I learned a lot, but I am a new person now. My life lessons are many and painful, but I am grateful for them all. I can say that now.

I was so angry at one point I took all Bob's designer suits and tossed them on the driveway, then drove the car over them a few times. I was broke and broken. My first step to growth was leaving my first husband. There was far too much domestic violence. I became a warrior for myself and walked right into freedom and possibilities.

But what now? What I needed was to become successful in my own right and I vowed to do that. I didn't know how or at what, but I just knew that my being successful would sting far more than a few dollars from him. And I found it. I really did. I committed to the hard work. I trained, got lean, ate clean, and began to tell that new story. And it was brilliant. That feeling of overcoming – it's good medicine. I fell too. Everything broke apart. In 2011 ... 2012 ... 2013 .... I had to start again. From zero.

My best work is yet to come because of a depth of internal wealth, an understanding of so many life experiences, that makes me more approachable than being the woman in a bikini and stripper shoes – I am just like those who read my books and follow me – peaks and valleys, perfectly imperfect. This is my story now. I'm happy that I am willing to show up, just as I am, and be ok with that. What I love is the raw stuff. The surprises. The me that will have a powerful impact on the world in a new way. She's a leader. A renegade. A pioneer.

To my younger self, I would say; continue to show up as this soul – you are needed, and your best work is yet to come. Never dim your light as I know you've done because others are threatened by it. The world needs you just as you are. Shine on. I believe!

Jennifer Henczel is an Award-Winning Leader, Author, Speaker, Podcaster, Producer and Founder of Inspired Influencers.

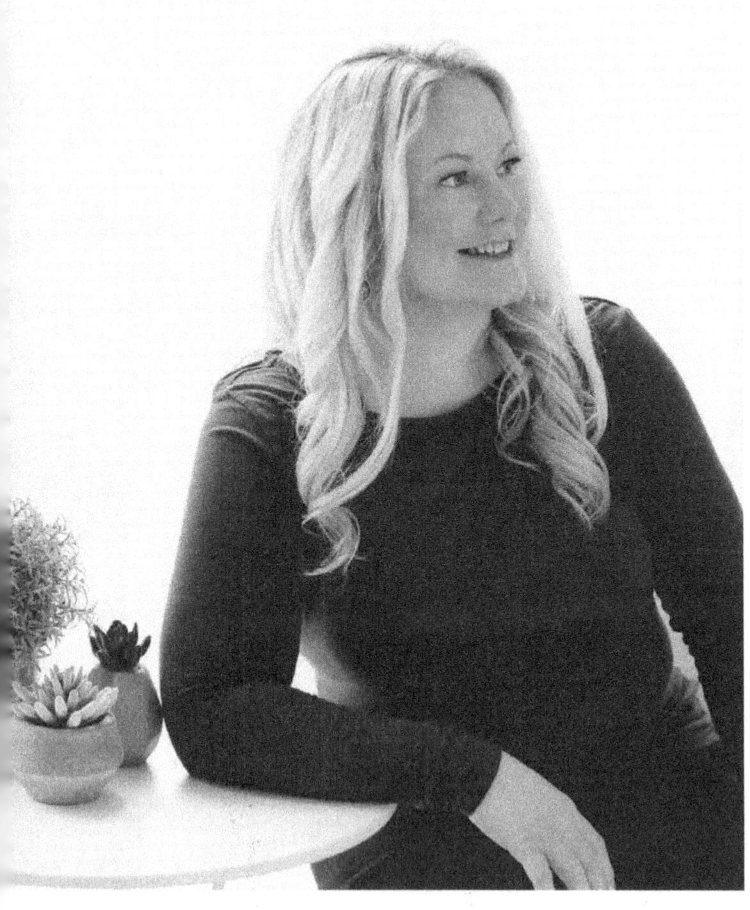

Jennifer Henczel

I love helping others with igniting their inner influencer, finding joy in their journey, and leveling up their lifestyle. But it's taken many steps to find my path.

Have you ever felt stuck? For many years I had become stuck in my life and business. After a life changing tragedy in my family, I discovered some major mindset shifts that made all the difference. I started by creating a community. It was a group for entrepreneurs, which quickly grew into a thriving business network. I found out that for anything to work, you need to be part of a community. You need to build your circle of support around you, it's not going to build itself. People will help you if you show up to be helped.

Since then, I've created many communities and helped thousands of entrepreneurs, coaches, trainers, and speakers to increase their impact and influence. I show them how to generate multiple streams of income from their expertise and start movements from their messages. I enjoy leading people through a process of creating harmony and abundance for themselves, while serving the world with their purpose.

In my podcast, I've had the honour of interviewing today's top thought leaders, storytellers, and legacy builders. Check it out on your favourite podcast platform to tap into timeless wisdom and get tools for transcending to new levels of success, happiness, and joy. I was able to turn my tragedy into triumph, and I want you to know that you can do it, too.
My communities continue to grow because people want to connect, and guess what, people want to connect with YOU!

I have fostered many joint ventures and love creating opportunities for leaders to cultivate meaningful connections and collaborations. Building a business or non-profit can be isolating. So, as you start each new day, I want to challenge you to show up! Be the change, be the solution, and be the leader you were born to be. I encourage you to reach out into your community. It's all about building relationships every step along your journey. We're better together!
You can book a strategy session with me, join as a member of my community and listen to my podcast at www.inspiredinfluencers.com.

Angela Feser is a Content Creator, Yoga Instructor, wife, mom of two, and lover of nature, paddle boarding, and her animals.

Angela Feser

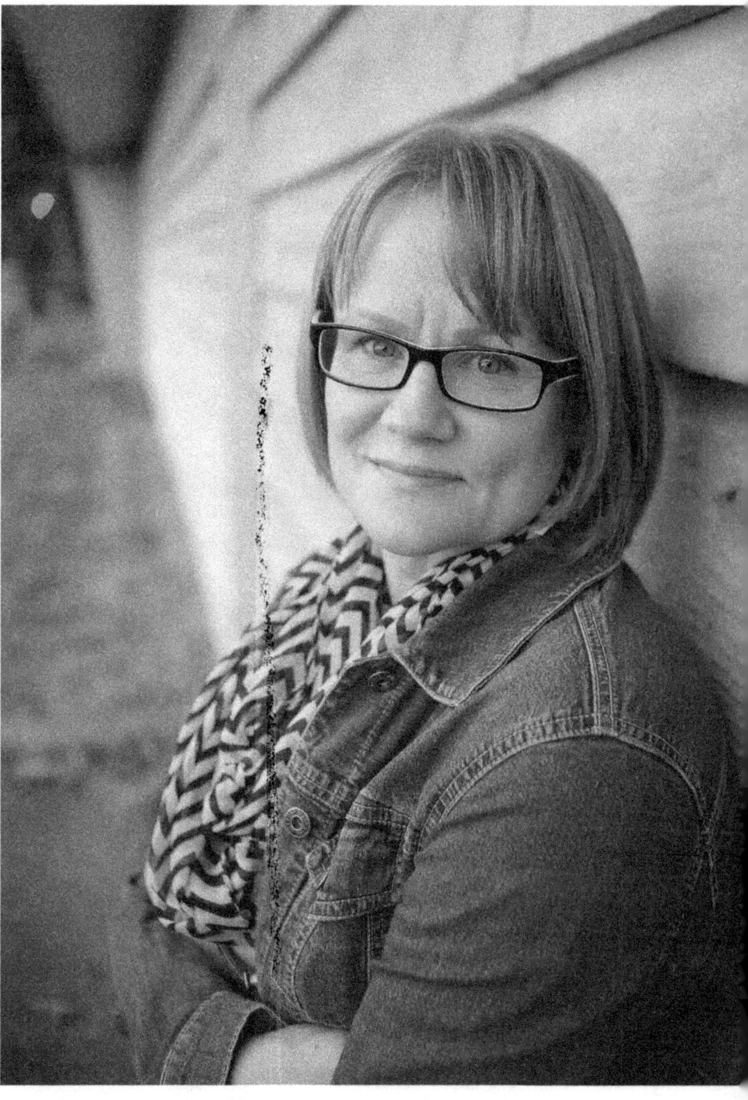

For a long time, I had a business idea brewing, but didn't know how to bring all of my passions together in a single offering that would serve the world in a positive way. I had a successful career before I had kids but being in a cubicle everyday was not satisfying. So, after our first child was born, I did not return to that cubicle. Instead, I wanted to find something that made me happy and fulfilled my passions.

As the wife of a first responder, I know what it means to sacrifice for your community. Celebrating every minute of life has become a way of life. After two back surgeries, I learned the hard way that you must take care of yourself before taking care of others, developing a deep appreciation for daily self-care. This is where my Yoga career began, and I became a licensed yoga instructor. As an organized creative, I wanted a way to more consistently express my creativity in my online community. All of these experiences have culminated in a new approach. Both yoga and online content creation have allowed me to practice creativity daily, opening my mind to new things, and thus has allowed me to expand my online world, helping so many different types of businesses and individuals. I love the variety this work entails.

This pursuit has resulted in an entrepreneurial adventure that has opened up the world in ways I never expected. I founded Angela's Social Bliss Blueprint, providing content creation and scheduling services to assist coaches, speakers, and other professionals. This allows me to express myself creatively while saving my clients time, so they can celebrate life in their own way. It's a win-win situation for all involved.

My clients rave about my talent and how they love my images. With my help they feel freer with their time and access a broader audience with ease, which enables them to focus on what they enjoy and do best.
Engaging with your audience regularly is essential for every personal brand and business today. Success to me is helping my clients achieve consistency, organization, and bliss in their everyday lives. I utilize all the tools of my yoga and meditation training, including balance and positive thinking, in every aspect of my life from parenting to content development, and beyond.

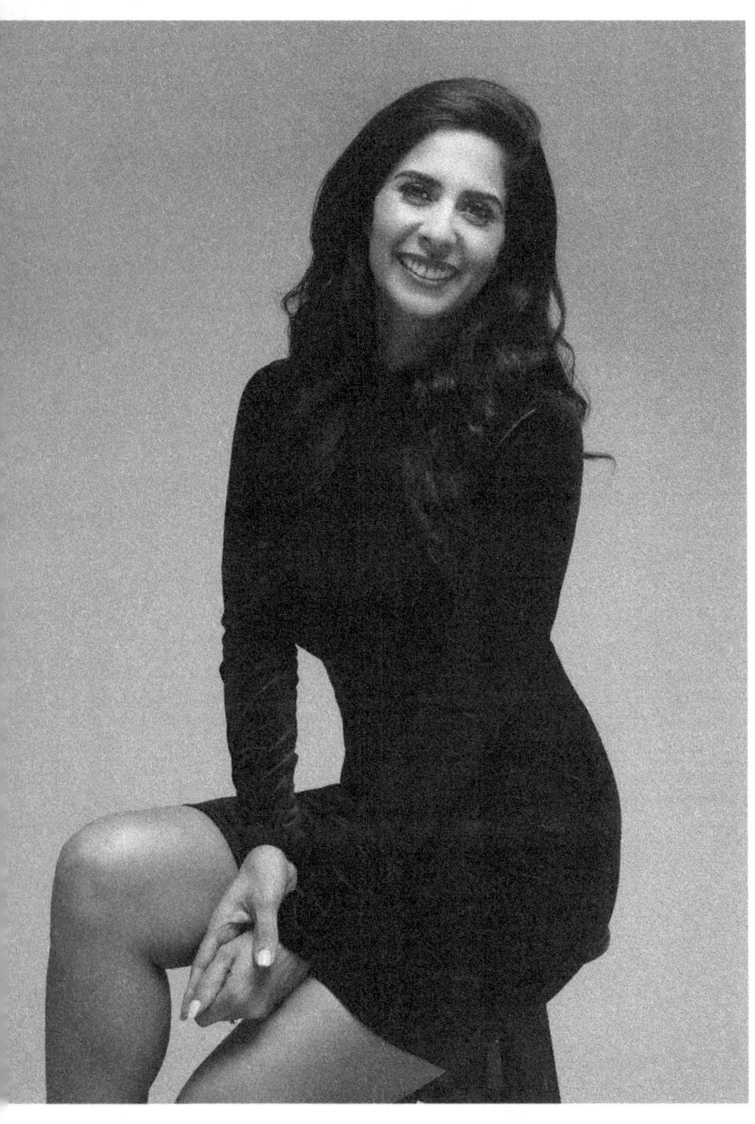

Nisha Khare BA, BEd, MEd is a Registered Clinical Counsellor whose continual growth stems from her personal belief that you never stop learning.

Nisha Khare

Through her work as a director/producer at Human Biography, she is passionate about weaving narrative into her documentaries, creating video content with icons like Katy Perry and Susan Sarandon, and channeling her inner strength as a "Woman of Wonder". She also partners with fashion, family and beauty focussed brands to tell their stories. While creating all this magic, Nisha continues to empower herself and those around her to move past the status quo and into the extraordinary.

"Women of Wonder" is a collective with the goal of connecting women to tap into their superpowers and elevate each other's lives.

It's an idea that has been manifested and curated in partnership with my incredible friend and visionary, Karly Neveu. Being part of creating this movement has ignited my curiosity and furthered my journey of self-discovery, while making connections within the incredible community of conscious women globally.

Through all the various projects, finding the potential for personal growth has been exceptionally gratifying. The unknown often leads to the greatest lessons in my experience. When speaking at the United Nations to share my message on "Powerful Partnerships", I was humbled with the knowledge that my ideas were being widely well received, and that something I created was having an impact on this world of ours. I was driven to do more and now I am proud to champion stories, ideas, and growth for a living. Some of the greatest lessons one could hope to learn are those that come from within, that come from my personal relationship with myself. Self-love is my answer. I was once blessed by the Dalai Lama, and while documenting his holiness, I realized in that moment that anything is possible. A small-town girl, from Prince George, British Columbia, who worked in a pulp mill now finds herself in perpetual spiritual discovery and striving for equanimity.

As a Registered Clinical Counsellor, I have created the opportunity to engage in fascinating exchanges in front of both live and digital audiences about mental health and spiritual growth. During my live online interviews, "Wellness Chats with Nisha" for the Stigma Free Society, I am also a part of the audience wanting to know how to inspire, cope, and grow through challenging times as a woman, a mother, a wife, and as a leader. The legacy of a person is dependent upon what a person does and creates, and I want mine to be of love, collaboration, and inspiration.

Jen is a problem solver with an insatiable desire to inspire others to chase their dreams as she chases hers.

Jen Govier

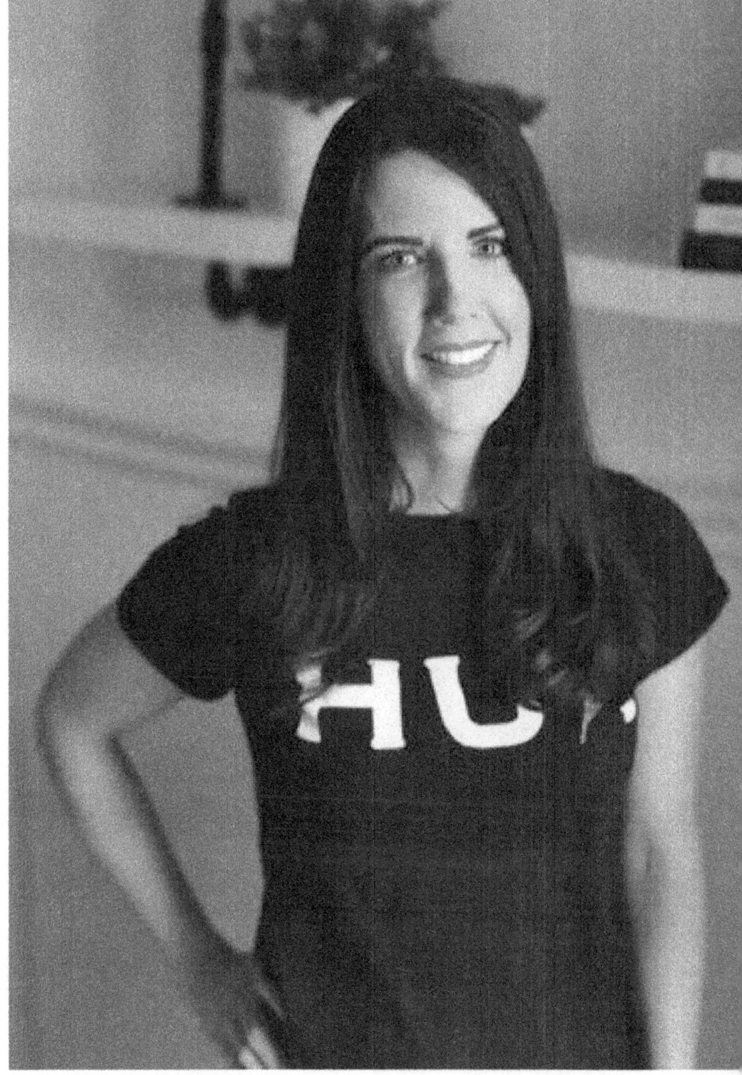

Photo Credit: Isabelle Mcmillan

I was always a dreamer! I remember tagging along with my Dad when he was cutting rich people's lawns and would pretend, I lived there. I would look through the windows and imagine myself eating popcorn on the big cozy couch. This was my dad's second job. He had ten kids to feed. My mom was a stay-at-home mom who made sure there was always a warm meal on the table. Both my parents knew what it was like to go hungry and ensured we never did. The greatest lesson they taught us, kindness doesn't cost a thing and yet the value it brings to someone is endless. My upbringing has shaped the way I see the world. I appreciate the little things and will take kindness over money all day long.

Interestingly though, I have worked in Finance my entire career. I have had a variety of different roles but loved most to inspire others to see their strength. I am a dreamer...I wanted to make a bigger impact on the world by helping others but wasn't exactly sure how.

The Universe has a funny way of making things happen! I was in the middle of a workout and got a glimpse of my unsightly camel toe...lol sorry, no better description. I immediately went on a mission to solve the problem. When I couldn't find what I was looking for on the market, I thought, why can't I invent it? So I did. That is how HUX ~ Helpful Underwear Xtreme was born.

It didn't happen overnight, and it wasn't easy. It has been four years in the making, 22 prototypes later, 80-hour work weeks, juggling two jobs, not having a clue what I was doing, raising two teenage sons with my husband, trying to keep doubt at bay and I am JUST getting started. While I have invented an amazing product that solves a real problem for women...HUX is about so much more! My goal is to inspire others to chase their dream. You don't have to have all the answers. If you take one small step every day in the direction you want to go...you WILL get there. Make the work you do about helping others and you will NEVER go wrong.

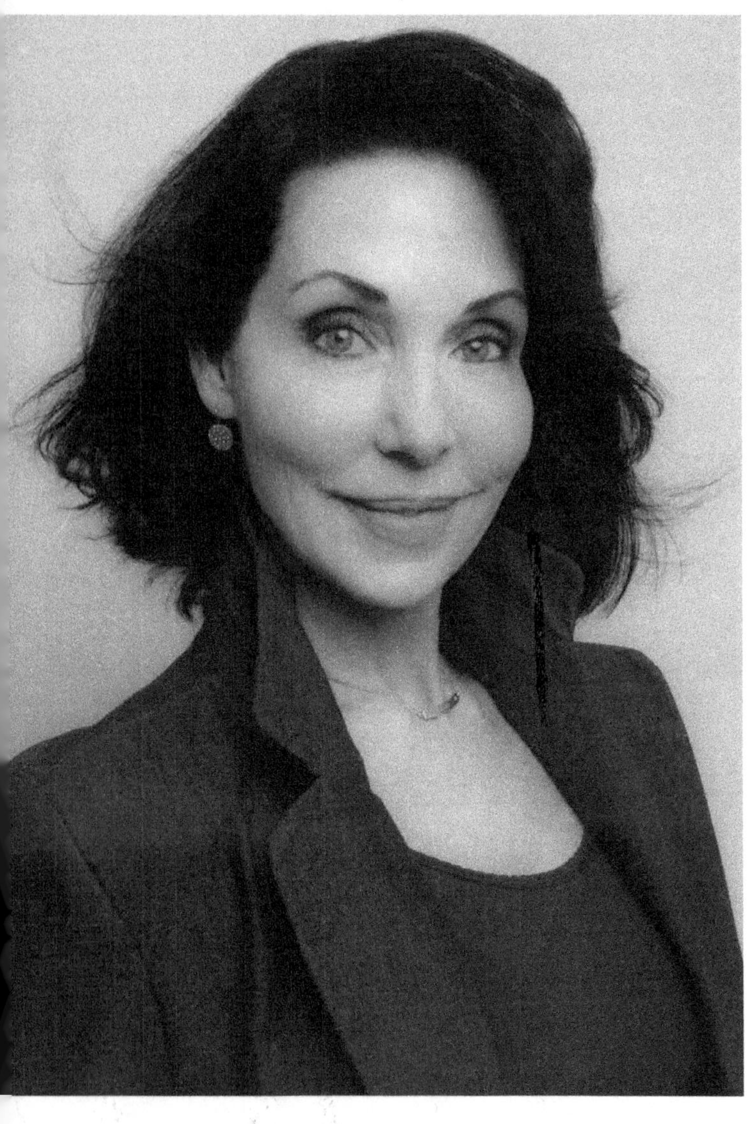

Alana is a mother, a fitness coach, a published Author of Strength Training Over 40, and a new business owner; all of which she achieved in her own unique (and some might argue, questionable) timeline!

Alana Collins

When asked by a friend to describe me as a child in just one word, my dad quickly responded, 'Defiant!' I was shocked! I saw myself as a conformist and people pleaser! How had I forgotten that feisty little girl and become so fearful of being different at the ripe old age of 25?

My dad's description of my younger self reminded me of that scrawny, little girl who was determined to never expose vulnerability, which I suppose could've been misconstrued as defiance. At an early age, I'd somehow decided that fairness was of paramount importance to me. I literally stuck my neck out in defense of justice like the 'Banty Rooster' my family often called me.

In retrospect, I'd prioritized the opinions of others over my own and transformed into the obedient girl I thought I was supposed to be. I had hushed my voice and had no clue where I stood. Yet more years would need to pass before I'd find a way to make peace with decades of marriage spent lost and alone.

Today I find myself negotiating my way through life as a single woman and parent, which has been a time of profound self-discovery and has allowed me to re-acquaint myself with the girl I'd left behind. I'm forever grateful for the stubborn, defiant, incorrigible girl who has emerged, with the rough edges softened by kindness, empathy, and the ability to keep an open mind. I've accepted that she's who I am and that I'm not meant to be everybody's cup of tea. I've learned that it's permissible, and sometimes necessary, to ruffle a few feathers!

I've also accepted that I'm on a different timeline than most people, exemplified by giving birth to my first biological child just days from turning 45, beginning a new fitness career in my 50's, and opening my Fitness Studio; a business owner for the first time at 63!

It isn't always easy living life out of sync with society's expectations, gearing up while most people my age are winding down. But the liberation of truly embracing who I am is utterly exhilarating, and I look forward to defying 'normalcy' for as long as I can!

Dannica Lamoureux is an award-winning Makeup Artist, National Trainer, and TV Spokesperson

Dannica Lamoureux

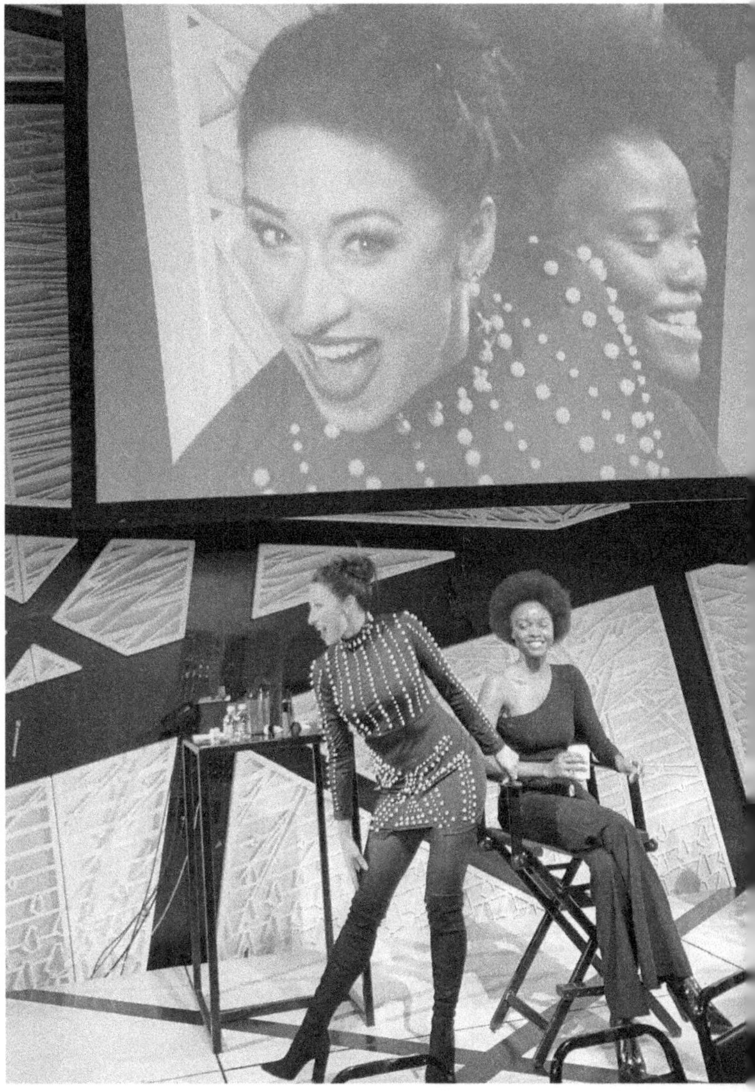

Dannica, spelled with two letter N's. Why, you ask? I was born in room 7, on the 7th floor of the hospital, on January the 7th, at 7:07 a.m., weighing 7lbs and 7oz. My parents realized my name needed seven letters, but they loved the name Danica, so they added another letter n. Lucky number 7 and an epilepsy diagnosis set the stage for the course of my life. During school, I developed mild seizures, which created learning gaps. The medications I had to take changed me from an active outgoing child into a couch potato. My mother decided to take me off the medication, but the learning gaps remained. There wasn't a lot of support to fill in gaps back then, so I became a creative and an outside-the-box problem solver. I was struggling to figure out what I wanted for myself until someone asked me to visualize what I thought success looked like.

Visualization is the key to future success! Closing my eyes and creating picture goals helped manifest the positive outcomes in my life. You must know what you want with details, feel the emotions that go with that, and then grit and persevere. While working at MAKE UP FOR EVER, I approached the company with my ideal job description and, after going back and forth, the woman I had visualized, wearing a suit jacket sitting in the super-elite airport lounge, materialized. I had become MAKE UP FOR EVER's Canadian National trainer and their representative on Today's Shopping Choice.

I have learned that life happens in moments that shape you, some difficult and some joyful. I choose to focus on the joyful. If you are self-aware and respect yourself and others you can be candid about joy and pain. Educating and working on live TV has taught me that words are important, be cautious and mindful of how you use them. Trust your intuition; if something doesn't feel right, you are moving in the wrong direction. Visualize and feel the emotions of achieving your goals. Trust yourself, know your worth, and you will get where you want to go. I did!

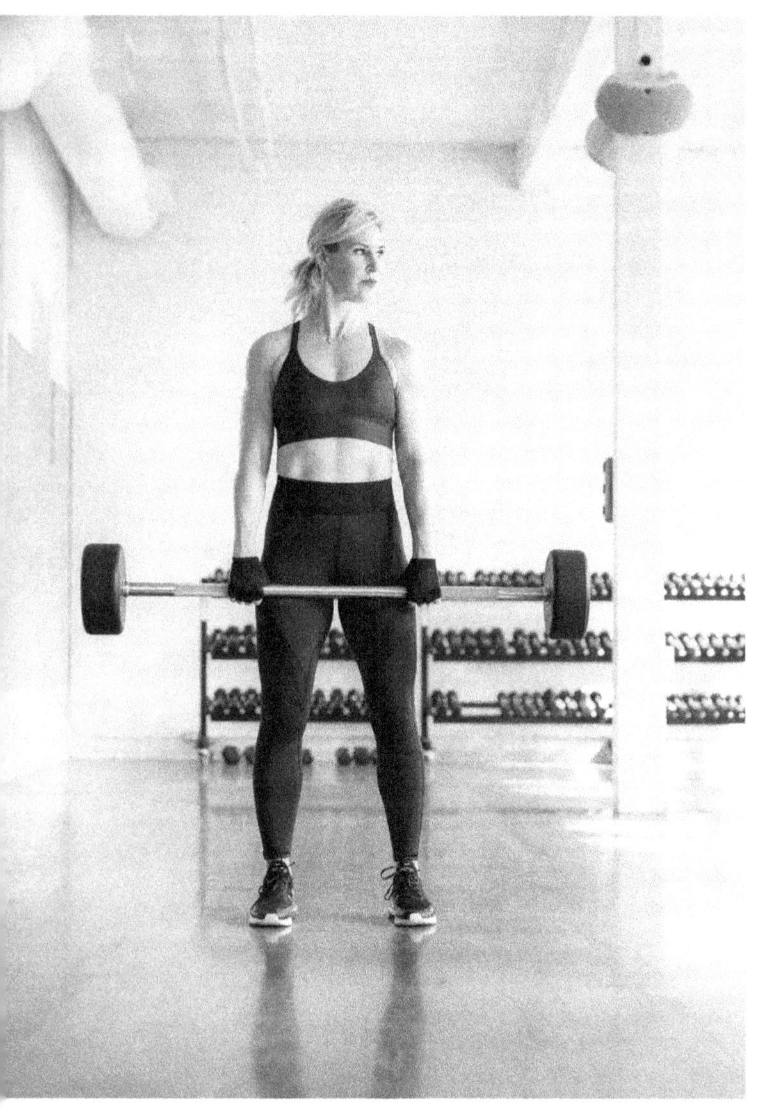

Michelle Epstein is the best friend you didn't know you needed, kicking your butt, encouraging you to push yourself to the next level, and changing your at-home fitness game forever.

Michelle Epstein

I got into fitness to bring women together and create a safe space. At the time there were very few studios for women-only that weren't focused on weight loss or quick fix classes. I helped develop a studio where the workouts were incredibly fun but effective, where women could socialize and connect, where the workouts were specifically formulated for women, but that didn't mean they were easy. What I am most proud of is the community that was built around Elle Fitness and Social.

I started behind the scenes, running the business, doing the books, managing the schedule and staff. Eventually, I started teaching classes, and that's where I discovered true joy. Simply put, I love making a difference in someone's day, make someone feel good, get them to move when they might not otherwise find the motivation. There is instant gratification from that in-person connection, that sweaty collapse after a crazy Bootcamp, that's what fills my cup!

In 2020, the unthinkable happened. We were forced to close our doors, and the in-person connection was gone. The whole reason I got into the business is taken away from me. What did we do? We pivoted and found a way to reconnect! People responded, and hundreds would show up and follow along with Instagram Live classes from home. Together, we found joy in that hour, sweating, slipping, and laughing. We realized quickly that the community we had built in-person was strong, and they weren't going anywhere.

A new business was born; Elle on Demand. The response was immediate and overwhelming. Somehow, we have been able to bring the same energy found at the studio to our online classes and the result is magical. Now, women from all over the world are discovering our workouts and joining in on the fun.

Being forced to pivot, to try and launch a new business while trying to save our current business has been incredibly challenging. Fitness is a passion – fueled by the feedback and results from our community, knowing you are making a positive impact on someone's day, helping them reach their goals and push their boundaries. Nothing will keep me from continuing to pursue this passion.

Iris is a visual artist based in Vancouver, who paints vibrant imagined landscapes as a means of healing from trauma

Iris Mes-Low

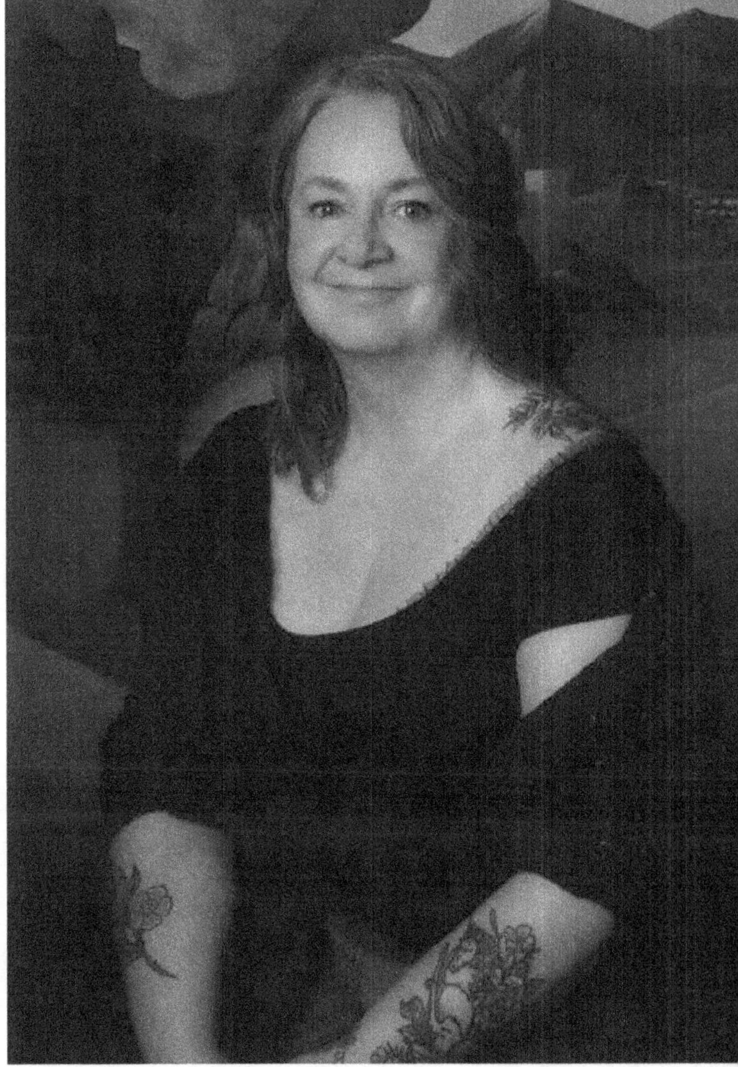
Photo Credit: Gabor Gastonyi

My work is a colourful, idealized version of the world I see. As a child, I watched my father paint, and he took the time to teach me a lot of what I know about art. I read artbooks, loved going to museums; Our home was filled with art and music and colour.

There has been a lot of darkness that I've fought through: depression, a PTSD diagnosis, the loss of my father at 14. These are the things that I put in a box in my head, to try to move past them. But you can't ignore that kind of pain – it breaks out in nightmares and moments when you're least prepared.

Painting has been the red thread that has run through my life. I lived more and more in my head, where things were bright and kind, and I could control the world around me. The colours were more vibrant, the trees more stylized. I started trying to bring that world out onto canvas. I carved out studio space in our home, bought art supplies on Craigslist when money was tight, painted on whatever surface I could get my hands on. I started to make connections with other artists, join arts organizations, volunteered at shows and craft fairs; I took every opportunity I could to showcase my work.

Having the talent is one thing, but doing the work is what makes an art career. I still read voraciously about the work of other artists, I practice my techniques over and over; I'll never be finished learning or improving. Now my work is in galleries, I sell my work and take commissions, but I won't ever stop working hard on it.

In painting the world, I sought solace in when the darkness threatened to take me, I've brought the damaged parts of me into the light. I used to try and paint the world around me but now I paint what's been inside me all along.

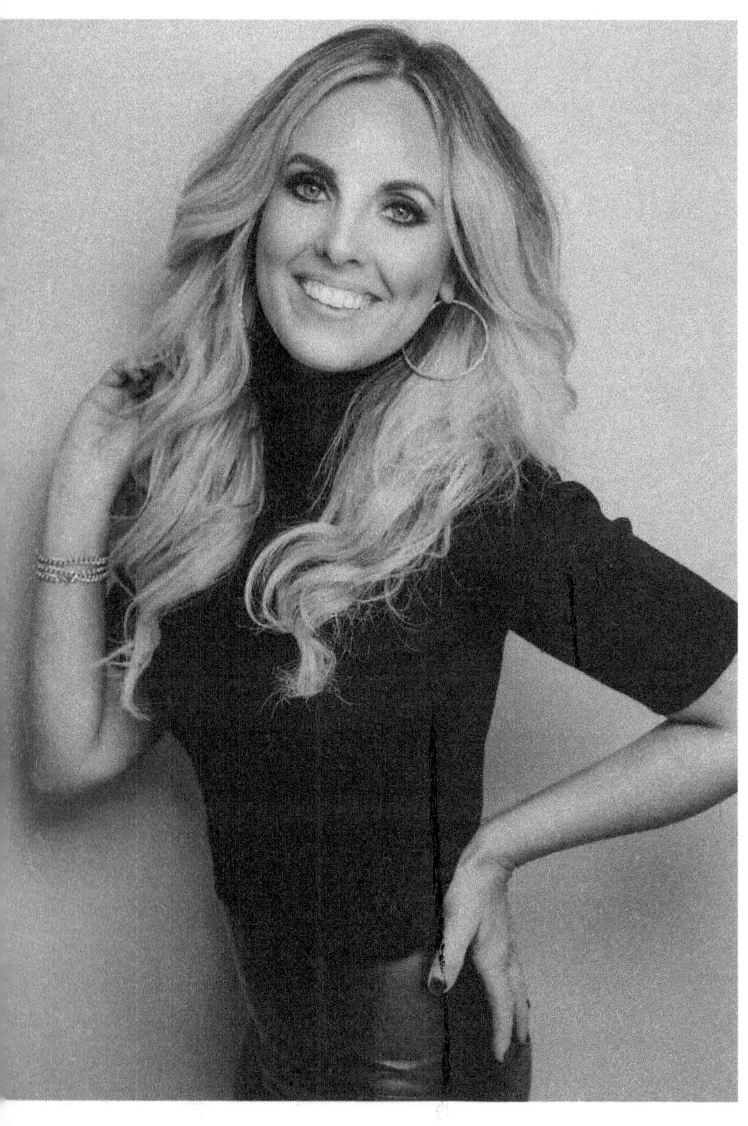

Holly Decker is an award-winning Makeup Artist, Beauty Editor, and creative mastermind.

Holly Decker

I woke up nine years ago, at the age of 36 - not knowing who I was or what direction my life was going in. I found myself in the middle of a divorce, no career, and the mom to three boys. I had been defined by being someone's wife or someone's mom. Now a newly single mom, with only a small resume of work I was faced with how I was going to reinvent myself.

Who was Holly Decker?
I had always been a makeup artist and took a few jobs to keep my toe dipped in the industry over the years - but now I was completely starting over.
When I would mention my dreams and goals of pursuing a career as a makeup artist, I was faced with criticism, gossip and doubt. Some things were said directly to me like "you will never make a living as a makeup artist" or "playing makeup isn't a real job." At times, I thought those negative comments might get the best of me, but instead it fueld my fire.

Reinventing myself at 36, was one of the scariest moments but something inside of me knew this was my path. I took the leap and went out into the world completely open to seeking and creating opportunities. There were many doors that opened and many that were closed. I realized quickly if it didn't open, it wasn't my door. A people pleaser by nature, I came to recognize that not everyone was going to like me. I learned that I needed to set boundaries and that words have power. With my success also came criticism, gossip and doubt. Things like "you are so lucky" or "must be nice " were said directly too me as well. When the hard truth is, I worked my ass off for this!

I have discovered my voice. I know that I am more than the stereotypical box I have sometimes been placed in. I recently had a pivotal moment when I was described as "smart"

A word I don't hear often when someone is describing me. That word shifted something inside me forever.
So now, I have finally chosen to turn off the noise, surround myself with my tribe - but most importantly I have chosen ME and there is so much power in that.

Barb Wallick is a mother, daughter, wife, and now businesswoman who is kind, loving, and wise – and always learning.

Barbara Wallick

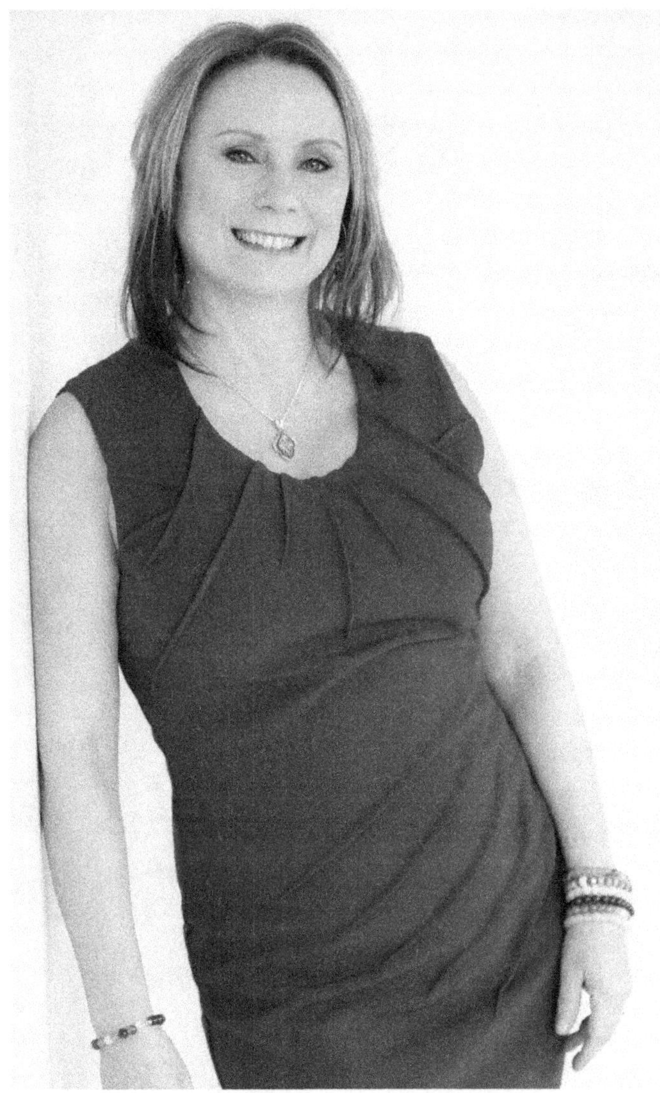

My life changed 20 years ago today, January 11, 2021. I became the mother to a fiery red headed premature baby daughter. Prior to experiencing this life altering high risk pregnancy and volatile delivery, I thought my life was pretty good. A successful career in finance, I was challenged and experienced life fully. I felt I was on the right track.

Becoming a Mother changed all of that. Experiencing near death changed all that. Suddenly I didn't know anything anymore. I became restless and started to question who I was. Who am I? A mother, career woman, daughter, wife, or was it something else? I became a seeker looking for answers. I suddenly realized there was more to life than what I had been taught in the traditional ways. I looked for answers everywhere, books, people, courses, and programs. My career in the financial industry no longer fulfilled me either. I didn't fit anymore, or so I thought.

Until one day I woke up; what I was searching for outside of myself wasn't there. What I needed was already inside of me. I was looking the wrong way, outward and I should have been looking within. The wisdom I was seeking was already there right inside of me. The ability to experience love and joy consistently was within me.

Each and every one of us is born with wisdom and over time it is covered up with teachings and learnings from our parents, teachers, and the outside world – mind blowing! The last 20 years I have been peeling back the layers to find myself, the mother, daughter, wife, and now businesswoman who is kind, loving, and wise. A woman who has taken back her power and realizes that when you tap into the wisdom within, you never run out of the joy and love of life. Seeking it outside yourself can be fun and wonderful, but it can also be fleeting.

I do not regret the experiences I have had along these very bumpy 20 years. They have gifted me with the skills to serve others in creating the financial success we all deserve, mind, body, and spirit. The pursuit is within.

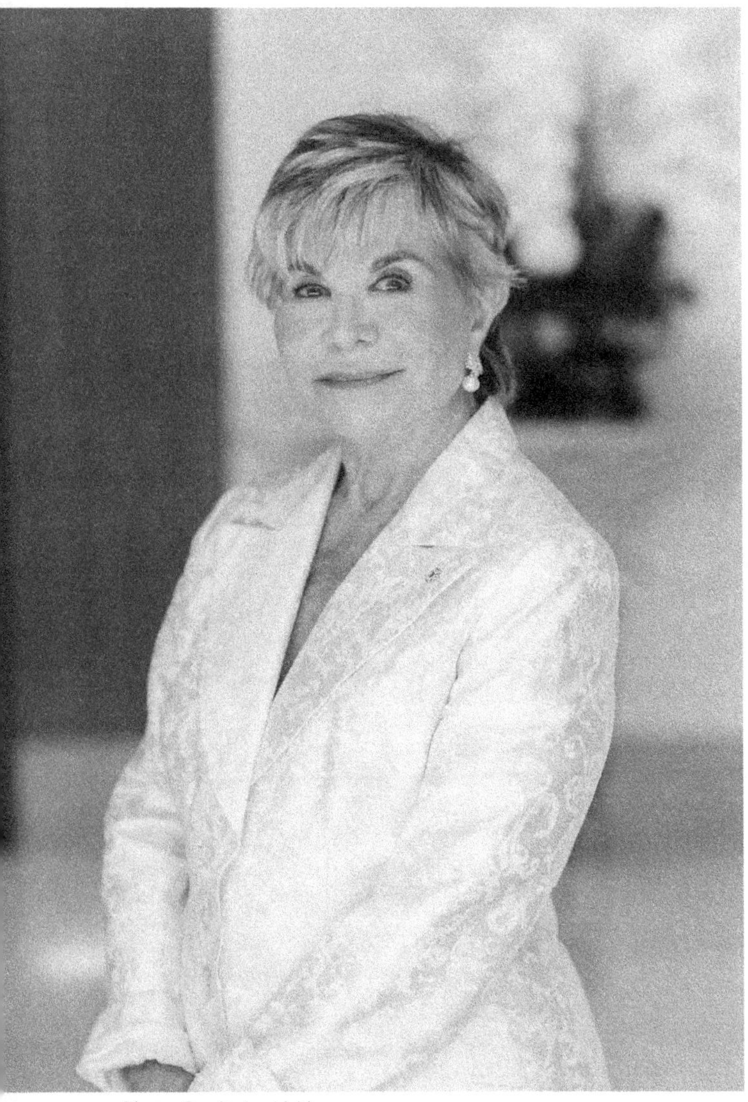

Photo Credit: Lori Miles

Leslie Diamond is a director of the Diamond Foundation, a founding member of the United Way's Women in Philanthropy, a member of BC Women's Hospital Council of Governors, and Women Moving Millions.

Leslie Diamond

You would think by now at my age I would have all the answers. I do not!!

Somehow, I have made it through an absolutely crazy upbringing, family addiction, breast cancer, another cancer scare, the loss of a child, and my greatest feat of all is still being married and in love (most of the time) for over 60 years.

How I have coped is mostly due to the fact that I only live in the now. My motto is that "this too shall pass" and it does. Leaving behind the tools to cope with Although you never get over losing a child, it just finds its place. I am in the last chapter of my life and looking back have accomplished so much.

I came to Vancouver as a young bride from Beverly Hills, California, and I still have trouble with all this rain – but love our city. I have volunteered with many charities working from the bottom up calling it volunteer employment. I now serve on numerous boards. I have learned so much from doing this. I received the Order of British Columbia a couple of years ago and I am very proud of the honour.

As I have aged, I realize that what matters is family. I am happiest in the kitchen making dinner for all my grandkids, great-grandkids, and my daughters and their husbands. Nothing could be better.

Try to enjoy every day which may be very difficult during this time. But "this too shall pass".

– Leslie Diamond

Amanda Da Silva is a personal development and lifestyle coach with a mission to empower women, and help them achieve their boldest, most ambitious dreams.

Amanda Da Silva

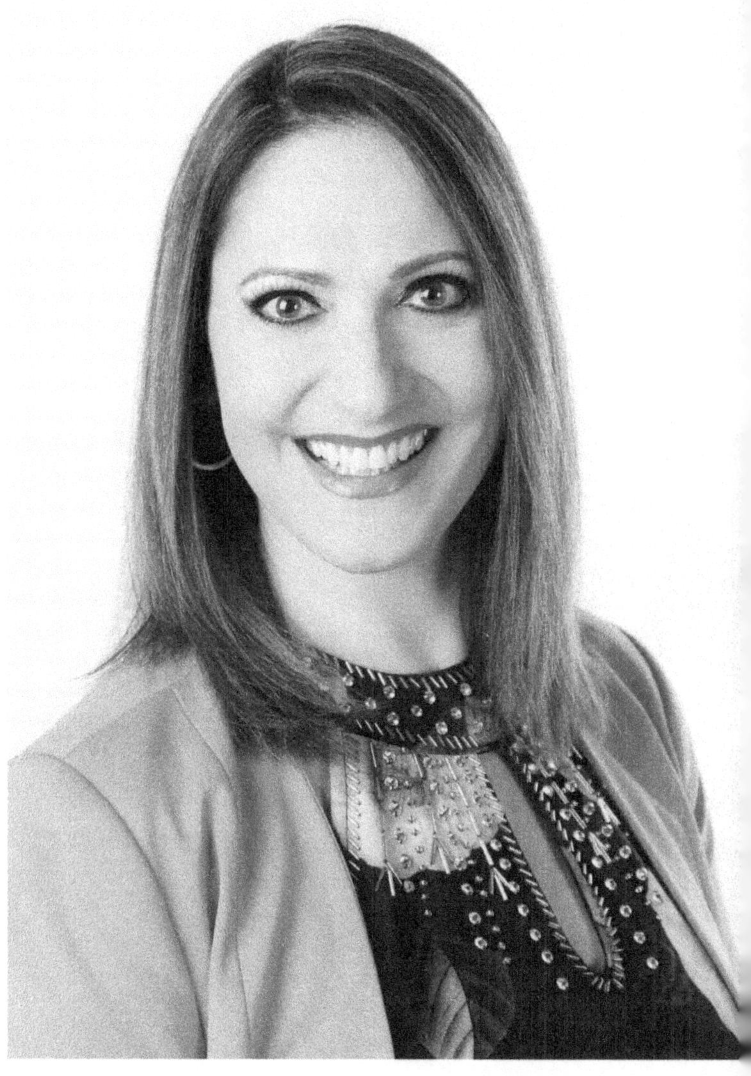

I believe in the joy of finding your true calling in life and, as I have found mine, I make it my goal to guide other women in discovering their purpose and unlocking their full potential to excel as leaders and entrepreneurs.

Career-defining moments are few and far between, but I vividly remember when my high school PE teachers pulled me into the office and told me 'you're a natural-born teacher and leader'. They encouraged me to get a degree in education, which is exactly what I did! I followed my passion and got my Bachelor's degree in Human Kinetics and Education, then a Master's degree in Leadership and Administration.

I've always been an avid student and a dynamic leader with a particular fondness for lifelong learning, which is why I started DS Education Group. I wanted to share my passion for continuous self-improvement and growth with other parents, educators, students, and leaders, all within a positive, inspiring, and supportive community.

This is still, to date, one of my greatest accomplishments, along with starting my life coaching business, all within 6 months. That and writing my own book! I learned a lot from my entrepreneurial journey; being my own boss allowed me to live my wildest dreams, but it also meant I had to be my own source of motivation. So, on tough days, I get myself out of bed and start my day because I know I have many goals yet to accomplish, fun, loving, memories yet to create, and wondrous adventures yet to go on.

I take great pride in empowering the people around me and making them feel understood, heard, valued, and cared for, but I'm also immensely appreciative of my amazing family for their belief in me. I wouldn't be where I am, nor the woman I am today without their unconditional love and support.

I feel humbled, grateful, and deeply honored for this opportunity to collaborate with powerful, kind, and passionate women who seek to elevate other women and support them on their journey to success.

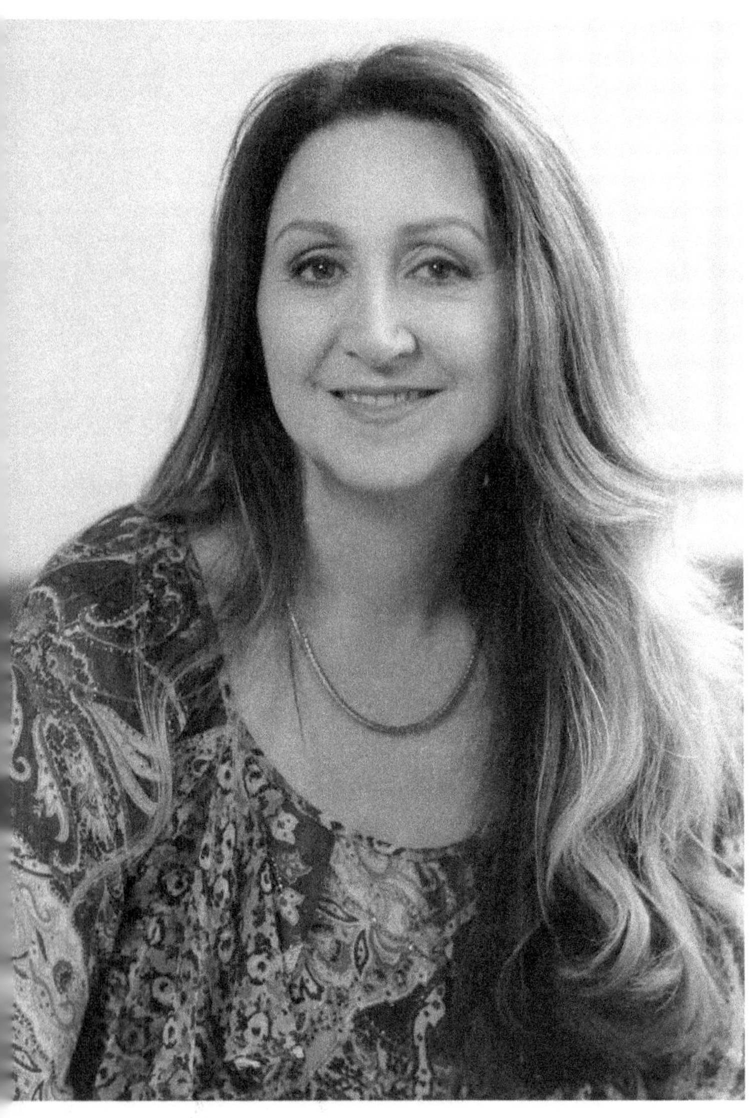

Estrellita's values on health and wellbeing guide her days and work as a fearless and Conscious Entrepreneur, politician, single parent, and in her newest adventure, as a digital wealth saver and educator.

Estrellita Gonzalez

I always knew I was destined to be an entrepreneur. I was exposed early on to entrepreneurship through my father and an Aunt. I saw a freedom they had that was appealing. At 24, I started my first company which had a disappointing end with a business partner. After years of working for others and then being laid off, I again decided to start my own business.

The motivation, then too, was freedom. I was a single parent and wanted a business that allowed for time freedom. I also wanted something that sprung from my creativity and values. So began the journey. I invested in myself through coaches, self-help books, and retreats. When I started my business, I doubted myself constantly. I really didn't know if I was on the right track and doing what I was supposed to be doing. But through "the work" I finally had my ah-ha moment which was so liberating, affirming, and empowering.

My journey revealed that my number one value was health and wellbeing. As I explored this and its meaning, I grew my brand from my initial skincare clinic to adding an online store, wellness centre, workshops, and writing, including four books. Getting clear on my values allowed me to get clear on my vision, why, and purpose.

As my business grew and I rolled with the punches, I kept at it though there were many challenges along the way. I never gave up because I was too stubborn to do so! I had a vision, and I was going to see it through. I also developed a visceral compass in my being which allowed for greater intuition, something I use in daily living and decision making.

In 2017 I had the opportunity to run for political office and have run in two successful campaigns since. I have created my life today through intention and understanding. Everyone is capable of living their dream life, you just need to do the work!

Julie Drapeau is a fitness enthusiast and the VP of Sales at Purity Life Health Products LP.

Julie Drapeau

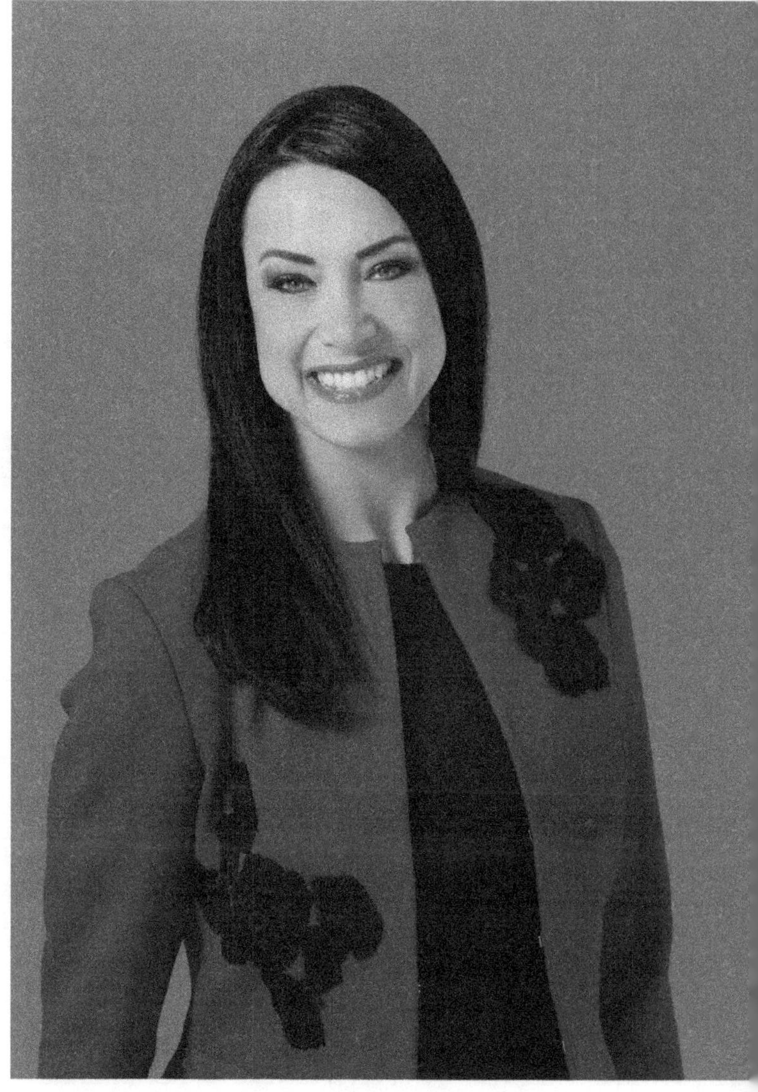

Hi there, I am Julie Drapeau, from Quebec City. I currently live in Guelph, Ontario, and have for the past ten years.

I often say to people you can take the Quebecer out of Quebec, but you can't take the Quebec out of the Quebecer. Because of this, I go back to Quebec every few months to get a refill of the spirit of Quebec.

My passion for life is based on living it with boldness and optimism. I feel so lucky to have been brought up in Quebec as it has provided me with so many opportunities well beyond what I thought was possible growing up in Quebec City.

I am passionate about Quebec and the opportunities that are available for Quebecers that also embrace a second language and the world beyond just Quebec. Quebecers have a serious advantage in North America with having a unique perspective on life and being able to leverage that for opportunities within Quebec and beyond Quebec.

With my passion for life comes my passion for fitness and taking responsibility for one's health. I spend a lot of time on my fitness enjoying building muscles and doing a lot of Functional Fitness. I consider myself an ambassador of health as I travel the world (when possible) and across Canada in my role as Vice President of Sales for Purity Life, a distributor of natural health products.

I do not look at life from a work/life balance perspective but instead as work/life integration. I love what I do and the products we distribute and the impact they have on people's health. It's easy for me to leverage my passion and drive to help motivate people to be better versions of themselves as it energizes me.

For me loving what I do, and where I am from, inspires me every day to be better and encourage others to do the same. For some inspiration, entertainment, and escape, connect with me on social media!

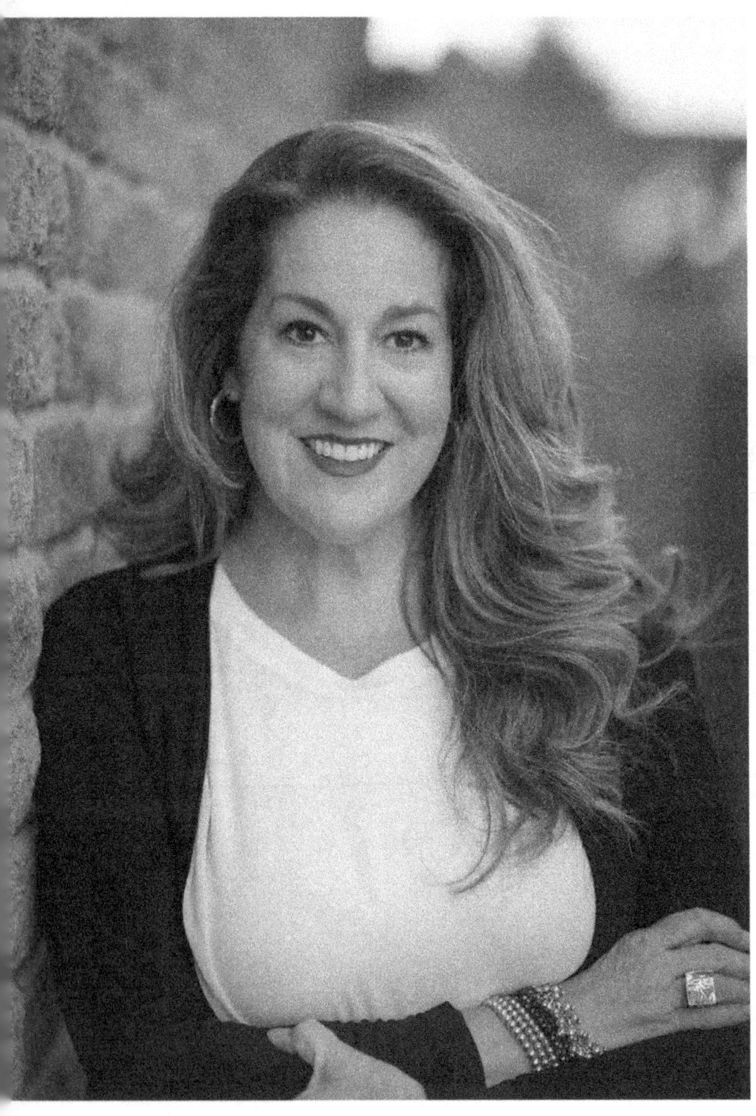

Julia Quinton Oosterman is an award-winning communicator, Chief of Communications & Public Affairs at Bluewater Health, and Inspirational Speaker

Julia Quinton Oosterman

Be Bold, be brave, be kind! Impassioned by these beliefs, I have shaped my world around them. They have driven my choices and led me to the full and happy life I now lead.

I was born a warrior, and at the age of 16 I boldly struck out on my own to make my way in the world. Along the way, I lived in socially assisted housing and worked various jobs in order to pay for my studies.

It was a challenging path that led to my graduating from university and beginning work in the communications field in Toronto. Over 26 years, I honed my skills and worked exceedingly hard to climb the corporate ladder.

I had four beautiful children and a solid career, but long days and hard work found me looking for a work-life balance. When an opportunity arose in Sarnia, Ontario to become an executive, Chief of Communications & Public Affairs for a busy two-site hospital, I took it. Ironically the move allowed me to find the balance I had been searching for and it took my career to new heights, winning the communicator of the year award and other global accolades. I also had more time to devote to my wonderful children and my husband.

I have discovered that work-life balance is more easily achieved when we learn to find internal balance as well. I feel strongly that my solid work ethic and need to achieve tangible results must be tempered with kindness and a willingness to allow others to shine too. Self-reflection is the key to developing a more encompassing leadership style that elevates and empowers others to reach their fullest potential.

As a leader, I hope to embody compassion, collaborative problem-solving skills, foster optimism, and a safe learning environment. One of the finest compliments I have received was from a member of my team who said to me that I have a very kind and caring heart. This made me feel like not only had I learned to find work-life balance, but I had also learned to balance the warrior with warmth and kindness.

I will always be bold and brave, but I will lead with kindness.

Deanna Rose is a functional integrative wellness coach and a desire whisperer, who focuses on empowering women to love and achieve their dream body, master unbreakable confidence, and create the life they are truly excited to live.

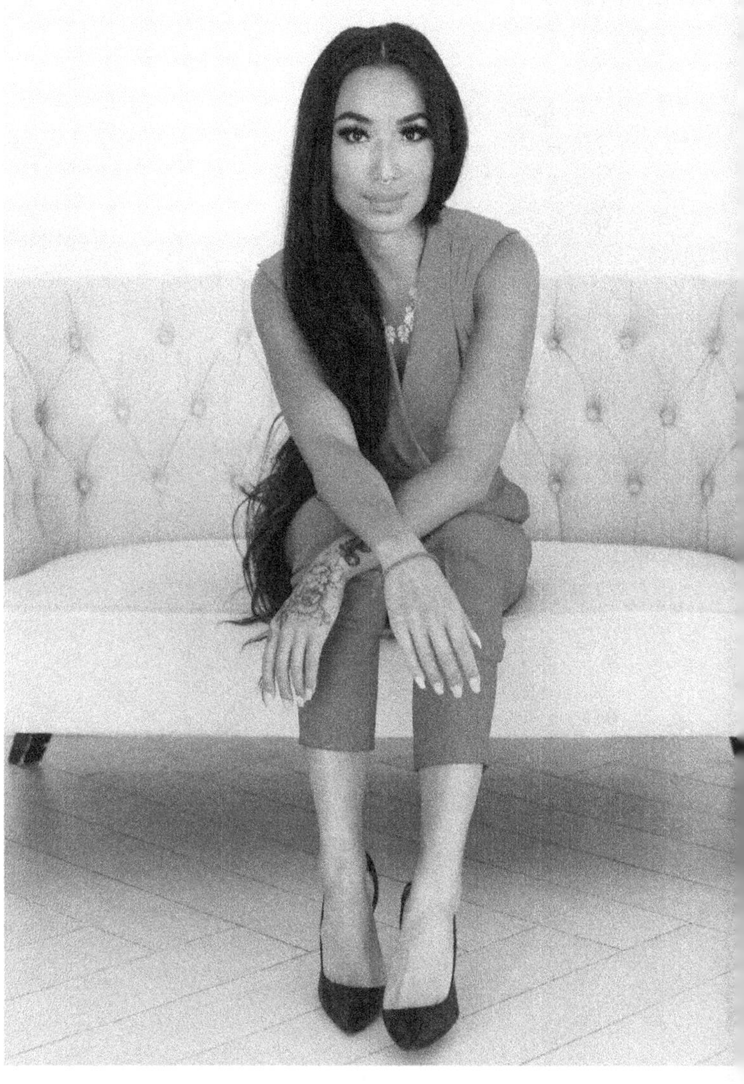

Deanna Rose

Most people cope through life, without realizing they actually never lived. We create our own physical and mental limitations on the daily. By breaking through those limiting beliefs, I help people reconnect with their confidence and freedom- the kind of life they never thought was possible. My life and career have been a series of bumpy rides with mixed emotions. When I was a child, I did everything I could to fit in. As I got older, I did whatever I could to be different. For many years, I felt trapped in my own body and mind.

I always felt there's so much more than what society told us. Everyone told me success means money and status. Nobody really talked about happiness or purpose.

I believe we manifest and are the co-creators of our own reality. Only when we dare to act from the heart, will we escape the confining social norms and society's imposed limitations. If we dare to walk the path our heart truly desires, we'll find freedom and happiness that set us free from the factors we perceive as bars on our illusory cells.

I feel like I've been chasing happiness and success all my life, sometimes without even consciously recognizing it. I've resorted to substances, people, experiences, and things. But nothing really lasted more than the amount of time it took to obtain them.

Lately, I realized I can't pursue the feeling of happiness or the status of success. Those are simply illusions we conjure up in our minds. Happiness or success isn't a destination; it's a part of the choices we make every single day. The beauty of life is we have the choice to live in those feelings every day like they are already part of our experience. We have a limitless ability to attract more of what we focus on.

Express YOU unapologetically and show up authentically, so you can make the impact you were born to make, live your purpose, and consciously create your Higher Self.

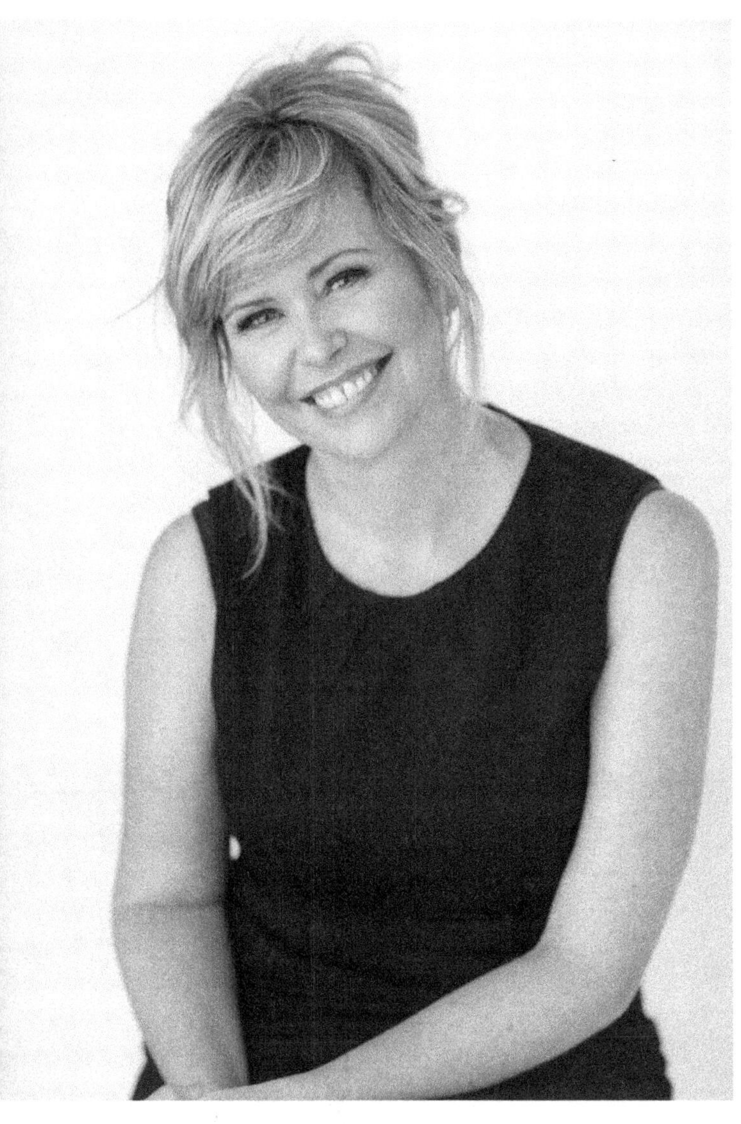

Danielle MacLean is a mother, partner of DCL law, and appreciator of wine.

Danielle MacLean

When I started out, I received all sorts of unsolicited advice. A disproportionate amount focused on what not to do, in particular, how not to "act like a woman" in business. I like to think that advice would be different today than it was back then. Just in case it's not, I make it a point to mentor new business owners.

I have lost count of how many times I was told to ensure I wasn't "too soft" or "too emotional." This led to second-guessing my instincts. What I've figured out is that you just need to be authentic. There is a difference between being compassionate and emotional. You can be assertive and still listen. These traits do not need to be mutually exclusive. A business will not be successful in the long run without the right people. This includes your staff, referral partners, service partners, and clients. Loyalty goes a long way in both life and business. So does trust (including trusting enough to delegate). My business grew because I developed a network that I could rely on, which at times included my competitors, and still does today, and not because I aggressively targeted my competition. Asking for help is not a sign of weakness.

One of the marks of a successful lawyer is the ability to recognize what you don't know and seek the expertise of another in the field. **Finding your people** is vital. Just as important is **learning the power of "no."** You cannot be everything to everyone. If someone isn't a good fit with you, they aren't a good fit for your business. This is a hard lesson to learn in start-up. It's difficult to turn business, and business connections, down. **Learn to trust your instincts.**
Surround yourself with those that you can learn from, and that are willing to teach you. Teach others what you have learned. Take insight from those starting out. Contribute to your profession. Learning is how you move forward.
Always be learning.

Be honest, be kind. Own your mistakes. Make it right. Strive for positive interactions.
Most importantly, **have faith in yourself.** You are tougher than you realize.
And please, filter that unsolicited advice!

Christine Monaghan's purpose is to grow into the next best version of self; influence others to do so. Her mantra: lead as you would like to follow.

Christine Monaghan

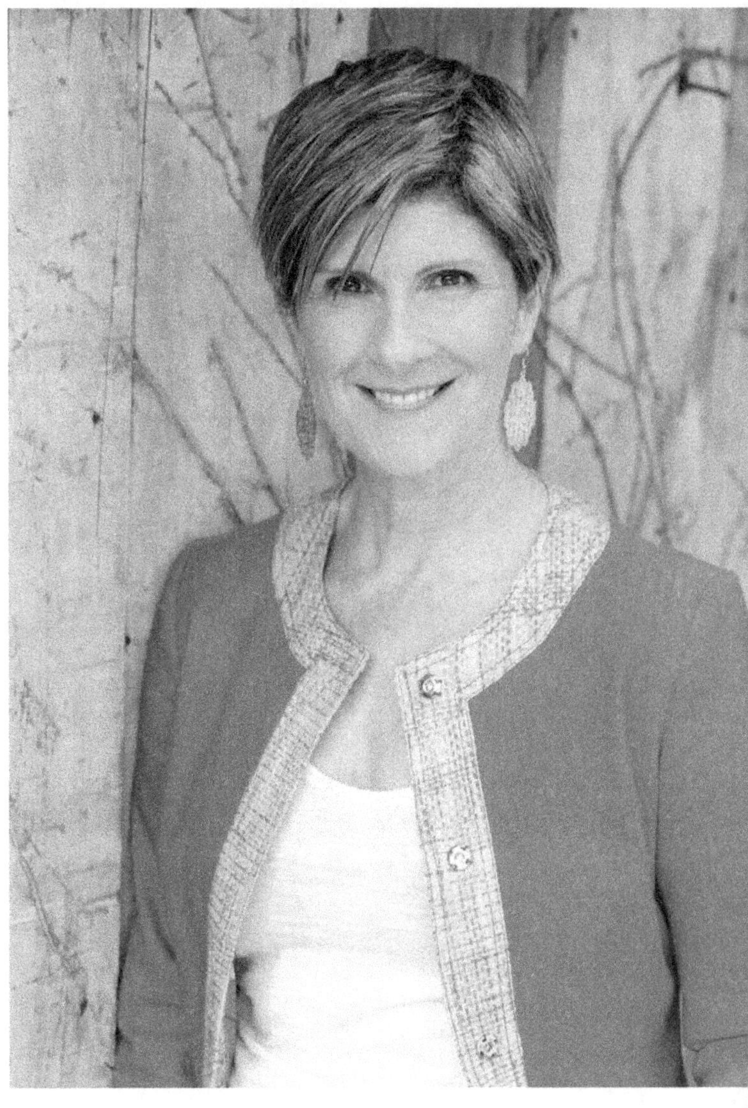

My what if warrior pursuit is about a mindset shift commitment from 'what if worrier' to 'what if warrior'. The choice is to surrender to sourcing quantum energy solutions, picking a lane and owning it with all ones' might, daily non-negotiables to top up ones' energy reserve, 100% focus on what you do want, replacing resentment with inspired-action, personal growth over attention on others' shortcomings, and befriending resistance - getting comfortable being uncomfortable.

Freedom through trial and error, outstanding wins, immense joy and love; I define freedom as liberation from internal limitations, creation of wealth on all levels, creating a life on ones' own terms, evolving a thriving business, optimum health and strength, love, knowing ones' constitutional rights, 'agreeing to disagree' conversations without toxic retribution, responding versus reacting; accepting 'what is' to surface possibilities.

Simple Riches 365 Fuel ones' being with: Biographies; gardening; a healthy lifestyle commitment, scrumptious meals; cashmere sweater, white tee, faded jeans; matcha lattes; crackling wood fireplace; raking leaves; beeswax candles; spirited potluck dinner conversations; wise minds; summer's first G+T; fresh aired linens; picnics at the ocean beach.

What I Value Loyalty; grace-in-action; understated success; elder respect; good ole door-opening manners; commanding monetary worth; fierce self-love; truth with detachment from another's acceptance; chivalry; silence; courage to stand solo from herd mentality; contrarians; working smarter not harder; rewarding accomplishments; pragmatic, intuitive leaders; street smarts; inquisitiveness; the power of RESET to slow down to move ahead.

Worldly Desires Seek to understand without trying to prove others wrong; listen to learn; accountability beyond apology; we solutions instead of them hatred; mindful business systems; leaving others with their dignity; stress is optional versus stress is normal leadership. Wisdom Allowing yourself to ASK, believe, allow, receive your truest desires, in the highest good of all, is your birthright. Lead as you would like to follow.

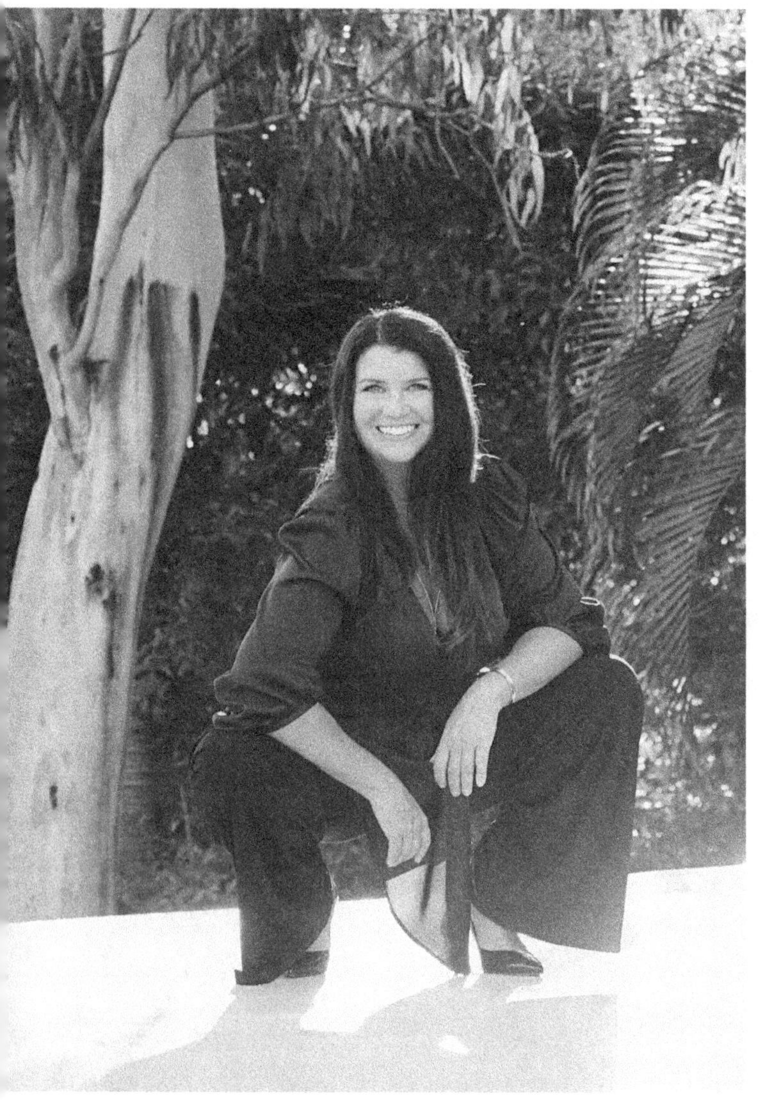

Jenny Gough is the founder of multiple businesses, a positive inspiration for change, and a friend.

Jenny Gough

"It's your life," was the doctor's parting shot as I left his office, my final visit for a tumour in my brain. I had accomplished my mission for the day - refuse chemotherapy, refuse any other treatment, carry on with life. It's my life, after all. The doctor said so.

I slid through grey-brown slush on the busy Toronto sidewalks, ice pellets biting my cheeks as the damp cold seeped into my bones, while I mulled over the doctor's words... "it's your life". Sounded legit - except I had the distinct feeling that it wasn't.

As 'Jenny the Engineer', I should have felt like a success. I was proud of my career progression, working my way through a variety of unique experiences, until hitting my main career goal – Consulting Engineer, and now heading up a company of my own. Others looked at me and thought, "Gee whiz, she's doing alright!" ... I looked at myself, and thought, "is this all you've become?"

It was scary to realize that if I could only choose one thing to remove permanently from my life, that it would be the career I had spent twenty-five years building, rather than the tumour that was causing untold health issues! I had become nothing more than a reactive slave to my cell phone and my computer, going through each day by rote. I was no longer proactively growing – not personally, not professionally. I wasn't loving life – heck, I wasn't even living life.

My internal, spiritual fight against these self-imposed obligations and responsibilities was making me physically sick, emotionally ruined, and less than a tenth of what I could be. You cannot fill from an empty cup.

I am so grateful for that unspoken final prescription from the doctor - "It's your life – so go live it!"

It's okay to want more; to do more, to learn more, and to give more. We are meant to elevate our thinking, spread kindness and knowledge, and leave impressions of increase with every encounter.

Turns out, the doctor was right - it truly is my life – to live joyfully, healthfully, to do my life's best work... which is to spread the word – IT'S YOUR LIFE – GO LIVE IT!

Mary Zilba is a TV Personality, Recording Artist, Producer, Entrepreneur, and Mother of 3 sons.

Mary Zilba

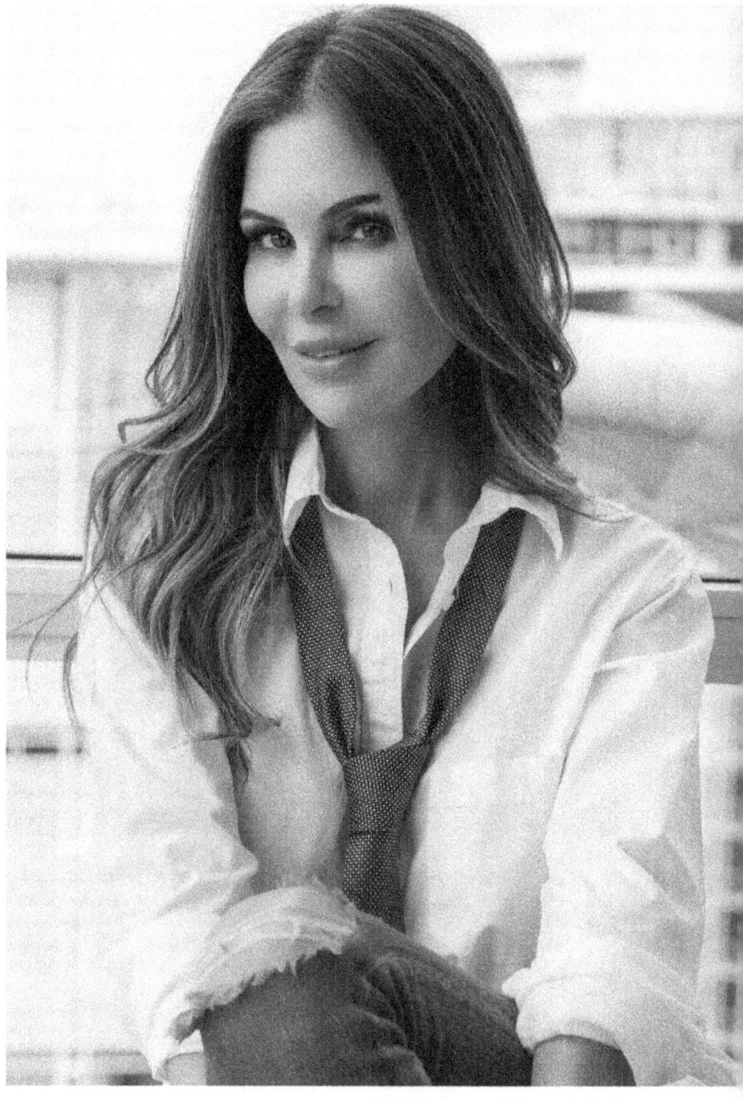

Alphabet Soup – that's what my life would look like if it were in a bowl. Some perfectly formed words and letters and others broken and scattered, all sharing the same broth. The broth represents my foundation of Midwestern roots and family values that have been the underlying fabric of my life, and the letters spell out all the choices I have made along the way.

Most people know me as a recording artist or as a cast member on the popular TV series, The Real Housewives of Vancouver. But few know me as the person behind the lens, who, like everyone else, has had my share of joyous accomplishments, devastating heartbreaks, insecurities, and a graveyard of failures. But what has it all taught me?

What have I learned?

I have learned so many things, but two lessons stand out the most: Resilience and Humour. Both have been the foundation of my existence. Having been raised in a large family with 7 siblings, resilience came naturally, but it wasn't until I became an adult that I fully realized how it has impacted my life.

I embrace the notion that "this too shall pass" and try to look at the glass as always half full. This has given me the marshal of strength that has allowed me to not only accept when setbacks happen, and people hurt me but that by reframing my thoughts, I don't allow myself to live in a negative mindset. One of my favorite quotes from Nelson Mandela, "Do not judge me by my success, but by how many times I fell down and got back up again".

While there is plenty in life to be serious about, I couldn't get through if I took it all too seriously, so throughout my life I have used humour as a daily vitamin. I have always been able to use it when life has thrown me curveballs and most importantly, I've been able to laugh at myself. A pinch of playfulness has always helped me get through even the most difficult of situations.

So, remember that sense of humour plays a huge role in your resilience. On your worst days, humour will help you bend without breaking!

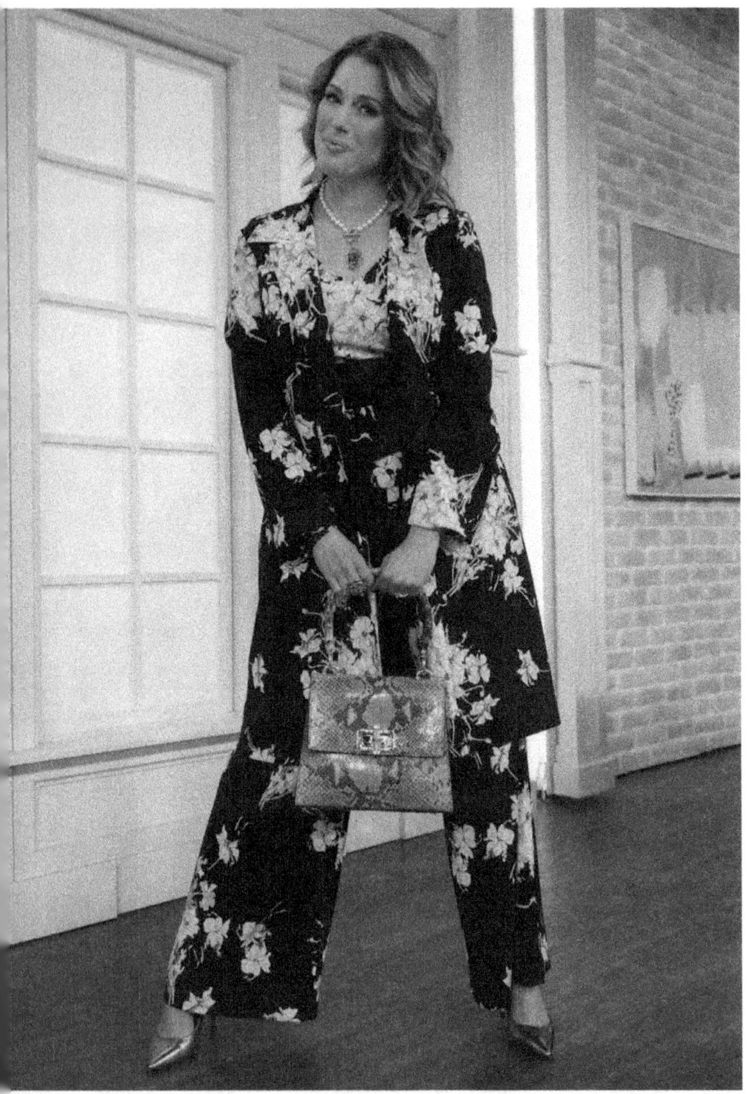
Photo Credit: Khalid Mahmood

Dawn Chubai is the Host on The Shopping Channel, former host of Breakfast Television in Vancouver, Award-Winning Jazz Vocalist, Actress, , Emcee and Spokesperson.

Dawn Chubai

She also serves as a Media Consultant specializing in On-Camera Training.

In my experience, the Universe will make room for your talents. The things you are good at naturally are your talents. In my case, it was my good fortune to be able to make a career out of mine. Even when I wasn't ready or didn't consider myself qualified; my instinct was always to say "Yes."

In high school, I was an average student, but I grew up with a strong work ethic which I learned from my hardworking parents. Whatever you do, do it well. How you do anything is how you do everything.

Every New Year's Eve our family would set our goals. We were encouraged to visualize our success in order to attract that which we wanted in our lives; the power of positive thinking. It is that mindset that allowed me to explore three careers, and all at the same time.

In 1998, when I was offered a weekly jazz gig on Edmonton's Whyte Avenue, I immediately said, "Yes." The fact that I didn't have a band put together was not a concern. I began singing professionally from that first yes, and I would later go on to win an ARIA Award for my debut CD, perform with the Dal Richards Orchestra, and later, the Vancouver Symphony.

In 1999 I was told that "everything I didn't know about being on television, could be taught," so I said yes to a job offer as the morning "weather girl." They said I had the one thing they couldn't teach - personality. Saying yes that day has allowed me to host a cooking show, a real estate show, a morning show, and work with the Vancouver Canucks.

While I am currently a Host on Canada's only shopping channel (TSC), I credit both my singing and broadcasting careers with propelling me to start my own business. Learning from my experience where "everything can be taught," I now work with and train those in the fitness, tourism, and hospitality industries to find their on-camera footing in preparation for television appearances. I believe we were put on this Earth to not only use our talent but to also share it and help others find theirs.

Diane Rolston is a Leadership Coach, the CEO and Founder of Dynamic Women® and she's on a mission to help one million women scale up their lives and businesses.

Diane Rolston

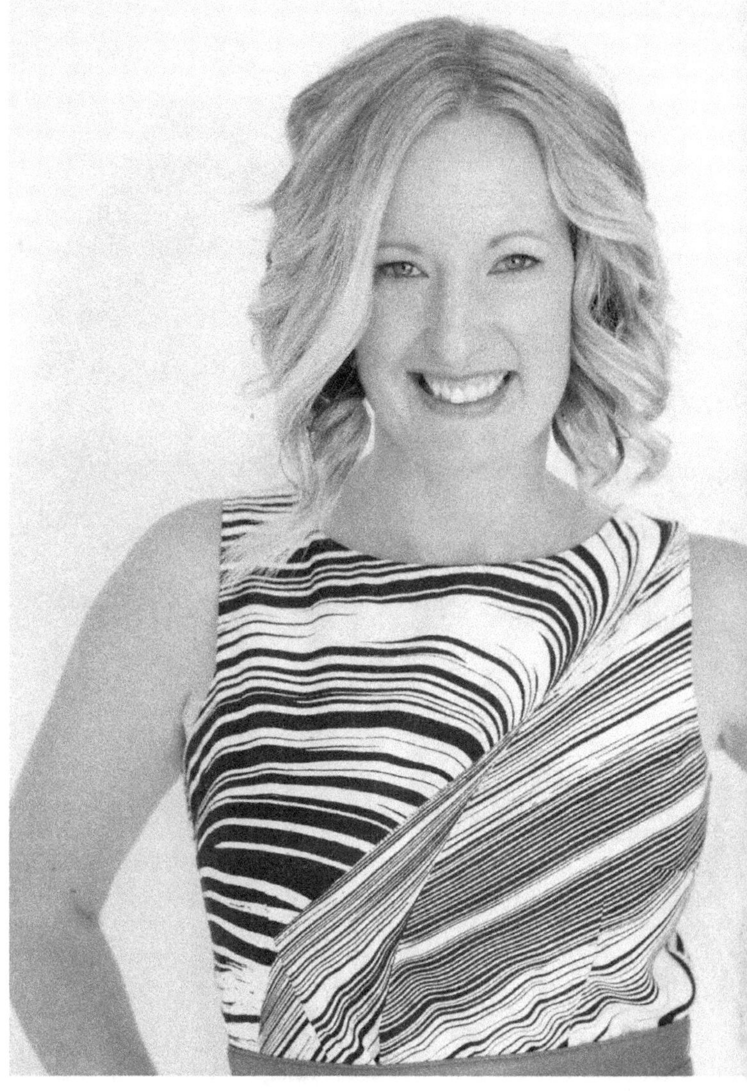

What are you meant to do with this one and only precious life?
It can feel like a BIG question. I didn't know at first, but others saw it in me.

Teachers sat me with struggling or new students to help them or be their friend. Sports coaches made me captain to champion my teammates to play their best. Friends came to me to talk things out, find a solution, and feel better. After high school, I couldn't find the right career. I jumped into teaching even though it didn't feel quite right. The beautiful thing is that every decision gets us one step closer to the right answer.

Ten years later, feeling unhappy and exhausted, I hired a coach. With powerful questions, she had me focused on what I really wanted in life, not just what the "high achiever" in me strived to accomplish. Coaching was the game changer to uncover my purpose and propel me forward. Because I had a coach, I finally uncovered what had been staring me in the face. Just like she was coaching me, I'd been coaching classmates, teammates, and friends for over twenty-five years to believe in themselves and step into their greatness. On a Tuesday, I admitted I wanted to be a coach. She wasn't surprised. Being so confident in the decision, I started my certification that Friday while working full-time and pregnant. Finally having clarity, was I done with my coach? Oh no! **With each level of success, you need a coach in your corner.** A year later, I left my 9-5, birthing not only a business but a baby.

Since then, I've hired more coaches for many areas of life and business: supporting me to be a Speaker, Author, Leader, Podcaster, and the CEO & Founder of the Dynamic Women® Global Club.

I feel blessed that I've won awards for what I love and have coached thousands of women to have Clarity, Confidence, and get into Action. They've opened businesses, left what's not serving them, made more money, followed a dream, and many other amazing accomplishments. Now I get to feature them on the Dynamic Women® Podcast and in my Dynamic Women® Secrets Books to impact even more women. My mission is to unleash one million Dynamic Women® with my one and only precious life! What's yours?

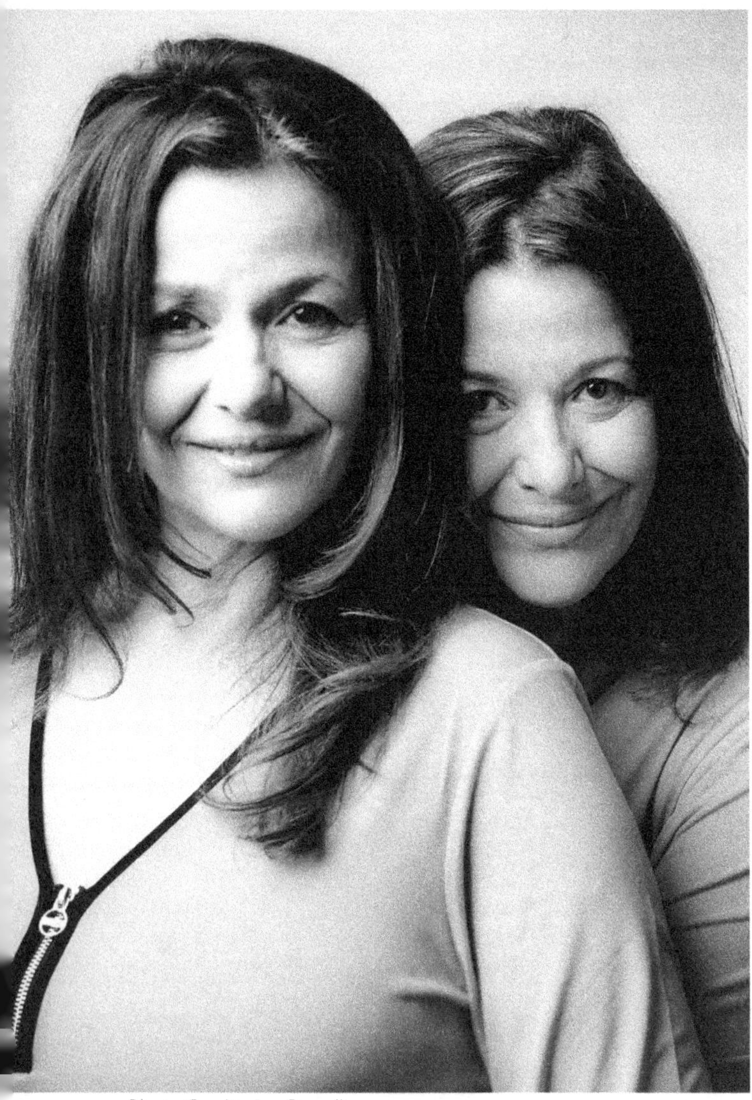
Photo Credit: Joe Borrelli

**My name is Asiza and I am a fine artist living in Vancouver, Canada.
My story sounds crazy—even to me.**

Asiza

When I was 35, my parents revealed a deeply guilt-ridden secret to me—
I was adopted and I had an identical twin sister half a world away in Romania. My twin, Gina, and I were separated at the age of 4. It would be 47 years before we saw each other again.

Growing up as an only child, first in Romania and later defecting to Canada at the age of 11 with my parents, I had always longed for a sister and I'm now convinced that my innate desire to draw female figures was a way of staying connected to my twin.

The thing that saddens me the most is that my sister always knew about my existence, butt I never knew about hers—I can only imagine how tormenting that was for her.

All those years, my mother had prevented Gina from contacting me and my sister suffered greatly as a result. Even after telling me, my mom asked me to keep the secret of my sister within my immediate family and for many years, I lived in fear of people finding out and judging my parents.
It was exhausting to hide behind the mask of their guilt and shame.

Although I love my mom unconditionally and appreciated all the sacrifices she had made for me to have a better life in Canada, it was difficult for me to forgive her for burdening me with her guilt and from knowing my twin sooner. Out of respect for her wishes, it wasn't until 16 years later, after both my parents had passed away, that I had the courage to start the healing process. Sharing my story through my art and pursuing my passion for painting was truly liberating. I am proud to say that I am a full-time professional artist now.

I do have regrets for not starting to paint sooner but I am living proof that it's never too late to follow your dreams. Gina and I still speak almost every day—she is the inspiration behind my art.

Mishel Schwartz is a celebrated painter specializing in abstract art, exploring the beauty of the natural world around her.

Mishel Schwartz

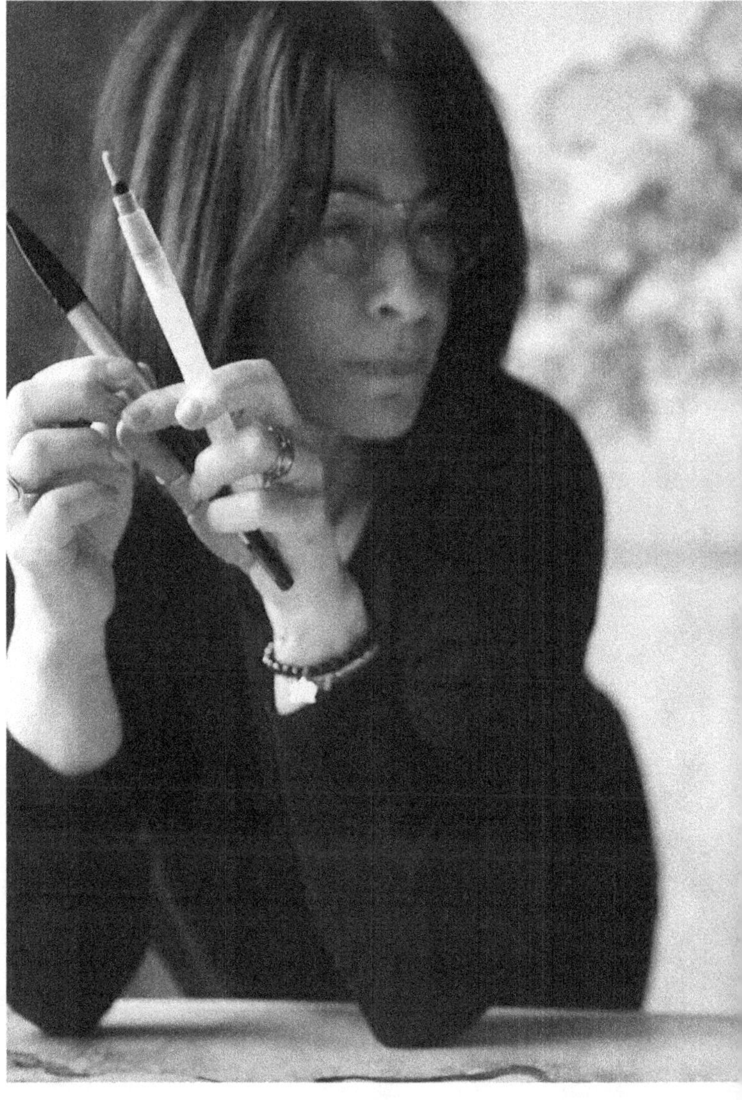

I often think of destiny, the destiny of an artist, and then survival, the survival instincts of being a human in this world. Are they mutually exclusive? Can one fulfill one's destiny and also survive? I haven't yet found the answer, but I know it is my destiny to keep searching for it in this life as the artist that I have chosen to be, at long last.

One of the greatest lessons I have had to learn in this quest is to adjust my definition of happiness and success. I've also had to come face to face with my fears - fears as they relate to success, but more importantly, the fear that I will have to relinquish my destiny in order to survive. And after more than twenty years of channeling my energy elsewhere, through forms of creativity that didn't exactly fit the bill, I challenged myself to step away from the status quo and jump headfirst into the unknowable life that comes with being an artist at heart.

Throughout this journey, I have often had to tune out the white noise of daily life and tune into the internal music of my true artist's beating heart. And when I finally took the plunge and said out loud that art would be my life; it eventually became one of my most grounding means of survival. Suddenly it was clear to me that with determination and self-acceptance, survival and destiny could coexist harmoniously.

Aside from my children, my family, and my friends, there is no force as great in my life as that which drives me creatively. Like maternal instinct, I have come to realize that an artist's instinct cannot be squandered. It comes with a certain responsibility, and you have to dive in with every ounce of passion and dedication available to you.

It also means embracing the unknown, trusting in myself, and taking the time needed to refuel my creative life with joy and appreciation in the little things, the daily tasks that once seemed so in conflict with my desires, and that today have become an integral part of who I am as an artist.

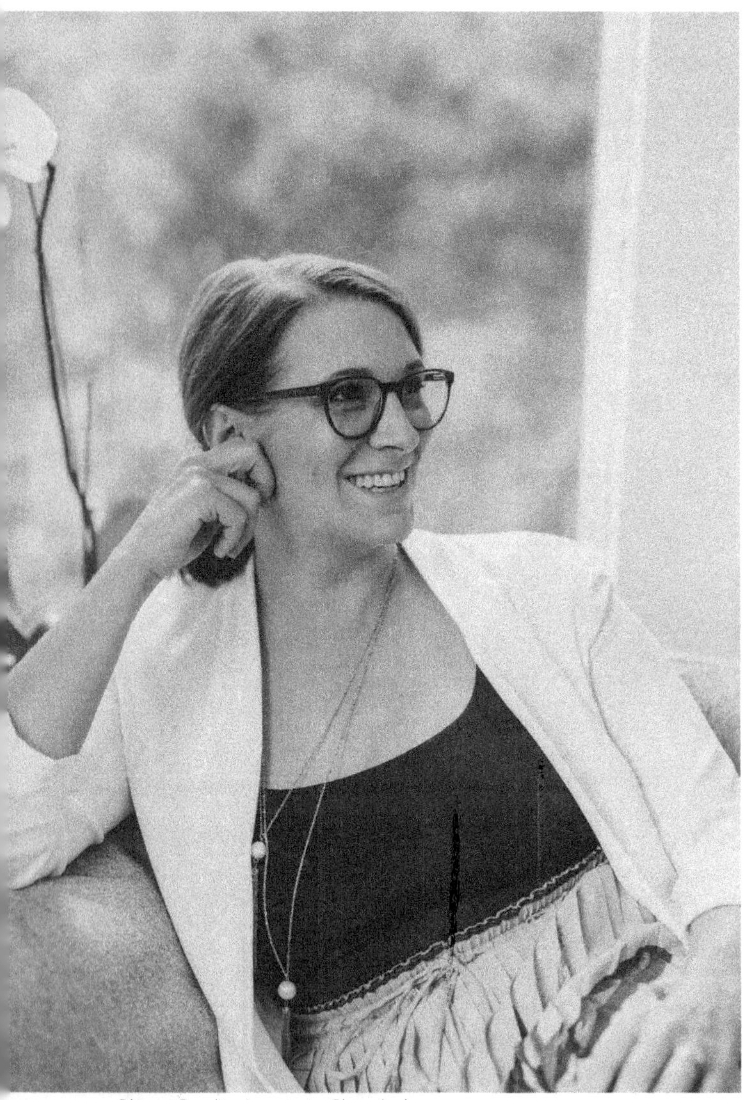
Photo Credit: Anastasia Chomlack

Theresa Lambert is a High-Performance Lifestyle and Success Coach, Speaker and Bestselling Author of "Achieve with Grace: A guide to elegance and effectiveness in intense workplaces".

Theresa Lambert

Theresa believes we get to have it all; teaching high-achieving women to succeed with more elegance and less struggle.

Much like you, I was a woman on a mission. I wasn't here to play small, I wanted it "all". You know - the title, the team, the growth, the recognition, and the self validation that comes along with all those things. I was ready to finally feel accomplished, powerful, and respected in a high-level career...and I was willing to do anything it took to get there.

Growth after growth. Promotion after promotion. Raise after raise. Until I reached the top.

When I got there, it didn't look the way I thought it should, and it felt even worse. I had become a woman I didn't recognize. I wasn't turned on in my marriage, I was disconnected from lifelong friends, and at the end of the day - I felt like a walking rolodex of financials, deadlines, and emails that I'd forgotten to send.

I was living proof that success doesn't always lead to happiness. There I was, perched atop the corporate ladder in my beautiful power suit and kitten heels, trying to figure out who I was these days. Had I become the woman I wanted to be? Was happiness supposed to feel this mediocre?

Did I even know what true joy felt like anymore? It got to the point where my success felt like a costume, and the woman beneath the expensive linen was longing to be heard, held, and brought back home to herself. I kept hearing this (small but always mighty) intuitive whisper saying, "You can have it all, and it doesn't need to feel like this. You can create success with elegance". So, I started making micro changes. Every day I journeyed back towards elegance. Tuning inwards. Surrounding myself with beauty. Returning to a present state. Welcoming rest. Nourishing my Self.

Every day I returned, just a little bit more, to the woman I desired to be.
And today, here I am. Successful & Elegant.

Catherine St. Germain is a vocalist, connector, and philanthropist. With over 40 years' experience in the music industry, her vast network of friends and colleagues has allowed her to connect people to help them achieve their goals.

Catherine St.Germain

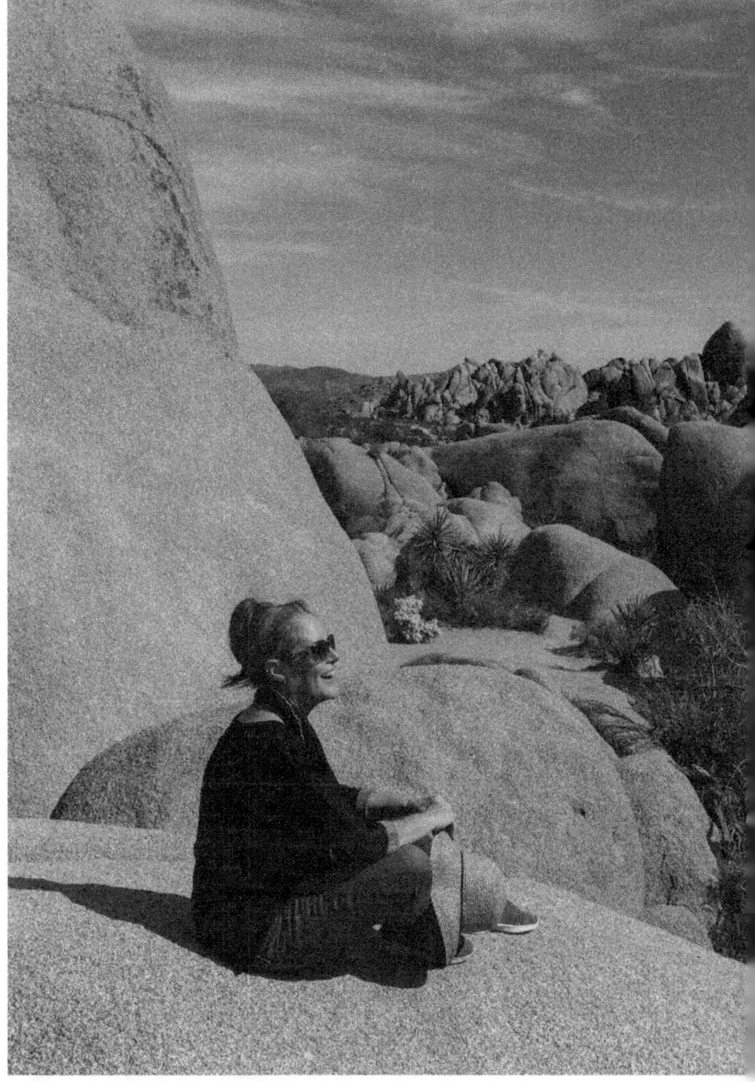
Photo Credit: Tammy Charles

Fertile at 50!!!

A few years ago, I discovered I was eight weeks pregnant!!! I know - 50 and pregnant. (It's all Mike's fault. Lol). I thought it was menopause! After the initial shock had worn off, we were excited. My HCG levels were solid, and everything looked great. Unfortunately, I miscarried the following weekend, yet my HCG levels kept climbing and were quickly through the roof. An ultrasound confirmed a "molar" pregnancy, a non-viable fertilized egg, which was growing aggressively, and an emergency hysterectomy was recommended. Molar pregnancies can invade other vital organs as cancer and must be tackled immediately. The news delivered on February 23rd was promptly followed by a chest x-ray and blood tests. At 7:30 a.m. on the 24th, a long talk with the specialist ensued, and as the cells had not spread to my other organs, we decided upon a D&C.

Although not as invasive as a hysterectomy, it was still surgery. By 4:00pm., I was in a hospital bed and awaited my husband, Mike Reno, arriving from California. My nephew Jeff was my taxi service, and two of my dearest friends tag-teamed the entire day, never leaving me alone. Emergency, busy as always, slated the surgery for 2:00 a.m.!

Mike and I, snuggled up on my single bed, were sound asleep when they came for me. Back in my room by 4:30 a.m., the surgeon assured us that the surgery had gone well. I was discharged by 9:00 a.m., and after being tucked-in at home, I slept all day. My blood was tested weekly for almost a year, as it took my HCG levels ages to zero out. After that year, it was tested every six months for the following two years.

What an emotional roller coaster! For someone without biological children, what appeared at first to be a miracle was more of a nightmare. Sometimes seeing a newborn can dishearten me, but I quickly snap out of it and realize it wasn't meant to be. My love is spent on all my wonderful nieces and nephews.

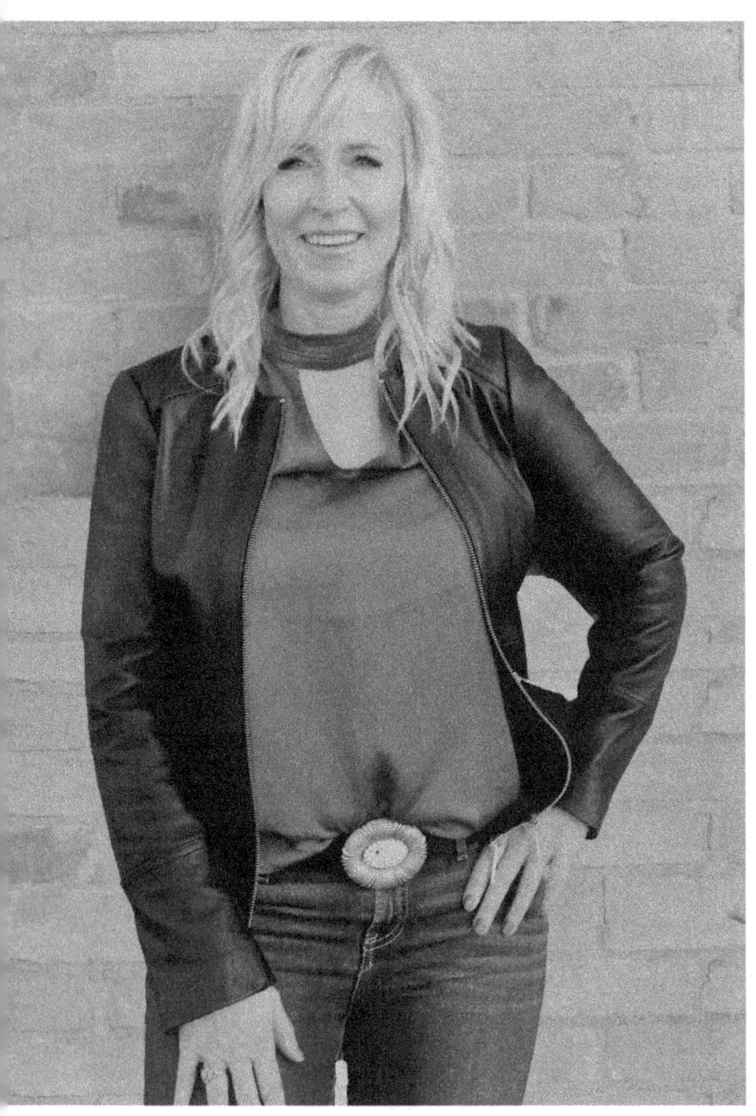

Robin Farr, Human Relations Project Manager for Kiewit Corporation, is an empathetic, courageous mother who has found her purpose in encouraging others to find happiness.

Robin Farr

Through empathy and courage, I've learned true happiness. We all know life is one hell of a ride, so hold on tight!!

The same year I was valedictorian, I also shockingly became a mother. Although my future had drastically changed, my son was the best love lesson I had ever learned. He taught me how to remain open-hearted. My calling has always been to help people. Nursing, an EA of special needs children, and assisting the visually impaired; I found my life's purpose. Eventually, I moved across Canada for a career change to teach in a men's maximum-security prison. This is where I truly found myself. The relationships I developed with the inmates were built upon respect, trust, and love. I became their mentor and helped over one hundred students to graduate and find pieces of themselves they had forgotten. I'm proud of the hard work, resilience, and teamwork that are the cornerstones of my journey.

An opportunity at a large construction company arose as a career change to be an event coordinator, headlining celebrities such as Steve Nash and Chris Hadfield. This was the most challenging experience of my life, teaching me to recognize my worth and believe in myself. It was a huge success!!

My life's purpose has always been to encourage others to be the best they can be. It's the reason I continued to follow my passion and became a personal trainer. Anytime I find a chance to help others or give back to my community, I take it. To me, living a fulfilling life comes with service and gratitude. Too many times, a missed opportunity, if not taken, could have been the lesson you needed for your personal growth. I believe when you are present, loving, and accepting, your path becomes clear, so be kind to yourself.

Through my journey, I have learned to follow my passions, fight through adversity, and always give back. This is the recipe I would share for true happiness. Be authentic, take chances and never give up.

Personal success takes 365 days a year of commitment & genuine self-love. Be patient, you're worth it!!

Valerie Blackstock is a dynamic, results-driven and creative marketing expert with over a decade of progressive experience in traditional & digital advertising.

Valerie Blackstock

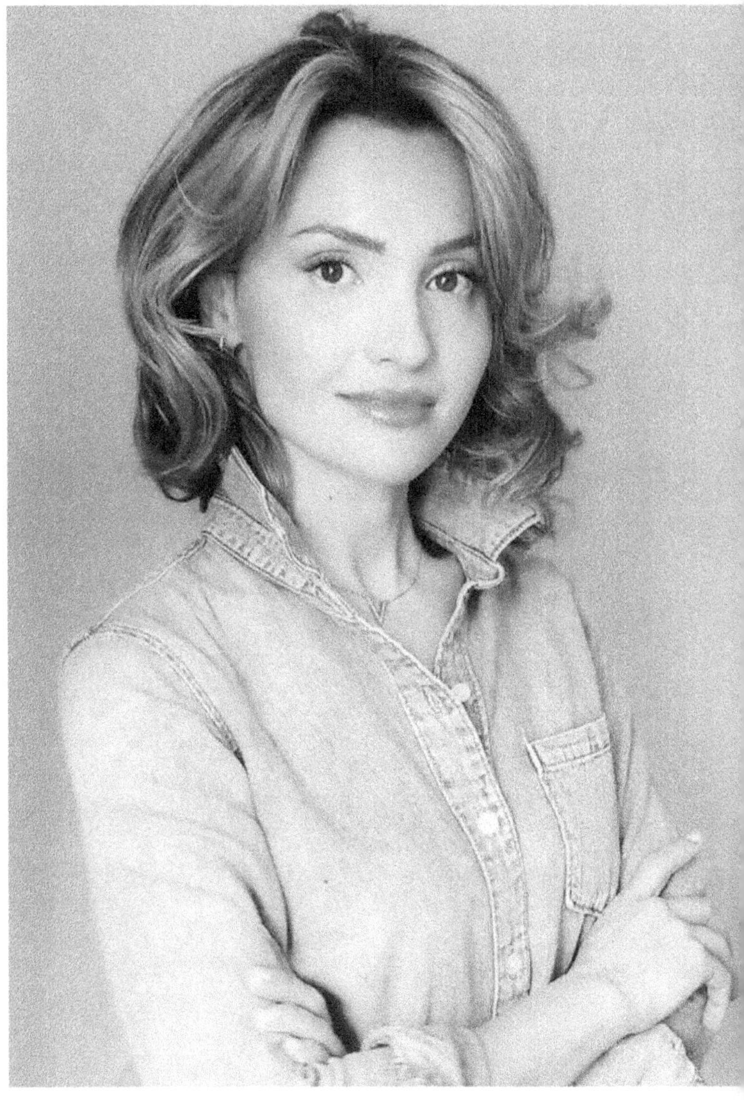

I have boundless imagination and twisted humour. Born in a small city located in the foothills of the Caucasus Mountains in southwest Russia, I have always known that I am unique. My homeland was notorious for delicious food, gracious hospitality, and unapologetic sexism. As a child, I caught on quickly to that last outdated convention and derived a plan of action. To assert equality, I would get all the girls to wear unicorn horns. My parents knew that local species taxonomy limited my opportunities, so they set their sights Westward to a land of better possibilities.

We immigrated to Canada in the winter of 1995. I was 15 years old and clueless. A tsunami of a culture shock swept right over me, leaving me lost and disoriented. To survive, I joined an elite swimming club called High School. Here, I was the new FOB on the block who did not speak a word of English. The training was brutal, to say the least, but I managed to graduate high school and moved on to college. I was an A-student during my first year, but by my second year, my poor choices caught up with me and my inner world collapsed. I was exhausted, and I did what Britney Spears would do years later - original trendsetter here - I shaved my head. Back then, it was still cool to label and ostracize people for breakdowns, so the consequences were abundant.

Still, I knew I would persevere, so once I overcame my setbacks, I took an evening marketing course at a university. I liked the discipline and decided to pursue it. It was difficult, but I worked hard and graduated with an undergraduate degree in marketing. This felt like a great accomplishment given my introduction back in high school. Bolstered by this newfound confidence, I decided to continue my studies and earned a master's degree. My education propelled me to work with various companies from start-ups to multinationals and after a decade of marketing for others, I started my own marketing consulting practice. I also accepted an offer to teach a marketing course at the very university where I took my first evening course, coming full circle.

Recently, I published my first children's book called 'Cherry Tree'. It celebrates a simple truth that our unique differences make this world genuinely beautiful and encourages everyone to be kind.

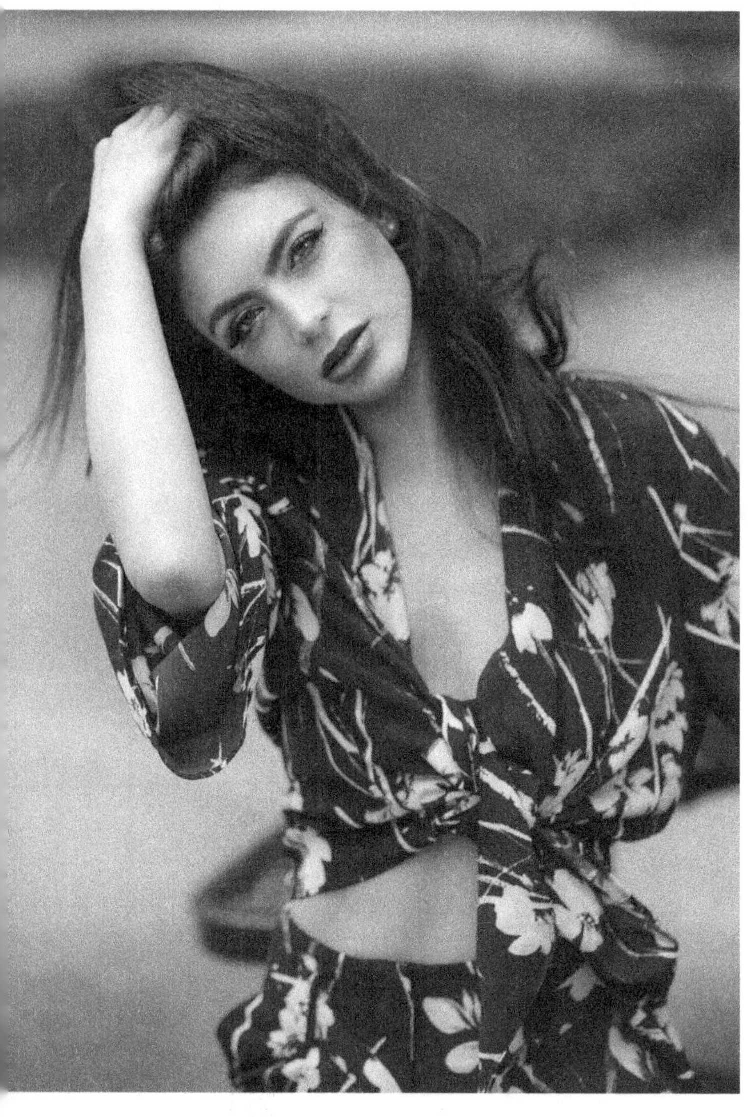

Ashley J. Hassard is a Canadian entrepreneur, teacher, publisher, photographer, model, motivational speaker, philanthropist, and overall life enthusiast.

Ashley Hassard

As an educational specialist with a background in human ecology and leadership development, she's a strong believer in the power of positive psychology and utilizes it to empower individuals and communities around her.

"It's funny how when you start to grow into yourself, the world starts to notice.

Really and truly though. The more you know yourself, the more people will start to know you; the more people who do, the more people who will want to. Once you get to know who you really are, you'll grow into a you that you're proud of, and once you start showing that real you off, you'll find that life will start complimenting you. While there's obviously no secret recipe to it, there are a few sure-fire ways to make it all a heck of a lot easier.

The first thing you've always got to keep in mind is: set goals, but don't stick blindly to them.
The vast majority of everything wonderful that has ever happened to me occurred not because I planned for it, butbecause I was willing to deviate from whatever "plan" I had.

Next, produce yourself.

Start right here, right now, with exactly what you have. Thanks to the internet we have so much power to promote, learn, and do. Figure out what you want, figure out what it takes to get there, build a website, promote yourself, and put yourself in the rooms of people who have done it before. Most people want to help you, and, if you let them, they will.

And finally, never forget that you are so much braver than you give yourself credit for.
So often in today's society we discredit that which we've overcome, things that we've done, or mountains we've climbed. We measure our lives by milestones, brush off the struggles, and gloss over the once scary details not realizing that it was in those exact moments that we showed our true strength.

Resilience is your superpower, and you have it in spades.

Suzanne Carter is the founder of M.Y.O Cosmetic Cases; she is a researcher, innovator, adventurer, and calculated risk-taker.

Suzanne Carter

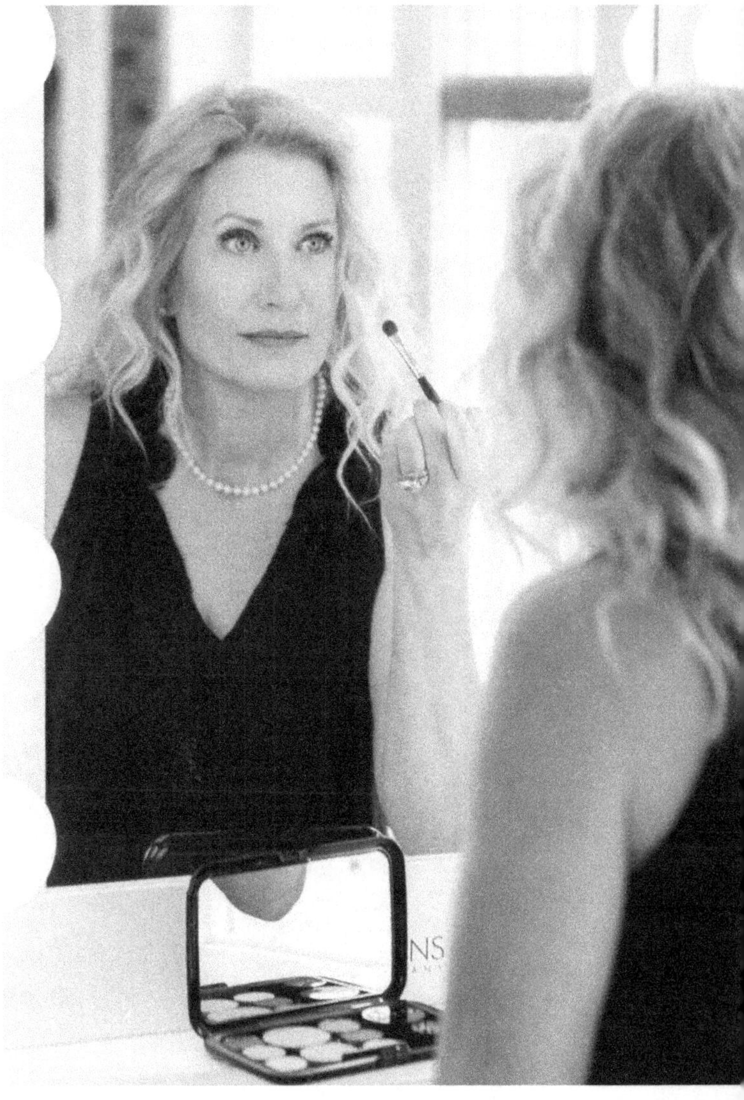

Growing up on a 25,000-acre dude ranch in the backcountry of B.C., bred a sense of creativity and innovation and ignited a thirst for adventure second to none. With over 300 cattle, 30 horses, and a multitude of other animals, every day was an adventure. Our holistic lifestyle included riding horses to round up cattle, breaking apart beaver dams that were flooding our meadows, and resourcefully using wine to color Easter eggs. Our cabins were made of logs, insulated with mud, and heated by a wood stove. These are some of the fondest memories of my childhood. On the ranch, being efficient was everything in getting a days' work one and dinner on the table.

With a ferocious appetite for adventure, by age 28, I had traveled to 28 countries experiencing diverse landscapes, architecture, people, food, and culture. Six months backpacking through Europe at age 21, you would find me volunteering in Italy at a rehabilitation camp for young people.

In my mid-twenties, excited to go back to school, I studied business, tourism management, and adult education. The blending of these fields decided my career path for the next 20 years; designing and facilitating corporate workshops, which I loved. Busy pursuing my dreams in my twenties, I thought about having a family but didn't get there until my thirties. Going back to my roots, my husband and I were able to give our daughters, our two most precious gifts, a small experience of the ranch life and its responsibilities with a horse through their teenage years.

My creativity, sense of adventure, and innovative thinking have driven all my decisions and gotten me to where I am today; an eco-conscious beauty brand owner of a product that's reducing cosmetic packaging waste, improving makeup organization, saving money, and increasing safety on set for Pro Makeup Artists. Knowing that I have created a sustainable efficiency tool that assists people at home and work brings me the greatest joy. My daughters motivate me to demonstrate what hard work can achieve and that we all have a responsibility to be part of the change we wish to see, ensuring a healthy planet for future generations.

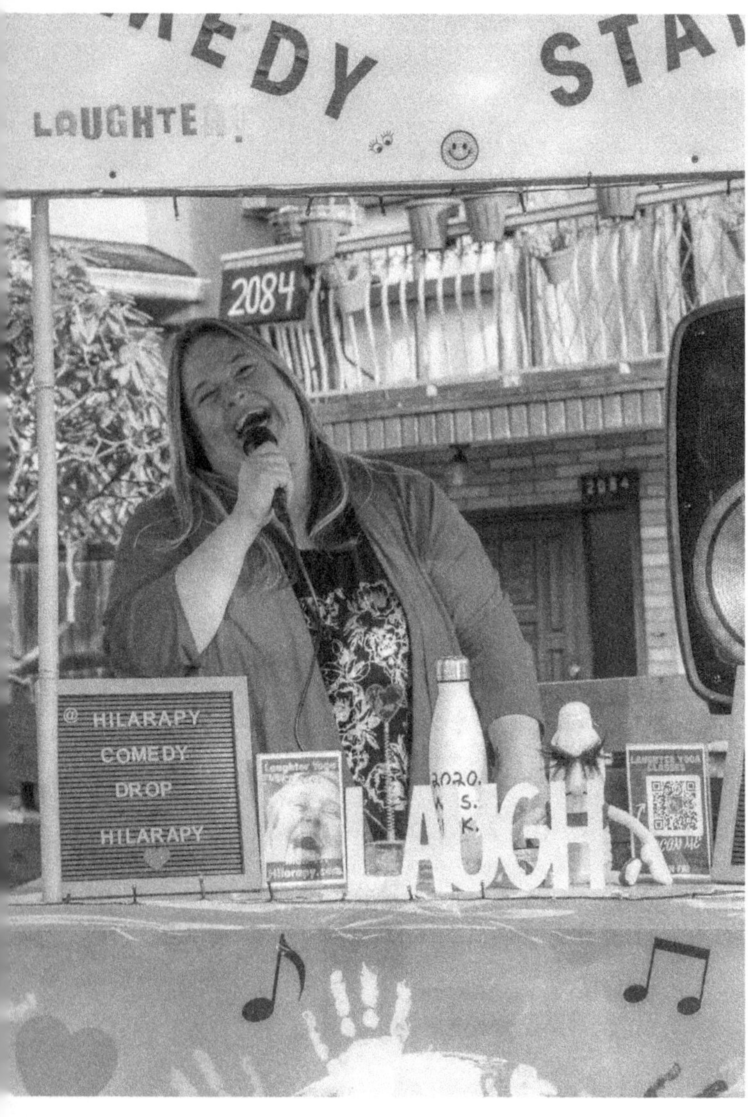

Tanya Horne is a mental health advocate, body positivity spokesperson, mother of three, and uses her voice to help change lives.

Tanya Horne

After struggling to raise three kids as a teenage mom, I found myself thrust into dealing with my own sexual abuse trauma when it happened with my children; I knew it was time to break these historical abuse cycles. I am a previously published author, an award-winning speaker, a coach, a lover of humanity, and a believer in strengthening the fabric of goodwill in the world through meaningful contributions. Yet still, after some levels of success, I could never seem to climb out from living my life full of apologies for being who I am. Recently, I decided that I was no longer willing to bend and hustle for other people's version of who they needed me to be.

The pandemic had us all switching gears, and I went from cleaning toilets to changing lives, starting with my own. I have always been a passionate contributor, someone who loves to feel included and connected with others. Unfortunately, my life was often plagued by other people's expectations and opinions of me. I found myself always living aligned to other people's truths and negating my own. I have always remained steadfast in my pursuit to "find myself" like I was on some cosmic search for how to be good enough; how to be someone important.

What I have found through radical self-love and acceptance in the past year is that all we ever need to do is be; be all of who we are meant to be. It is with this recognition that I have allowed myself to really step into the spotlight of my own life, to take up the space that I require to be seen, to be heard, and to know that I know that I matter. After a lifetime of living behind the scenes, I decided to step into the spotlight and own my story. This is where my comedy career as the Sit-Down Stand-Up Comedian, a mental health advocate, and a body positivity spokesperson came to be. This soul spark ignited my ability to be all of me through my stand up, laughter yoga leading, and my contribution as a Core Community Connector with Hilarapy.

Shana Recker is a business and mindset coach who empowers people to take action on their biggest dreams and desires. Founder of the Pursuit Elite Mastermind, the Dream Hustle Academy & The Pursuit Podcast

Shana Recker

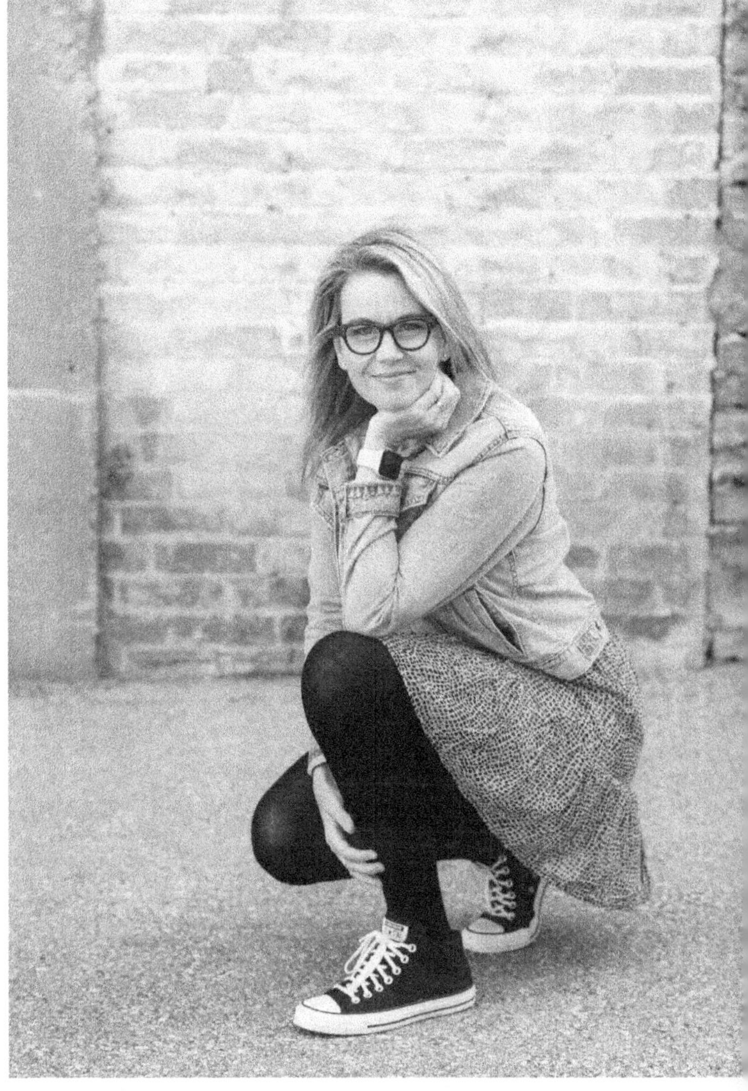

I've come face to face with many setbacks and roadblocks over the years, the biggest one being my own thinking. For starters, I put off starting my online coaching business for a full year because I felt like I "wasn't ready," but in all honesty, I was scared. Most people knew I didn't go to school for coaching, I just had my own experience in my niche, so I figured people would think I was a fraud. I was worried about what others would think of me.

That's when I invested in my first coach. He helped me understand my experiences were worth just as much, if not more, than any coaching certificate. He was right, and I got started.

Building my own successful online coaching business taught me many things, the biggest being the only way to make your desires come to life is to TAKE ACTION! Bold, scary, action! The path to your goal unfolds as you take the steps. It's impossible to have it all figured out before you move.

Since that big, bold, first step, I've created a six-figure coaching business and have helped hundreds of new entrepreneurs get over their fears and pursue their online business dreams! I have a natural ability to activate people to take action on their passions. Because of my own experience, and helping so many others, I know the fears that are holding them back. I help push through their own mindset blocks, map out their strategy, and feel confident about their actions. One of the biggest lessons I teach is that our thinking creates our results, and obstacles are our biggest gifts. The roadblocks and challenges are here to help us. Looking for the positive in every situation moves you closer to your goals faster than worrying about what's going wrong.

There is freedom in knowing we create our own results through our thinking. When it comes to achieving our goals, we can get caught up in the strategies. Actions are important but having a clear understanding of how your mindset impacts your results is just as important.

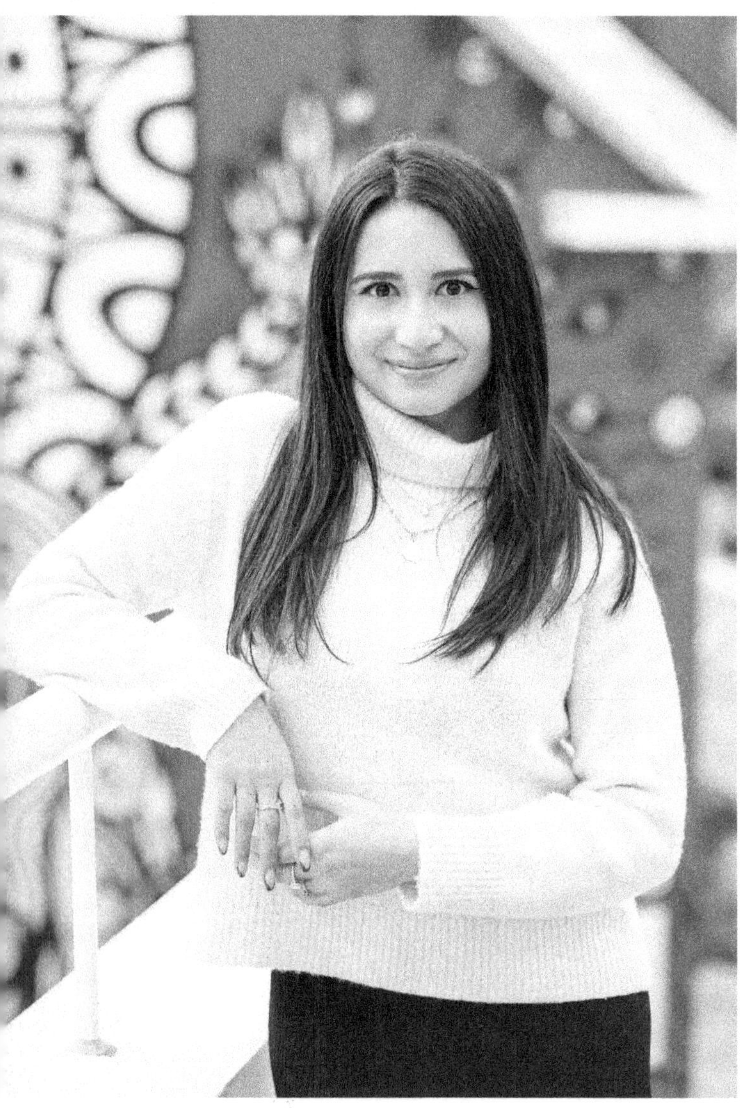

Gabriela Trujillo is a Life Empowerment & Emotional Healing Mindset Coach and Speaker who focuses on helping women find alignment in life with spirituality, mindset techniques, and neuroscience for overall well-being.

Gabriela Trujillo

My dearest family and friends tell me that my greatest strengths lie in my pursuit of empowering others, with my upbringing and healing being my most outstanding teacher. May that be with my honesty, my positive determination, authenticity, intuitive observations that drive my soul, and a free spirit kind of motto with unwavering faith to walk my light. I should let you know that I shed countless layers to break down to be who I am today, and in hopes to share that light amongst many to join forces with me to make that change for them too.

You'll be sure to know, the pursuit of happiness means depending on who you ask. I'm in my mid 20's, and to me, when I reflect on my life and career, where I went entirely right was my utter faith in presence, intuition, and the conscious-subconscious mind for internal transformation.

I have not walked a typical life since my childhood. After living in a toxic household until early adulthood, I lived with depression, anxiety, trauma, and PTSD. I became ever so proud to break through the healing within five years of that chapter ended. I moved to Toronto with my can-do spirit, started living in my dream apartment, and got rid of the car that gave me freedom. I took the real change that had come from conscious efforts evoking massive transformation to break down many of the ups and downs in just a matter of years; you can do it too. I promise!

Each step, whether it's working the odd jobs here and there in between cities, learning the unspoken life lessons no one told you about or meeting people from different walks of life in separate chapters, stand tall and proud of where you come from, where you've been, and where you will be. I've discovered with more knowledge and experience, that with a leap of faith, it's possible to always prioritize your well-being as the greatest gift to yourself and your future - your truth matters.

Ami Mckay is the top Vancouver interior designer and creative director at PURE Design Inc., an award-winning, internationally published interior design firm.

Ami McKay

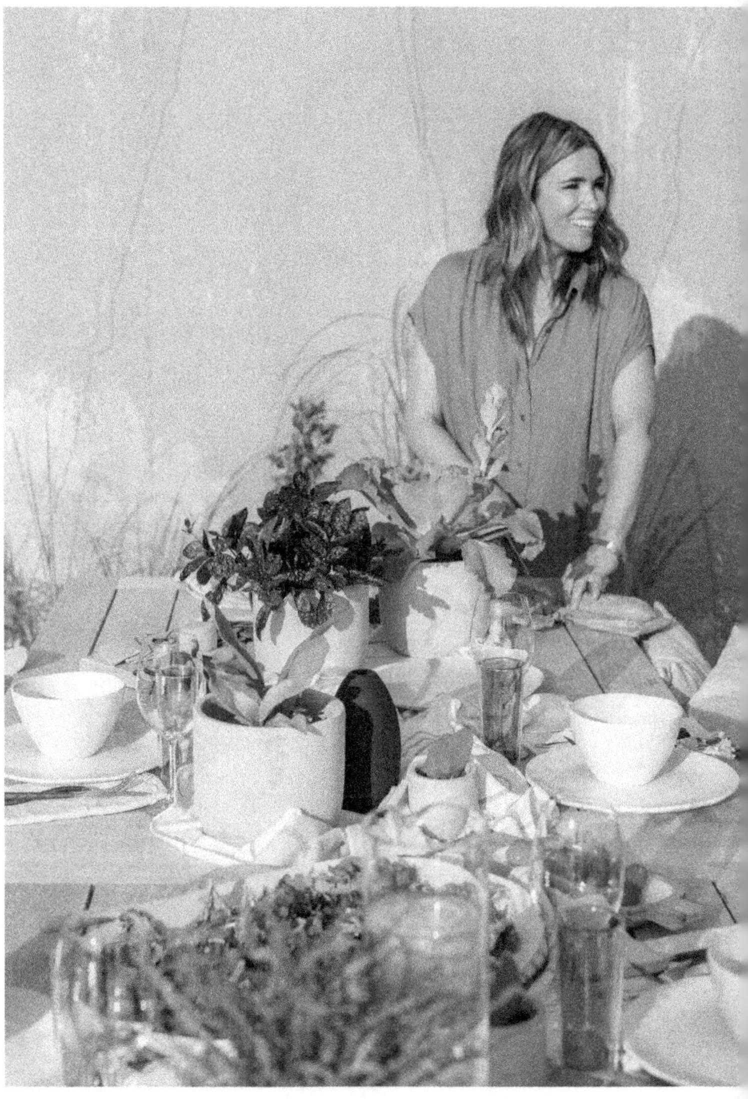

When Ami McKay was 18 years old, a newspaper reporter asked her what she wanted to be when she grew up. Her answer?

Run a successful design firm and be happy.

Today, as the Owner and Principal Designer of PURE Design Inc., an award-winning, internationally published Vancouver interior design firm, it's clear that young Ami would be proud. Not to say the journey to this point was always easy. Like most business owners, the early stages of building PURE were filled with many obstacles, challenges, and failures. To overcome these setbacks, Ami continuously reminded herself that life's journey is never linear, and that failure is inevitable. In Ami's eyes, if you have the strength and courage to get back up each time you fall, you'll always finish standing. This is sometimes hard for Ami as she was diagnosed with Ehlers Danlos Syndrome, which knocks her off her feet.

It's this perseverance and passion that Ami tries to instill in those around her. She is the first to tell you that PURE is successful because of its amazing team and that it wouldn't have been possible for her to do it alone. Ami recognizes that creativity rarely happens in a vacuum, and so she's worked her entire career to build a network that is supportive and empowering, both for her and for each other. Ask anyone in Ami's circle, and they'd be quick to tell you that her superpower is the ability to make those around her feel good about themselves. And it is this esteem and empowerment that has allowed Ami to build a world-class team at PURE that continues to take her business to heights she never imagined.

While most may think that building a successful design firm would be enough to satisfy 18-year-old Ami's goal to "be happy," it's only one half of the equation. For Ami, true success (and true happiness) can only be achieved when you share that success with others. That's why PURE was built to put people over profits. Because numbers come and go, but you will always remember the way someone made you feel.

For Ami McKay, true success is leaving every person she meets feeling better than she found them.

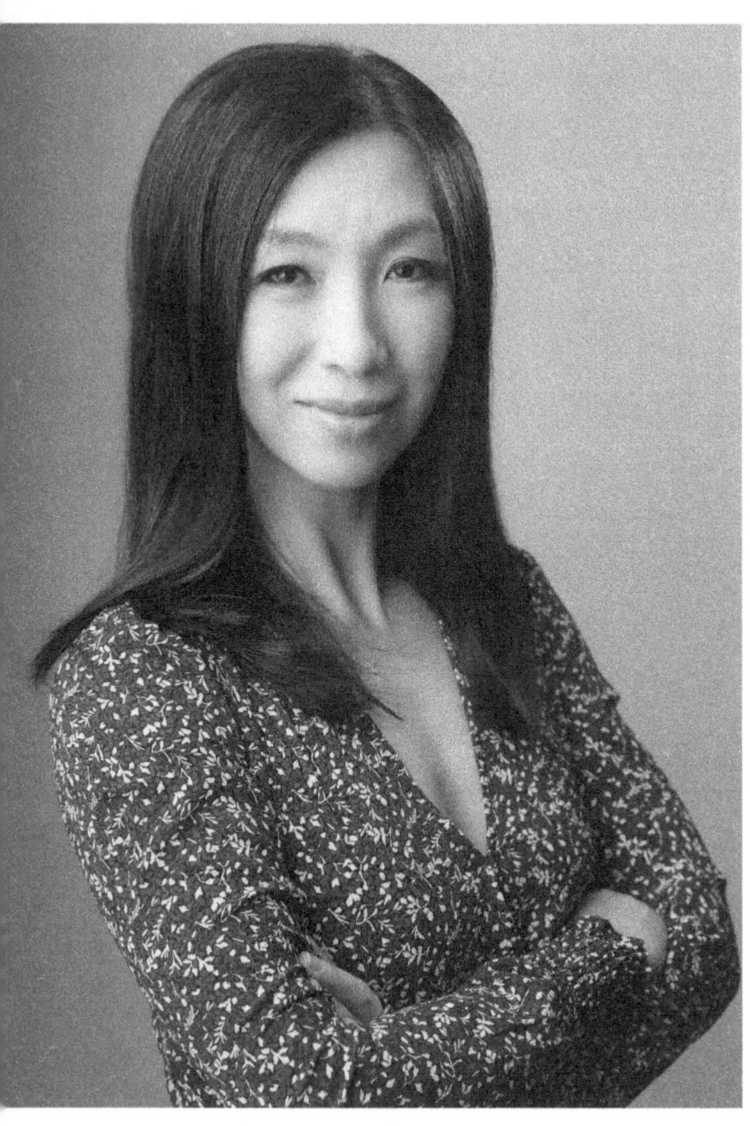

Lily Yuan is a producer, artist, art instructor, mother of two, and Canadian bodybuilding competition medalist.

Lily Yuan

Many people find it difficult to ignore the discourse of others! Their words, their views, and their attitudes can lead to self-evaluation and inordinately impact one's mood or behaviour. Many people will adjust their lives according to another's vision of them. I am not one of those people.

Born with an artistic nature, I longed to explore all life's avenues and adventures, being bored with the status quo. I enjoyed new ideas and anticipated the puzzling challenges that might lie ahead. A true artist is often a perfectionist and has the patience, determination, and diligence to achieve the highest standards in their work. I view life's twists and turns like a new work of art.

The beauty and excellence of a new painting is attainable but requires devotion, practice, repetition, endless thought, and ample time. It also requires you to follow your own heart and make sometimes difficult decisions.

My life decisions are divided into two categories, business-related and personal. Business-related decisions are made based on what the market will bear; what is needed. Your personal judgment is essential but predicting and understanding the market's demands are vital to a guaranteed success. Personal decisions are likened to a painting that portrays your own story, designed with your own elements. Personal goals are equally as relevant as business goals. They must be given equal time and commitment, for they round out your life and make you feel whole. Too much passion and obstinance can be harmful when making business decisions, but personal goals cannot be achieved without them.

Surround yourself with like-minded professionals that have the required skill sets and the same passion and energy as you. We learn from everyone, both colleagues and mentors. My path has been guided by many mentors; masters in their fields. I cannot thank them enough. This quote sums it up for me, "A conversation with a Master is worth ten years of reading books." Pursuing my dreams can sometimes be lonely and time-consuming, but life is short, and there is nothing more important than living every moment and creating the change you wish to see.

Randa Derkson is a Certified Holistic Nutritionist and Certified Sports Nutrition Consultant, recipe developer, and mom of two littles.

Randa Derkson

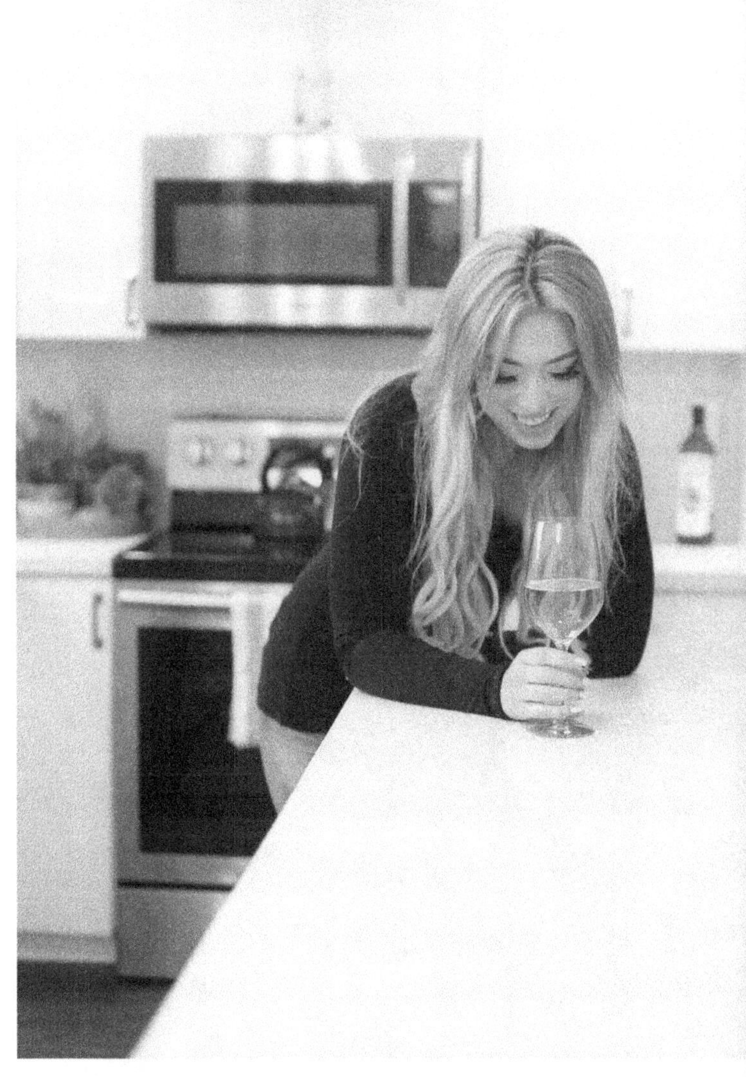

Basically, my life revolves around food. That being said, I love pizza, tacos, chocolate, and red wine. So, it's my mission to teach nutrition without a deprivation mindset because let's face it, diets don't work.

I'm incredibly passionate about helping moms escape dieting because I was that mom. The mom who only ate "clean," who would have a treat and feel like she failed, the mom who would binge after said "failure," only to restrict my food the next day and start the hamster wheel all over again. After years of dieting, deprivation, and being hungry to be "skinny" my physical and mental health hit a breaking point.

I couldn't do it anymore. I knew I couldn't continue like this, if not for me - for my kids. I didn't want them to see a dieting mentality, and I knew I had to break the cycle. I started after my daughter was born in 2018. Instead of seeing my large arms and focusing on that, I started to lift weights to be strong (and be able to carry that car seat!). I looked in the mirror daily and praised myself, praised my body for being able to haul a car seat and baby around all day, and gave myself grace. That's when it changed. I saw food as fuel, not the enemy. That's when I knew I had to share this with other moms. After a lot of work and education, I help busy and overwhelmed moms get out of the diet cycle and see calories as fuel instead of the enemy.

No more end dates, no more restrictions. Just a healthy lifestyle that includes balanced nutrition and chocolate. I want to help you to take charge of your health, use what I give you as a template, and build a healthy lifestyle into your life, not your life around a healthy lifestyle.

Let's ditch the fad diets (been there, failed at that), calorie deprivation, and restriction around our favorite foods. I'm here to teach busy moms realistic nutrition that you can apply to your family because no one wants to eat a salad while their family enjoys pizza.

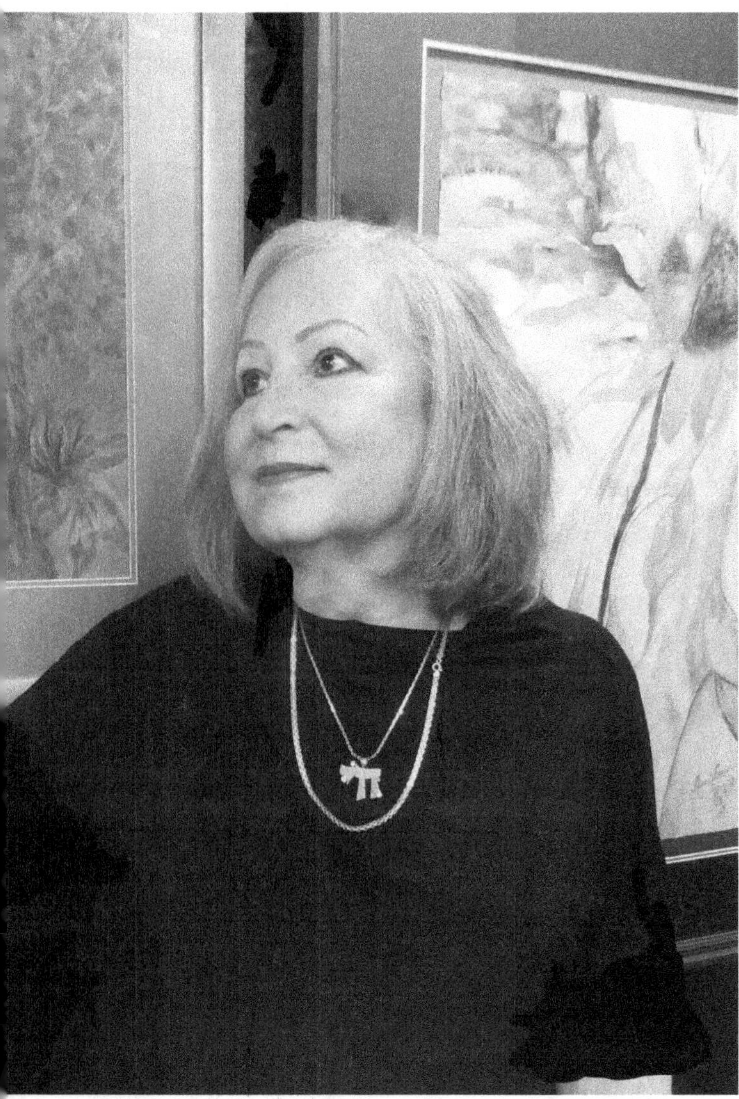
Photo Credit: Dr. Teri Fisher

Ava Lee is a highly original and imaginative thinker, who graciously shares her creativity and knowledge through multiple media, including music and fine arts.

Ava Lee Millman Fisher

MTA, BMT, LMus, AMus, DipEd

I am grateful! I am appreciative of the myriad of opportunities with which I was, and am, presented, and of the combination of choices that I have made. When I take a long glance over my shoulder, I recall that as a young child, the arts were emphasized in our family home. I joyfully participated in Hebrew lessons, piano, ballet, tap, art, and drama classes. My Dad was of Jewish origin, born in Poland; he emigrated to Montreal as a young boy. My Mom was born in Montreal to Jewish parents who had emigrated from Russia. Judaism glowingly enveloped our lives. I intuitively garnered from the totality of my background the understanding that through my life's journey, I should and would be morally required to give back.

Early on it was recognized that I exhibited an obvious delight in all that was artful. With maturation, I continued to demonstrate a developing interest in the arts and pursued them in the spirit of adventure and exploration. I also studied the past with an emphasis that was constantly alive to the treasures of my religion and my culture. When it came time to pursue a university education, I had serious debates with myself about whether to proceed with music or fine arts. The debate ended when I had a vocal audition at McGill University, and won a vocal prize. In the Faculty of Music, I reached for a career in opera and the classical art song. I also studied a vast repertoire of Hebrew and Yiddish songs. I received my teaching accreditation from MacDonald College. However, I never gave up my love of painting. I took numerous lessons and classes and could be caught in the act whenever I had spare time.

Marriage and motherhood followed, with the birth of my four fabulous sons. Life was very hectic! Nevertheless, when my boys were all in school full-time, I decided to return to university to pursue a degree in Music Therapy. Upon graduation and accreditation, I worked for over twenty-five years with those suffering from mental illness. My rewards were profound! Gradually, as my spinto-soprano voice declined with age, my love of painting moved dominantly into the foreground. Today, creating works of art is my visual voice.

Elise is an entrepreneur that is passionate about creating, personal growth, justice, and sustainability.

Elise MacDonald

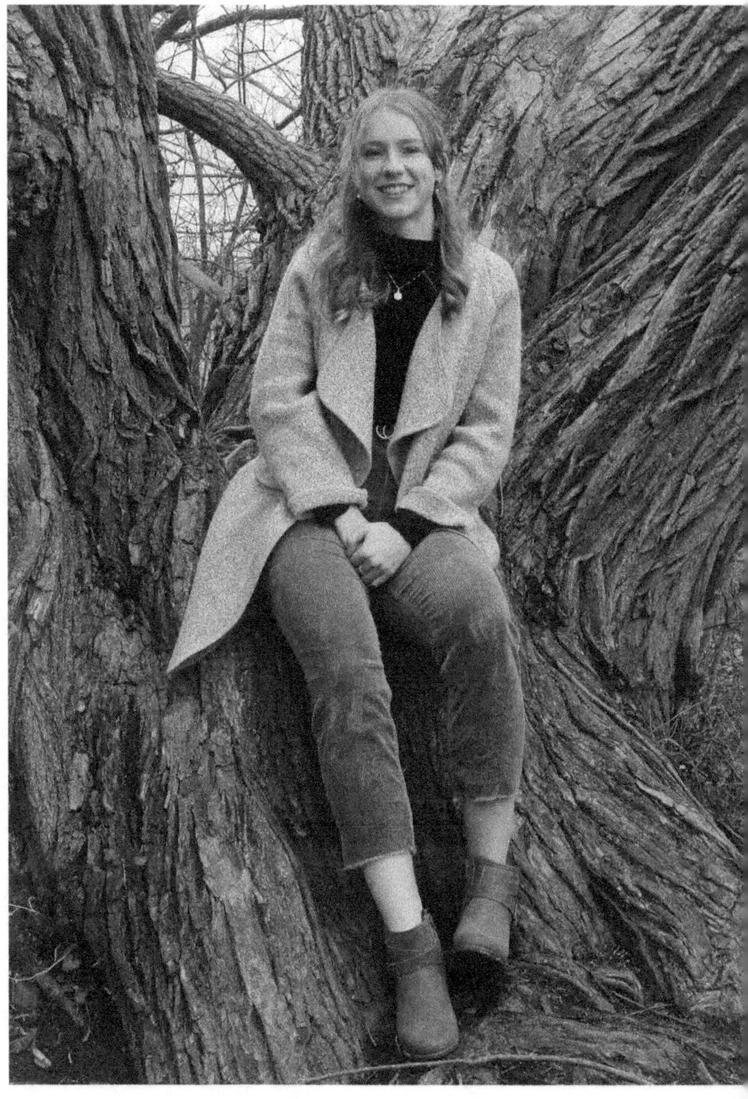

In my pursuit of happiness and success, my greatest lesson has been to believe in myself. It took me a long time to realize I have something important and valuable to share. Growing up, I was often the kid in the background. Very shy and quiet, reluctant to share my opinions because I was nervous about how they would be perceived. This mentality is something that I have struggled with in many facets of my life. Through building my own macrame business, I've proven to myself that what I have to put out into the world through my passions that inspire me are important, and there is value in sharing them. Alone I can do great things! I think for young women, this is a realization that is so important.

Taking steps to become confident in yourself to the point where you can stand alone and believe in a vision only you can see is so powerful. It is transformative regarding how you view yourself in the world and how you represent yourself to the world.

I try to represent the truest and best version of myself through business. To me, this means incorporating aspects such as social justice and environmental justice into my platform to make a positive impact. I aspire to create something bigger than myself by taking small steps and using them as a catalyst for change.

I want to leave this world having inspired and empowered others and fought for justice. These are goals I continually strive to incorporate into my business.

I started my business when I was 18 years old to make some extra money on the side. I wasn't sure if my creations would be something people would like. I remember wondering if I would ever get an order. At that point, I wouldn't have believed that four years later I would be asked to be part of a women's empowerment book! If you have a vision, belief in your ability, are patient and persistent, you never truly know where your passions may take you!

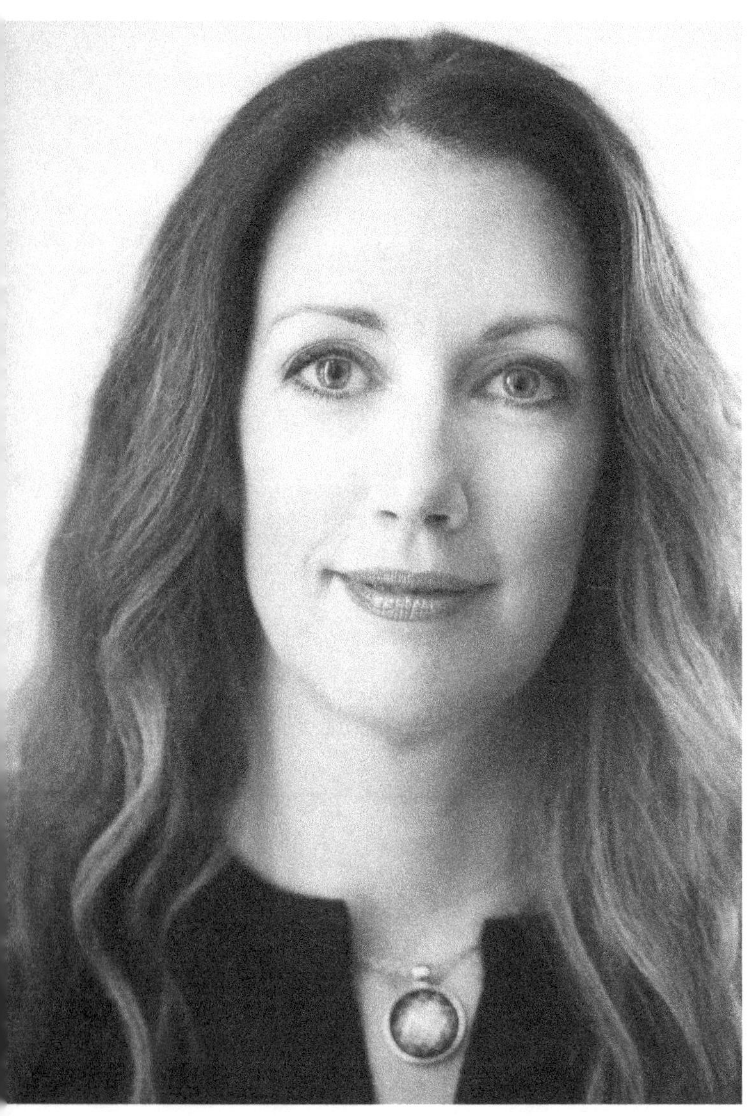

Tanya Farlinger is a dynamic small business owner, a champion for her all-female staff, and a leader who now follows her own dreams.

Tanya Farlinger

I did everything I was supposed to. I got an education, started at the bottom, and worked my way up the ladder in my chosen field of Aesthetics. I successfully led cosmetics teams, day spas, and even a Caribbean destination spa resort. Specializing in the beauty and wellness industry, employee productivity, training and development, social media, and marketing, I built solid relationships with staff members, industry distributors, and my local Chamber of Commerce. It wasn't until a cancer diagnosis at thirty-seven that I stopped to look around. I came up to breathe, and I realized I'd been killing myself for someone else's dream.

When's the last time you stopped? Is your life what you envisioned, or have you been too busy sacrificing, raising a family, and working to even think about it? That was me.

Cancer was my wake-up call.

I was raised by a driven family and urged to work hard to succeed. I was grateful to be alive and now healthy, and less than a year later I dove headfirst into giving back, so much so that I changed careers, and experienced complete burnout managing an integrative cancer centre. It was too much. Another wake-up call.

After a long talk with my Nonna about what I truly valued in life, I awoke, and this is when exhālō Spa and my true purpose was born. To lead and empower women, spread joy through the power of touch, and create a healing space with positive vibes for all to enjoy. She encouraged me to move forward.

The word exhālō is a play on the words exhale and halotherapy. Our lovingly created watercolor mandala logo centers and calms the mind and features the throat chakra. Eminence Organic Skincare and Hair Design services are built surrounding our healing & immune-boosting Salt Therapy Room. I now work daily alongside the most supportive group of positive women - my Dream Team, and after three successful years, we've opened a second Ottawa location.

Now when I stop and look around? I smile, and even though she's no longer with us, I know my Nonna is looking down on me with pride, light, and love.

exhālō, the spa that feeds your soul. Simply exhale, we've got you.

A dedicated Realtor who believes in the power of positive thought.

Amaal Ebrahim

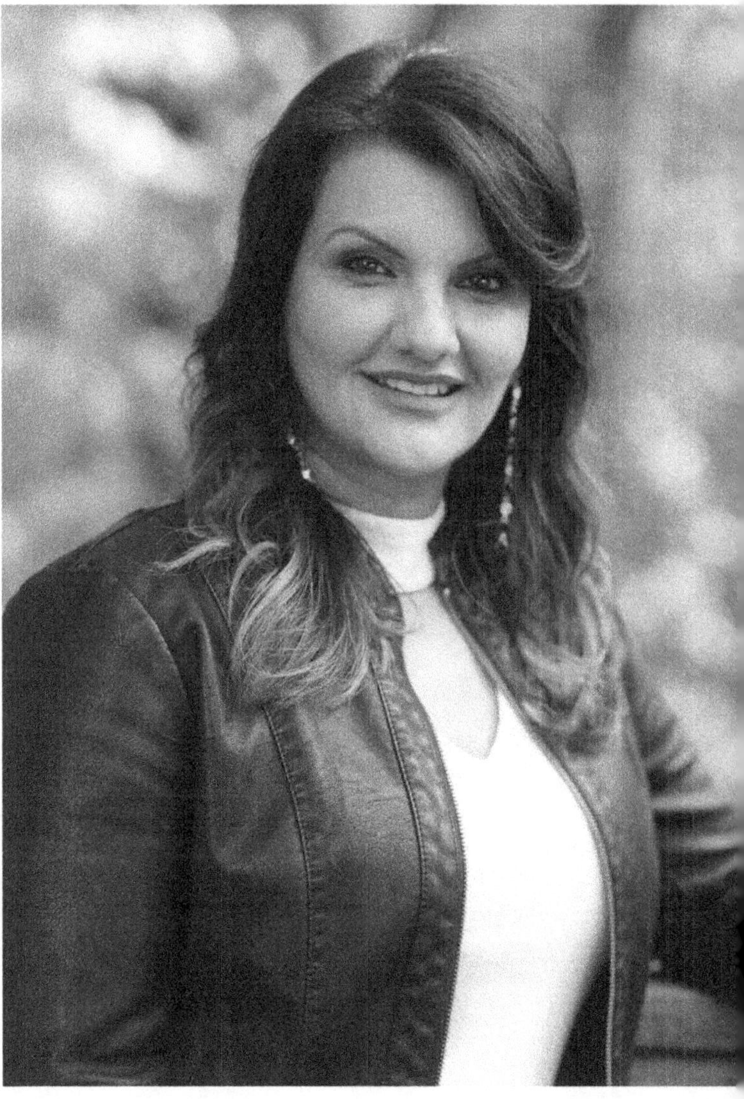

As I watched my daughter on stage at McMaster University, I fought hard to keep the tears from running. My only child was openly expressing herself with grace and confidence. I had released my desires to the Universe, and the Universe delivered. I believe that what you put out there does indeed come back! After many years of hardship, our lives were finally in a place of safety and abundance; we weren't just existing anymore, we were living meaningful lives.

As a child, I moved from home to home and country to country between parents, finally returning to Tanzania from Congo, at the age of 18. At 24, I married a man that was not suited for me.

A year later, after giving birth to our child, we got divorced and I embarked on a new journey. My late mother was my sole support system during those trying days, and even though it was exactly what we needed, I still yearned for the freedom and independence to make my own choices and decisions for me and my child.

With nothing but a high school diploma, I moved to Toronto. My new adventures with my 4-year-old began with learning how to drive, to cook, to make it through winters, to make my own decisions, and to make it here without any family support.

Through the tough days and lonely nights, I maintained a strong sense of positivity and kept my inner self grounded. I have no regrets; the experiences made me stronger, more resilient, and taught me the life skills that I could then impart to my daughter. Over the years, I have learned to maintain a positive attitude, harness my intuition, allow my inner voice to be louder, and to treat myself and others with respect.

I absolutely LOVE what I do for a living because I understand how important a home, not a house, is to my clients.

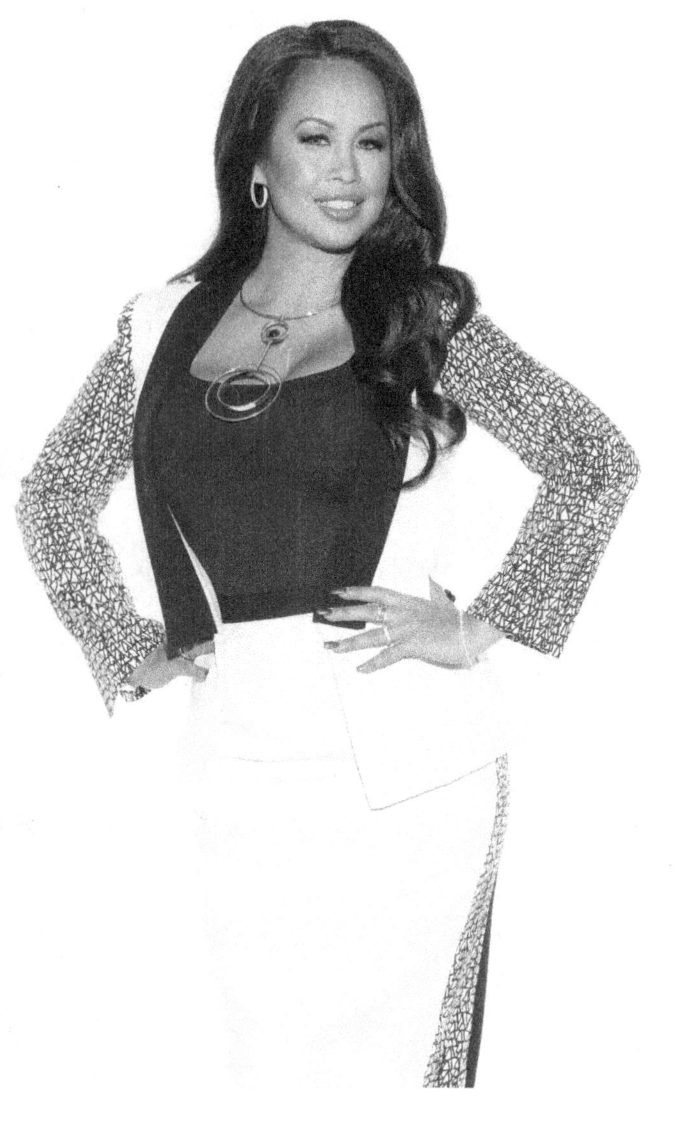

Carmelia Ray is an award-winning Celebrity Matchmaker, TV host, producer and online dating expert. She supports some of the most successful singles in the world to find love. Camelia has been dubbed, "The Most Successful Matchmaker" among leading entrepreneurs and thought leaders. Her mission is to connect her elite clients with their soulmate through her tireless ability to collaborate and network in high-level social circles.

Carmelia Ray

I worked at the first dating service in 1992 in Canada, interviewing singles who shared their struggles of finding love in a pre-digital world. Fast forward 28 years and singles are struggling to date in a pandemic with isolation and depression at an all-time high.

I've seen remarkable changes in the dating landscape as more and more singles are turning to dating apps, and digital platforms to find a life partner. I've interviewed over 65,000 singles on the challenges of how to date, meet and keep their match in a competitive and busy dating landscape.

As a serial entrepreneur, I thrive when working with peak performers who work hard, play hard, and are ready to meet their match. I'm a "Mompreneur" raising three kids at home. I'm the daughter of immigrant traditional Filipino parents and the middle child between two boys. My parents taught me the value of hard work, resilience, never giving up, and having an attitude of gratitude.

I'm a frequent media contributor on multiple media platforms and have had my dating advice featured in notable outlets. Mentions included are on CNN, USA Today, The Morning Show, AskMen, Variety, The Hollywood Reporter, OK! Magazine, Global News, The Washington Post, The Marilyn Denis Show, CHCH News, Elle, and countless others. My experience has attracted in-demand partnerships with major dating companies, brands and Celebrities. I've been the Host of my Reality Dating Show Mom vs Matchmaker for 4 Seasons with multiple guest appearances in other TV shows.

I recently launched my relationship podcast Better Love. An online Matchmaking Academy to certify new matchmakers and dating coaches. I'm the Chief Matchmaker at Censio, a premiere Matchmaking App. As well I've just launched a professional Livestream and production studio called MXL Live Lofts to help entrepreneurs share their message with the world with video content!

Sarah Khan is a business acceleration strategist and the CEO of Linchpin Virtual.

Sarah Khan

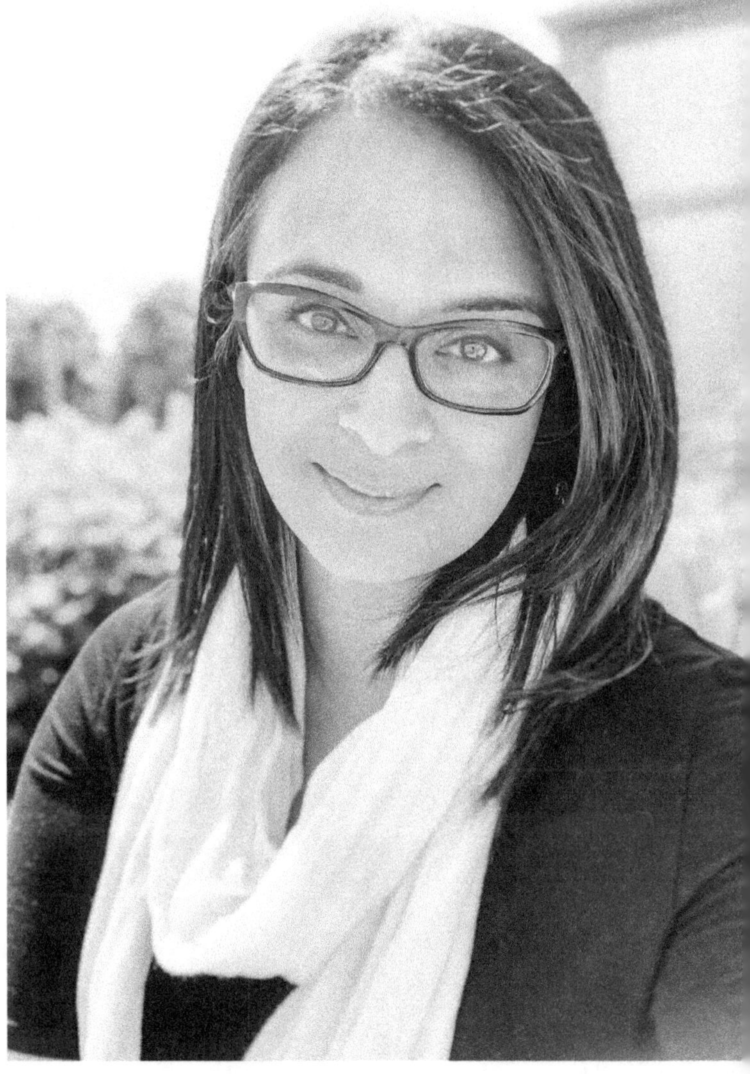

They say if you chain a baby elephant to a post, it quickly learns that the length of the chain is as far as it can ever go, even into adulthood. So, it never tries to break free and go beyond the length of the chain.

I never wanted to be an entrepreneur.

The idea of working for myself was terrifying. The uncertainty and the hustle were not for me. Entrepreneurs work more hours a week than the average employee in a business. I liked my set hours. I didn't mind the occasional overtime. It was liberating to know someone else worried about quotas, sales, networking, and recruitment. I just went in, did my job, and went home.

I was a model employee; loyal, driven, incredible work ethic. I followed the rules, I toed the party line, the proverbial Kool-Aid was my drink of choice. And yet, the older I got, the very things that had once given me security and structure became confining, stifling, suffocating.

As time went on, being okay with things simply because "that's the way they've always been" or "that's just the way things are" didn't feel okay anymore. Not because I had some grand awakening in my 40's but because the very machine I had helped build and keep running for years suddenly turned on me and slowly started eating me alive.

Walking away from all I had ever known was gut-wrenching. Starting my own business was not the exhilaration it is for some. It was a necessity, a lifeboat keeping me afloat in the waves of uncertainty. Because in the early days as a business owner, I was still playing by the rules I'd played by my whole life.

Until, like the elephant who finally realizes it's stronger than the post, I realized the rules were my chain.

So now I'm working on shifting the paradigms we exist in as women, mothers, business owners... busting the chains of traditional marketing, strategy, and growth. I help other women do the same in life and business. Because the very chains we are told are there for our protection are the ones keeping us from truly stepping out into the world.

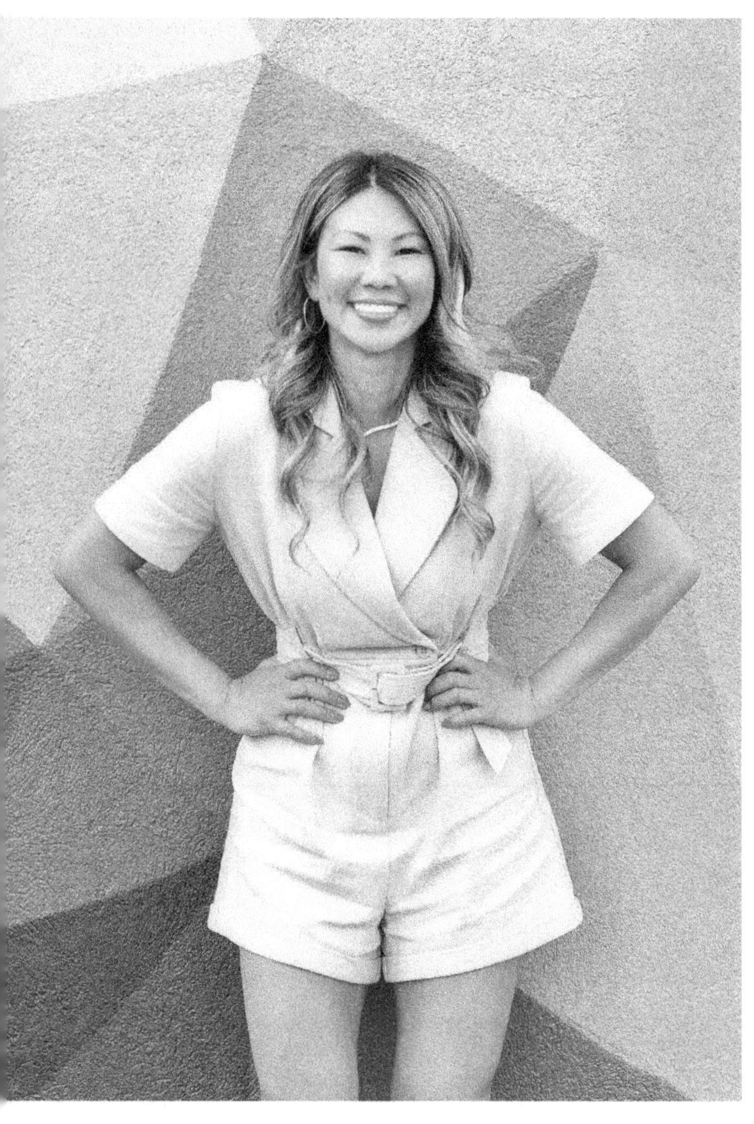

Jenny Wun is a real estate professional with almost two decades of experience in the industry. A serial entrepreneur, she founded West One Real Estate Marketing and Parallel Project Marketing while leading a top producing real estate team in Metro Vancouver. She frequently acts as a guest speaker on matters relating to women leadership, the local real estate market, and new home construction trends. She also co-hosts a podcast, "In The House with Toni and Jenny."

Jenny Wun

This woman, a stranger to me until that day, showed me photos, and therein the proof, my partner of almost a decade, her partner for almost as long.

Here is where the kind of woman I am, shaped what I did next. I walked away, maintained my integrity, and accepted my past. I forged onwards with the person who I always counted on – myself: she who is steadfast, driven, and industrious. Through my financial acumen and fierceness of character, I rebuilt. I committed to living a life of my own design, all about creating success on my own terms and committing to going after my goals strategically, ambitiously, and unapologetically. I am that kind of woman.

As a champion of women, I want women to go after the big deal they might not otherwise feel qualified for, the raise they might not ask for, the partnership they might not feel they have permission to pursue. I help women learn how to kill it in this industry.

It is not about competition, as I hope so many women have figured out. It is about being the best version of myself and wanting the same for others. I help women build those unshakable foundations, knowing how essential mine has been for me. Call me a mindset maven. Through my initiatives and conscious dialogue, women find their freedom through confidence, mental wealth, and emotional agility. Women must own their self-worth.

You, yes you have permission to love yourself, to honor your value, and to build your own life and redesign as needed. It is our time – through collective voices – to rewrite the rules.

I am that kind of woman. You are that kind of woman. We are those women.

Amanda Asta is a breathwork practitioner and the founder of Transcend Academy, one of the world's most robust breathwork training programs.

Amanda Asta

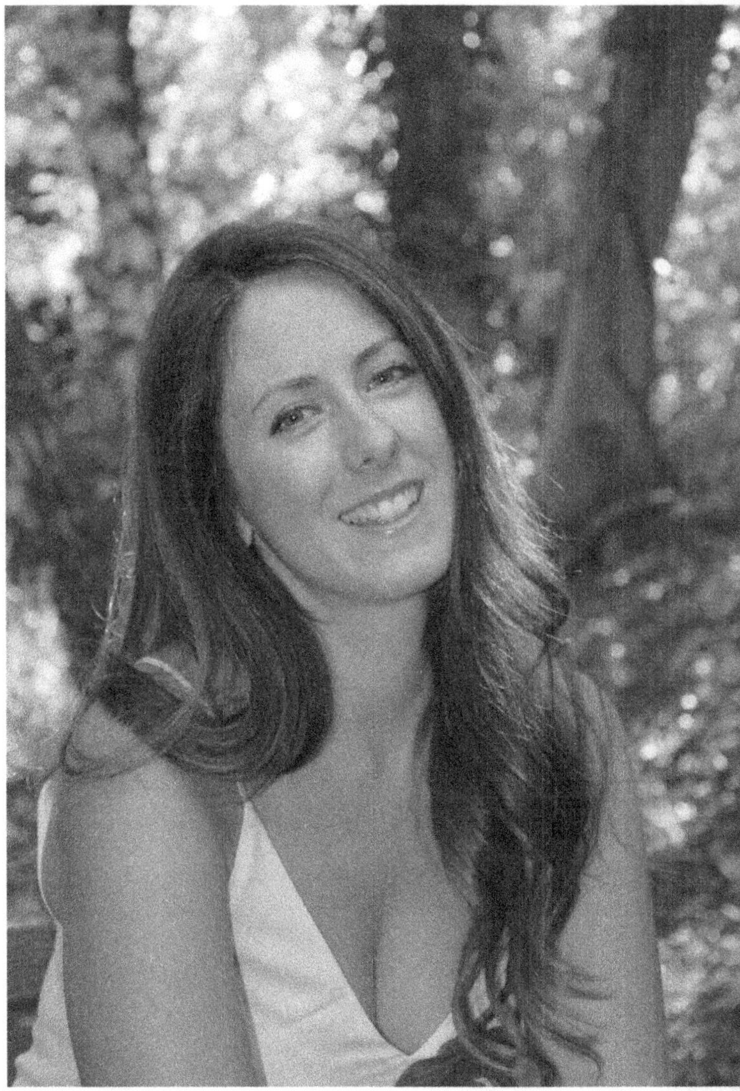

Breathwork has changed my life for the better. I was fortunate enough to discover it by chance in Peru and have seen and experienced incredible transformations with breathwork ever since.

It integrates beautifully with my passion for civil liberties, human rights, and collective evolution as a species to bring about greater fulfillment and joy to our lives. I believe "the root of all evil" isn't money but the unhealed ego.

So, my mission begins one person at a time, doing the inner work to evolve past our traumas, limiting beliefs, and patterns passed down to us through the generations.

If we can clear the slate for future generations, we can revolutionize the flawed systems that perpetuate inequality and environmental degradation. This is the passion behind my service, and my modality for achieving this is Breathwork.

I founded Transcend Academy, one of the world's most robust breathwork schools, to train people from all over the world to share this modality and manifest a tidal wave of healing. Every student will impact thousands of lives in their communities. Throughout our training, I have been so inspired by all of the incredible students in the program. It draws people who want to change lives, see and feel the meaning in their work, and know that breath is the key.

I knew breath was the key the first time I tried it. Having tried several other healing modalities, including plant medicines, I was shocked by what happened to me during my first breathwork session. I gained access to so much clarity and had a massive emotional release. As I turned over the first time, the first thought that came was, "I have to share this," and it's been my passion ever since.

Hosting workshops and retreats in Bali, New York, Vancouver, Costa Rica, working with CEOs and men's groups, I've seen breathwork change the minds and hearts of people in profound ways. It's remarkable and empowering what we can do with our own bodies. That is another passion of mine, to empower both clients and students.
To me, that is the truest essence of leadership, and a worthy pursuit.

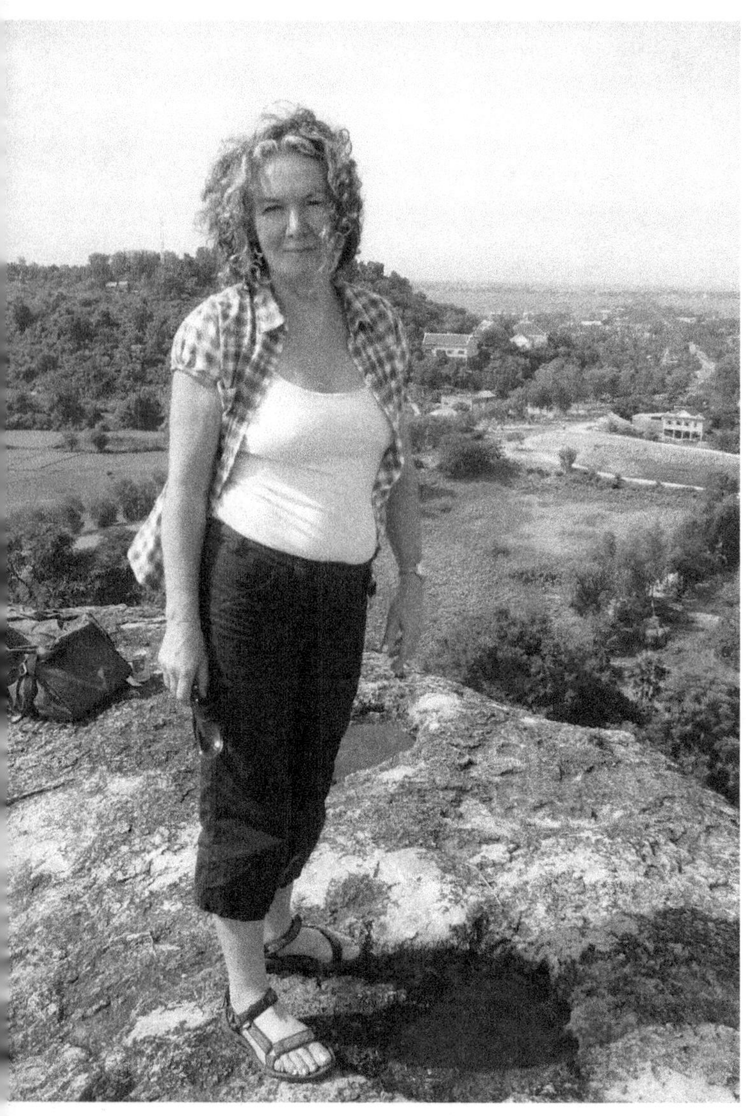

Joy Peirson is an artist who has exhibited her work in many shows around the world, including the Middle East and Canada.

Joy Peirson

The most recent of life's more difficult hurdles happened to Joy in 2012. She was diagnosed with Parkinson's. In disbelief, she sought the opinion of several doctors after the first one told her to go home, make her will, and get her affairs in order. Fortunately, her experiences with Parkinson's since then have not been quite so dire.

She has concentrated on activities that make her happy and avoided events, people, and pursuits that are not so positive. She took up all kinds of exercise to delay the increasing symptoms of Parkinson's.

She rented a studio to pursue her passion for painting. On July 18th, 2015, she remarried and is very happy with her new husband. To make things even better, her children are also very happy with her new husband.

Happiness, she has concluded, is often a choice of outlook and expectation. It's not whether one has a glass half full or empty but whether one has a glass in the first place. She is now 70 and has had a fair amount of time to test this theory. As her birthday approached, she decided it was worthy of celebrating so, she hired a lovely hall, the Vancouver Rowing Club overlooking Coal harbour, a wonderful caterer, and best of all, a great band who played songs everyone could sing. There was a huge mix of people and family, and everybody danced.

Since her Parkinson's diagnosis Joy has chosen to make her Art Career take off. Her studio in the Eastside Atelier, on William & Clark in Vancouver, is a refuge and bolthole, but most of all, a never-ending source of delight. Imagine; a place all your own to Paint and Draw, surrounded by like-minded souls, and other artists. People come to buy her artwork, and she finds it such a pleasure to experience that sharing.
Without that reminder of mortality, the diagnosis, of Parkinson's, would she have had the courage to pursue a lifelong dream, however late in life?

Robyn Marshall is a lover of arts and anatomy who found a unique and profound way of providing a life-changing service that channels both of these passions.

Robyn Marshall

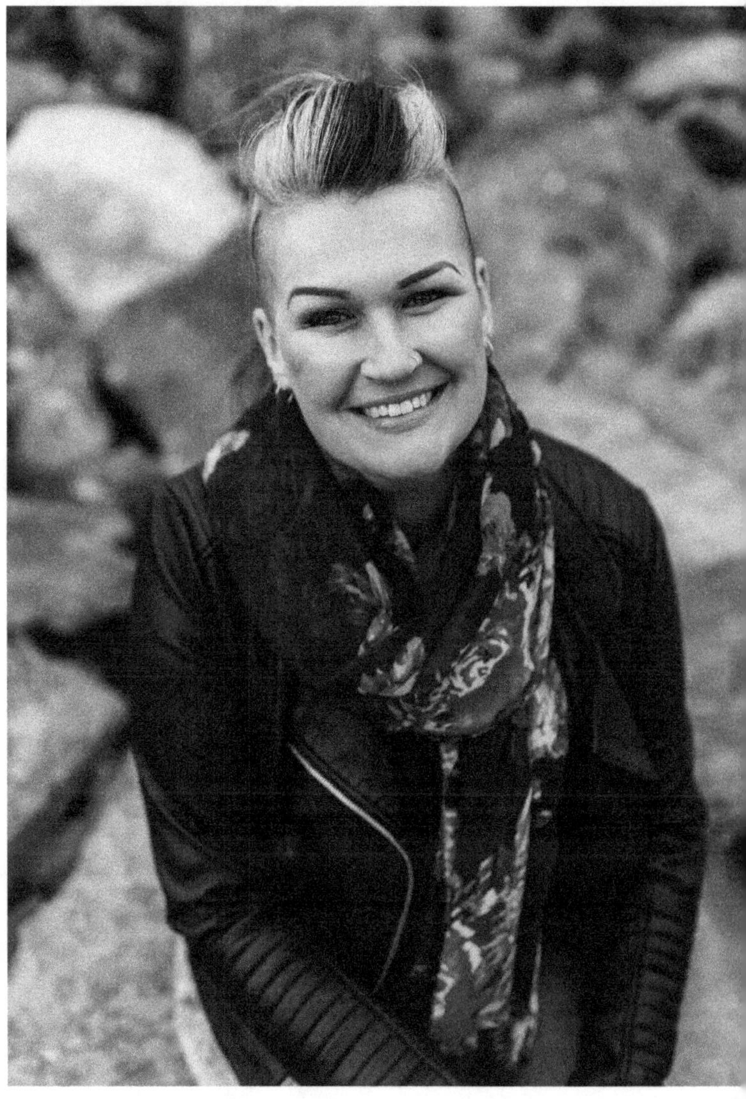

At a young age, I had the dream of being a medical illustrator. I would spend hours learning how to draw anatomy by copying drawings from the Grey's Anatomy book given to me by my dad. Although I have had no formal education, I was able to fulfill that dream by drawing large scale skeletal drawings, four feet by four feet, and selling them to doctors' offices across North America.

I have always been drawn to using my time and energy for the betterment of the communities around me. From volunteering in soup kitchens in Vancouver, BC, to working with the homeless in Little Five Points in Atlanta, Georgia, my heart has always been geared to helping those in need, no matter what that need has been. Until I began tattooing, I had never found a way to blend the dream of using my gift of art with my desire to make a difference in people's lives.

When you think about how art can help people, we often think about inspirational or emotional revelations or soothing responses to beautiful paintings, music, or sketches. Art can be life-changing, but it's a different kind of A.R.T. that I've been called to for the betterment of the communities I serve. A.R.T. in my work also stands for areola restorative tattoos, and for breast cancer survivors and the Trans MTF/FTM community, it is a restoration of self-image, comfort in one's own body, and so much more that I seek to provide.

As the first Canadian tattooer to offer phalloplasty tattooing, I am able to add colour correction and vein detailing to give a more realistic look. This is a life-changing service I am able to offer that until now, has not been provided to the transgender community.

I am honoured that I am finally able to use my art to make such a life-changing impact on people's lives, helping them feel better in their skin.

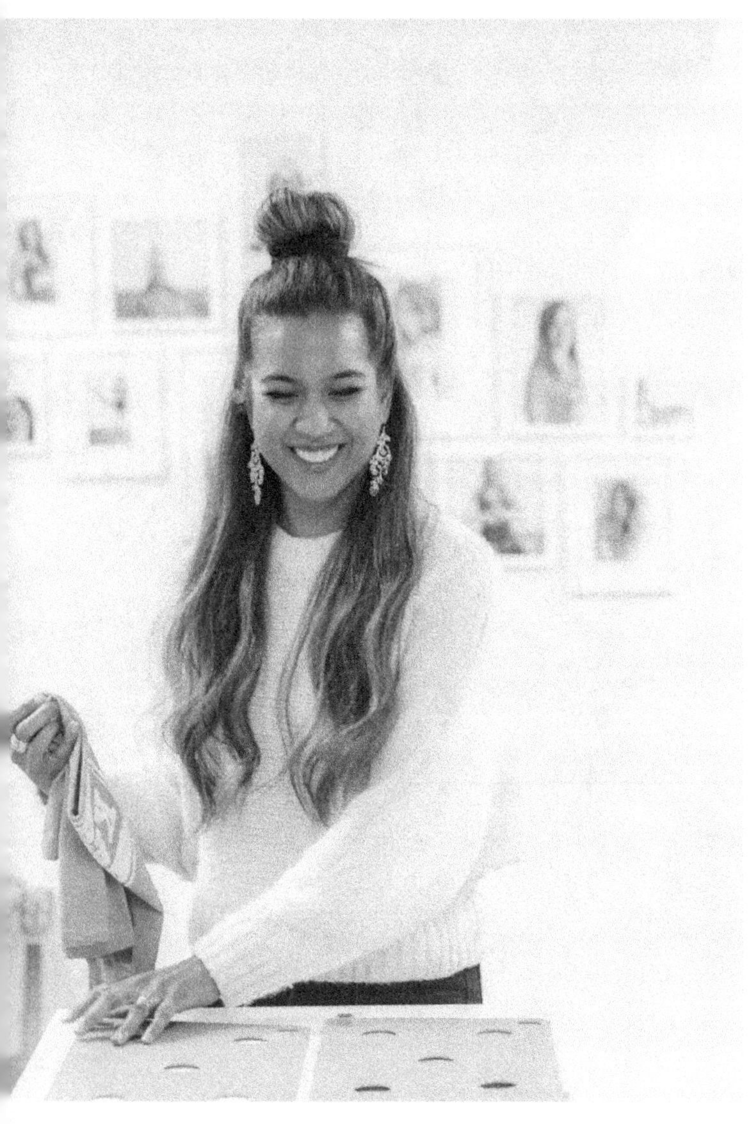

Henrietta C. Devine is the enabler of all good things and the Founder and CEO of TAGULAN, a lifestyle apparel company, and the author and podcast host of Play Love Magic.

Henrietta C. Devine

Imagine what it feels like to be in a state of relaxation, a state of ease, of joy, of happiness, in the state of gratitude, of wonder, and awe, continuously cultivating this higher state of being in alignment.
What if we stopped and existed truly in the present moment? Is it enough to just **be?**
Aligning to my heart, I feel ease, calm, joyful, loving. For each of us, getting to this place of alignment will look different. For some, it's art, or music or dance or writing or singing. It doesn't have to be one thing forever; it can be multiple things.
Finding the state of flow is ideal alignment.

Life is not supposed to weigh us down. Our life experiences will bring us to feel lower vibrations since it is necessary to go through and process these emotions of shame, anger, grief, fear, worry, etc. However, we aren't designed to stay in these lower frequency emotions. We know this to be true since science has proven our physical bodies, mental health, and emotional well-being, become unwell and dis-eased when we stay too long in frequencies that are less than positive of our highest self. Surrounding myself with a lot of space and beautiful textures, scents and nutritious food, physical activity that makes me sweat and meditation daily, ambient music with binaural frequencies, being outside in nature and in the sun as much as possible, helps my process of energetic alignment.
It is ongoing and persistent growth of learning about myself, my strengths and weaknesses, and developing without judgement of where I am on my journey. Studying martial arts at a very young age taught me the outcome of practiced discipline over a sustained period of time. My confidence builds as I develop self-trust through my actions in keeping myself safe and cared for. Every experience in my life has been an opportunity to loosen my attachment to expectations and to surrender more deeply to the freedom of cosmic flow.
Find your state of alignment and pursue to take action to all that calls you, and in the pursuit of creating beyond your own desires, with a purpose greater than yourself, you'll find the universe will respond to co-creating truth with you and for all those who come into your world.

Maxine Cunningham is an investment banker turned economist, turned environmental economist, turned startup founder and CEO of Pick My Brain.

Maxine Cunningham

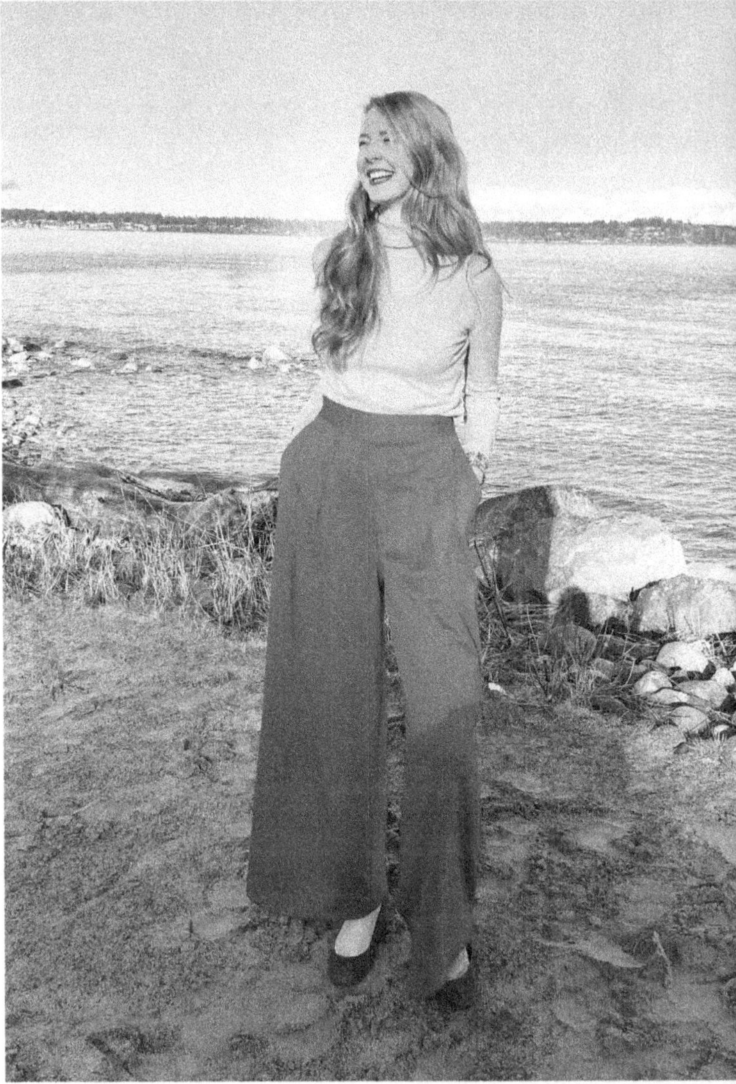

Five years ago, I took a very big leap. I quit a job I genuinely loved as an environmental economist at an international think tank. I left a city I fell for and a group of friends I had developed deep relationships within Ottawa. And I asked my boyfriend, at the time, to quit a job that he was paid really well for to come with me. Why? All because a company called Airbnb showed me the power of what was possible when you combined tech and peer to peer marketplaces was unlimited.

This is what I told people before I quit:

"I want to quit my job, and I want to take one entire year off. But I don't want to call it a "year off" I want to call it a "year on." I want to make my own university schedule. One where I get to study peer to peer marketplaces the entire time. I want to drive across Canada and talk to as many people as I can about what they do, what they love, and what they want to do more of. I also want to fly somewhere warm for one month and read 20+ books. I know if I do this, I'll find what I know I need to find. Do you want to come with me?"

I jumped. He jumped. And we both left our worlds as we knew them in exchange for one year to think, be, explore, and adventure. Little did we know how much the world would open up to us in ways that we never even knew were possible.

Enter Pick My Brain; an online platform that is helping unlock value in totally new ways. Just like Airbnb did, only instead of monetizing a shared space, we are monetizing people's knowledge. But even more than all of that, we are pursuing a mission that makes us more alive than anything else we've experienced, and I wouldn't give up anything for that feeling. The world is our oyster, and all we have to do to open it up is to not ignore the moments when we know deep down, we need to leap.

I leap, you leap. You leap, we all leap.

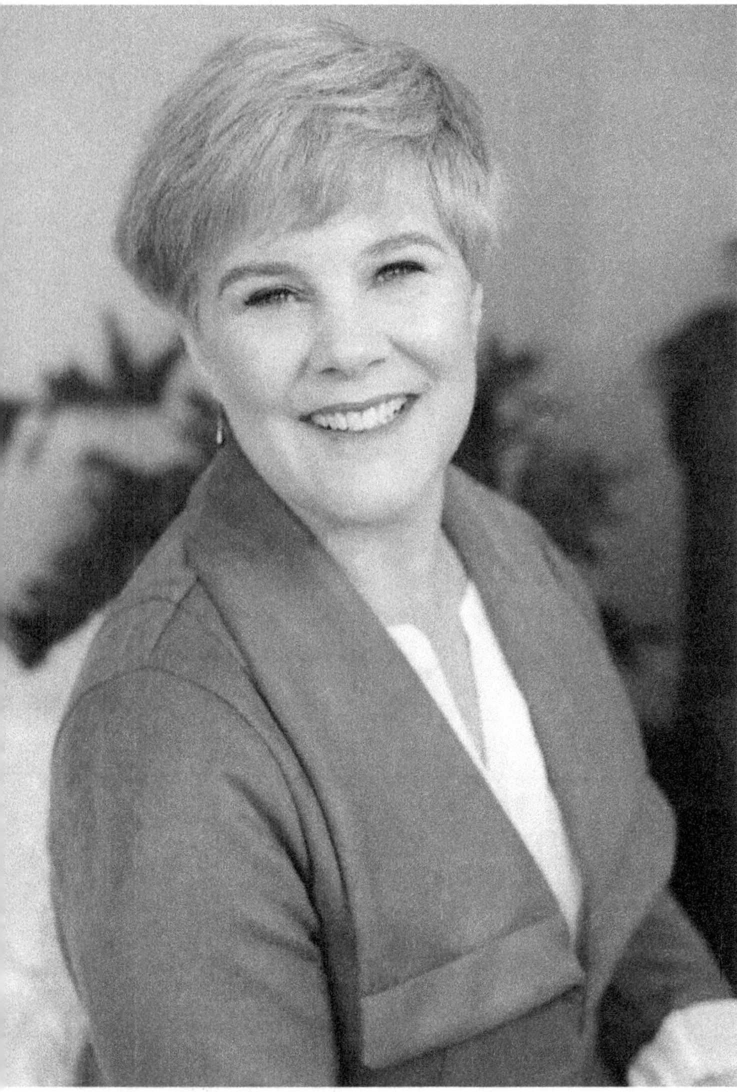

Photo Credit: Kristy Powers

Cathy Derksen is a financial planner and a mindset coach who is dedicated to improving the lives of the women in her community.

Cathy Derksen

I am creating a cycle of wealth and success among women around the world! This goal excites and inspires me every day! Over the past ten years, I have been on a journey of personal growth and evolution. I have completely reinvented my life in order to remove myself and my family from a very toxic situation, including an abusive marriage, and I started a completely new career.

Making these huge changes in my life took courage and years of determination. In creating my new life, I recognized I was inspired to help other women create a life they love.

My current career in financial planning has allowed me to help women shift their lives and feel more confident about their future. I love this work, but I realized that there was a critical step missing. I could give people all the information they needed to make good financial choices, but in most cases, their situation didn't change.

I realized that without a shift in mindset, people will not change their reality. If they grew up with a mindset of 'never enough money,' their behaviour will continue to create this reality. If they have the mindset that they are 'too old' to change their life or that they are 'not smart enough' to learn new skills, they will subconsciously stop themselves from moving forward.

The focus of my new project is to lead women through the process of discovering the mindset that keeps them stuck and to build the personal tools to create a new reality. As women, many of us have lost track of our own goals as we got busy in life as mothers, caretakers, dedicated employees, and business owners.

When you feel that life is drifting past, it's time to take a leap of faith and create a life that brings you joy. Give yourself permission to think about yourself and where you want the next chapter of your life to lead.

What brings you joy? What's next for you? Follow your heart, and don't let a limiting mindset stop you.

Dr. Divi Chandna, MD, is an Intuitive Coach, teacher, author, and speaker.

Dr. Divi Chandna

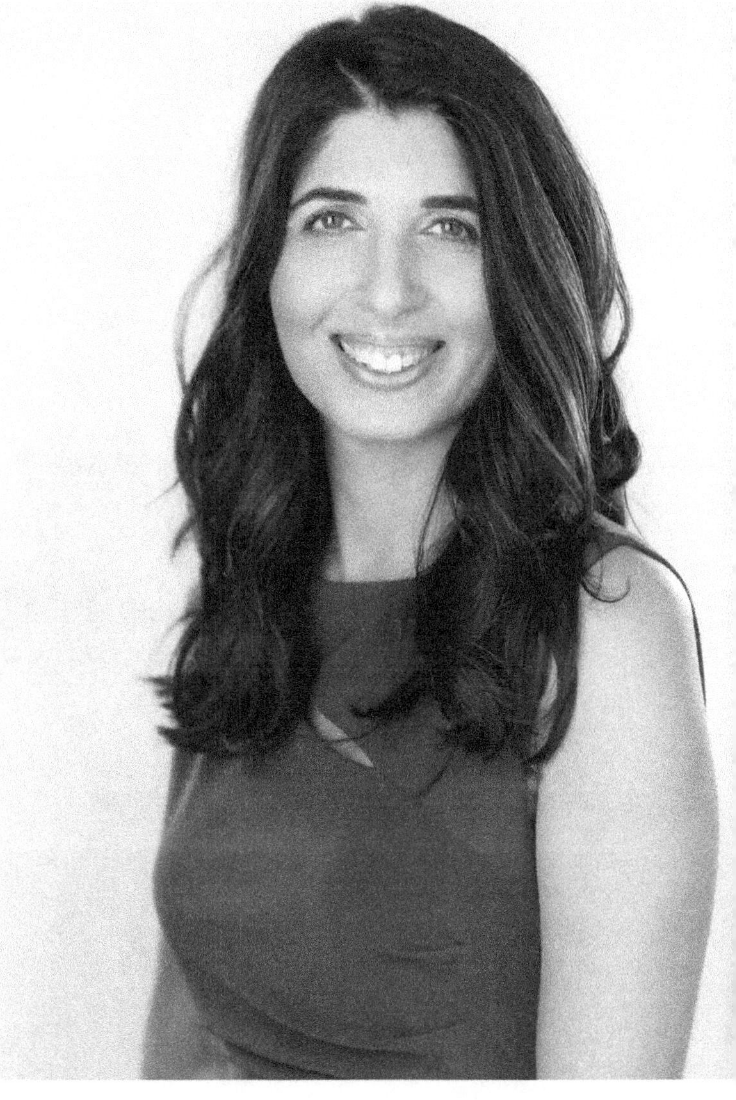

I love what I do! This often entails asking myself if I feel good in this moment doing the task that I am currently doing. I am adamant that an element of joy must be present in even the most mundane tasks. My most deeply held belief is that joy and love are our natural set-points, and our minds are instrumental in getting us into total alignment. Practicing specific habits of mind and emotion can lead us to an authentic place of love.

My parents trekked across the globe from India to make our home in Canada. Higher education was my prime focus. At age 25, I had graduated medical school and was out in the world trying to save one patient at a time. Then, in my 30's, chronic pain became an excruciating part of my life. My waking moments were taken up with my medical practice and illness. This couldn't be the way things were meant to remain, so I began a voracious study of the link between disease, stress, emotion, and the mind. Chronic pain and working with various patients gave me a front-row seat in the theater of life!

The journey to health, a winding road, led me down a path of study, training, and acquiring credentials as an intuitive coach. Truth is a person's intuition, their soul knowing it is at peace. I was impassioned by helping others discover their inner truthsSounds a little hokey right? As a scientist and medical doctor with a great understanding of the physical body, my own journey to find health and that inner light clearly defined the link between mind, body, and spirit.

Living life with passion is about living from the heart, which means living from the soul. Connecting with the soul is to by-pass the mind and truly get in touch with our bodies. We are each imprinted with a roadmap to our careers, success, and gifts meant for only us in this human realm. Locating that road map means healing the mind through the unpacking of our stories and viewing them through the lens of the soul.

This is where forgiveness, love, and healing live.

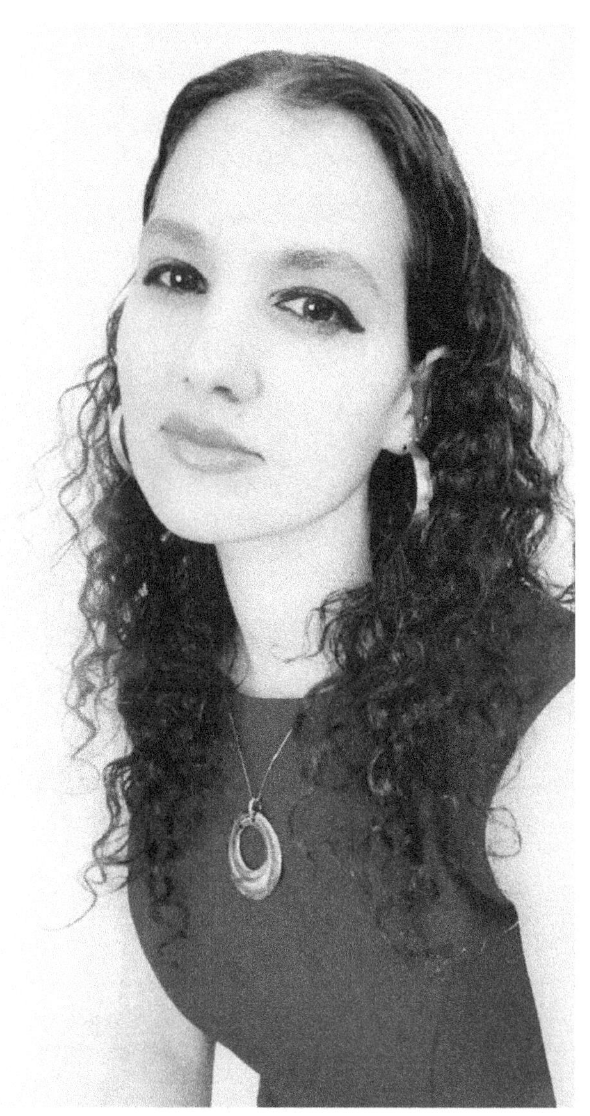

Lia Murrain is an award-winning entrepreneur and the owner of B Snug Inc, 2012 Ltd & London Kids.

Lia Murrain

"I don't know what it means ... but I want to be one". I remember that thought vividly from when I was ten, and the word "entrepreneur" jumped out at me from the pages of my book. It was intriguing and fancy, and it represented the story of a famous businessman. The spark was lit. I could do this. After all, I had made my first dollar when I was three, and my mind would spin as I eagerly pocketed the bills, experiencing this concept called business.

Twenty years after my first money-making experience and straight out of an English university with my master's degree, I was hired by a world-renowned investment bank. The wheeling & dealing was exciting, and the vast number of zeros on the end of a deal were thrilling, but the buzz wasn't mine, the hustle wasn't mine, I wasn't the boss. This clearly wasn't me.

The excitement from those early years continued to be a backdrop of my life and my goal remained; to be an Entrepreneur. My first company, a retail venture, saw me win several entrepreneur awards, highschools & universities invited me to lecture, and London's Telegraph ran a full page story. Was I an entrepreneur yet? I wasn't sure ... so I kept hustling. My second company, a spin-off distribution company which is still thriving seventeen years on, kept me busy but I needed more.

I started admiring a multi-award-winning brand and dreaming; complete with presentations and designs of what I would do if I owned the company. Amused friends would ask why I wouldn't create something similar, and I would reply that I didn't want something similar - I wanted to own the company.

Years later without hesitation, I boldly reached out to the company knowing I wanted to take it to its next phase. Twenty years after the **Buggysnuggle™** company had first launched, I acquired it and my years of subconscious acquisition had been realized.

Thoughts are creative, and our power is immense if we visualize the things that we want as already ours.

Paula Skaper is an entrepreneur, speaker, gifted strategist. Paula always has a plan for growth. She never has a plan for dinner.

Paula Skaper

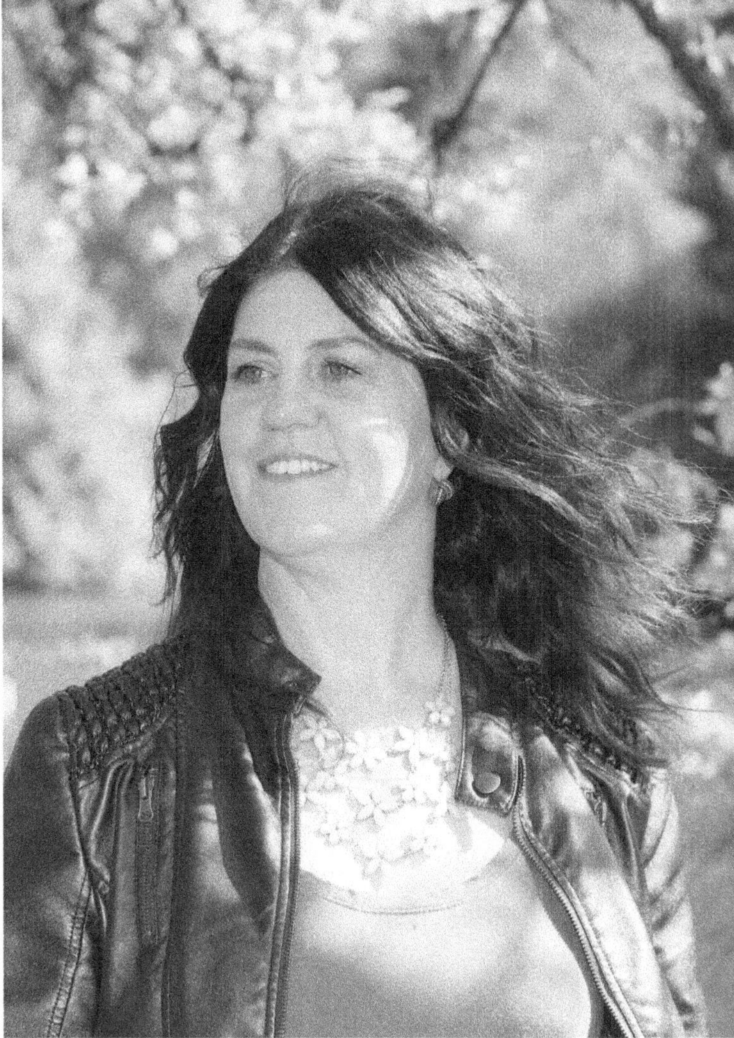
Photo Credit: Viktoria Skaper

Their Opinions Don't Matter.

My husband was on the floor playing barbies with our then 2-year-old daughter. I didn't waste time with hello. "I quit my job today."
He looked up and raised his eyebrows, saying nothing.
"I want to start my own company." I held my breath, waiting to be talked out of this crazy idea...

It didn't happen. All he said was, "I'm sure you'll do fine. What did you have in mind for dinner?" Then he went back to playing barbies.

It was that easy. Decision made; I knew I'd figure it out.

And I did. For a while.

A few years, a mortgage, and a second child later, it had been a difficult year. Sales were down and I was out of ideas. I turned to a fellow entrepreneur for advice. He told me to pack it in and get a job.

We sat at my kitchen table while he rattled off an endless list of reasons why I wasn't going to succeed. Instead of helping me look for solutions, he laid out why I, as a human being, didn't qualify to be an entrepreneur.

- You're not cut out to run a business – you don't have the right 'background'.
- Your parents weren't entrepreneurs, and you don't have the connections it's going to take.
- You're female, a mom with a young family.

I got mad. Then I got busy. I hired a part-time nanny, doubled down on my sales efforts, cut expenses, prayed for a miracle, and somehow turned things around.

Two decades and countless challenges later, I'm still growing and learning every day. None of us wakes up knowing what the day will bring. We each must play the cards as they are dealt, one card at a time. But you, and you alone, have the power to choose how you will show up in the game.

You are defined by what you do, not what anyone else thinks. To succeed in life, there are really only two things you have to do - decide what's really important, then trust yourself to figure it out. Everything else will fall in line.

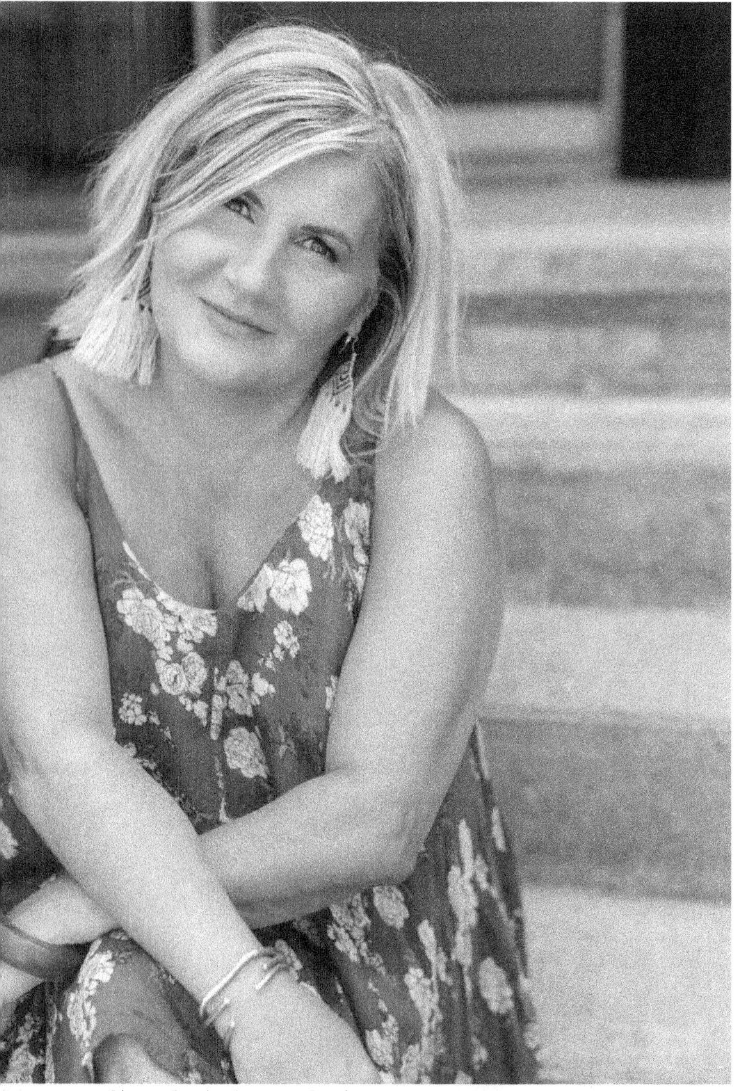
Photo Credit: Brittany Gawley

Oresta Korbutiak is a holistic aesthetician and the founder and owner of ORESTA organic skin care.

Oresta Korbutiak

I believe that a woman can achieve and maintain a healthy and radiant complexion at any age, naturally.

My skin care journey began when I struggled with adult acne in my twenties. Desperate to clear up my skin, I overspent on an overabundance of abrasive acne products, medications, and harsh chemical treatments. With little success, I then incorporated a holistic approach that, much to my surprise, cleared up my acne and led me to pursue studies in skin care.

Upon graduation, excited to pursue a career in natural skin care, but without any job opportunities, I created my own opportunity.

In 2001, I founded ORESTA organic skin care, Ottawa's first clean beauty boutique and holistic spa that has grown to three brick and mortar locations. In 2004, I established an e-commerce clean beauty store on Shopify. It was store number 39 of now more than one million stores.

As a holistic aesthetician for over 20 years and now in my 50s, I understand skin issues and concerns that women experience at every age and how to successfully address them. While the mainstream beauty industry directs us to 'miracle products' promising a youthful, radiant glow, the truth is that without a holistic approach to beauty, you will never achieve the results that you desire. Skin will not perform optimally with topicals alone. It requires healthy self-care rituals, nourishing products, self-love, and self-acceptance.

I am passionate about healthy beauty and radiant aging and in supporting women to reclaim their radiance and be the best version of themselves!

Jackie is inspiring and selfless. Her positivity reminds you that there is more to life than challenges, illness, and adversity. There is hope. The director, host, producer, and founder of eveRIAthing TV, and the newly launched motivational platform, The Real Diy. Jackie is strength and positivity personified.

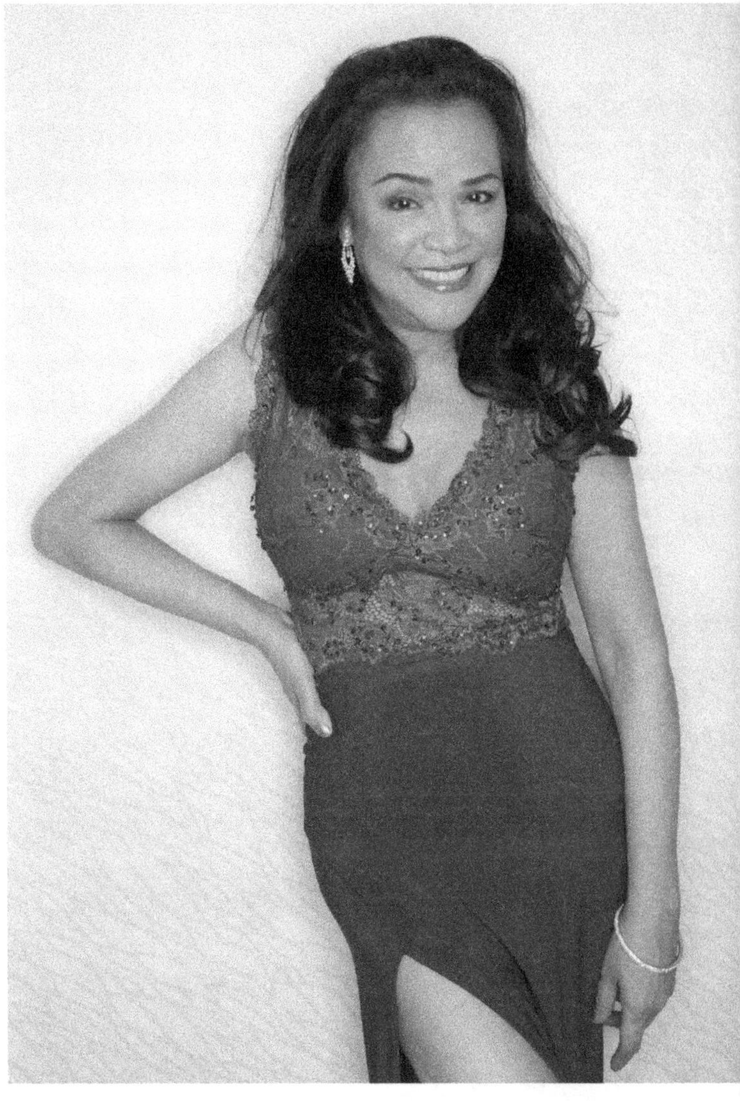

Jackie Diy

I am a mother of two wonderful girls whose stories make me who I am. My eldest, Deanne, suffered from viral encephalitis when she was four. As my husband and I watched her slowly drift into a coma, we held on to God and one another. At the hospital, I'd talk and sing to her and read her nursery books as she lay unconscious. Our source of strength was our faith in God. Like a miracle, Deanne later regained consciousness, but she was blind, lost mobility in her right extremities, and lost her speech. One thing kept us hopeful: she was alive and not a vegetable as the doctors warned. She regained her vision, but with her overall aptitude affected, she was bullied all of her young life but with her determination, she now has her own small business, and I am a proud mom!

Living with crippling anxiety and anorexia nervosa, my Ria, multi-awarded TV host, musician, and songwriter fell into depression in 2017. As she started to lose all hopes in life, I called on to God, "Lord, not a second trial, please, but I know that you allow these things to happen because we WILL get through them. I trust in You." My past relived itself as I watched Ria cry every day. Except for her sobs, the house was quiet. She has stopped singing but we never stopped praying. Raffy and I once again drew strength from each other as we helped our girl hold on to whatever hope she had left. Like a phoenix, Ria rose from the ashes in late 2018, started singing again, and launched her new music in 2019.

Faith and family. Love and gratitude. These are why I want to inspire others to never give up, to be grateful for what we have, and to remember our blessings when times are tough. We will rise after every fall.

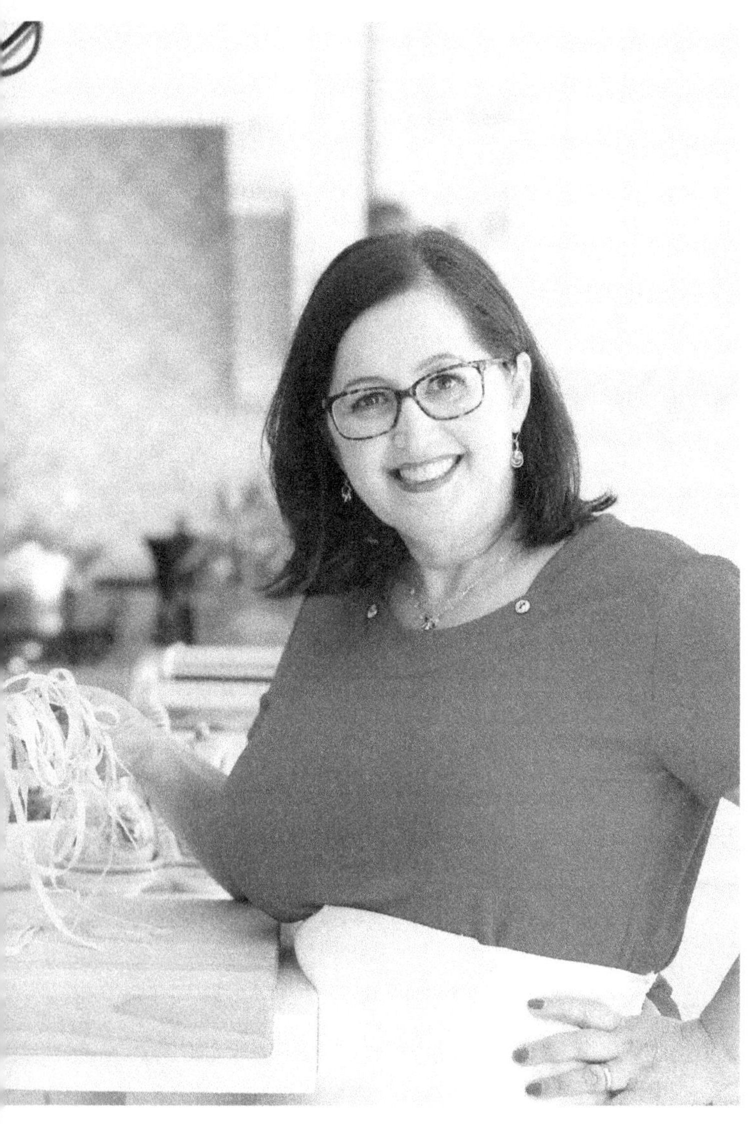

Marzia Molatore is the founder of Bella Cibo's Italian Cooking Classes and recently published her first cookbook, "Cooking with Mamma Marzia."

Marzia Bellotti Molatore

Buongiorno Friends!

I was born in Naples, Italy, and grew up in the Valtellina region of Northern Italy. I grew up with amazing females in my life who nurtured my love of food and cooking. Cooking wasn't just an activity but a way of life for myself and the women in my family.
My passion and love for cooking emerged from spending endless hours in the kitchen with the most fantastic cooks I could imagine; my mother, my Nonna, and all of my aunts. In 2003, I took a leap of faith and moved to Vancouver to join the love of my life, my husband, Dan. We have two beautiful children and have surrounded ourselves with wonderful people who helped us find a new community here in Canada.

Sometimes life throws opportunities to you when you least expect them. In 2013, a group of my Canadian friends wanted to learn how to make one of my most staple recipes, lasagna - from scratch, of course! From that moment, I knew my destiny was to inspire others to make homemade food and share my Italian culture and recipes with the world!

From that night, I started Bella Cibo cooking school. What began as a fun hobby grew into my passion and career as a business that hosts multiple classes per week. Bella Cibo has won awards and got local media attention and has inspired so many families to cook and spend time in the kitchen together.

A few years ago, I wrote down my business goals, and one of those goals was to write a cookbook. When my mother-in-law passed away in 2018, she gifted me her notebook with all of her recipes. This gift from her, and the support from my family, gave me the adrenaline and inspiration to write my first cookbook. This book is dedicated to my family and all the women who have ever moved to another country in the world, found their passions, and fought to keep their traditions alive through food, family, and a sprinkle of love.

Denise Dupré, a passionate expressionist abstract artist, paints from a well-grounded, spiritually connected space of love.

Denise Dupré

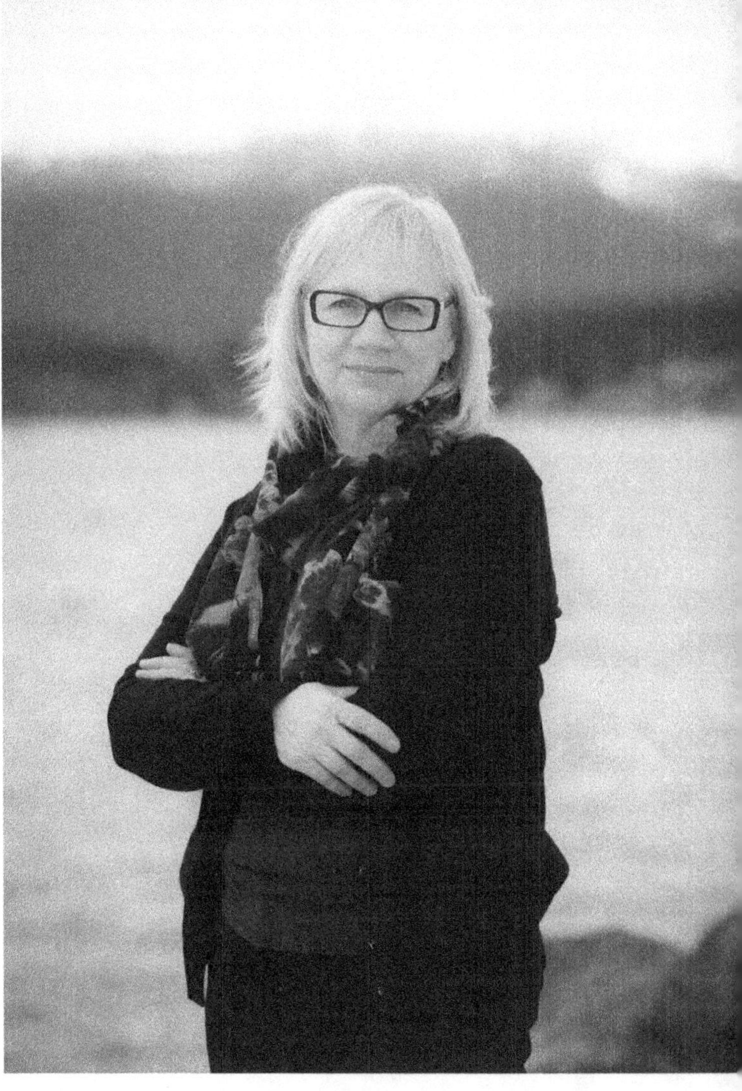

As an artist my desire has always been to create art empowered with a sensual expression and spiritual connectivity. I aspire to produce work worthy of bringing joy and inspiration to others. My happiness and success have had much to do with finding my calling. We must eternally strive toward our callings as they are how we actualize and experience personal happiness and limitless fulfillment.

During early adulthood, my decisions often resulted in less than satisfactory outcomes leaving me with self-doubt and unhappiness. My attempts to follow a path of my own choosing were compromised by internal struggles and self-sabotaging decisions. I grappled with emotional instability and personal insecurities stemming from a lack of trust, thus drowning my life's potential, my purpose and ultimately my own happiness. Self-reflection, introspection and hard work coupled with a yearning to fulfill my potential and become the person I was meant to be, drove me to take stock of what was getting in my way and actively work toward changing it.

Being grounded has been the key in getting to a place of trust. Support from my loving and unwavering husband and our three amazing daughters has been and is still essential to grounding my soul. I am grateful for my closest family, friends, and professional mentors throughout my life who have guided my skill development and supported my dreams. Self-acceptance, short-comings and all, has taught me to value humility, patience and forgiveness. I maintain that holding those we love close, with sincere respect, lifts our souls toward love and enlightenment. We must treasure our community of persons.

My belief is that hard work and inspiration are crucial in reaching our goals. Being resilient enough to persist on a chosen path, clear or unclear, is necessary for success. Reflecting on defeats and conquests, valuing our inner voices and ignoring our voices of self-doubt allow us to facilitate a path and develop flourishing careers. We must learn to trust and listen to our soft inner voices. Recognizing passion, value and truth gives true purpose and allows us to live meaningful and authentic realities.

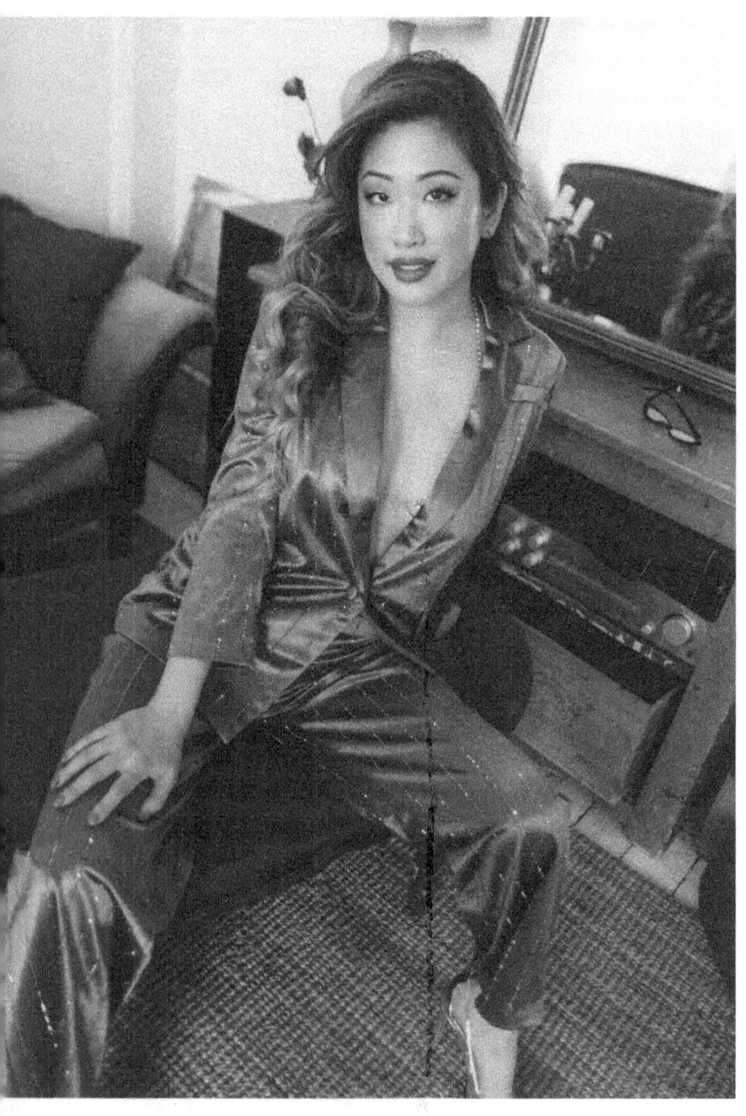

Betty Lam is a beacon of positivity, a magnet for women who are passionate about life, and the owner/founder of Betty Glam Boutique.

Betty Lam

My greatest lesson in my pursuit of happiness is that you should never downplay your happiness to make others feel comfortable.

Questions that I dreaded answering in a difficult year are the usual, "how are you holding up," followed by, "despite everything?" During the second lockdown of 2020 - an old high school classmate messaged me saying "Betty I am going crazy. I'm losing my mind. How are you doing?" I felt guilty for saying "I'm great!" while others are struggling or hurting. Even though I missed having a social life - for the most part, I was still happy and always found reasons to be grateful.

I had exciting opportunities come up during the pandemic, but when people ask, "what's new with you?" I was compelled to downplay it and say, "not much," since the world was in chaos.

Happy people tend to live in the moment and acknowledge what is happening around them. A facet of mindfulness is acceptance. When you practice acceptance, you welcome your experiences, feelings, and thoughts by looking at them with kindness, grace, and an open mind.

During the pandemic, I went through my very first breakup. I had anticipated the day when I would break down and become a hot mess post-break-up, but that day and those tears never came. I promise I'm not heartless. I love and care deeply, but I also know how to pick myself up and go from being okay to being happy again in a short time. The only part I didn't like, was knowing that I had hurt someone I loved. Aside from that, I was still a happy-go-lucky girl who lives her life with grace and gratitude.

Another key to happiness is seeing the world in a positive and hopeful light, even during dark and challenging times. Let's normalize not feeling guilty for being happy. And don't ever downplay or apologize for your joy and success. You deserve all the great things that are happening to you. If you have good news don't be afraid to SHARE IT - shout it from the rooftops, celebrate yourself, and allow yourself to absorb those joyous moments!

Isabelle Mercier is a 'no-nonsense' dynamo, born to catapult heart-centered entrepreneurs and leaders to build impactful brands, businesses, and lives – she is also French, therefore, very passionately direct.

Isabelle Mercier

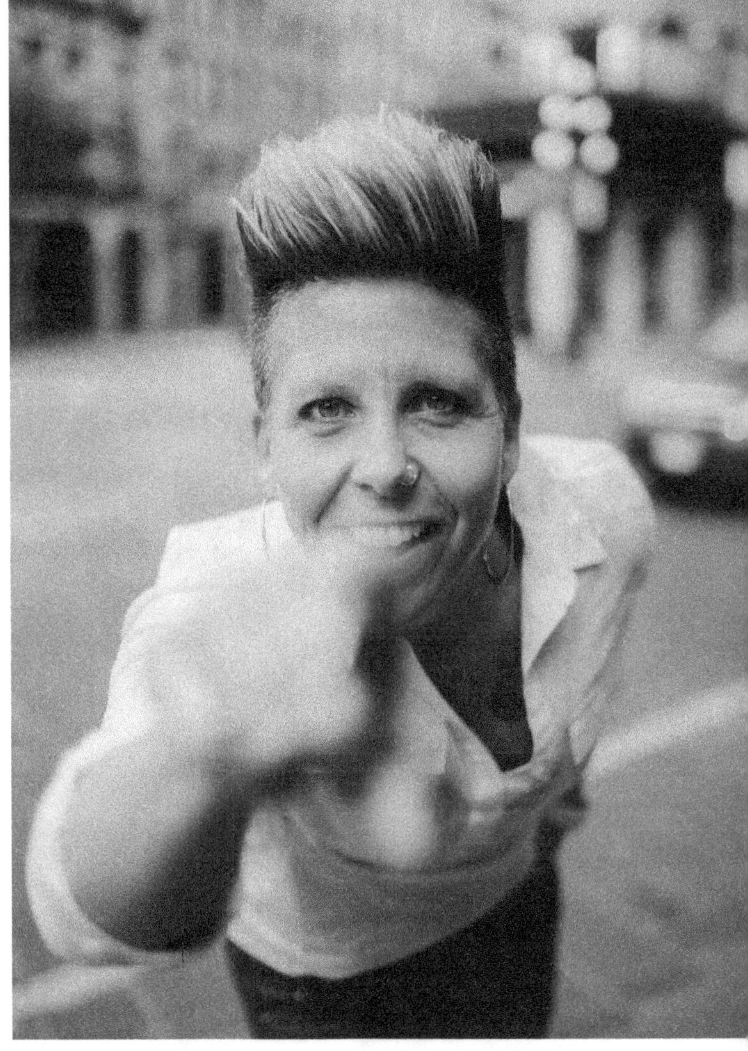

How direct am I?

Well, in my industry, I am known as the Simon Cowell of Brand Positioning and Business Growth and yes, I choose to take this as a huge compliment because this guy can sure spot and catapult talent forward. I am just a hell of a lot kinder and let's face it, more fashionable!

My friends and family often lovingly brace themselves every time they ask for my opinion and will say, "I should have asked for the sugar-coated version," to which I reply, "That was the sugar-coated version!" Despite my directness, I do try to deliver with kindness.

Why am I sharing this? Because to me, happiness is when what I think, say, and do are in harmony.
Thank you, Gandhi, your words have elevated and continue to elevate my life every single day. I believe in these words so much that I have them tattooed on my left arm.

Aligning these three simple words together – Think, Say & Do – seems simple enough right? Think again. It takes a lot of guts, courage, and most importantly, a healthy dose of compassion to be able to consistently be and stay in alignment with this little threesome of awesome.

I am clear that my purpose for being on this beautiful planet of ours is to empower people to truly be themselves and own their badassery.

And as long as I am doing that, I am rockin' life!

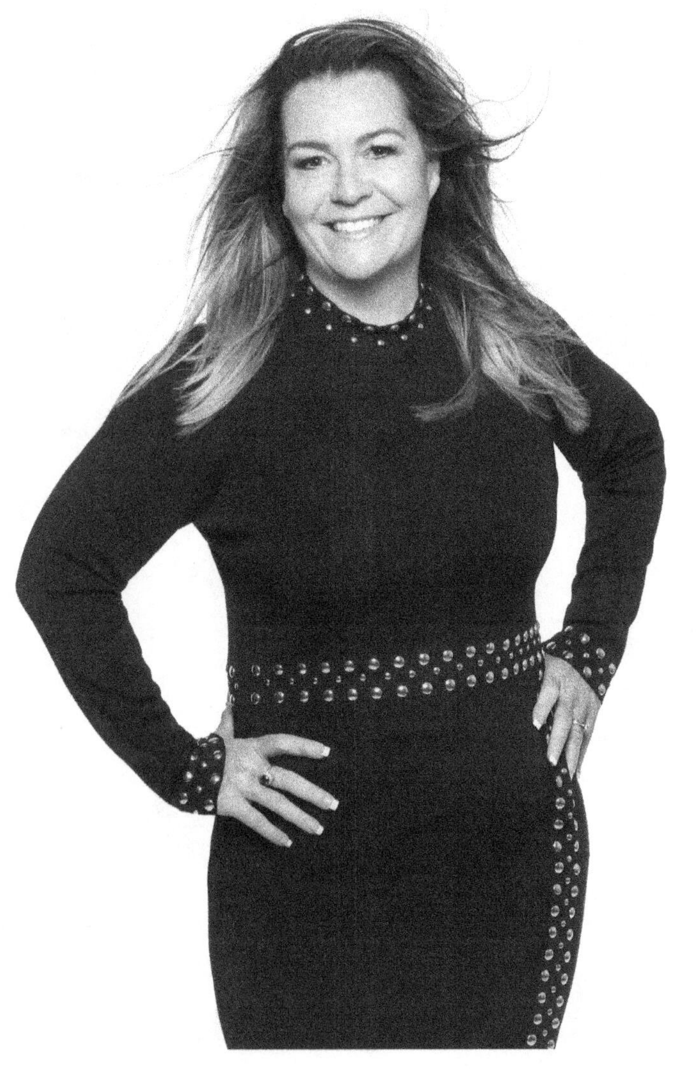

Leanne Myles is a Senior Mortgage Advisor and an advocate for a can-do attitude to achieve great things!

Leanne Myles

The first time I ever walked through fear, I didn't really know that that was what I was doing. It hasn't been until my early 40's that I am now realizing what I have done. I have recently hired a coach and believe it or not, her coaching is helping me in every aspect of my life. Through the exercise of noticing and naming, I am beginning to see some extraordinary things about my life, both good and bad.

But the ability to realize what you have come through is no easy task. Walking through the fear is something that has almost come intuitively to me, as I have just had to what seems like "live this way."

Growing up in small-town Labrador City, most of my adult life has been walking through fear. I left that town at 17 and went to boot camp, you want to talk about culture shock? From that day forward it's all I have ever known; see something, want it, get uncomfortable, and get it. I have since that time worked many life decisions this way, my divorce from my children's father was especially difficult, and I probably stayed longer than I should, but again, I saw a path, got uncomfortable, and then got what I wanted.

This very simple thing (which isn't so simple I am told) has carried me through all facets of my life. When it came to goal setting, again, see what you want, get uncomfortable, and then "get what you want."

I also know this is all about the story we tell ourselves, the daily story of can or can't that lives in our minds. When you actually believe you can, you can move mountains. To date, I have been through every life event there is; marriage, divorce, job loss, illness, Bankruptcy, and through all of it, I chose happiness because it's not about where you are today, it's about where you know you can get.

Today my struggle is with food and health, I am seeing it, and I want it, and I am about to get real uncomfortable. I can already tell you it will work out fine!

Marilyn R. Wilson is a freelance writer, published author, speaker, and passionate interviewer who loves giving wings to others' stories.
She is a lover of old things, sees the beauty in imperfection, and has a deep connection with nature. In fact, nature is where she goes to heal – sometimes by standing barefoot in the dirt.

Marilyn R. Wilson

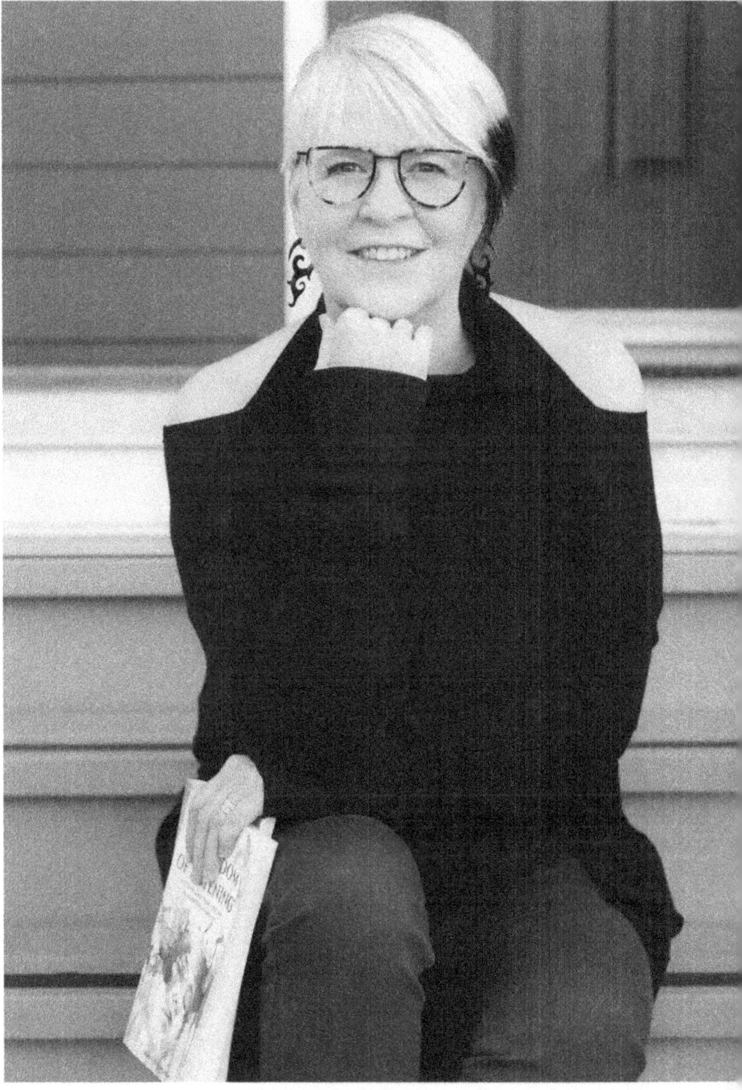
Photo Credit: Kristy Powers Photography

Growing up, I simply didn't fit in. Everyone else seemed to manage, so I assumed I was broken and hid my true self deep inside. Then, at age 50, I made a leap into the unknown that would change everything. With no experience and no idea what I was getting into, I submitted several ideas for articles to an NYC magazine. This was done on a whim with no expectations, so I was shocked when I heard two were accepted.

The world shifted during my first interview. I realized I had found a passion that brought me joy: I loved hearing people share their stories. That didn't mean my journey would be easy. In fact, it proved to be very challenging.
To book interviews, I had to publish articles, which meant figuring out how to write. There were sleepless nights, intense anxiety, and many tears shed as I learned and made mistakes - in the public eye.

Interviewing brought me a great sense of fulfillment. In addition, writing freelance articles led to me becoming a co-owner of a local magazine and publishing two books. Through it all, I loved hearing how unique every life was. I was also stunned to realize how much I was being changed just by listening to the wisdom these people shared.

What lesson had the most impact? The very things people wanted me to change – my intense focus, my racing mind, my insatiable curiosity – were actually my talents. I was not broken; I was exactly who I was meant to be.
Learn to love and embrace your own uniqueness. Give yourself the freedom to embrace others just as they are.
Revel in being surrounded by diversity. More than anything, ignore outside pressure to step into a box that doesn't fit.

Choose to live your best life and live it without apology.

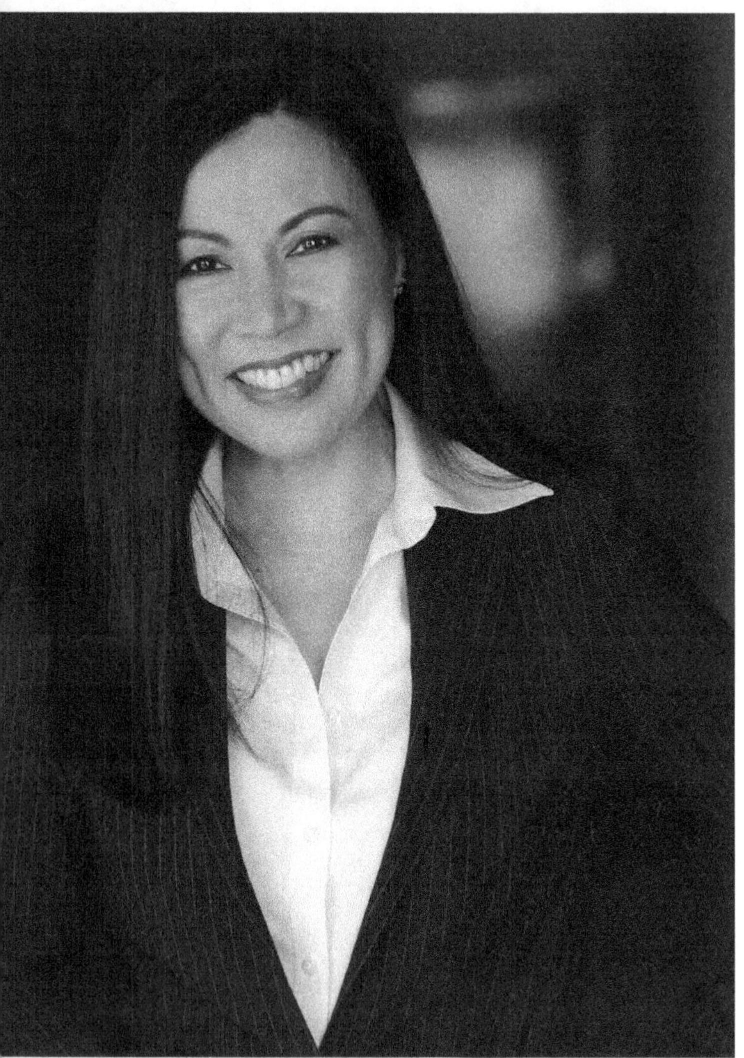

Photo Credit: Gordan Dumka

Brenda Wong is a preeminent talent agent who loves the challenge of negotiating contracts while passionately promoting her clients.

Brenda Wong

Brenda grew up in East Vancouver, a lower-income neighborhood. She didn't realize they were poor because her father provided richness in life and unconditional love. He fostered self-acceptance, hard work, to never take a handout and never pick a fight, but if you're in one, finish it.

She learned to be tough and mature at a very young age in order to survive; her father died suddenly when she was 12 years old. Finances became tight, she landed her first job at age 13, then she worked in the entertainment industry as a teen actor, later as a stunt performer.

Wong even stepped into the role of Academic Director, twice, both times excelling in managing higher education. However, it was her transition to becoming an agent where she found her purpose. Rising up from hardship, and having faced racism and sexism in the workplace, she founded MVM Agency and set about making her mark.

The business grew over the next 20 years to become a strong reflection of her core values. It now leads the entertainment industry in offering an atmosphere of inclusion, booking work for clients regardless of race, age, size, or gender orientation (male (he/him), female (she/her), transgender, non-binary, BIPOC, and LGBTQ+).

Strong bonds are developed with each client and over time they each become a part of her extended family.

"I treasure and value the mentorship of young adults, especially young women. What inspires me is to strive to be a better person. I grew up having people I didn't want to be like and seeing situations I never wanted to be in. I knew not all of us are dealt the right cards, but that doesn't mean you can't reshuffle the deck for a better outcome."

– Brenda Wong

"Our deepest fear is not that we are inadequate. Our deepest fear is that we are powerful beyond measure. It is our light, not our darkness that most frightens us. We ask ourselves, Who am I to be brilliant, gorgeous, talented, fabulous? Actually, who are you not to be? [...]"
- Marianne Williamson

Stephanie Lehr

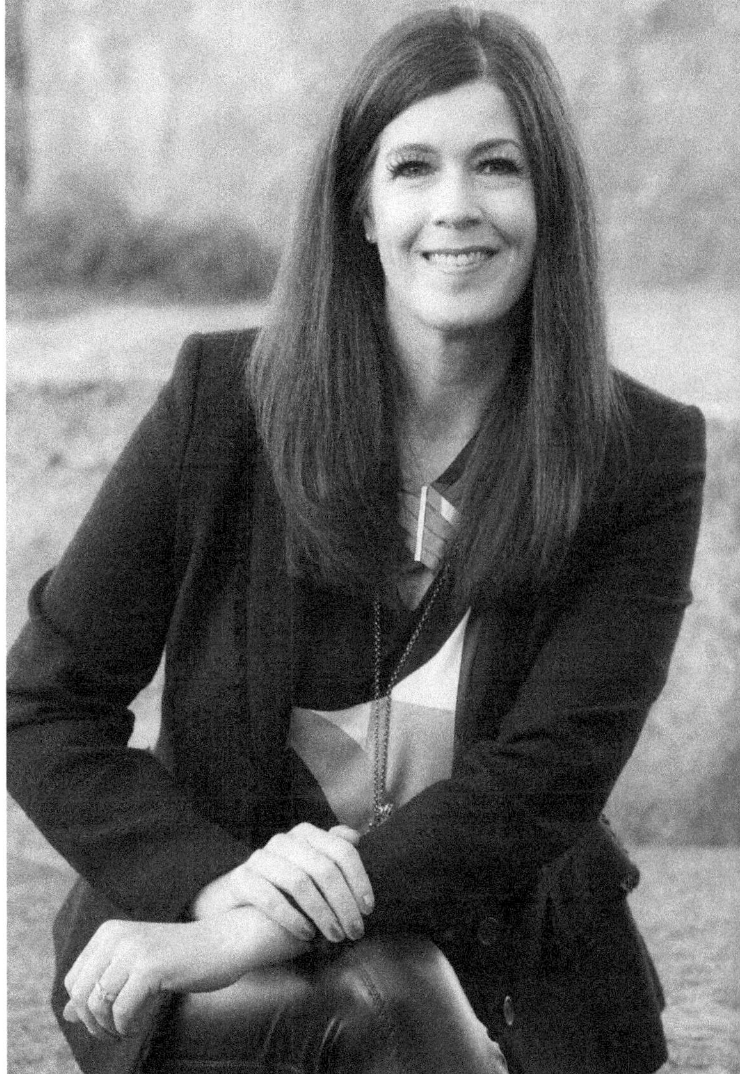
Photo Credit: Dawn Stenzel Photography

This quote reminds me of my beautiful, endless possibility. It gives me permission to show the world my extraordinary gifts regardless of others' opinions. This is true for me and this is true for other women, women like you. I'm a Certified Life Coach Practitioner specializing in empowerment, divorce, and career. I help you find your footing to get back on your feet and into your high heels again! I help you to gain clarity, confidence, and connection to your values and goals, envision your dreams, and help you move forward to create and live your Next Best Life.

When I work with you, I imagine that I'm holding space for your next level self. Even when you don't believe in yourself, I believe in you and your greatest life vision. So, come with me on this visualization, and let's imagine 365 days from now and see what's possible for you. There's a momentous celebration happening. You can see bright, colour-bursting balloons and beautiful streamers in all your favourite colours filling and framing the effervescent lit room. You notice the massive, elevated sign, "WOW, YOU REALLY DID IT!" You can hear energetic music transcending, flowing, and hugging the space, and all who hear it, connecting people, creating treasured memories. All your cherished friends are smiling and singing your praises! They're raising their sparkling crystal flute glasses to you and your incredible success! Feeling overcome with joy, you leave the party room to an adjacent room to collect your thoughts. From here, you can hear your friends toasting you.

What is it that you would want them to say about you?

What is it that you would NOT want them to say about you?

What do you want to achieve and avoid a year from now?

What are your next steps to march forth and celebrate an elevated 365 days?

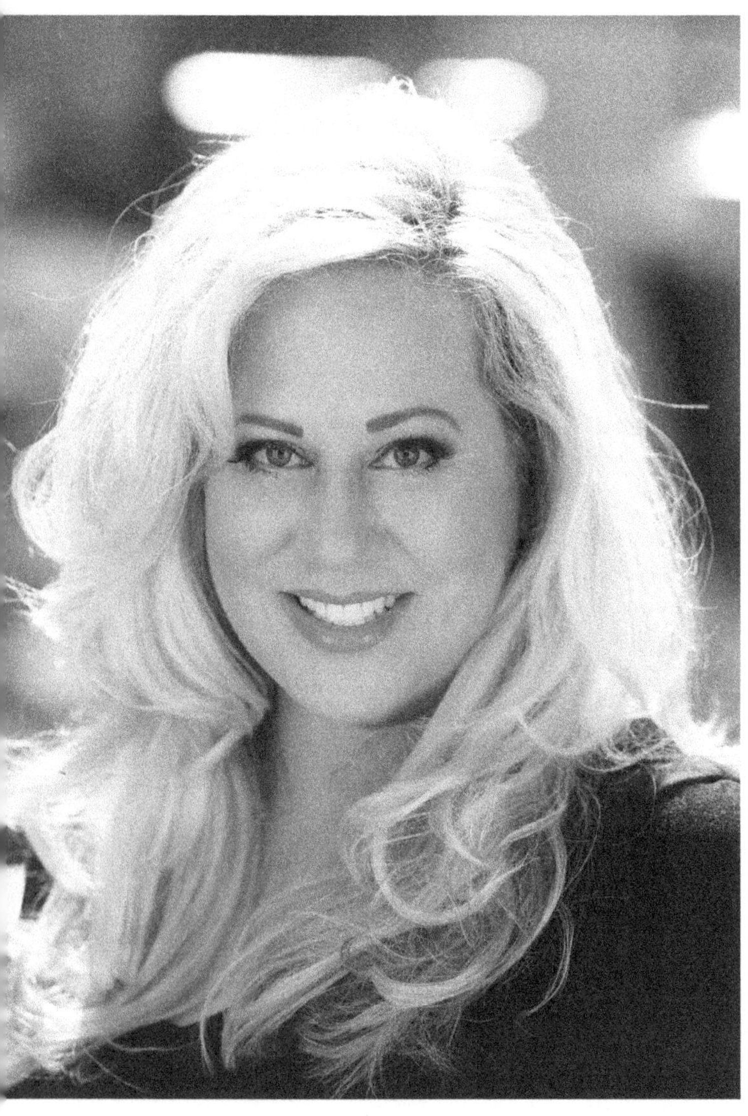

Colleen Kirk is the founder and CEO of 3 Graces Beauty, a brand that celebrates the beauty of the Human Spirit.

Colleen Kirk

The Beauty of Grace

I come from a small town in Nevada, the youngest of five, raised in a very conservative household. I was the silently rebellious one. Forbidden to wear makeup as a young teen, I quietly developed my secret passion to be a makeup artist. At nineteen, I moved to Los Angeles set to make my dream a reality.

I started with a sales job for a small beauty brand at Nordstrom while continuing to hone my skills as an artist. A promotion led to being mentored by one of the greats in the makeup business, who opened doors for me as a makeup artist in the Entertainment industry, working my magic on the faces of celebrities. This small-town girl could have never imagined it. Was it luck? Maybe. I think it was the grace given by the mentors that helped me.

I spent the next decade traveling to 42 + countries training makeup artists, educating people on how to use and sell beauty products. I met amazing people from different cultures, backgrounds, and circumstances. Their stories both humbled and inspired me. I saw that beauty is not simply our western ideal, or a "look," or an impossible standard to strive for, it is as diverse as the people I met. To me, beauty is so much more than a pretty face or great makeup, it is the kindness, wisdom, joy, and grace so freely expressed by people I met.

This experience was life-changing and gave me a far different perspective of beauty than the one I had known in Hollywood. It also gave me the courage to create my own beauty brand.

3 Graces Beauty is a culmination of all that I have learned from those I've met. It is driven by the philosophy that true beauty is interconnected with grace. Makeup can transform a face, give you confidence, and express your personality, but it does not define who you are. Nor does your age. True beauty is rooted in the human spirit, and our mission, along with clean beauty products, is to create little moments of grace that celebrate the beauty in all of us.

As an entrepreneur several times over, and a mother, Dawn Reid loves creating the meaningful, intentional business, ZenWand, with her family.

Dawn Reid

I guess you can call me a woman who has followed her heart. Over my life, I have experimented with several businesses, finding new passions and getting ever closer to finding my soul's calling.

I grew up in rural Quebec, and as a child, I worked with my Dad at our family's apple stand, making pies and jellies. In 1978, when I was 18, I opened a boutique that featured local artisans. Here I found my passion for creating, curating, and heart-centered-business. I moved to BC, and while raising my children, Morgen, Marylottie, and Jason, I launched a successful business, Kate & Mo Christmas Stockings. In my forties, I guess you can say I woke up. In my dreams, I was gifted the idea for a company called ZenWand to create tools for mindfulness, healing, and meditation. This was quite a new concept for the general public at the time. When my daughter, Marylottie, joined me at ZenWand, we created a fundraiser in memory of her close friend. We started designing and handcrafting gemstone bracelets, researching and learning about the unique healing properties each stone has. Through this Love Project, we were eventually able to put up a gazebo in his memory. We saw that we had tapped into something bigger as we started to receive interest and orders from all over. Many people seemed to understand there was something special about the energy and intention behind these bracelets.

Presently, ZenWand is a successful online retail, wholesale, and fundraising business. I love to see the joy that our bracelets bring to people. When I feel my best and most successful is when I can give back. For this, we created our Just Because program where we are gifting gemstone bracelets to anyone needing a little extra love.
Now at 61, looking back on my life, this I know:

I love working with my family. I love designing and creating. I feel best when I'm following my heart - and I never give up. What brings me the most joy in life is giving and helping someone feel loved. Our world needs more love. I know now that that is my life's work.

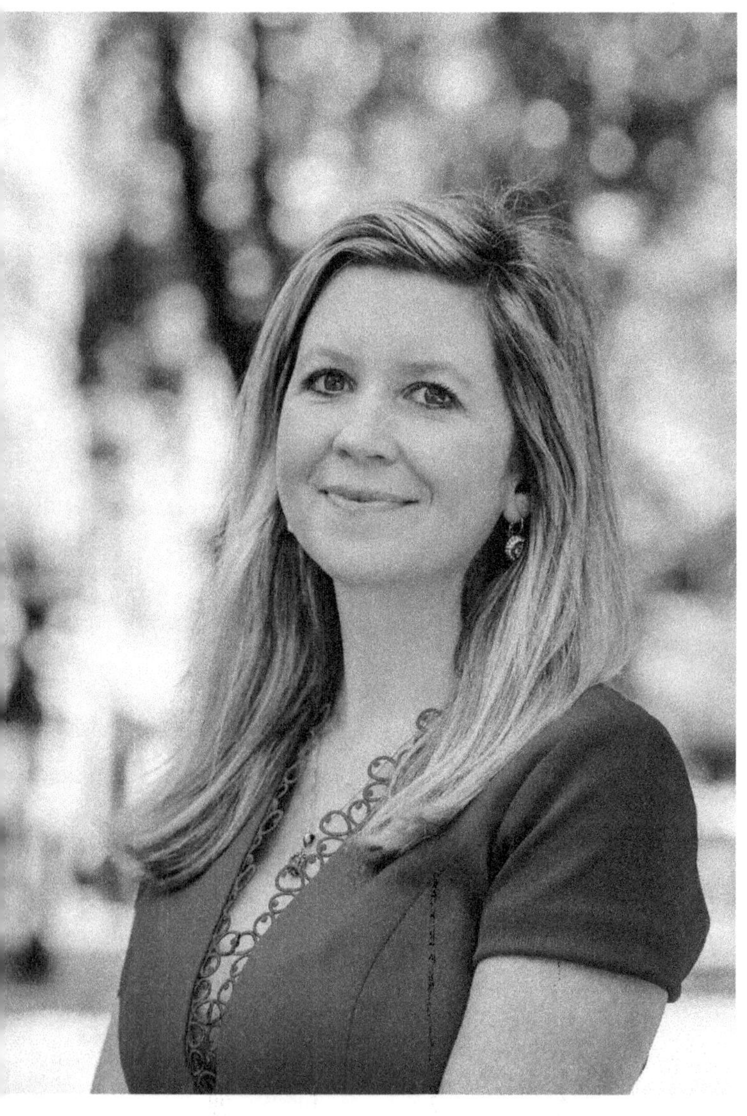

Talia Beckett Davis is the Founder of Canadian Women in Public Relations, American Women in Public Relations, and President of Pink Pearl PR, an agency specializing in luxury female marketing.

Talia Beckett Davis

She is the host of the Fempreneur Podcast, author of several public relations e-books, and editor of the Fempreneur.com blog.

When Talia first became an entrepreneur, she moved to London, England from Canada to follow her dreams of working in international business. In Cardiff, Wales, she wrote the business plan for Pink Pearl PR on a cocktail napkin. Then, Talia landed her first PR client and went on to work with leading brands across the globe, helping them to get featured in high profile publications. Talia felt a calling to give back to the PR industry and help other women in PR succeed.

As the Founder of Women in PR North America, she works to help others move into leadership positions and get a seat at the boardroom table. The movement that she wants to make is for employers to recognize that the gender pay gap that exists in the public relations industry is affecting not only women but their entire family's finances.

Talia believes that to be successful as a female entrepreneur, you must take the time to make yourself visible. She works with female entrepreneurs who want to create a profitable brand image and need a plan to stay focused. When her clients implement Talia's publicity roadmap inside the Public Relations Academy, they can build their influence and confidence. Confidence comes from taking action and helping others.

Focus on how you are going to help the person you are teaching in your online course, or how much it will help not just your client, but other members of the team if you get your project in on time.

Success does not happen overnight. The most successful female entrepreneurs are not the ones that instantly succeed. They are the ones that get up, take notes of what did not work, brainstorm, and keep going. True failure is never trying in the first place and you cannot build a successful career or business if you give up too quickly.

Alanna Falys is an entrepreneur, passionista, and nerd. Most of all, she is what she never thought she would be - a teacher.

Alanna Falys

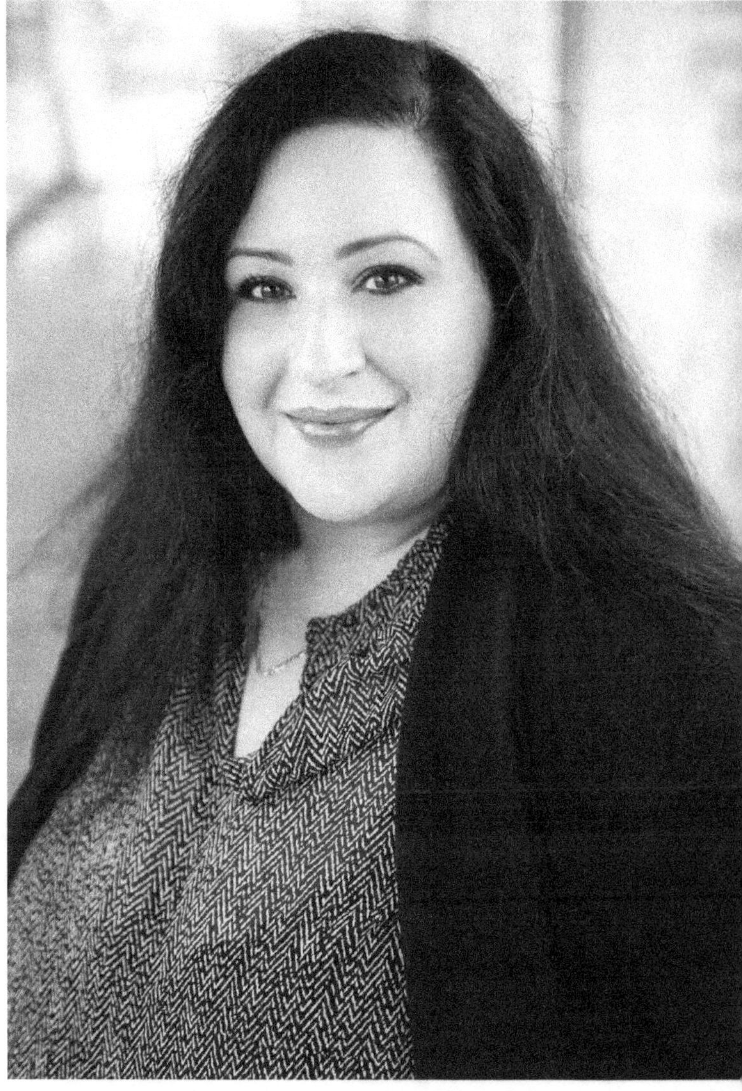

I never wanted to be a teacher. I wanted to be Oprah... or Prime Minister. Growing up, I was always the precocious one. I was always the one raising my hand and asking too many questions. I took risks- some worked out well, some *ahem* didn't. I was brave, and I put myself out there. I was fortunate to be given chances. These chances changed my life.

I come from a long line of teachers. Both my mother and grandmother were teachers. I didn't want to follow in their footsteps, but the road less travelled led me up this path.

My calling chose me. While studying towards a career in law, I fell deeply in love with the transformation education facilitates, and like any great love, I fell hard.

As a single mom, I knew I wanted to fiercely show my girls what is possible; I studied relentlessly, and I took a chance and started my own company bringing my passion to life.

In the same year, I was given a chance to be an Olympian - well not literally, but sort of. I was given the chance to be the Sr. Project Manager of Training and Development for the employees of the Vancouver 2010 Olympic and Paralympic Games; the glowing hearts who supported Olympians, and the champions who cheered them on. This chance, this magical opportunity, propelled my esteem, my confidence, and my utter perseverance to live to the fullest.

PRIMEtuitive stands for Positive Results. Innovative Mastery Education... intuitively.

I am deeply passionate about quality education, as I have learned that education is not created equally. That passion has evolved into manifesting an organization that brings engaged, impactful and proactive learning to everybody.

What I know for sure is that by taking a chance on yourself, and believing in the possibilities of the unknown, the road less travelled will navigate you to your highest self.

People took chances on me, and I know that because of them, a little serendipity, and a lot of hard work I was able to navigate the road less travelled and I made it my own.

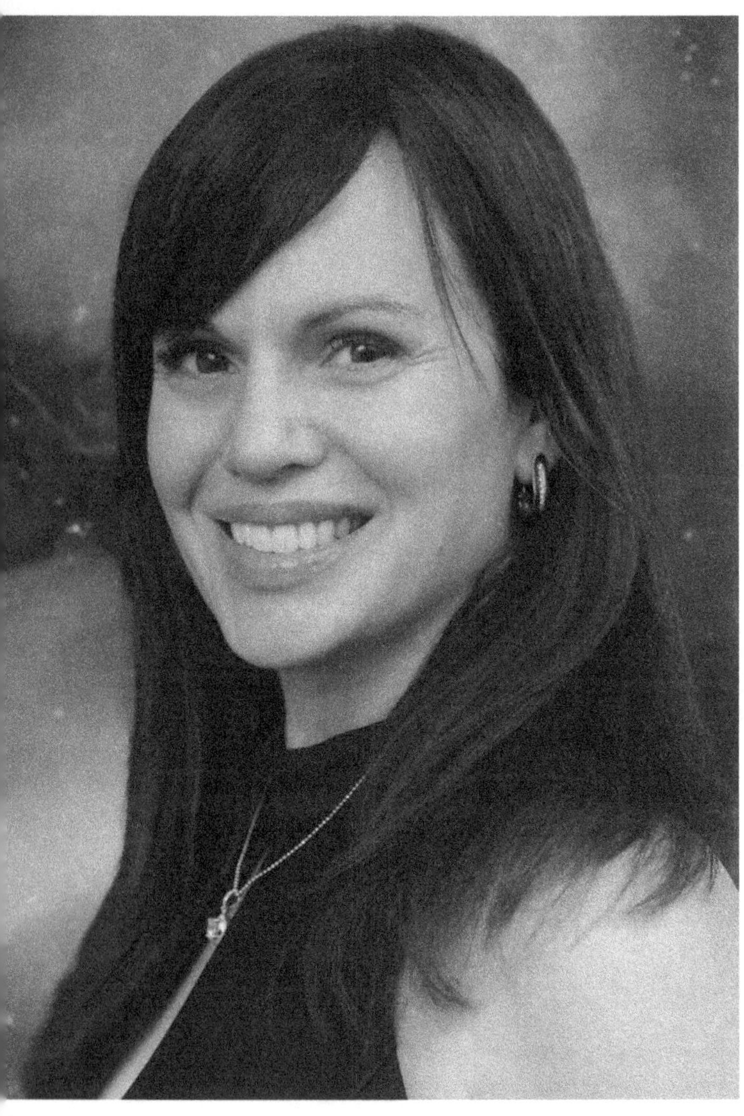

Sheila Neufeld is an immensely talented abstract painter, a world-traveller, and brings a sense of adventure to everything she touches.

Sheila Neufeld

Throughout my life, I have always felt that my ability to grow and adapt is important and learning to follow my intuition was part of this. I have chosen to expand my horizons by travelling the world and experiencing other cultures. This has increased my confidence and has brought me meaning, depth, and compassion.

One of the trips that brought the most to my life was also one of the most challenging. In my twenties, I backpacked India for four and half months, half of it completely on my own. When I first set out to do this trip, I was told India was a dangerous country. Of course, those who told me it was dangerous had never been there themselves.

I was excited and nervous about this new adventure. I arrived in India and, by the second day, I got dysentery that lasted for six weeks. I stayed in some places with friendly cockroaches; sometimes I stayed in Ashrams. I saw the most extremes of riches, poverty, and illness beyond what I had ever seen before. I also saw more smiles and more generosity than I ever have seen in North America. People on the street would look at me and wait for me to ask them for directions as they were excited to help. I threw my Western schedule out the window, as in India, time is very flexible, and rules are constantly changing. I had to adapt. There were times I wanted to come home; however, I stayed, and I am so glad I did.

When I travelled on my own, I followed my intuition because I had to. I became more confident and able to handle situations that would have normally scared me. At the end of it all, I returned with an appreciation of the privileges of my life, and with the knowledge that I could handle far more than what I thought.

So, when anyone gets an opportunity for a unique travel experience, I tell them to go for it! Be safe and plan; however, also ride with the unexpected. Follow your intuition!

Melissa Rosas is an event planner specializing in entertainment, film production management, digital marketing, and publicity. Melissa Rosas never once thought she would be an entrepreneur.

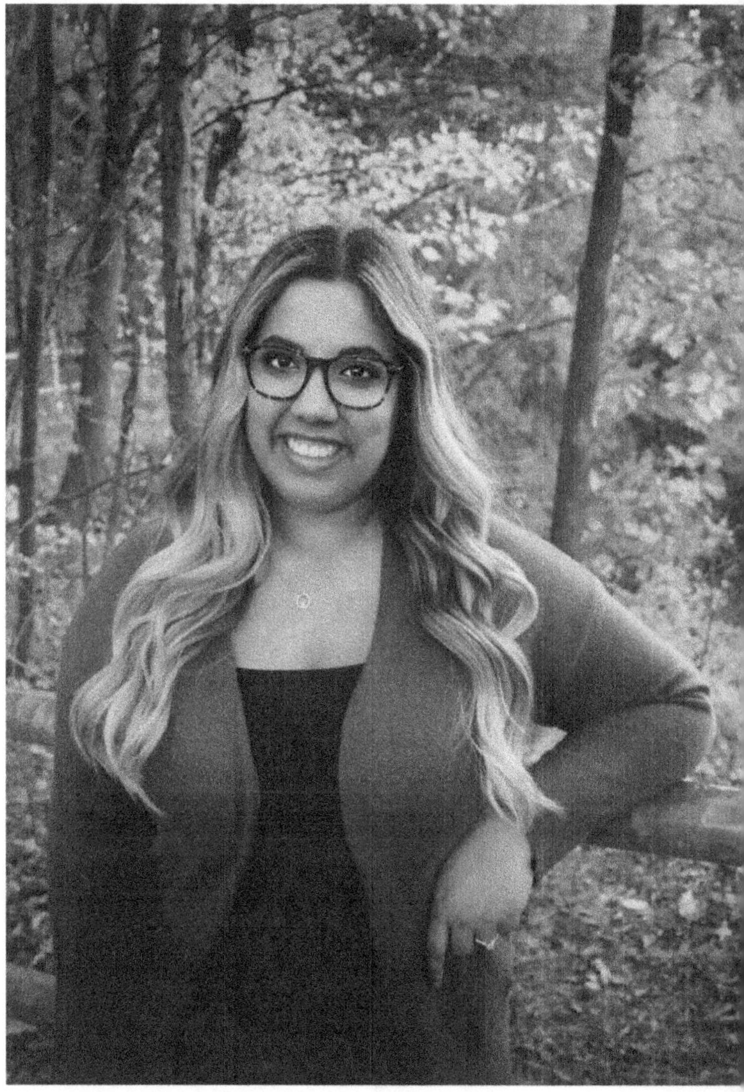

Melissa Rosas

I never in a million years thought I would own a business. I grew up comfortably with the conventional mindset that after I graduate from university, I would become a teacher. At the time, it felt like an obvious path for me to take. While being an educator is an incredible and commendable profession, I didn't want to do what everybody around me was doing. I'm outgoing, opinionated, strong-willed, a travel bug, and most of all – a people person. I love life, I love hard, and a lot of my best decisions were derived from, "f*ck it, let's do it." I never want to do anything the easy way because to me, that's boring. I always have to find a way to make it bigger and better.

Life has a funny way of pushing you to where you need to be. During my university career, I fell in love with public relations and media, and found myself feeling enthusiastic for immersive experiences. Then, all of a sudden, I was registering my business, producing events, billing clients, and I just thought, "How did I even get here?" It was truly an amazing feeling.

Looking back, I don't even know why I wanted to be a teacher. I mean, I would've rocked it, but I can't imagine not doing what I do now. The specific type of problem-solving that goes into planning and executing live events is my world, and I love every part of it. Life doesn't have to be conventional, and I truly believe life is what you make it. Just because I'm a woman, it doesn't mean I have to live a cookie-cutter life. By the way, I did apply to teacher's college. I didn't get in, and while for some, that would have been a negative experience, it was the biggest wake-up call I've ever had. It ultimately led me to my true passion. The universe clearly had other plans for me.

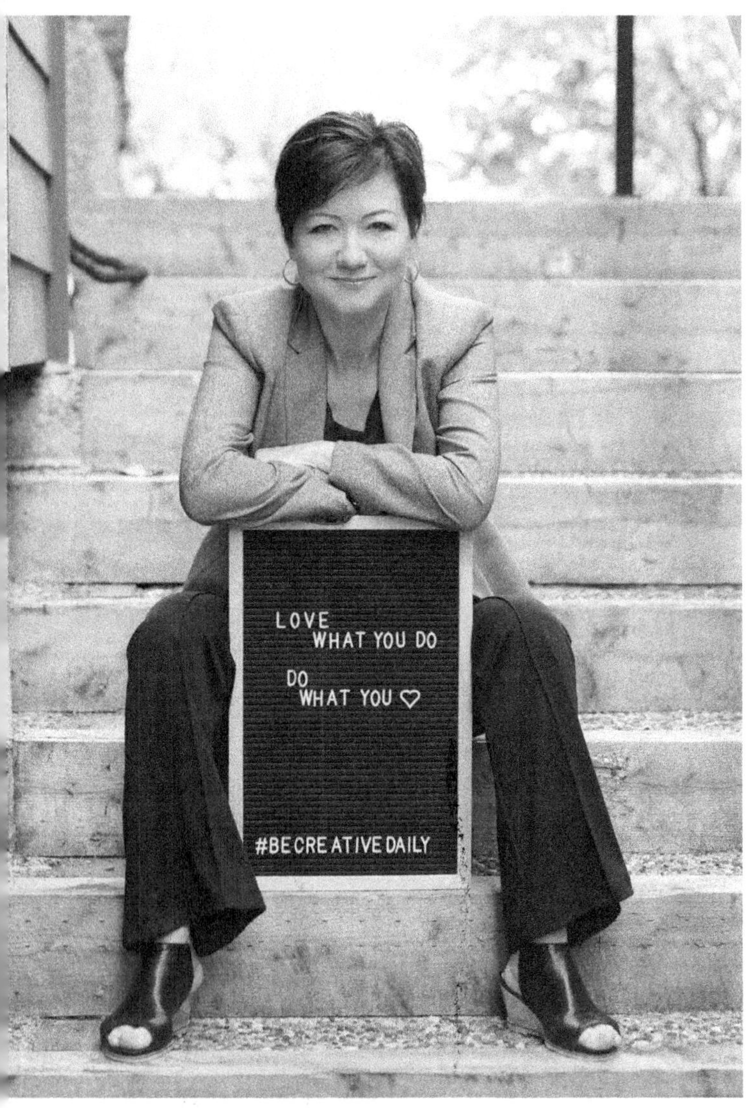

Michele is an award-winning business owner, public speaker, acting coach and arts and culture advocate.

Michele Partridge

Things I wish I knew in my 20's as a young entrepreneur:

1. Business: Don't go into business with someone you can't have a coffee or beer with. Otherwise, that relationship will never be at the level you want it to be. This is true in business and in life. Listen to your gut. There have been times that I thankfully listened to my gut, and there have been times when I didn't listen. Let's just say, it took a few times for me to listen.

2. Listen: When I was a young twenty-something entrepreneur, I was a bit arrogant. Ambitious and arrogant. The best thing any entrepreneur can do is listen to those who have done what you want to do. Listen to your mentors. If you don't have a mentor, find one. Ask them questions. Then listen. Record their sage words of advice. Then pay it forward for those who come to you for advice.

3. Strengthen your Strengths: This one is borrowed from my friend Kathryn Ritter, and I love it. Yes, it's important to always work on your weaknesses, but it's important to keep those superpowers you have in check as well. Be known for those superpowers, and don't be afraid to 'toot your own horn' about it.

4. Filter Your Thoughts: This one is a goodie. I no longer send angry emails. Yes, I write that email, but then I EDIT it and find more professional ways to explain my points. Take the higher ground. As Michelle Obama says, "When they go low, you go high".

5. Look at the Big Picture: I find as I get older, I don't sweat everything anymore. Take a moment, breathe, look at all sides. Be rational. Don't let emotion dictate situations. This takes practice. At least for me it does. But I'm getting better at it.

I'm a 52-year-old entrepreneur and have had many careers in my life. I've worked in fields such as film and television, video gaming, hospitality, customer sales, public speaking, business management, and education. I've learned many valuable skills along the way. Those skills have led to my latest business venture. I am now a confidence coach.
Ready for the next adventure.

Cara Thien is the president of Aaxll Brands Company Limited, Co-Founder of Balance CBD, and an accomplished entrepreneur.

Cara Thien

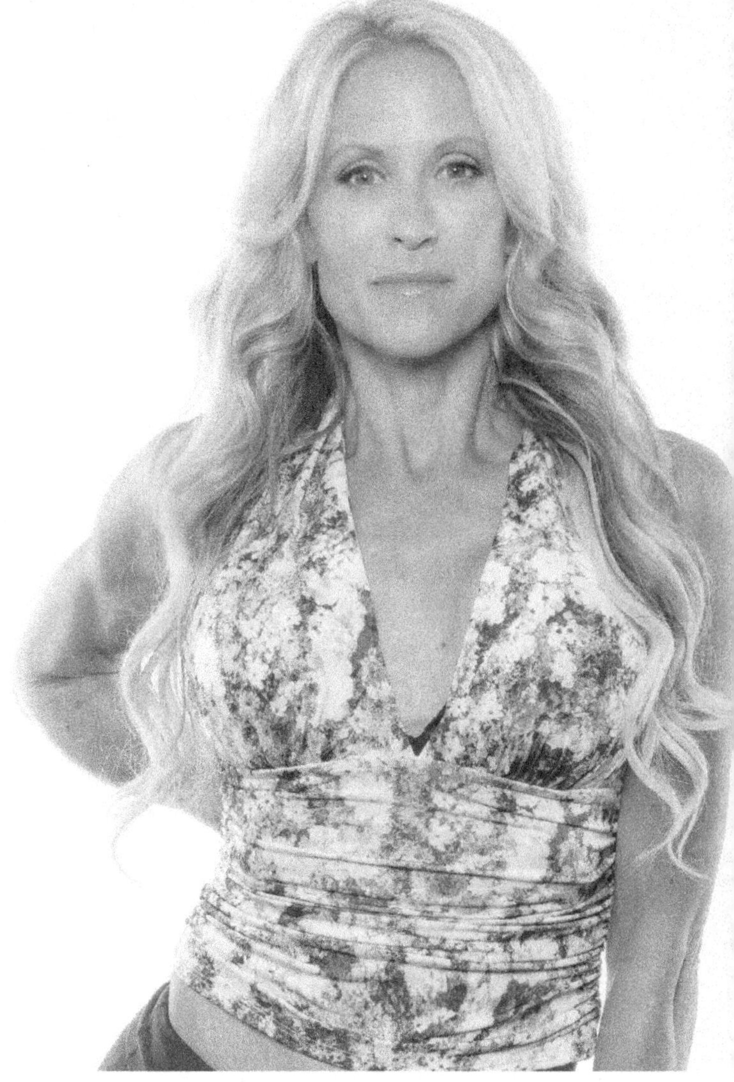

As a motivator, public speaker, philanthropist, model, and fitness enthusiast, she brings a fiery passion to every endeavor. Whatever she takes on, she succeeds, each high achievement a testament to her fortitude, intelligence, and charisma.

As president of Aaxll Brands Company Limited, Cara has developed top-selling brands in the USA and continues to innovate and disrupt the status quo. Cara started a beautiful family and began another personal journey of excellence, competing as a fitness athlete at the age of 30. She harnessed her success to open a fitness studio, and her drive elevated her to the top 5 in North America at the prestigious "Arnold Classic" and the GNC North American's. Following her eighth year of competing, Cara's health began to wane as her physical and mental health broke down. She sought out help from medical professionals and was diagnosed with chronic fatigue, fibromyalgia, menopause, and severe anxiety. Despite her diligent search for a solution and experimentation with numerous medically advised remedies, Cara's health continued to decline. It was at this time that she decided to take her health into her own hands and began exploring CBD and its benefits.

Resilience and perseverance are in her blood. She now works tirelessly to bring products to market and brands to life. Once involved, Cara will not stop until her vision is fully realized. Currently, launching Dani Pepper L'olio in the USA while adding an additional three products to the already successful Balance CBD line, 2021 is proving to be another virtuoso year.

Cara has a passion for the formulations, the package, the symphony of players it takes to get the brand to market. She is a maestro of motivation, a catalyst for collaboration. She loves forming a team of professionals and watching the magic happen. With sales of over 1 million in their first year, Cara has created a formidable force in the industry and left an indelible mark on everyone with whom she has worked.

Never resting on her laurels, she continues to finesse and refine. Ever committed to self-improvement and the betterment of others, she has evolved from one market to the next showing the grit and grace of a true leader.

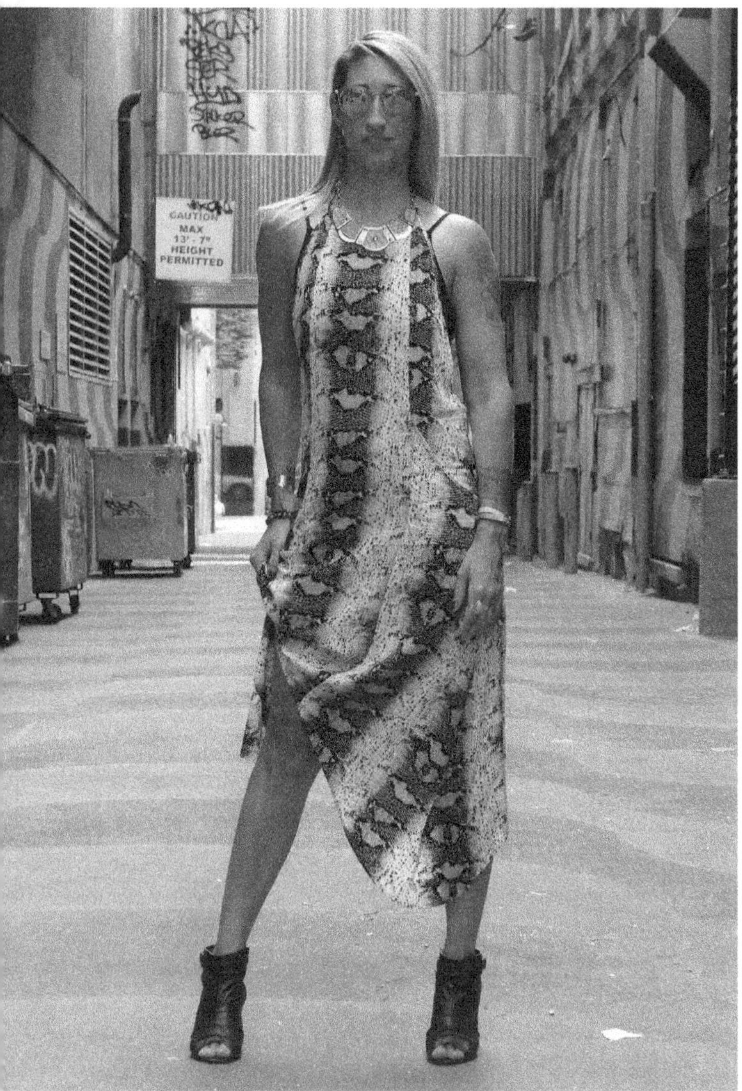

Photo Credit: Dan Galic

Nicole is a wife, mother, animal lover, tree hugger, art enthusiast, graphic designer, but most importantly - one-of-a-kind.

Nicole O'Keefe

There is one trait that has stayed consistent throughout the chapters of my life - being authentic. Ever since I can remember, I have been a free-spirited individual who expressed myself through fashion, accessories, ever-changing hair colours, and my love for the planet.

Yes, I was that shy, quirky kid in school who strived to look different and supported causes my friends never heard of. I am not sure how I survived my adolescence, but I stayed true to my creative personality all the way through college and into a career in graphic design.

This authenticity turned into my brand.

I refuse to change my behavior or ignore my values and beliefs in order to be accepted by anyone. Whether it be a personal or professional relationship, I believe you should never change or mold yourself in order to seek the approval of others. A loving shout out to the employers, friends & family (especially my supportive husband) who have embraced my authenticity and made me who I am today.

In 2015, I learned that life is shorter than we think. A true Pisces at heart, I dream big, and enduring the loss of five family members in one year pushed me to turn dreams into realities.

If there is a passion or hobby you have been wanting to try, stop putting it off until tomorrow. In the past five years, I have challenged myself with a yoga teacher training certificate, metal forming jewelry classes, pole dancing, acro yoga, learning Spanish, creating a blog for eco-warriors, and working my way through a marketing management certificate at BCIT. Travel has become a priority for me, and it doesn't matter how old you are – never stop learning.

Over the past twenty years as a graphic designer, I have built up an extensive list of clients based on genuine connections. Amazing skills and work ethic go a long way in my career, but having clients refer you because of your transparency and outside the box personality really shows that being authentic in every aspect of your life is important. Just be you!

Mariah Owen is a retired world champion athlete turned award-winning actor, filmmaker, writer, and entrepreneur, who founded her boutique production company, GTE Productions when she was twenty-one. She's been lucky enough to work with some of the biggest names in the biz and had films premiere at festivals around the world such as SXSW, Cannes & Sitges.

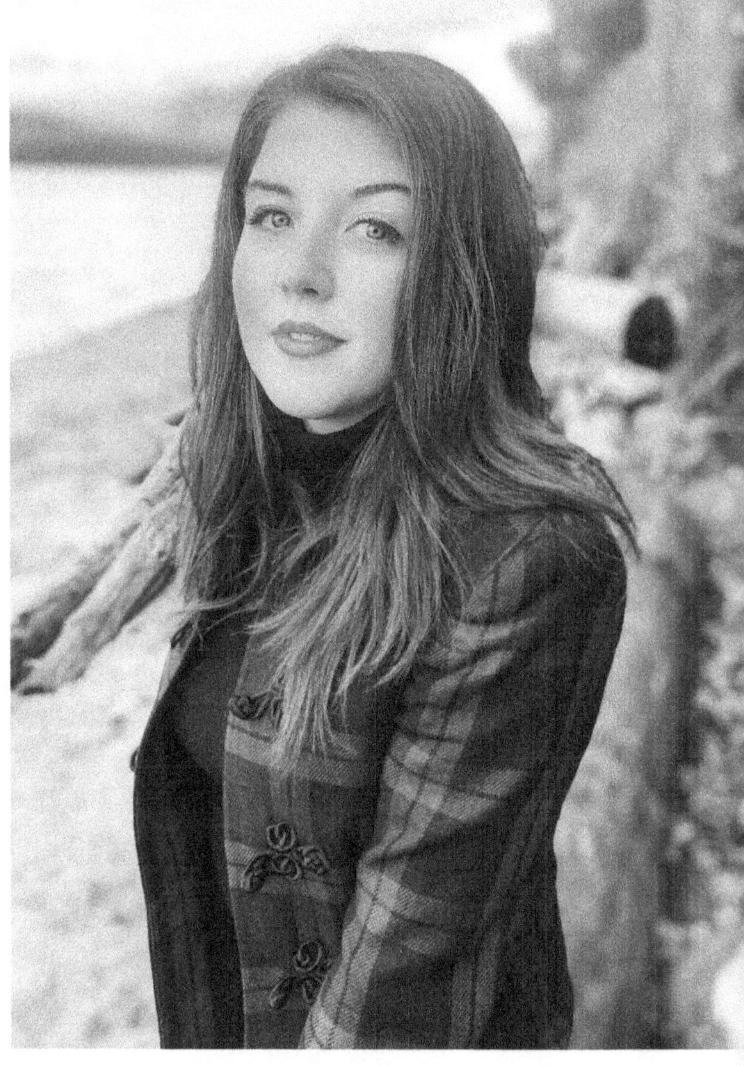

Mariah Owen

When not making movies, I can be found chasing after my very sassy and beautiful rescue puppy named Mammoth, named after one of my favorite places to ski, Mammoth Mountain. She has helped me during one of the biggest transitions of my life, career, and the 2020 pandemic.

I believe in being good to people and helping them shine their brightest. I like to do this by holding space, reminding them of their strengths, and giving support to them to keep moving forward. I am definitely a hard-working individual yet love collaborating and being inspired by others on a team.

The hardest part about getting started is just that - starting. I honestly ran before I could walk out of necessity to get things made with my prod-co. I wasn't getting the opportunities I craved, so I decided to make them. On the tough days, I go back to that moment and think about all of the awesome people who helped me get here. My friends, mentors, and family continue to believe in me, even on the days that I don't believe in myself. I am so grateful for them and their unwavering support.

As a storyteller, I am used to creative blocks, my remedy is to get outside in nature or do an activity that I enjoy without any type of judgement. I calm my mind and find that's when inspiration sparks. Another remedy is to just do the damn thing. Discipline is not a gift bestowed to some of us; it is something we must fight to achieve!

My mantra when things get tough is "everything will always work out for me." I hope you'll use this mantra too and know that you can achieve anything when you work really hard and are kind to others.

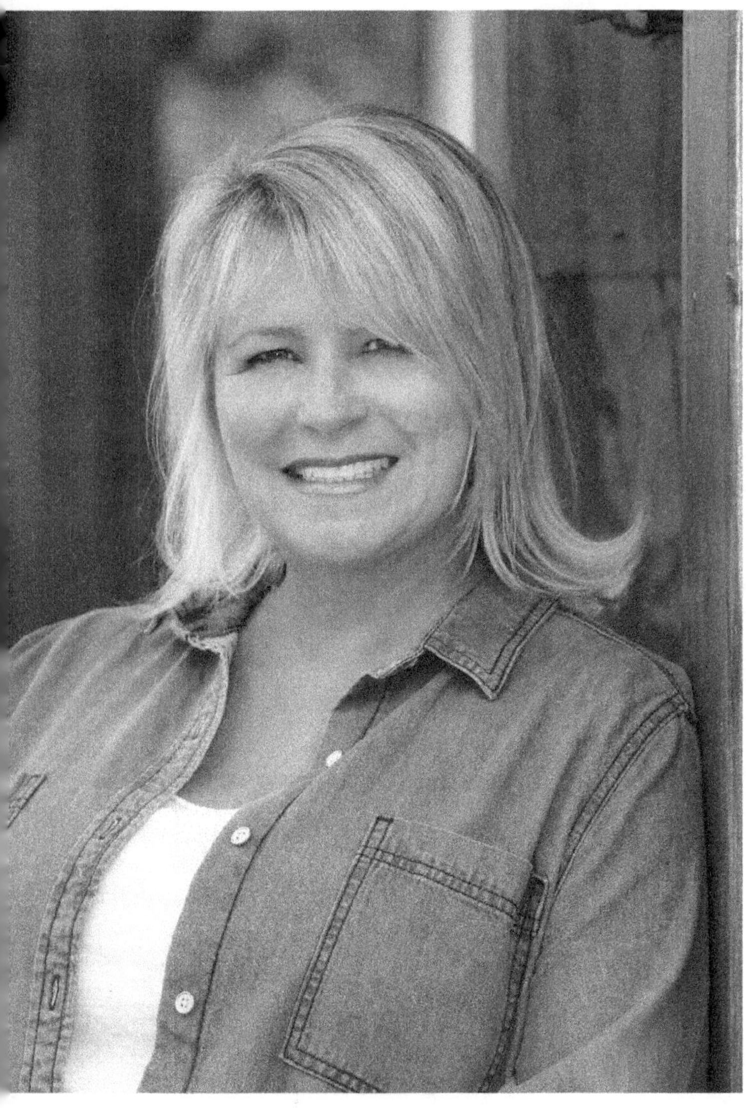

Katherine McEachnie is a Wine Scholar and #1 Best Selling Author.

Katherine McEachnie

The key to life is having the right attitude. I learned early on that "your attitude is your altitude."

I did not have an easy life growing up. I lived on my own at age 15 and put myself through high school working evenings to afford my apartment. My motto is to never give up. Being diagnosed with invasive cancer in my twenties and told I had three months to live, I fought the fight of my life, defied the odds, and kicked cancer to the curb. My favourite quote is, "There is no chance, no destiny, and no fate, that can circumvent, hinder or control the resolve of a determined soul."

After sipping the most flawless glass of wine, I started educating my palate, immersed myself in studies, and travelled to world wine regions quenching my thirst for wine knowledge. Graduating at Guildhall in London, UK was a highlight in my life. Cooking school in Italy was another.

I found a man with forever ingredients, and we have been each other's rock. We both loved and lost with cancer, which is what ironically brought us together, and for that, we share a profound love. My dream of owning a vineyard came true in 2017 when my husband and I bought a ten-acre private estate on the Naramata Bench in the Okanagan. When I stood in my vineyard for the first time, I cried. My realtor said she was a conduit between the universe and my destiny. It is a culmination of all my wine & viticulture studies coming together. I live an inspired life amongst the vines, and I share my passion as a wine educator in our community. We are blown away at the exceptional quality of wine being produced in BC.

vWe grow four different grape varieties, have fruit trees, and a beautiful vegetable garden. I am a home chef, inspired by nature's bounty all around me. I spend most of my time in my country kitchen, cooking for others and hosting vineyard gatherings. I am about to release a cookbook with all my most-asked-for recipes, entertaining secrets, and wine pairings. We love our Okanagan lifestyle and wake up every day with an abundance of gratitude.
Dreams do come true; I am living proof.

Janet is a naturally curious creator, photographer, and photo educator. She has a knack for making every person she meets feel welcome by her genuine, bubbly nature.

Janet Pliszka

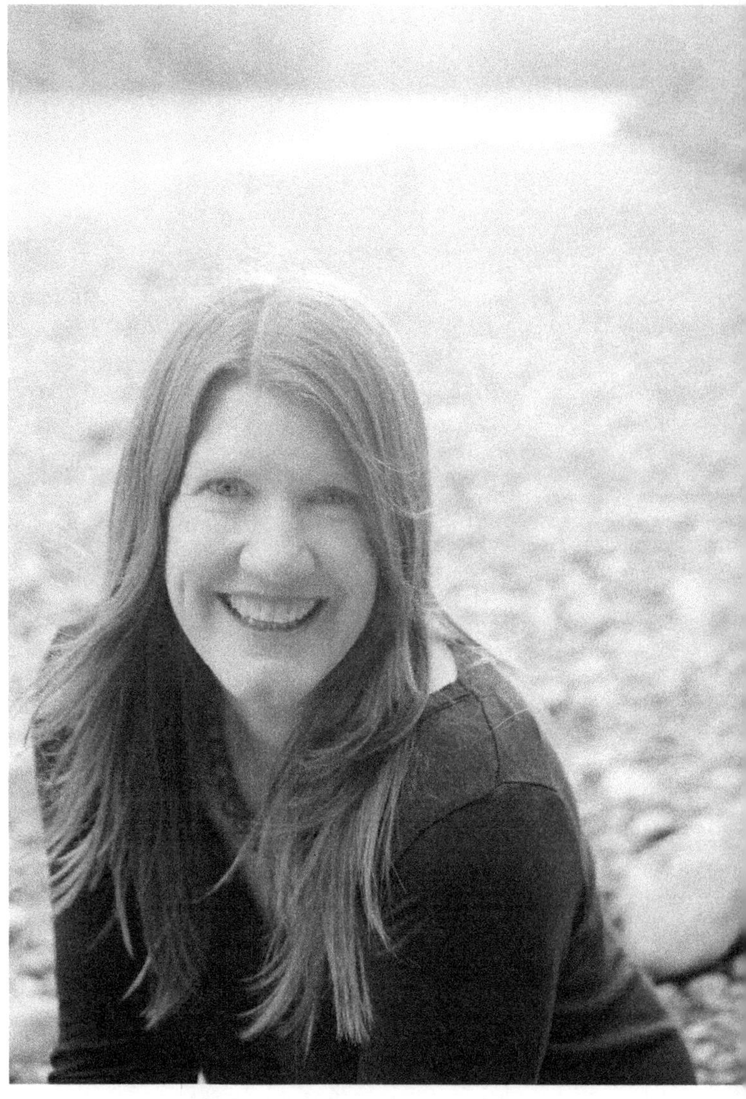

Hello! So great to meet you! One of my greatest joys is to help others see beauty in themselves and the world around them. I know I am here to show people, young and old, that they belong and they matter.

Photography is my gateway to inspire others to know how amazing they are. Whether I am behind the lens taking photos or in front of a group teaching them how to take their own, my purpose is to prompt individuals to see themselves and their surroundings in the most positive and interesting light (figuratively and literally, of course).
I love, love, love spending my days with other people. They fascinate me, and I love their stories!

You will often see me trekking out in Alberta's outdoors, encouraging families to be their best, imperfect selves doing what they love together. Or you will find me seeking eclectic gathering places with gorgeous light to capture the true essence of family. My mission is to have families say "that is so us!" every time they see their gallery. And they do.

As an entrepreneur, I'm equally motivated to amplify business owners' passions for their work and embody the essence of what they do and how they do it. Nobody wants "just another headshot". With my eye for all things that feel natural, I capture the spirit and spark that fires them up!

And, oh man, nothing fires me up more than witnessing a kid's world open up before them as they connect to themselves, others, and the universe around them with a camera in hand. Through Kids' Photography Academy, I encourage youth to see usual things in unusual ways, to see beauty in the different and unique, and ultimately to share their own voice in the process. Bringing kids together to celebrate their art, adventures, lives, and each other is a mission of inclusivity and self-love that is so important.

Photography is my channel to fun, healing, joy, and connection. I am so grateful for it. Helping someone else feel connected to their own story is what matters most.

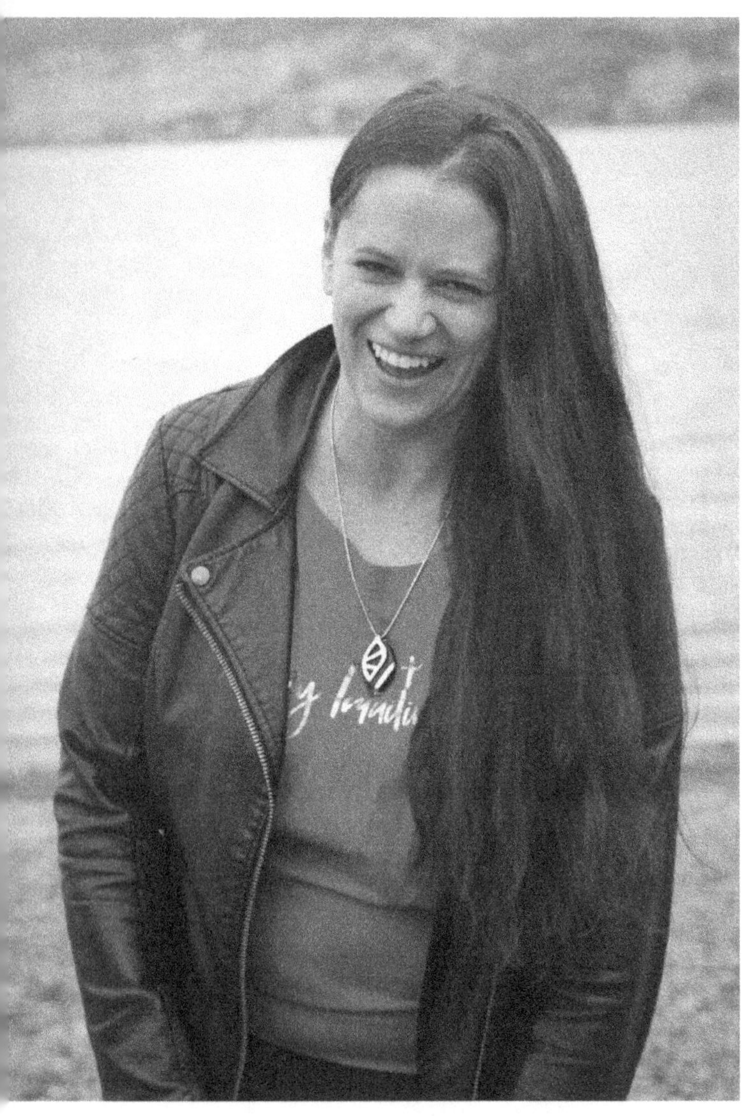

When I was five years old, I climbed a mountain with my Dad. Little was I to know this mountain was about to become a metaphor for my entire life.

Cindy Van Arnam

I used to believe that life was all about climbing the mountain. That hard work, effort, determination, and a stubborn mind were what brought one to success. That recognition for a job well done came when you got to the top of that proverbial mountain.

When I started my business four years ago, I created a 'mountain'. I became a workaholic, I took on clients that were beyond challenging, and I made my work hard. At the time, I 'knew' in my mind that in order for my business to be successful, I needed to work hard, hustle, grind, and get shit done.

I was working seven days a week, sometimes fifteen hours a day, living Paypal to Paypal, just barely making ends meet.
I believed that was how it was done.
And then I learned a new way of doing things...

It is clear that our world is in the midst of a radical transformation as old paradigms crumble, and we are exposed to the truth; that our old business models aren't working. I believe it is our responsibility to lead the way in this transformation by doing things differently, more consciously, and in alignment with our higher purpose.

The materialization of our desires now depends on a different form of leadership, financial stewardship, and personal accountability. As I learned to focus on my own personal power and discovered how limitless we truly are, I finally understood that hard work isn't the answer.

As I reclaimed my power and developed a deep inner knowing, it became clear to me that it is our Divine right to receive and to show up in service to the redistribution of wealth on the planet.

Today, I am passionate about leading emerging entrepreneurs to fully discover their own limitless power so they can create sustainable wealth through their passion and service to their higher purpose - minus the hustle, the grind, and the mountain.

Tammy Bailey

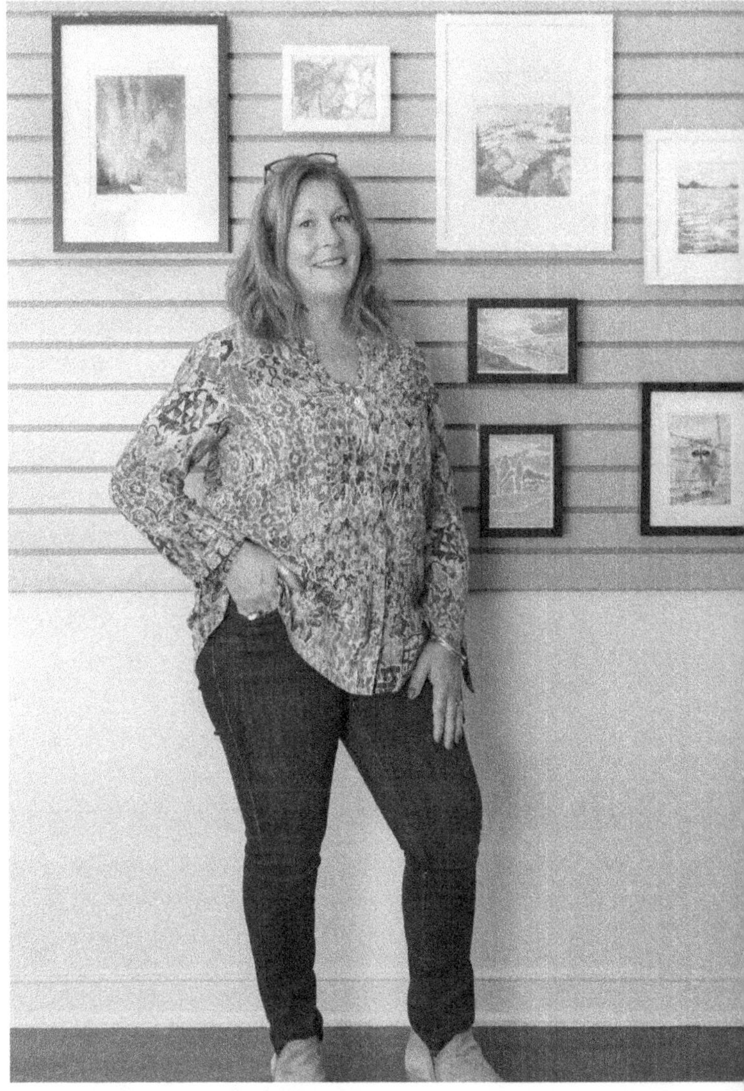

I have been sober since March 18, 2004.
I used to say that my family growing up put the fun back in dysfunctional. Truthfully, it was not fun. Both my parents were stunted by alcohol. Anger, verbal abuse, physical abuse, and emotional loss were my childhood. I learned a fear-imposed, unrealistic standard of perfection. Be good or else! And I feared the or else.

An alcoholic home of, don't think, don't speak, don't feel and whatever you do, don't tell the neighbours! I carried this shame for many years. Painful events that had not been processed in my past were my undoing, but they were also the gift of a new beginning.

One truth that has been consistent throughout my recovery journey is that my past is my ally and incentive. It has reminded me daily to work on the present, so my future and my family's future is better. Sobriety has graced me with a gift of a new legacy.

A legacy that is one of healing, not harming because I have learned from my parent's and my own personal addiction that alcoholism is a family disease. Painting has been one of the many discoveries and gifts I have been given through recovery. This is where I have been able to express my passion, playfulness, and deep soul joy. This quiet time while creating takes me on this incredible journey from my head to my heart, allowing me to share the joy and beauty that inspires me while painting in my home studio. I am discovering that happiness is within me.

Today, I am sober. Understanding that my attitude is more important than my aptitude. My best is good enough, and some days my best is not so good. And I am okay with this. I have a choice today to live in the moment with a willingness to learn from everything that has happened. I have been taken on this amazing journey called recovery, with all its sadness, joy, inspiration, and love. I am authentically me, good and bad, and that is success.

I am grateful to be able to continue this pursuit of self and art discovery by sharing a brief part of my story. Knowing it is okay to think, speak and feel. Understanding there is no shame in telling.

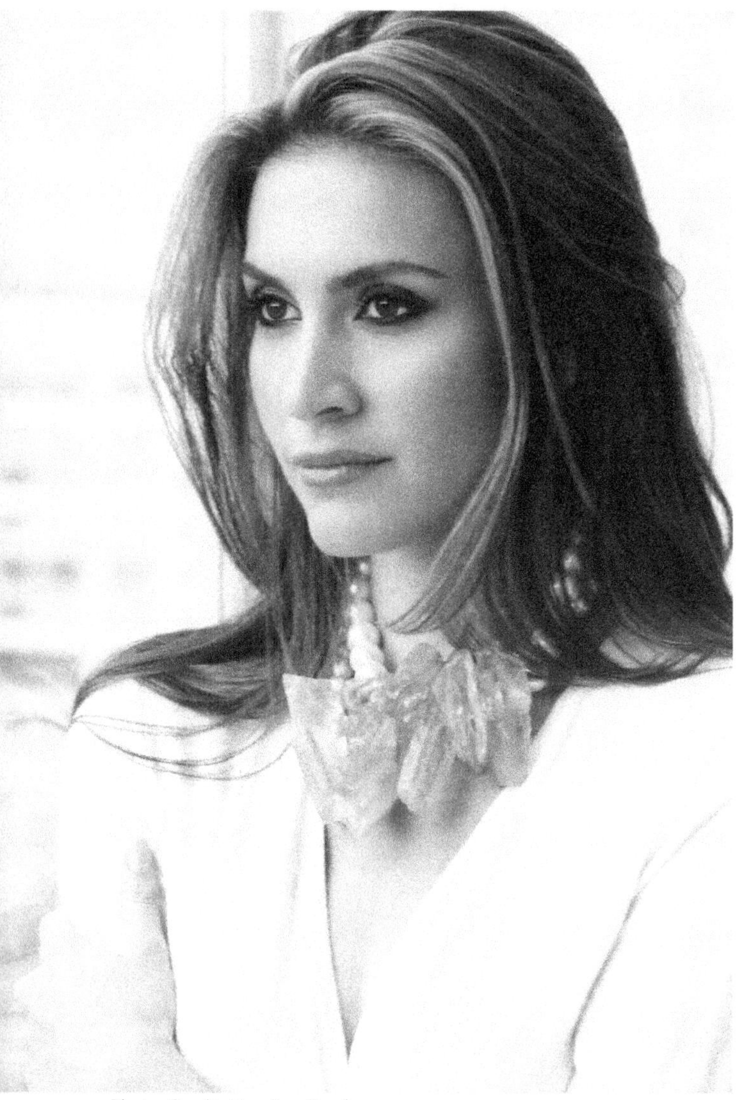

Photo Credit: Karolina Turek

Nazanin Afshin-Jam Mackay is a Human Rights Activist, Co-Founder of Stop Child Executions and The Nazanin Foundation. She is an author, singer/songwriter, Miss World Canada 2003, author, and public speaker.

Nazanin Afshin-Jam

In 2006 I was living a comfortable Canadian life. I was pursuing a career as a recording artist when I heard by chance a tale that both chilled and stirred my soul. In a short time, I found myself leading a campaign to help save the life of a girl in Iran, who shared my name, and who had been sentenced to death for stabbing one of three men who attempted to rape her.

For defending her life, and that of her niece, she was facing the death penalty, placed in solitary confinement, sleeping on a thin blanket on the cold, dank floor, living among rats and cockroaches, tortured and isolated. At any moment, she could have been executed.

There was as if a part of me was awakened. I was driven to do all in my power to stop this misery and secure her freedom. I told my music manager that night that I would have to follow this higher calling.

What motivates me most is fighting injustice, ending suffering, and seeing people, especially youth, live full and meaningful lives. This cause to which I was drawn gave me energy and focus. Her circumstance could have easily been my fate had I stayed in Iran after the revolution and been subjected to its draconian Shari'a laws. I was grateful to be living in Canada, a free democratic equitable county with the rule of law.

I had a mission to do everything in my power to see this girl through the injustice of her situation to save her from this horrible fate thrust upon her by this evil regime. Thankfully, through perseverance and the efforts of many like-minded people, we were successful, and she was spared the hangman's noose, freed from jail, and is now happily married with four children.

We must all check in with ourselves from time to time to consider whether or not we are living out our calling, utilizing our blessings and abilities to the best purpose for the betterment of others.

If you have a dream... make it a goal. Find the confidence to be the best version of yourself and all the world will benefit.

Sandra is an award-winning realtor, innovator, and devoted mentor.

Sandra Pike

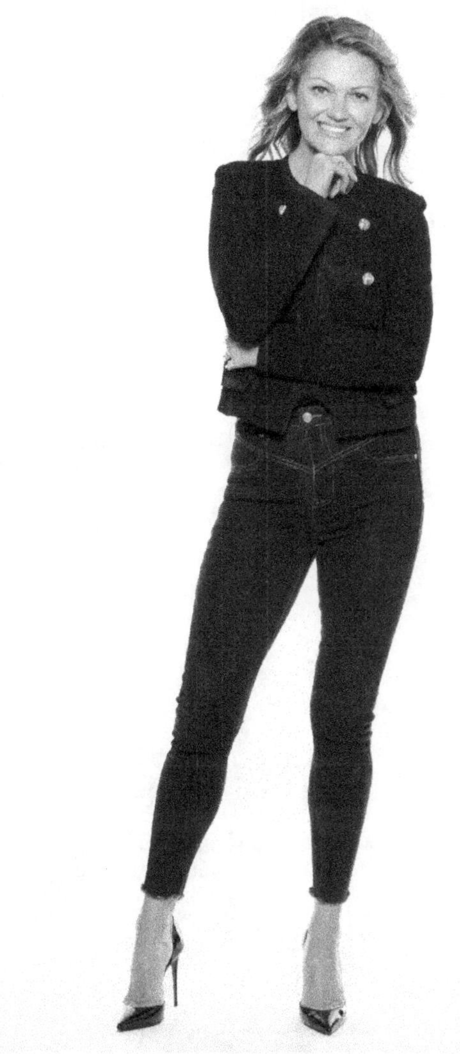

Actions define us. They make what we believe, known to others, and are our shining moments. Whether my parents are aware of it or not, their actions determined my future. Their hard work, generosity, and unwavering belief in me set the stage for how I would live my life. I don't think that on the day they gave me, their only daughter, a substantial amount of money to get back on my feet, that they knew they were giving me and those in my future a gift of incalculable value.

After a poor relationship choice, I was left in debt. The money was to renovate my home and install a small apartment that would supplement my income and help me stay soluble. We agreed I would pay them back when I eventually sold my house. My parents, of moderate-income, had worked very hard for their savings. Their trust in me defined them as people and parents. Believing in me, allowed me to believe in myself.
They led by example.

At the age of 40, I picked myself up, dusted myself off, and began to build an extraordinary life. My deeply ingrained work ethic, drive, and collaborative nature fostered relationships with many talented and like-minded individuals. With an eye on innovation, I built an award-winning team with whom I am so proud to work. Mentoring others is a passion. Seeing people believe in themselves and their skills is so gratifying. We must lift each other up! I get fired up about innovative ideas and technologies and have paired with prominent companies that allow the team to help families locate homes that enhance their lives.

Success, stability, and a belief in myself enabled me to take my parents on two cruises and travel to other places of interest. Future trips will include Dublin, which is a long-standing dream of my fathers. Still, one of my proudest moments will remain the day I was able to call my father and tell him to check his bank account. His loan was returned prior to the sale of my home, and his faith in me had not been misplaced. Actions matter!

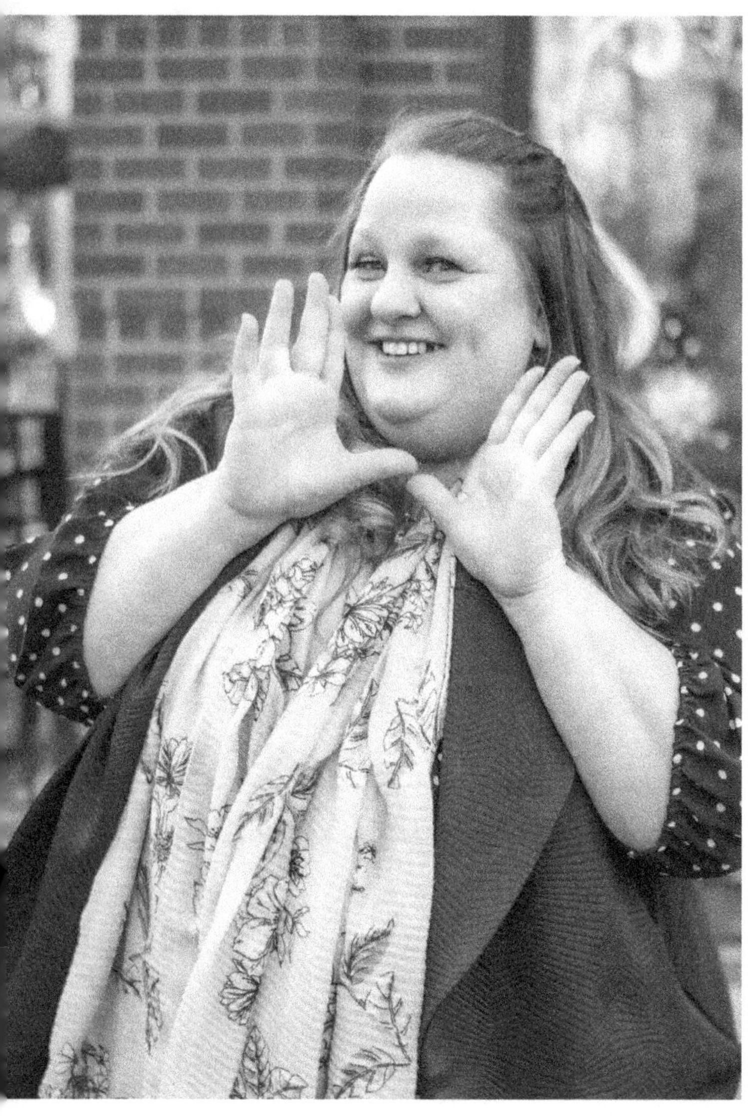

Suzanne Fleur de Lys-Aujla is a Co-Founder of Women in the Mortgage Industry, and Vice – President of BC Lenders Group.

Suzanne Fleur de Lys-Aujla

As a young girl, Suzanne struggled in school and always felt a little different from others.
She didn't know it growing up but found out later in life that her academic struggles were the result of dyslexia. Since her learning disorder was undiagnosed, she was labelled a poor student and frowned upon by teachers.

She recalls a defining moment from her youth when a schoolteacher cruelly stated that her future would most likely be limited to marriage and children because she didn't have the capacity to excel in the "real" world.
It was hard and painful growing up as an underdog, feeling alone and misunderstood in her struggle.

However, Suzanne had a tenacious spirit and was determined to succeed despite the odds. Even though she lacked a support network at the time, she refused to accept the limiting beliefs that others tried to impose on her. She knew she could make something more of herself; why not go out in the world and surprise people?!

As luck would have it, Suzanne was introduced to a woman through a mutual friend who offered to be a mentor. This touch of kindness was all Suzanne needed to lift her spirits and get her up and off to the races. She began to believe in herself more and took consistent forward action towards her dreams. Within a few years, Suzanne established herself within the financial industry and built a respectable career. Having finally arrived in a happy and successful place, she felt an innate desire to help others. With her natural gift for building relationships and supporting people, Suzanne became a trusted friend and mentor to many industry peers. She's been recognized countless times for her numerous contributions over the years and is most proud of the Michael Ellenzweigh Outstanding Service Award, where she was applauded for demonstrating exemplary service, integrity, and value within her industry.

As someone who has overcome numerous challenges, Suzanne feels her purpose now is being of service to others. Mentorship has made a profound difference in her life and she is paying it forward, spreading her kindness and supporting those in need so they too can recognize their value and succeed.

Jan Rankin is a visual storyteller who enjoys creating beautiful pieces with paint.

Jan Rankin

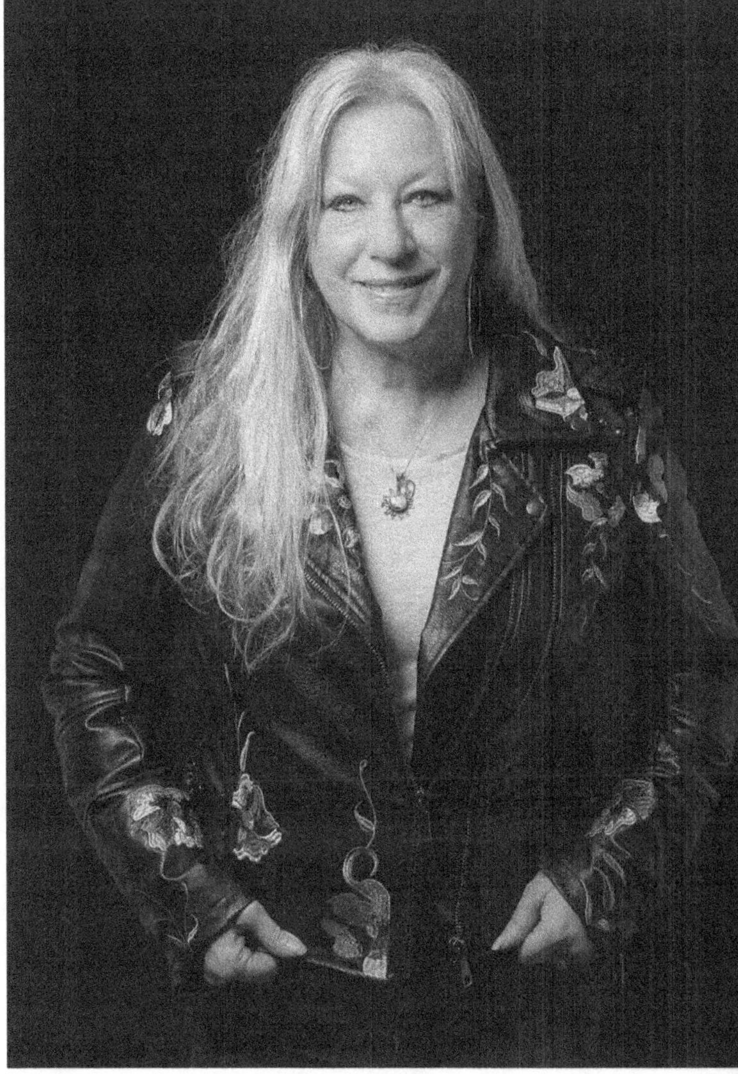
Photo Credit: Radina Photography

Once upon a time, like young girls of my generation, I believed in fairy tales for all things in love and life. And as happens, my illusions were frequently shattered through my teen years and early twenties. Until I met a man when we were both twenty-three who would change everything I held to be true about living as Ron was dying a young death. We were married at twenty-five, and by twenty-six, I was a widow.

An aggressive illness was stealing Ron's body. He endured painful procedures and treatments that would have destroyed anyone. But he was one of those magical people who found something to laugh at every day. A reason to smile. A gift to give to another, even if it was a song on his guitar. Our time together was short, chaotic, sad, joyful, and so much more. Throughout his illness, he always called the shots and lived each day on his terms right to the end.

What I received was an incredible gift of seeing clearly how to live a life on my terms. To not stay in relationships of any kind, marriages, friendships, family, clubs, that only take and don't give back. Not that every moment will be shrouded in "happily ever after," but I'm not willing to continue to invest where any joy cannot be found. I tend to listen to that small inside voice (that sometimes gets really loud!) as it leads me in new and interesting directions. I have loved and lived in many different career paths and been polished a bit smoother by all of them as well as raising my sons for many years alone.

Now, as life allows, I am able to shift more inward and I am gifted with a reintroduction to my creative and spiritual artistic self of my youth. A journey of painting and writing that has shown me new and exciting paths to interpret and share my world on canvas and paper, building on skills learned through life to work alongside other artists and bring together their collective talents. I am writing my own story on my own terms in real-life every day. No fairy tales.

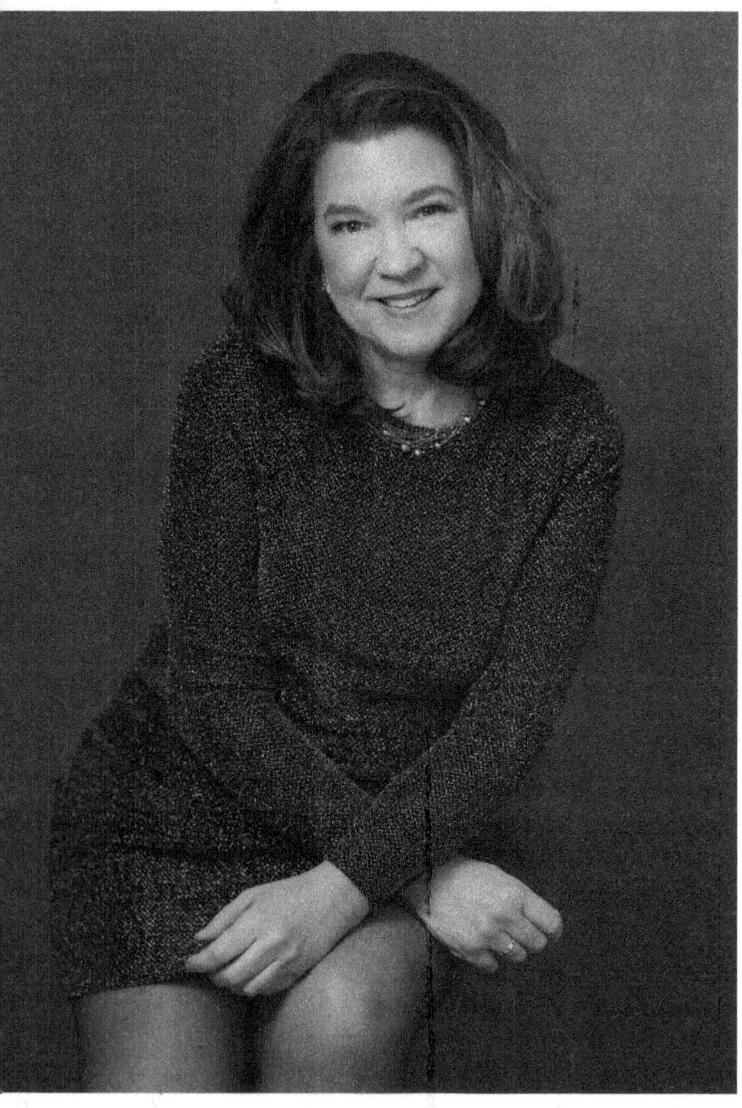

Jill Ganton is a mother, pianist, interior designer, and businesswoman - and is unafraid to speak up.

Jill Ganton

"You can't be brave if you've only had wonderful things happen to you." - Mary Tyler Moore.
Suffering in silence while the mind is unyielding in its constant clamour of disbelief, questions, fear, despair, shame, and yes, psychological evil is unbearable.
It was Spring of 2020 that I had been "captured" for seven weeks by an online sexual predator.
I must speak. How could this have happened to an educated Christian woman, single mother, a retired teacher, musician, artist, and owner of an online interior design business? But it did. Out of concern and care, some didn't want me to write; to forget this ever happened, that it would be erased from my memory.
I cannot do that. This is the beginning of my story.

THE GREEN DINOSAUR By Jill E Ganton (aka Ms. Jillie)

Green was my favourite colour. The many green shirts and my well-worn khaki sofa attest to that.
It's been three weeks. I should've started writing earlier... it's too late now... I'm in the abyss, deeper each day.
I'm writing this now before I lose all my sanity, dignity, self-worth, and identity, for I do not know how to get out – safely.
My son, my lovie! Will you be ashamed of me? You'll have questions as I do... How did this happen? Why did you let him? Why did you not fight hard enough?
Yes, why I didn't fight hard enough against this skilled and manipulative man indeed!
"Indeed" was one of his words. There's a chill when I read that now.
It took only three weeks to fully submit to him, to which he boldly stated, "You are MINE"! Yes, he capitalized the word "mine." It was as if Satan himself had reached out and pulled me beneath the pages of discernment, level-headedness, and rationale. This was the first red flag I ignored. Really, it wasn't.
It was when he asked me, then later insisted, then consistently trained me to call him "Sir." I addressed him no other way; he was a man of influence, power, and high intelligence.
This would be the pattern. The pattern I resented, hated, loathed, grew to accept, counted on, and eventually needed.
Did I say he was a married man and, if that weren't enough, a grandfather?

Linda Bickerton-Ross is an artist and photographer, and one of the founders of the Langley Community Music School.

Linda Bickerton-Ross

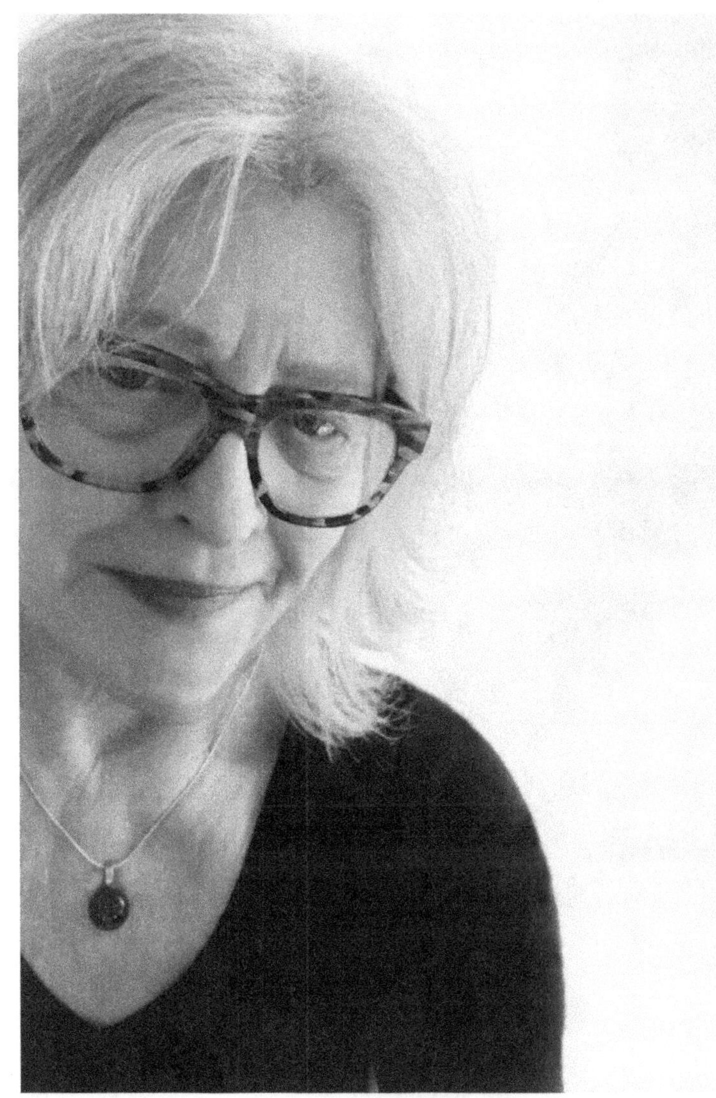

On a West Coast spring day, I stood on the stage at Kwantlen Polytechnic University. As I gazed down at the engaged faces of my two accomplished sons and beautiful 99-year-old mother, my heart was filled with love and gratitude. Along with four colleagues, I was receiving an honorary doctorate for founding the Langley Community Music School four decades earlier.

A lifetime ago, my mother had made that day possible. Although she had a new baby and four older children, she returned to work so that I could pursue advanced music studies. I enrolled at the University of Toronto, then later studied in New York. My vision of a musical career was bright and within my grasp.

But life took another path. By 1969 I was, instead, a young mother at home with one small child and pregnant with another - my musical career seemed a million miles away. I struggled with the daily tedium of small-town life, housekeeping and loneliness, desperately missing my music. Sharing this frustration with a friend, he asked me what I might do to gain greater fulfillment. With burgeoning excitement, I described my dream for this rural community; to establish a music school where faculty and students could work collaboratively teaching, learning, and performing.

Inspired by my enthusiasm, he passed me the phone number of a woman who, like me, was a classically trained pianist. "I think she might be interested in your venture," he said. Marilyn Lamont and I arranged to meet that afternoon, and over numerous cups of tea and hours of animated discussion, we birthed the beginning of the Langley Community Music School. The school was soon established and gradually evolved into one of the largest non-profit music schools in British Columbia. Winning national and international acclaim, it is considered one of the finest music schools in Canada, providing innovative and exceptional experiences for students of all ages and abilities.

My involvement with the school continued throughout the years, enhancing my career in public education and my life as a single parent. I never lost my creative roots as a working artist. Eventually, I went on to pursue my current passion, the art of photography.

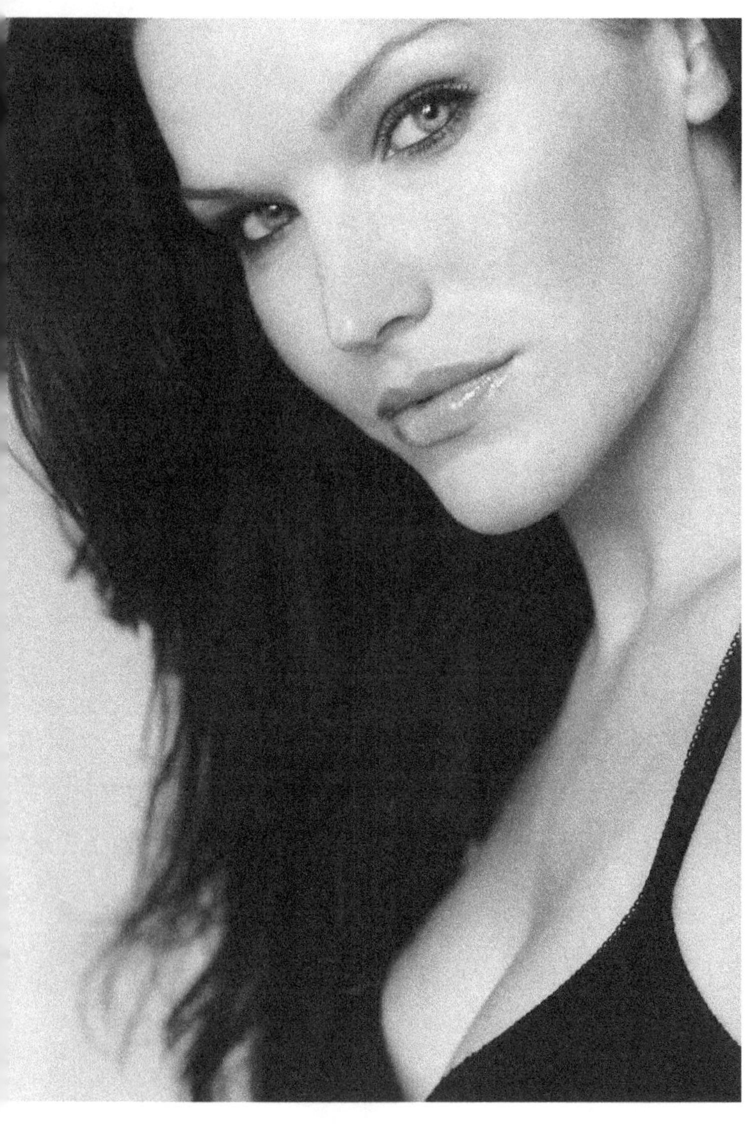

Karen Cliche is an actress of twenty-five years in tv, film, and radio. Her love of marketing led to a side career in event management and brand representation with a passion for women-owned businesses.

Karen Cliche

I recently got a tattoo on my left arm that says, "No dress rehearsal," which is a lyric from a Tragically Hip song, but I got it as a reminder to myself that life is a one-shot deal. You don't get a second chance, so live it to the fullest! I have felt this way since I was a kid. Some parts of my childhood were difficult, but I used that pain to try to change the injustices I saw, particularly when it came to women's rights.

I started volunteering at the Montreal Women's Centre when I was eighteen and have continued on that path ever since. Even my dream to become an actress was partly so that I could have some kind of positive influence on girls and amplify my voice. When I had my daughter, I chose to be a stay-at-home mom and put my acting career on pause. I also found myself wanting to try other things in life. So, I gathered up the courage to start from zero and dive into a whole new industry that I had no experience in. I interned for no money, I did door to door and cold call advertising sales on commission only, I worked twelve-hour days at hot dusty festivals, and eventually, I started managing those events. I never once thought, "I am too good for this," I just said YES to every opportunity that came my way.

I wanted the experience, I loved the challenge, and I saw it pay off. I felt such a sense of pride and accomplishment. I highly recommend getting out of your comfort zone and saying yes to things. You never know where those doors lead!

So now I fill my days with parenting my amazing daughter, Sienna, acting in films, doing voice work in radio and TV, getting hired for freelance sales, managing promotional events, and volunteering at Harmony House women's shelter in Ottawa. I remain open, never wanting to regret passing up an opportunity to grow and be brave.

Life is not a dress rehearsal - it's showtime!

Joanne Patenaude is a proud French Métis woman, an artist and the founder of C'est ta Vie Jewelry.

Joanne Patenaude

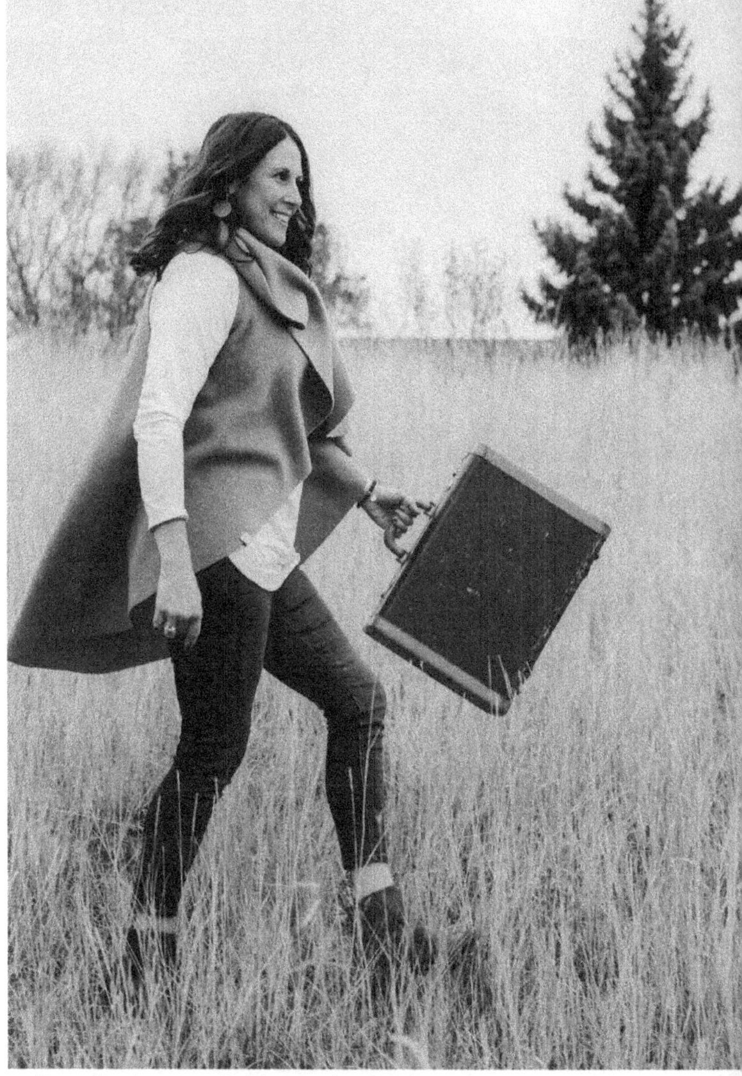
Photo Credit: painted by the sun photography

I am a proud French Métis woman. I was born and raised on Treaty 1 Territory – the original land of the Cree, Ojibway, Dene, and Dakota peoples, as well as the homeland and birthplace of the Métis Nation. The water I drink comes from Treaty 3 territory of Shoal Lake 40 First Nation and our electricity comes from Treaty 5 territory.

My familial lineage stems from the Cree and French peoples of the Red River. I was told that my great grandmother would use white powder on her face to hide her identity, so I wasn't raised with Metis traditions. I found my way through my Uncle Aimé, who shared his knowledge of our family history.

Year after year, I celebrate my culture and heritage at the largest and longest Winnipeg Winter festival, Le Festival du Voyageur, through fiddle music, dancing and jigging, and bright, intricately embroidered clothing, beading, and sashes.

Upon entering the Festival grounds, you distinctly smell the bonfires, hear the clack of the Red River Jig danced on a wooden stage, taste the sweetness of maple taffy on snow, and marvel at the detailed ice sculptures created by artists from around the world. I have been attending this festival since I was a young girl, even before I knew of my family history; yet, intuitively, I knew it was part of my fabric, I felt a deep sense of belonging.

In 2016, my life came full circle when my business, C'est Ta Vie Jewelry, became a vendor at the Festival. My creations were amongst all the other artists' works, and I truly felt at home. I was honoured and felt valued. Today, I am a vegan – for the respect of all living beings.

I also embody the values of the Seven Grandfather teaching – wisdom, love, respect, courage, honesty, humility, and truth – all of which are essential to living a full and healthy life in one form or another, as a moral steppingstone and cultural foundation to which I live my life every day.

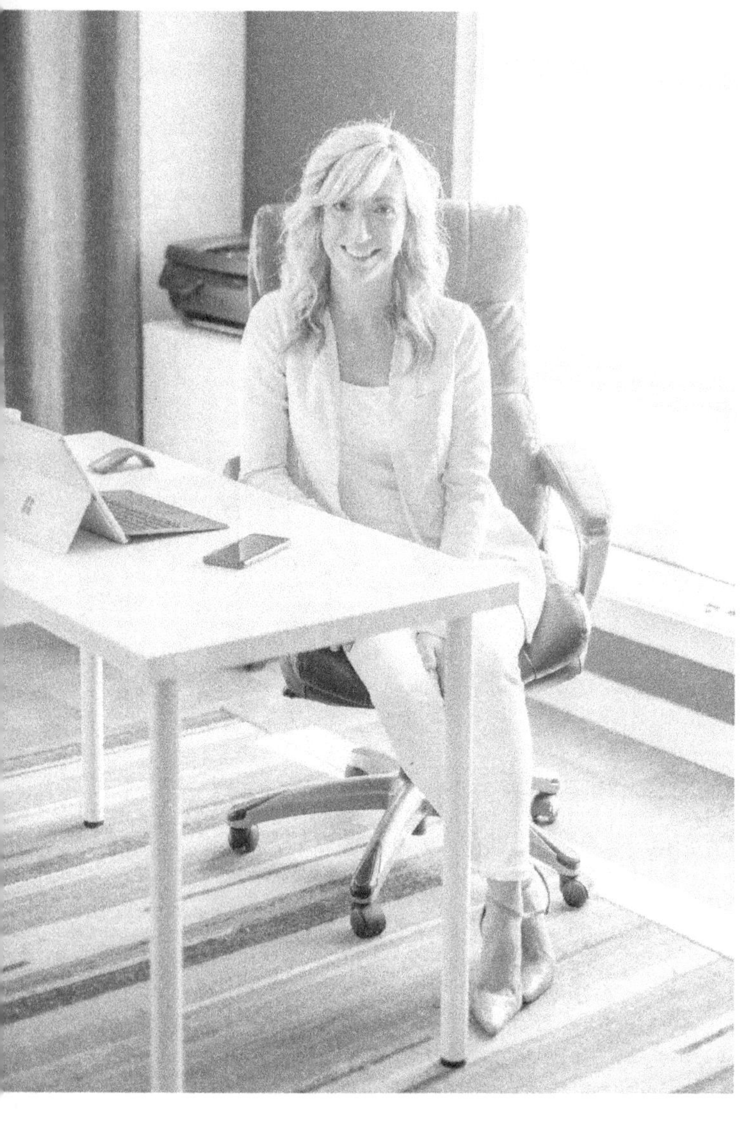

Lynne Roy is the resilient founder of elleRoy Consulting.

Lynne Roy

I've often said I'd write a book about my life. Not only could I fill the pages with stories of setbacks, turmoil, and past relationship traumas, but also stories of overcoming obstacles, healing, and triumph. Perhaps one of the more relevant stories to tell is one of perseverance, determination, and resilience – it is my home-buying journey.

I have struggled financially my entire adult life. From raising my now sixteen-year-old son alone, with little to no financial (or emotional) child support, to paying off post-relationship debt, and then accumulating student debt after going back to school to get my degree in marketing, saving for a down payment was one of the biggest challenges of my life. It took fourteen years of paying off debt, rebuilding credit, and saving every penny I could, to finally qualify for a mortgage on my own. But I did it. Financially, I was ready.

At the time, my mom was in her second round of chemo in her battle with cancer. It was an emotional time for our family, and it hardly felt like the right time to buy a home. Yet something kept pushing me to reach this goal now.
I wasn't really looking to buy a condo, but from the moment I saw it, I knew it was meant for me. My son and I were living in a small, two-bedroom apartment that we had desperately outgrown, and a new place would provide the space we needed to grow and evolve.

Surprisingly, the home buying journey unfolded with little to no challenges or setbacks. I had exactly what I needed right down to the last penny, and with a quick possession date, it was almost too good to be true.

Three weeks after we moved in, my mom lost her battle with cancer; and it was suddenly clear why the universe had guided this process when it did. She needed to know that her middle, rebellious daughter was going to be ok without her.

It was through this perseverance, and her unconditional support, that I finally have a home to call my own – to continue healing and growing into the brave soul I came here to be.

Katie Allan is a fiercely independent engineer and project manager for Kiewit Construction.

Katie Allan

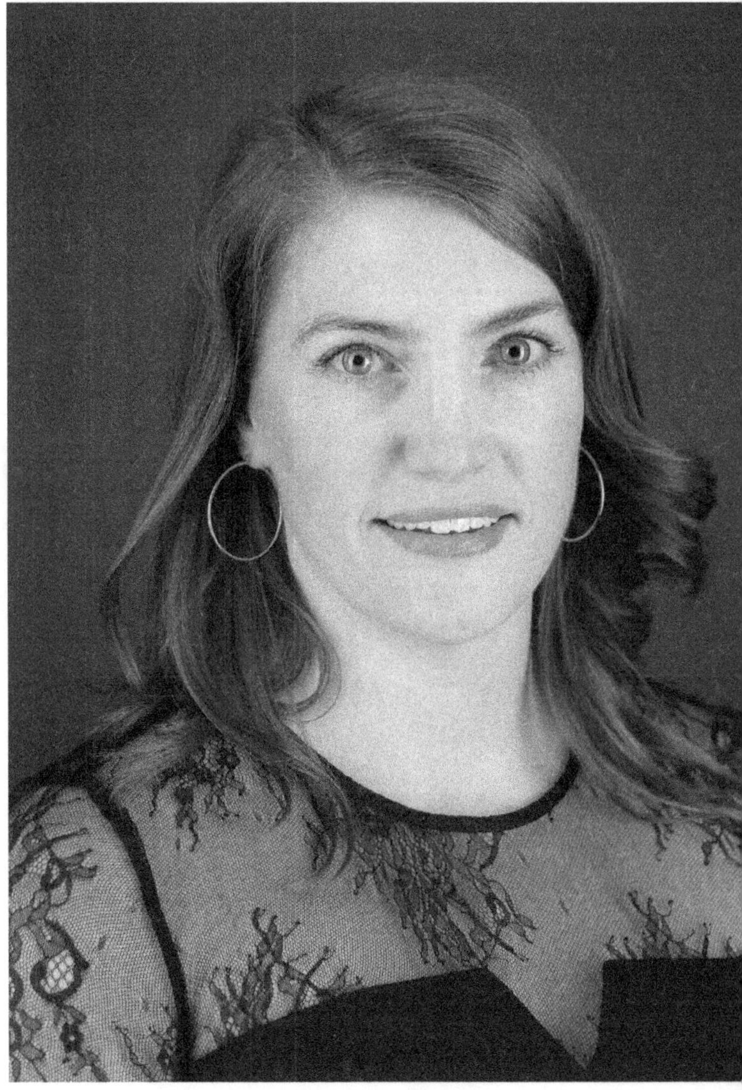

I have always been fiercely independent. In fact, one of my mom's favorite stories is about my first morning at daycare. As she dropped me inside the center, while the rest of the kids were crying for their parents to stay, I put my little hands on her bum and physically pushed her out the door. This independent streak was also demonstrated in my constant need to outperform my older brother, during our youth. It really didn't matter what the topic was - mischief, academics, or sports. I often found myself, along with a few other girls from high school playing soccer against my brother and his teammates. Rest assured, there were no special rules for the girls. We were all just players held to the same standards and rules.

Finding my own path has always been a driving force and choosing an educational path only to find my original plan wasn't for me encouraged me to switch gears. Being resilient, I have always believed my future is in my control.

Completing my engineering degree, while bartending taught me how to prioritize my time. I needed time for fun, school, and work, which didn't always produce stellar results or make me top of my class, but it did allow me to stay afloat and move forward. Finding balance in life allows one to enjoy the journey.

My intense self-determination and skillset led me to the construction industry where I currently work with highly driven achievers who compel me to put forward my best efforts. Construction is demanding yet exhilarating because the outcome of your efforts quickly takes form in outstanding physical accomplishments – a bridge, highway, structure, etc. The complex projects I've worked on, need a whole team to succeed but allow individuals to shine in their areas of expertise and see their individual contributions.

Historically male-dominated, I am currently witnessing the exciting evolution of the construction industry which is becoming more diverse. I am proud to be part of such a dynamic and growing field that is continually adapting and changing.

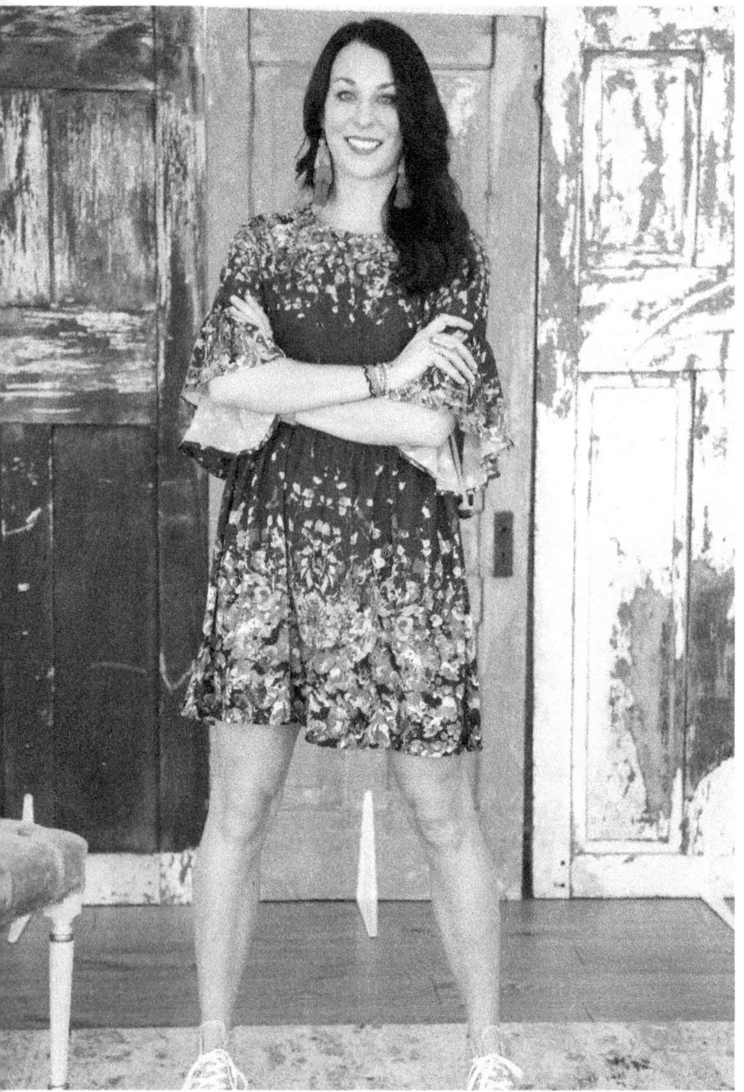
Photo Credit: Greg A. Sager

Sarah Jansel is a creative, fashionable, workaholic whose superpower is her ability to simply get things done. Sarah was a twenty-year corporate veteran, having left her career as a VP of human resources for the e-commerce entrepreneur life, she hasn't looked back since. Sarah is a spirited go-getter who tackles new challenges eagerly.

Sarah Jansel

All my life, I've been incredibly resourceful when it came to overcoming life's hurdles. You may call it "middle child syndrome," but sitting still has never been a part of my life. Some people tell me I should stop and smell the roses. Others say I have too many irons in the fire. None of that resonates with me; I have too much drive to succeed. I love the rush I get when creating something new: a business, a recipe, even redecorating my house. When I'm creating, I'm thriving.

I spent years training for my VP role like an Olympian, but in 2019 I began questioning my path. While laser-focused on my corporate career, suddenly like a Mack truck coming at me, I knew I needed more. Throughout the years I had always kept a foot in creative spaces because, deep down, I knew I had another calling beyond the corporate world. My closet is full of fabulous outfits; I even acted and modelled on the side. I procured a unique collection of jewelry from all over the world. These artistic passions craved to be unleashed, so that same year, I opened an online fashion boutique, Sadi & Sari. Opening the boutique has only been the beginning of getting creative with e-commerce, and it's picking up speed.

In 2020, a shift in our economy presented another opportunity for me; I began showing others how to create online stores to fulfill their e-commerce dreams. My business background, and skills I acquired through launching my own boutique, serve me well and fire me up to help others carve their own paths. Being an entrepreneur was in my blood, and the two keys to my success are resourcefulness and creativity. Not only can I help you successfully bring your own business online – I make sure you look fierce doing it.

Rosie Abigail Smith is a gifted performer and budding entrepreneur, with the perpetual goal to empower those around her.

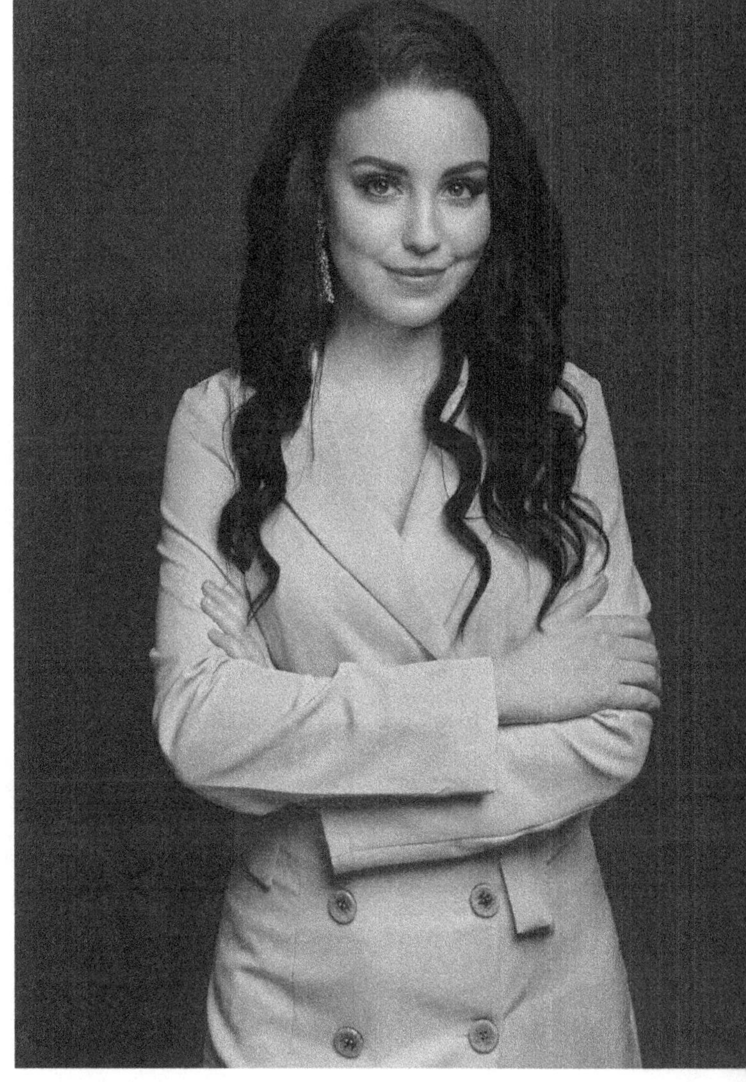

Rosie Abigail Smith

I was both entrepreneurial and very theatrical from a very young age. As a little girl, I would create random "businesses," like making bracelets out of strings and beads, and sell them to my family and friends in the make-belief store of my bedroom closet. I remember keeping a DIY cash register and printing "customer receipts" on my mother's old typewriter. But I was also always an entertainer. I would steal my father's VHS camera and film myself acting in my own "shows" where I would play all of the characters, as I switched wigs and costumes and spoke in different voices.

As years passed, it all made sense when I took a personality test in college and found out I was equally right-brained and left-brained. I felt I had to make a decision as to whether I wanted to pursue my dream of being an entrepreneur or become an actor.

I decided to move to Toronto and chase my goal of having a successful acting career. I knew this was Canada's casting central and was where I would have a real shot at success. Moving to a new city all by myself did not scare me; I never lacked ambition. As time passed, with a lot of excitement, auditions, new relationships, jobs, and challenges, I realized I wanted more. I wasn't going to wait around for auditions while serving tables like the average actor. That is when I decided to dive into my other long-time interest: entrepreneurship.

I launched my e-commerce company, Bion Express, to create a stream of income and enable myself to attend auditions without worrying about a set schedule. For a while, I felt like I was cheating on one dream with the other, consecrating my time and energy on building the operation. It's only after I realized I can be both an artist and a businesswoman that I allowed myself to truly dance between both of my callings.

No one is just one thing. I encourage everyone to explore your talents to live up to your truest potential, and I aspire to see more women in business, cinema, and decision-making positions.

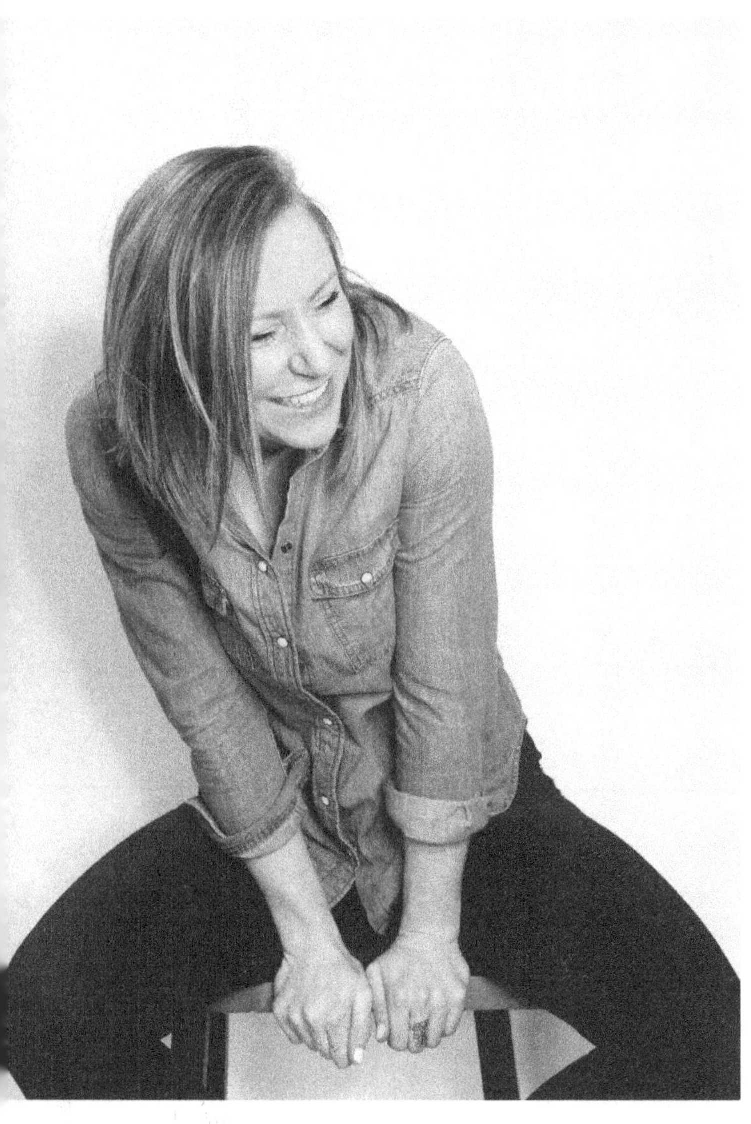

Krystal Gabriel, MBA, is a Professional Integral Coach, Certified Love, Sex & Conscious Relationship Coach, NLP Practitioner, Emotional Intelligence (EQi 2.0) Certified, and is completing her Human Design training.

Krystal Gabriel

Type A. High-Achiever. Ambitious. Alpha. Aries. Go-Getter.

I used to wear these as badges of honor. They got me far: NCAA Division I athlete. MBA top of the class. Award-winning businesswoman. Travelling the world working with some of the most purpose-driven and progressive companies, teams & leaders... everything looked good.

Then, my world stopped at 33. Breast Cancer. I was in shock, but I wasn't completely surprised. I had been speeding past warning signs for a long time, too busy chasing achievement and maintaining the perception that I had it together all the time. Cancer wouldn't let that continue. The diagnosis gave the muzzled parts of myself a megaphone. Turns out they had a lot to say. I hadn't been ready to let go of the superwoman complex and perfectionist tendencies I was certain had led to my success, even if it was killing me. I was hiding from my own truths because facing them meant I had to change some things. Maybe a lot of things.

I had to understand my true motivation for over striving. I had to let go of trying to do everything at the highest level all the time. I had to let myself be human and be helped. While my inner warrior allowed me to face these uncomfortable truths and advocate for myself in my journey, slowing down, trusting, and finding peace in uncertainty largely saved my life. In that, I started to ask myself different questions – What if Superwoman was as dedicated to softness and vulnerability as she was to being a warrior goddess? What if she embodied all parts and knew when to call each one forward? And so, the work of becoming an integrated and fully expressed "soft and solid" woman deepened and continues. Strategy and soul; structure and flow; discipline and play; action and stillness. Neither at the expense of the other. Not anymore.

I still have big goals, ambitions, and dreams - I'm an Aries, an Ox, an Enneagram 3 after all - but I no longer believe I have to sacrifice vital parts of myself to have everything I want. I can lead and love with all of who I am. I can succeed and be healthy, fulfilled, and deeply connected in my relationships.

I believe all women can have this.

Jonica van Rikxoort lives in the beautiful Okanagan with her husband, family, and their velcro pup, Dutchie. Although surrounded by world-renowned wineries, she still prefers a martini! Jonica's hobby is chasing rainbows.

Jonica van Rikxoort

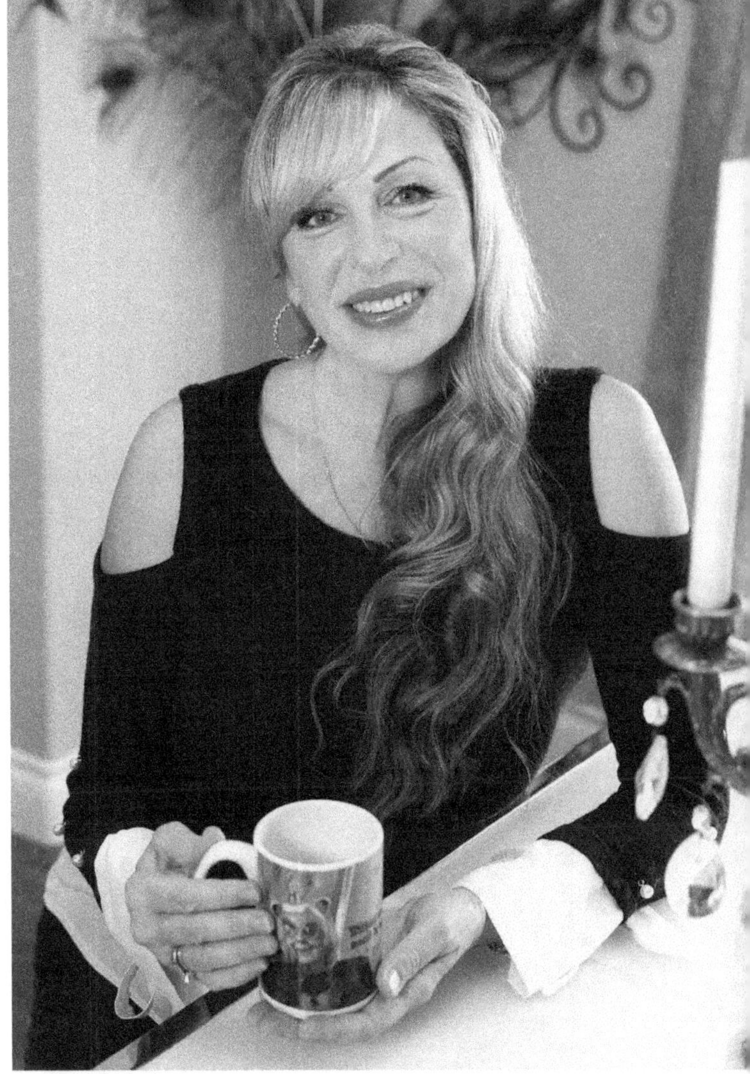

Photo Credit: Douglas Earl Brown

From Playboy Bunny to fashion TV host, I never in a million years thought that at the age of 61, I would be known for publishing a children's book about 'square poo' with my 90-year-old mother, Teri Baker.

In 2009 during a TV interview, I made a promise to help publish one of my mother's many stories to leave behind her legacy, and though I had tried on many occasions to find an agent, the stars did not align. In 2018 Teri was diagnosed with stage four cancer with only three weeks to live, so my husband financed the book, and we became self-published.

With time against us, I stepped up the ante and collaborated with the talented animator/illustrator Izabela Byzmek. Though not exactly the most enjoyable conditions, we ploughed through. If I'm to be blatantly honest I was never much into poetry, but here I was the co-author creating our first children's book, 'What if Bunny Poo was Square?'.

If you believe in miracles, I can tell you that God was on our side. With the aid of medicinal cannabis, we were granted 20 months. During that time, we had an amazing whirlwind of adventures from photoshoots, and book signings to television interviews. Where Teri would normally say no to the limelight, she agreed to absolutely any suggestion. Those times together were beyond the most precious, and I will cherish them forever.

My mom's legacy will live on through her family and those who knew her! She had a passion for life and all creatures big and small, not leaving out the unicorns! She was truly magical and one of a kind.

We grew up on Mom's theory that even on a rainy day we'd see a rainbow. So now, whenever we see one in any shape or form, we know she is sending us her love! So, if you were wondering why I chase rainbows, that would be why!

Quote: Without unicorns, there would be no magic!
~ Teri Baker ~

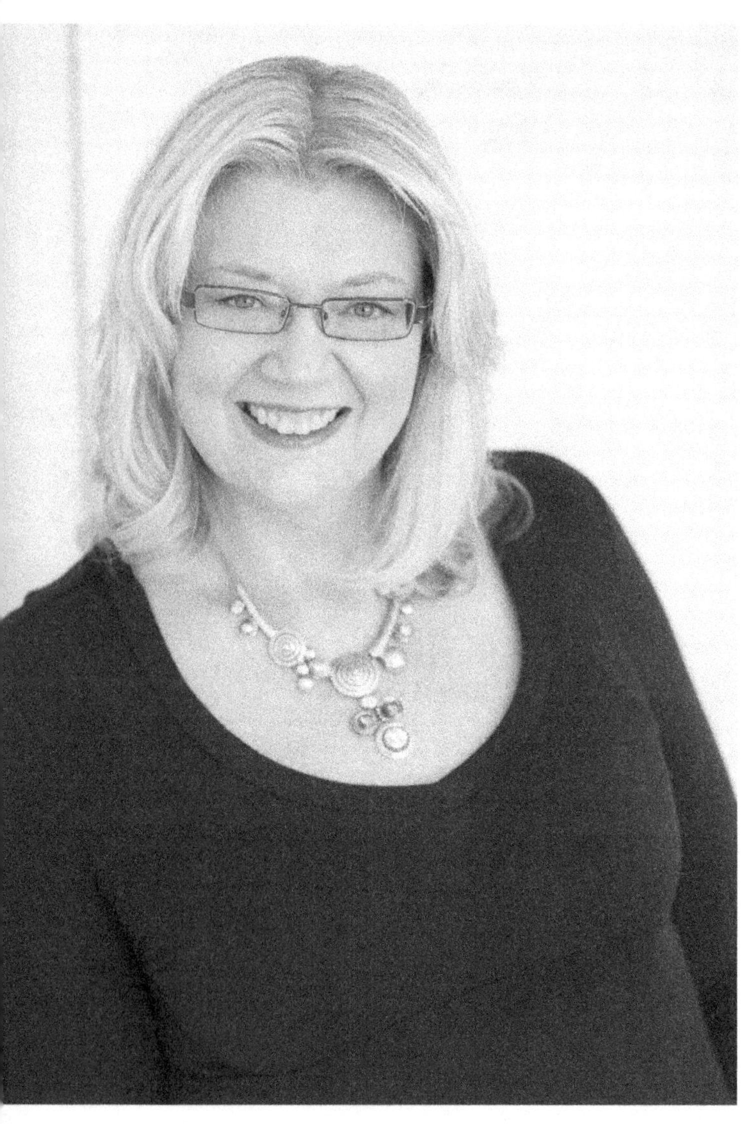

Alyson Jones is a therapist, educator, writer, speaker, and business owner.

Alyson Jones

"You cannot be both perfect and fabulous – so I always chose fabulous!" - Alyson Jones

Welcome to my page. I am Alyson Jones, and I am thrilled to be a part of Pursuit:365. I am President and Clinical Director of Alyson Jones & Associates, a large counselling centre with several exceptional counsellors who are reframing mental health services to be more accessible, practical, and resource-based.

I have developed the MORE philosophy for living, in which I celebrate exceptionalism, not perfectionism, and I want to share a little about that with you on this page. This philosophy has benefited my clients, my associates, my family, and myself. Basically, we are talking about a methodology I have developed for living in the moment, that I use in my own life, and to guide my clients. No matter what situation is in front of me, I run through my list of core words, "Movement, Opportunity, Reality, and Exception." First, I look for circumstances or challenges that need to move; second, I assess the opportunities in front of me; third, I observe the reality of the situation; and fourth, I commit to a path where the first three factors can lead to something exceptional.

An exceptional life is a choice we make. It is important to understand that an exceptional life has nothing to do with perfecting your life. An exceptional life can be highly imperfect. In fact, it must be imperfect. We must choose to be imperfect, and allow the learning that imperfection brings. To accomplish an exceptional life, we need to let go of perfectionism. Why? Because it is getting in your way, and if you take a perfectionistic path, you will never become fabulous! The two cannot exist together.

Perfectionism is the arch-enemy of an exceptional life. Perfectionism can never be accomplished, as perfect does not exist. Perfectionism is the antithesis of the MORE philosophy, as there is no reality in it. It only discourages us and makes us feel small and inadequate. Unlike the frustrating path of perfectionism, the path of exceptionalism is achievable and real. Being fabulous is all about MORE and it leaves room for us to celebrate our quirks, learn from our mistakes, unleash our creativity, experience joy, and find meaning while being present in our exceptional lives.

Dr. Allison Patton, ND is a West Coast mother, Naturopathic Physician, and Politician.

Dr. Allison Patton BSc., MBA, ND

*Services of naturopathic medicine provided by a health profession corp.; Ardour Wellness Inc.

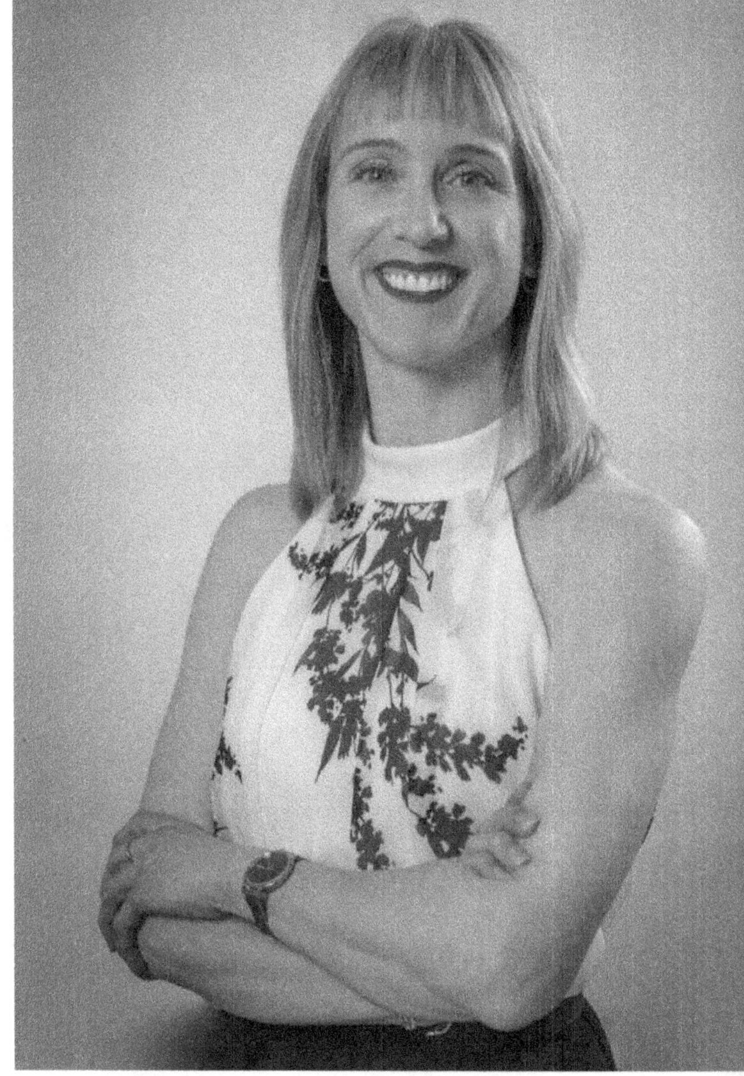

I am a high achieving, high energy, loving, creative woman who thrives on collaboration and challenge and who enjoys being a naturopathic physician, a mother, and a politician.

I have discovered over time that I experience deep meaning and purpose in my life when I find myself on the other side of an achievement that, at first, I utterly feared.

For me, living equates to helping. My best self comes forth when I can be there for others and do things to make them feel better.

As a healer, I need to work very hard on my own personal growth. I am only able to help to the level I have evolved. To follow the challenging path of personal growth is an honor and privilege that allows me to be a more compassionate and caring naturopathic physician.

Leadership, at its core, is about helping and serving others today and imagining a new way forward tomorrow. As I work through the challenges of proactive personal growth, I have noticed that my methods of demonstrating my style of leadership often seem unorthodox and chaotic as opposed to organized and calm. During the most chaotic of these times of transformation, I try to practice self-love and self-care, and if I cannot, I reach out to my small, trusted circle and ask for help.

Currently, I have the immense pleasure to participate in life as a mother to an energetic, intelligent, and deep-hearted athlete and daughter. I am a Naturopathic Physician in my new modern centre of excellence in naturopathic medicine, Ardour Wellness, which means the passion of life. I also serve as a Councillor elected in the City of Surrey.

At the end of my days, if I can reflect that I have loved courageously, that I said yes to helping others, that I contributed to my community, that I healed wherever I could, and that I took as many opportunities as possible to jump into the abyss and shine, then I will deem that I have lived my life on my terms, and I will be at a place of deep peace and gratitude.

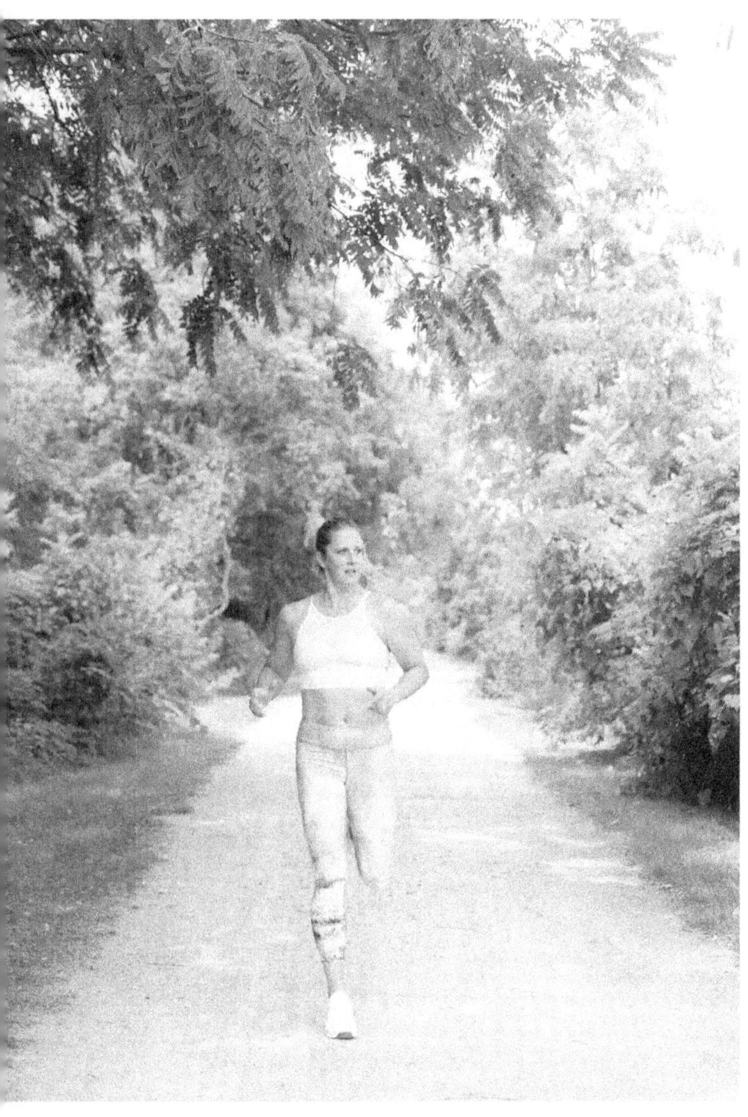

Moni is a respected athlete and sought-after performance and fat loss specialist who works with busy, active women over forty to help them lose hormonal inches and reconnect with who they really are.

Monika Tupholme

There have been many times in my life when I've felt as though I've lost myself...
Having kids at thirty-eight and forty-one, the reality is, the majority of my life I spent only having to take care of one person: me. My focus was on what I was **doing** (playing professional volleyball), where I was **going** (travelling everywhere), and who I was **being** (trying to figure out who I was without athletics).
I'm a competitive work-horse by nature.

I learned early on that failure was a part of success - you can't have one without the other. Every time I failed, I would mourn, dust myself off, learn, and get back at it. Then family life came, and failure took on a new meaning - it wasn't just about me any longer. Unconsciously I keep myself in a "safe" place. If all my thoughts, emotions, and efforts go towards my family, then we will be ok. They will be safe and happy, and so would I, right?

Wrong. In the process of feeding that control, **I lost myself.** My goals and dreams no longer took center stage. I didn't know how to make myself a priority anymore in a way that didn't make me feel guilty.
That competitive, single girl that loved a challenge, growth, and running ~~naked~~ free was still there but was afraid to come out. I missed my old self - like missing the university friend that used to make you belly laugh so hard that you wee a little.

Then it happened. Someone asked me the simple-yet-not-so-simple question: **"what makes you happy, Moni?"**

I tell myself; the answer may not come overnight, but it is a first step.
Now it's just time to get in the driver's seat and go. The destination is not the cheesy find yourself diner, but rather the beautiful hills of Tuscany, where you truly feel connected and confident with yourself and what you are still capable of physically, mentally, and spiritually for decades to come.
And don't worry, there will be a great bottle of wine open when you get there.

Dr. Allana Polo is a Naturopathic Doctor, business owner, and mom of two young boys.

Dr. Allana Polo

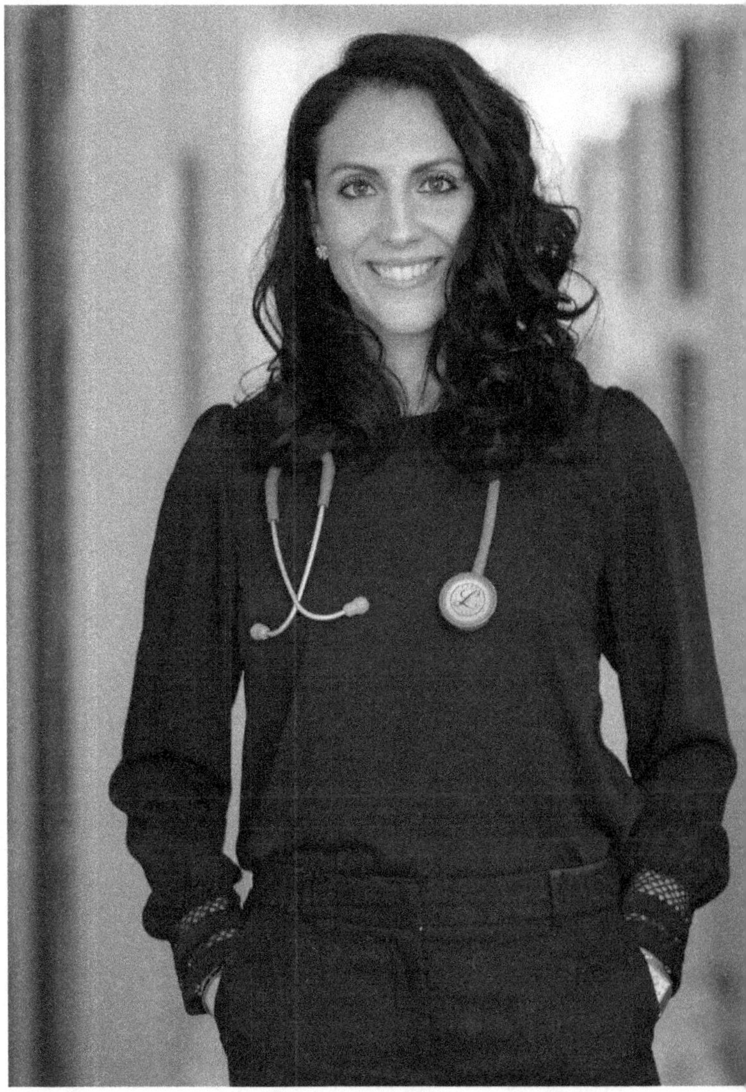

Women are burning out. Recent stats confirm, that 52% of us are burning out from the weight of household responsibilities alone. Combining the mental stress of home with the stress of work, no wonder women are at risk for burnout. Burnout has become so 'commonplace' that it has now been classified as an official medical diagnosis by the World Health Organization. Most professionals and parents alike, have felt it; exhaustion, lack of focus, apathy, chronic stress, and a lack of pleasure from things that used to ignite.

I've definitely been there, haven't we all? We live in a society where being burned out is a badge of honor. We have endless to-do lists and plates piling up. The irony; everything put on our plate was put there by us.

As a Naturopathic Doctor, business owner, and mom of two, I know burnout well. I work primarily with female leaders, busy moms, entrepreneurs, and professionals. I witness burnout on the daily. I see chronic and deep fatigue. I see how this manifests as physical symptoms and imbalances.

Women who are emotional, yet the rock. Tired, but keep going. Worried, but full of hope. Patient, but impatient. Overwhelmed but never quit. The women who think something is wrong with them because they are so tired. A voice telling them they need to "work harder."

Until, that powerful raw, and real moment, where I can look in their eyes and gently say, "you're just burned out." That sense of relief, to hear that kind of validation, that nothing was wrong with them. That they were in fact strong enough. They had the ability to handle what they could, but not the capacity for more.

In a society where we want to do more, we have to do less. How can we support our bodies to be the strong, powerful, resilient women we are? No amount of supplement, pill bottle, or diet plan is going to help with that. It comes from a place of putting yourself first, your oxygen mask on first. You can't show up for someone else, if you haven't shown up for yourself, fully, and unapologetically.

So, this is your sign. Know you have the power to say no to what doesn't serve you. Less shoulds. Less to-do's, more ta-da's. More meaningful and purposeful connections. More water, less coffee.

The beautiful thing, most beautiful of all, is that burnout is reversible.

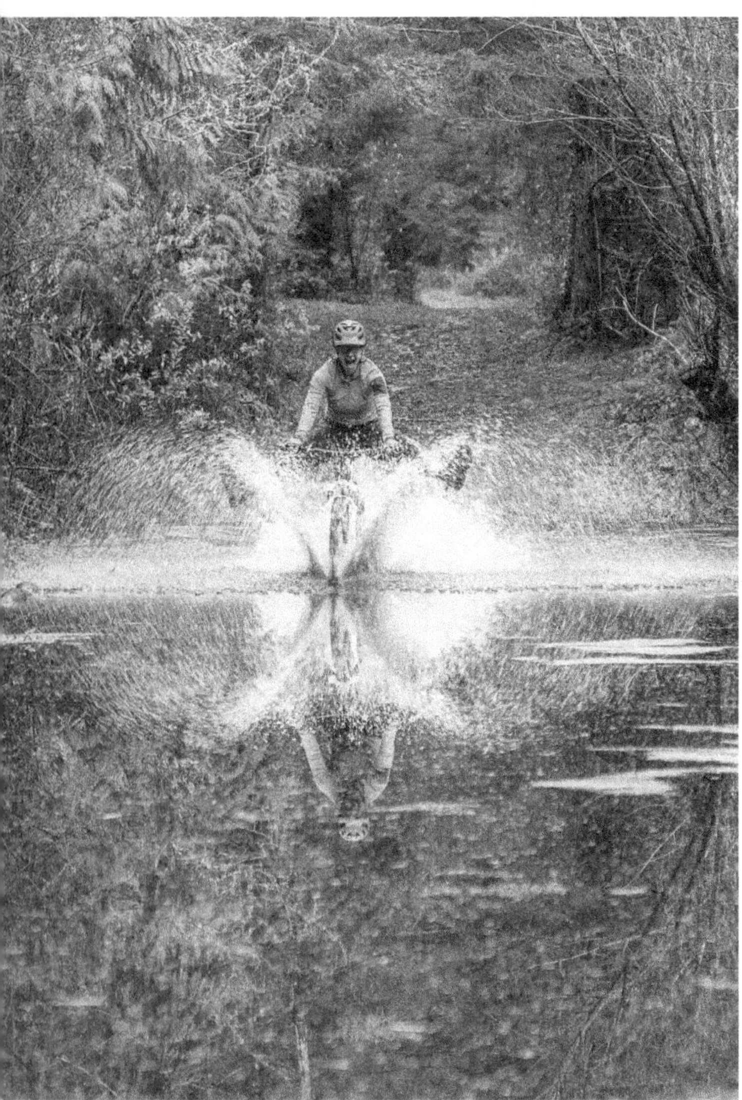

Photo Credit: Linda Mackie Creative

Carmel Ecker is a life coach and the creator of Single Parenting Made Simple, a coaching process and community designed to help single parents rise above their challenges to write a new, more empowering story for their future.

Carmel Ecker

I didn't think I could do it.

A 350-kilometre, seven-day mountain biking stage race on some of the best trails in southwest B.C.

It seemed crazy and impossible that I would ever be fit enough to do it. But somewhere between when the first racers dared to place their knobby tires on the start line and the race's eighth year, I started to think it could be within my reach. This made no sense. I was a single mom with a three-year-old son by that point. I was mountain biking once a week at best. The odds of me finding time to train — beyond my daily bike commute — were slim, and the race fee would eat up my entire vacation budget. And yet, not far from the finish line of that eighth race, in Whistler's Olympic Plaza, two girlfriends and I giddily typed our credit card numbers into a laptop in the back of a white cube van. Among the first ten people to sign up for a 600-person race that sells out every year, we celebrated our collective insanity.

I had no idea how I was going to make this happen, but I'd committed about $2,000 to this adventure, so I was damn well going to find a way. I'd worry about logistics—childcare, transportation, training—later. I'd just told myself, "Yes, I can!" and come hell or high water, yes, I would. I would fight through injury, 40-degree heat, 6-hour days in the saddle, chafing, and long segments alone in the forest to become one of 531 people from 33 countries who finished that year's race.

I was proud of myself. I'd lived my belief that when you step outside your comfort zone, you grow to meet the challenge. And I'm told I inspired others to do the race the next year.

Since then, whenever I doubt my abilities, wondering if I have what it takes, I remember the "impossible" race and change the story.

Jessica September Buchanan is a Canadian independent perfumer based in France.

Jessica Buchanan

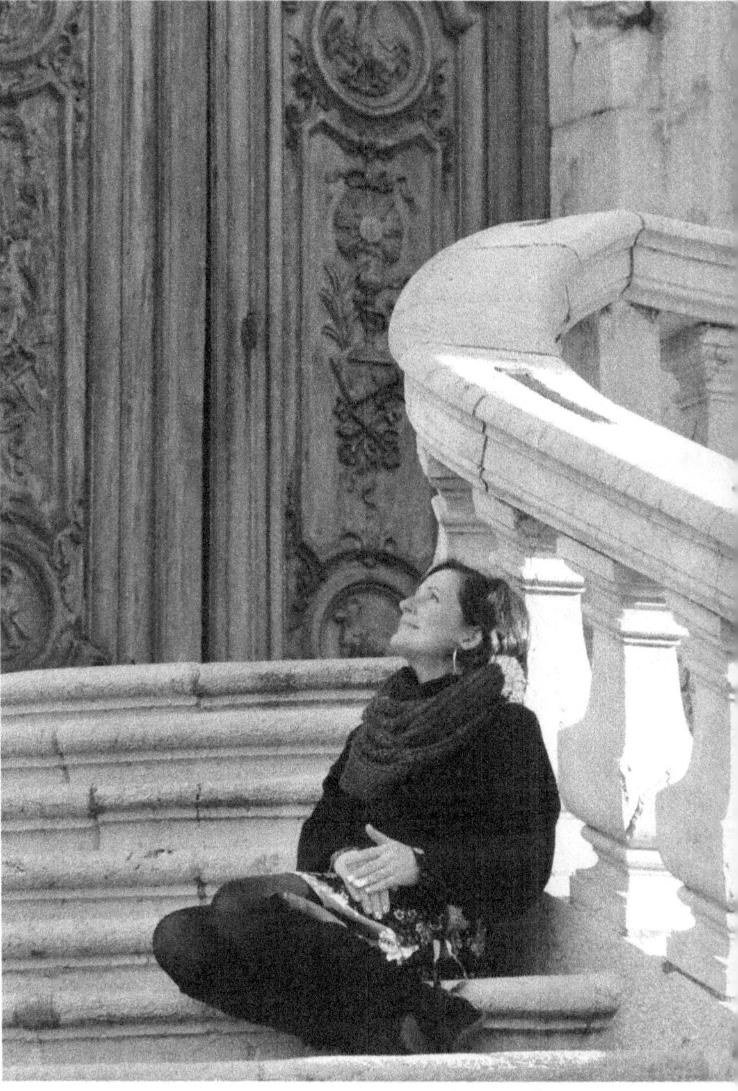

Since a young age, I have often felt like I didn't quite fit in. Maybe because I grew up in rural Canada, homeschooled until grade nine, close to nature, but apart from society. I wonder sometimes if this made it easier to move alone to a foreign country where I didn't speak the language and end up staying- a place where I could feel comfortable and valued for being different.

That January day that I lugged my suitcases into a tiny Parisian boutique hotel room and sat down on the tiny bed after selling my house, and travelling to France to attend perfumery school, I thought; I might as well be on Mars for all the context this has right now.

People say I am courageous, but I don't always feel that way. I have always put one foot in front of the other, sometimes anguishing over decisions; to stay in France or not, to open a boutique in the old city or not, to continue my life on the path less travelled, or not. And yet, thirteen challenging years later, I am still in France and have learned to cultivate happiness over time. I have learned to tell myself - and believe - that I am amazing, courageous, talented, and endlessly creative. Even when the well runs dry sometimes, with that infamous "writers' block," or when I am feeling like a failure. When I am terrified that the spring has run dry and I will never create again, or even survive another day, I find a source even deeper and find a new vein of energy, of beauty. I have learned to be frugal in trusting others and to always listen to myself first, because at our source, only we know best and have our own best interest at heart.

I have learned to make friends with that inner voice, the good one, the calm one that tells me true and honest things, and to weed out the other ones that push me to do impulsive and destructive things that usually lead to bad decisions. Also, and maybe most importantly, I have learned that things can't be rushed, that they happen exactly when they are supposed to.

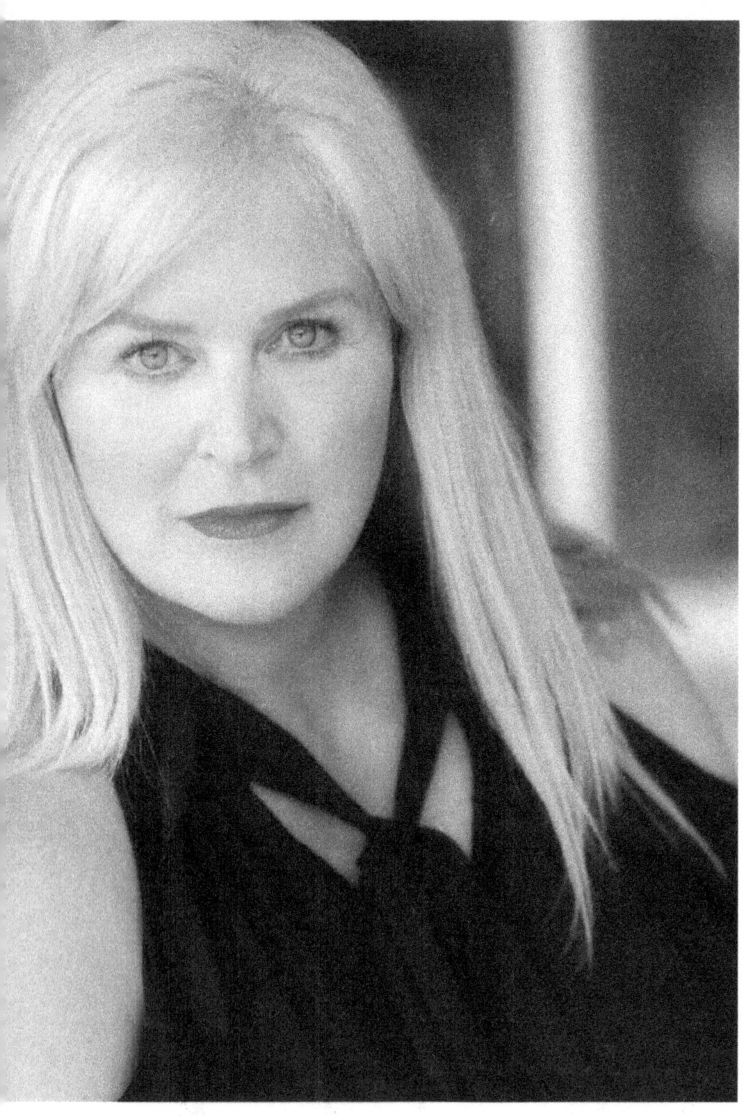

Jacqueline Fowler is an academic, a mover, a mother, and a thriver. A newly budding yoga teacher, she is a physician that retired early due to spinal injuries and has found her light and joy while moving through loss and pain.

Jacqueline Fowler

When I cast my mind's eye back on the woman I was ten years ago, there is almost no recognition. I was a healthy mother of two with a busy medical practice. My interests and activities were wide and varied. I loved mountain biking, snowboarding, surfing, and pretty much anything associated with an adrenaline rush. You name it, I tried it.

My life changed forever - twice. Once in 2012 and again in 2015, both at the hands of inattentive drivers. In those moments, that person I had been was altered in almost every way. Physically, I was changed. I struggled to sit up, lie down, stand, or make myself comfortable. Mentally I struggled with memory and fogginess. Emotionally, I was depressed and frustrated. Finally, after years of painful immobility and following two rounds of neurosurgery, my physical condition is improved. I lost the ability to practice medicine, and with it came crushing grief. I grappled with the concept of "if I am not a doctor, then who am I?" I had trained for many years and worked so hard so that I could serve people.

I decided to find joy in the uncertainty. I had my self, and that's all I really needed. So, after the long recovery, I began to rebuild my life anew. The landscape of this new life is different, but it is equally as beautiful. It's just different. Change is inherent in all things and embracing the impermanence of things allowed me to be present in my life now.

Today I am taking a new path. A yogic path. A route that I never thought I would be travelling. I am now a slightly dented mother of two with a busy study in the practice of yoga and a passion for supporting mental health and resiliency. I love road biking, snowshoeing, and snorkelling - anything not associated with an adrenaline rush. I am still me. That white light. The one permanence in a world full of evolution. I feel joy in what is now, and I'm grateful for it.

Michelle Chapin is the passionate and energetic founder and SHE-EO at Campy Home.

Michelle Chapin

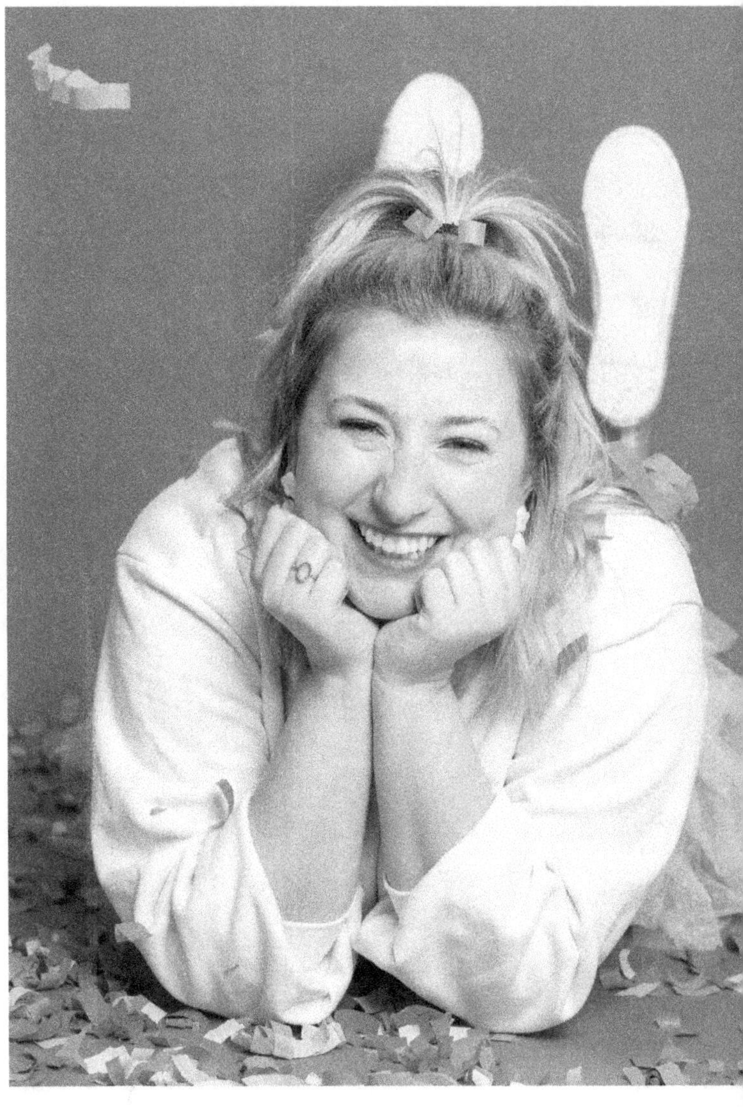

As a little girl, I always knew I would grow up to be my own boss one day. Flash forward twenty years, with lots of trials, tribulations, and tears. The road to owning my own company, Campy Home, was a bumpy but entirely necessary journey. Through all the tough times, the moments of asking myself "what am I doing?", stepping out of my comfort zone, and taking risks, I helped myself to gain the confidence and drive to run my own company, on my terms, with my vision in mind.

When I purchased Campy Home a few years back, I struggled with imposter syndrome. It was my first time investing a lot of money into my own business, I was new to the world of candle making, and I had this company that didn't feel like me. I felt lost and way in over my head. I made it through my first year of business and made big goals to really make this company my own. The past year has been all about injecting myself into my brand and recreating something I could be proud of. With the help of Ruby & Parcel Co, I have completely rebranded Campy into a fun, cheerful, and energetic brand, just like myself!

Campy has been able to do a lot in a year. We've donated to various charities such as Dress for Success, Rainbow Railroad, and Interval House of Ottawa. We've created over seven new products that have been a huge hit. We're finally owning our social media game and establishing an engaging presence online. It's been a big year for us, and I think the coming year will prove to be even better.

Oftentimes I've found the recurring message in life is that we go to our job every day, and it doesn't matter if we like it or not. It's a part of life, we must do it. I refuse to accept that for myself. I believe that we all deserve to work at a job that we love. A job that ignites our passions and makes us feel fulfilled. Find what you love and run with it.

Xo, Michelle

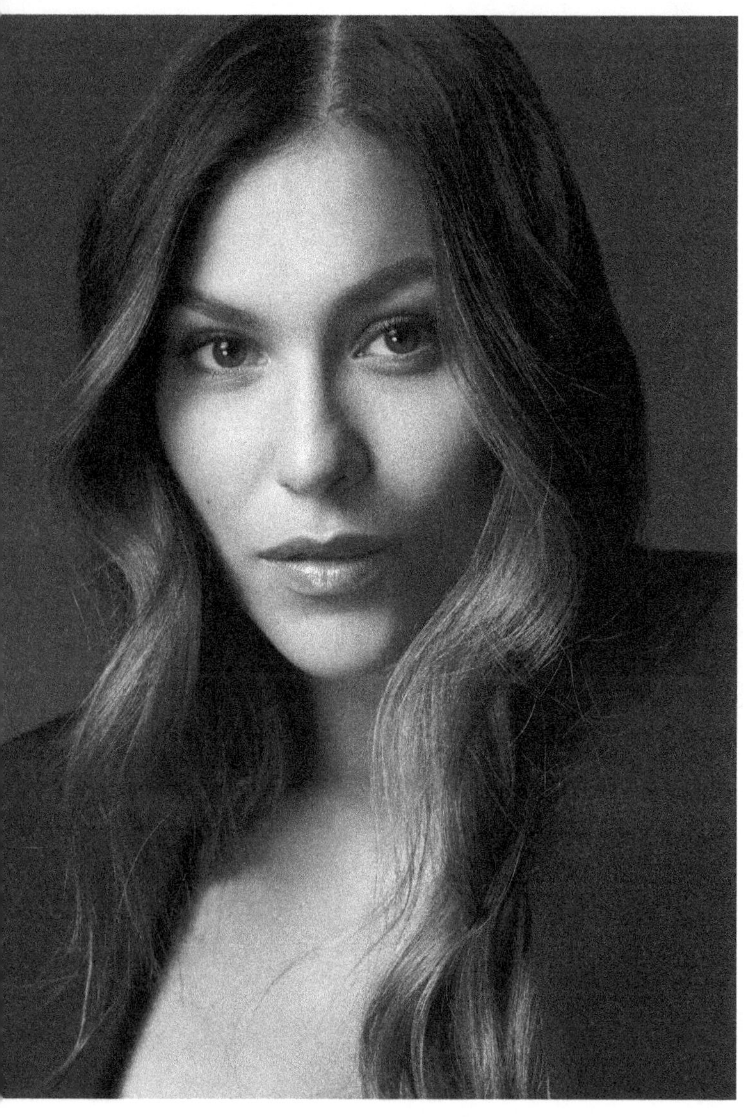

Working in film, television and fashion for over a decade, Michaella Shannon's mission is to change how Indigenous Womxn are portrayed in the media.

Michaella Shannon

I have learned that the key to success is transparency and if I am being honest, I am having a really difficult time writing just one vulnerable and authentic story in 365 words about myself. As an Indigenous woman, when I am called to these spaces, I feel like there is pressure and responsibility to say so much.

I have been walking in both worlds my entire life. Sometimes I am too "white" for my Indigenous community and sometimes I am too "native" for my non-Indigenous community. I see, feel and understand both sides of the "spectrum." On the surface, you will see a TV host and personality, a model, an actress, a writer, a facilitator, a student, and a mental health support worker.

But if you were to take all of that away, you would see a Nehiyaw (Plains Cree), Lakota, and Irish woman who has taken it upon herself to overcome bullying, racism, discrimination, sexual abuse, domestic abuse, depression, anxiety, PTSD, oppression, and trauma.

Most people see "success," but those titles are just words from a colonial framework. And regardless of these successes, I am 3.5 times more likely to go missing or to be murdered for being an Indigenous woman. At twenty-five years old, I have already experienced two attempted kidnappings. As I try to make it in these mainstream industries of the dominant society, I have taken it upon myself to break cycles, break stigmas, and break barriers. Indigenous people may carry intergenerational trauma, but we also carry intergenerational knowledge.

I was asked to share something vulnerable, but to be honest, I am trying to change the way Indigenous women are portrayed in the media. We are often portrayed as weak, vulnerable individuals due to the media around MMIW and it has been my goal to flip that narrative.

I've turned many negatives into positives. I walk in both worlds, so I must do the work in both worlds. I'm doing the work in my community to help others overcome the oppression, racism, and intergenerational trauma that still exists today. And I am fighting to make it in these mainstream spaces, so that young Indigenous girls and boys feel like they matter, belong, and are valued.

Vancouver-based abstract painter, Donna Giraud, is an internationally collected artist. She creates paintings that will make your other walls jealous and is an eternal optimist, an ambassador of kindness, and a painter of positivity.

Donna Giraud

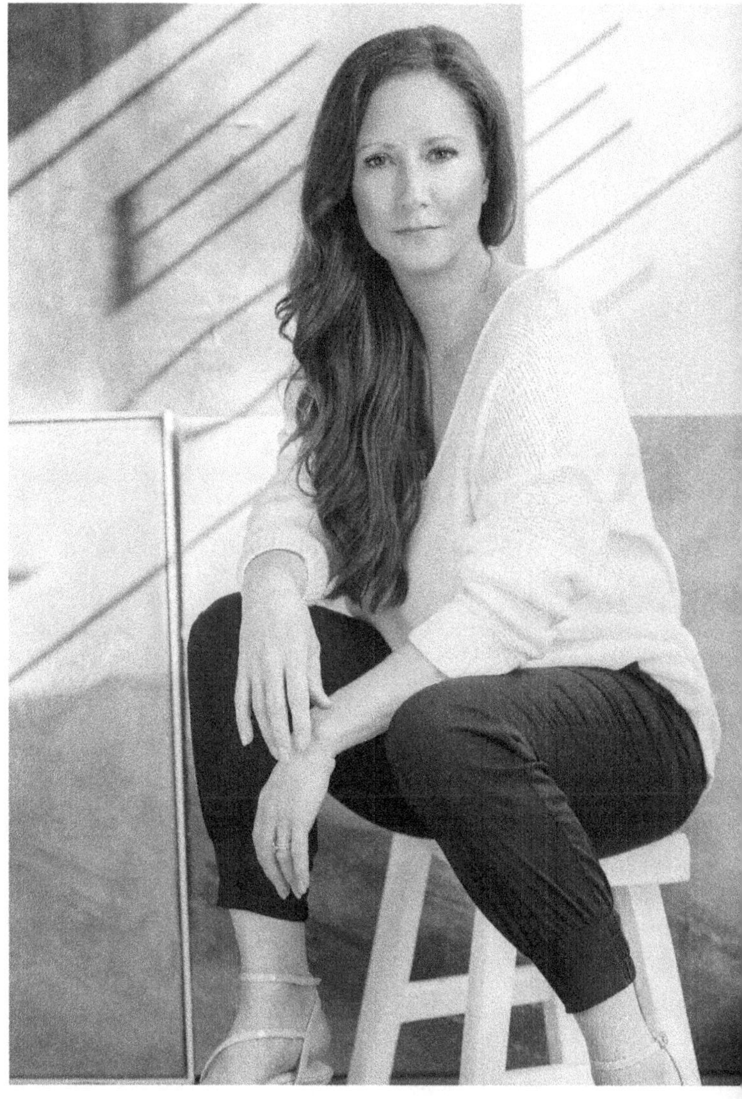

I am that person who knows the entire life story of my Uber driver before the end of my ride. I am that person who says hello to every human and dog I pass on my early morning walks, and I am definitely that person that isn't afraid to mentor and share all of my knowledge because I am confident there is room for all of us to succeed.

I can thank my dad for my unwavering gift of the gab and relentless energy. I grew up seeing the power of treating everyone with respect and how a conversation with a stranger can be both silly and full of connection at the same time. I learned that fostering relationships is the backbone of a fulfilling life, and that I was capable of leaving a highly respectable and honoured career as a Head Nurse to discover the voice of my then passion, now career, as a painter.

Being an artist is hard. Not very many of us can say we make a living out of the art we create. With this career choice comes an enormous amount of competition, constant rejection, and the many societal opinions.

I believe, now more than ever, that people need a reminder that goodness still exists. Over the years, I discovered I could tell stories through texture, where there is a world thriving because of love, hope, and togetherness. I figured out how my paintings could create visceral emotions and challenged people to reimagine a future free of chaos and destruction, a time when we could pause and reconnect.

Whether it is with a piece of art or with my actions and words - to positively change the trajectory of someone's day is my ultimate goal. As I reflect on the journey my artistic path has taken me, I can confidently say the combination of tenacity, kindness, and optimism has been the secret to my success.

My hope is that the next time you find yourself passing a stranger on the street, you look up and simply just smile. I am almost certain it will change the trajectory of both of your days.

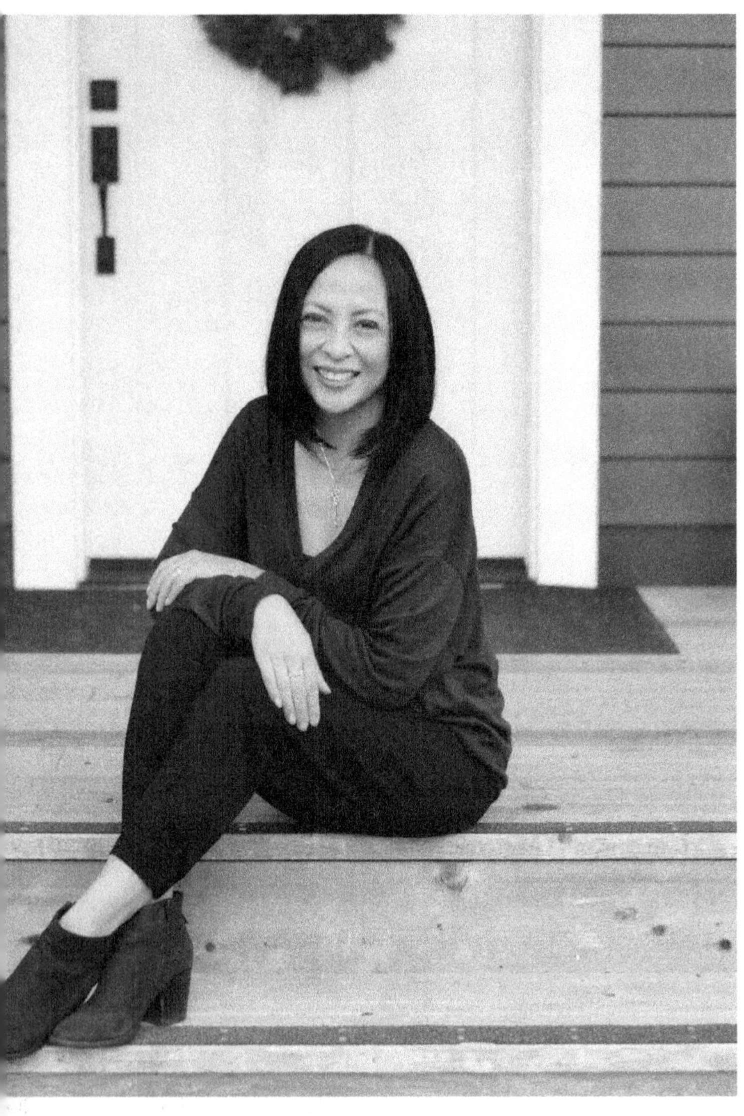

Adina Neufeld is an advocate of clean beauty, a Discover Your Sacred Gifts™ Guide, a recovering perfectionist, and joyfully obsessed with appreciation practices.

Adina Neufeld

There is no behind.

If I had a magic wand, I'd use it to share that message with my young self. It would've saved me a bunch of misery. Mind you, I've always been stubborn, and I likely wouldn't have listened.

I wish I could say there was one defining moment in which I got it all together. It could've happened in the aftermath of the destruction of my childhood family unit, the death of my mother, health issues, or a robbery in my home. The truth of the matter is, there was a series of moments, both dramatic and subtle, that brought me to the feelings of success I enjoy today.

Let's rewind. From the start, I received the message that I was behind, and somewhere along the way, it became the lens through which I saw the world. As a child, I was told I was behind in elementary school; behind in developing as a teen; behind in getting a degree; behind in landing my ideal dream corporate job; in having babies, in having babies that could do all the things according to a certain schedule, behind in hitting "good motherhood ideals"; behind in re-entering the workforce, becoming an entrepreneur and in reaching the top level of my company.

Can you see the pattern?

The funny thing is I couldn't see it... until suddenly I did.

Abandoning the long-held belief that there is such a thing as behind and that I was in that category, was cathartic. It's allowed me to better appreciate the wonders of life and feel true satisfaction. Redefining "success" and focussing on intentionally feeling joy and gratitude on a regular basis brings more ease and external success. It's manifestation in progress. And it's ongoing.

So, if you've ever felt behind, let me tell you - You are doing great. Wherever you are on your journey, you are not behind. Your road may not look like anyone else's. It's supposed to be different. Keep going and remember to appreciate the little things along the way.

Kim Drury is a mother, daughter, and sister, who instinctively took on the role of anchor when her family needed it most.

Kim Drury

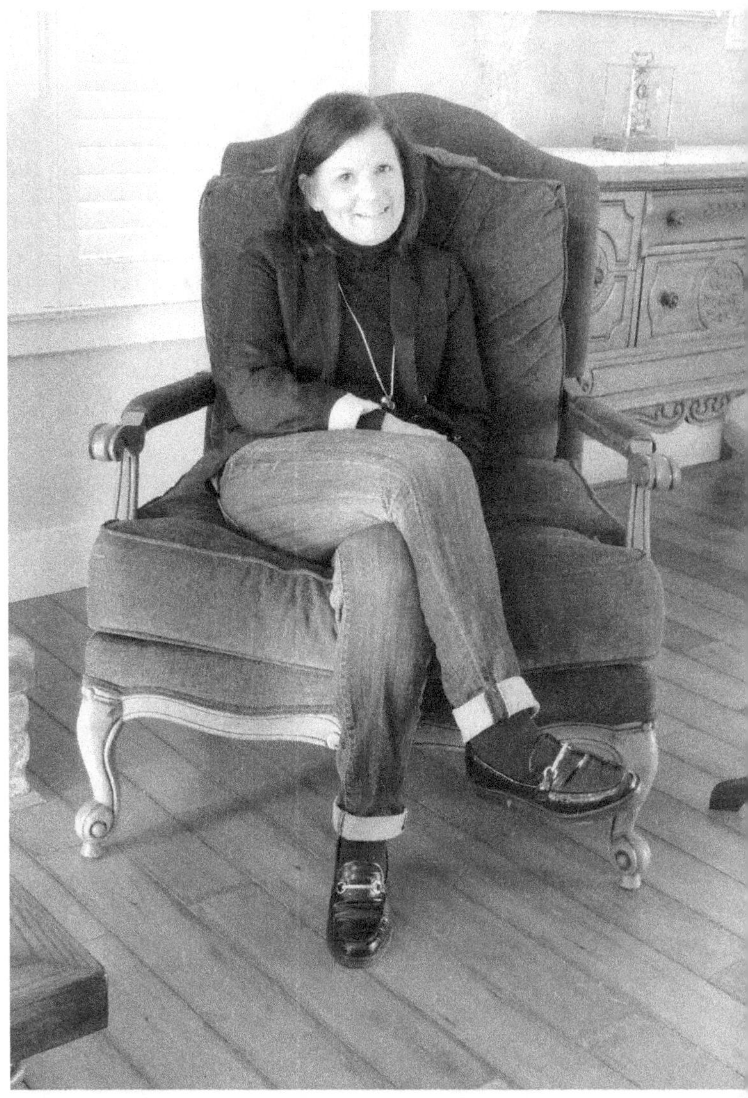

A retired professional hockey player. A gay son. Small-town Ontario, 1970's. My dad was 34, retired and unemployed in 1976. Alcohol began to be a daily habit, then, a lifelong medication. My Mom tried to hide the battle zone we were living in, my brother struggled with who he was, and I was trying to stay out of everyone's way.

Being the anchor really isn't something you choose, it evolves. Bob was my first and only friend for a long time. In late September, starting at yet another new school, we stood waiting for the bus. I was eight, heading into third grade, my older and much more confident brother was heading into fifth grade.

Right there at the bus stop, Bob eyed up a set of twins. They appeared to be about his age. He said, "hey" the boys came over. It was that easy. He never forgot about me, "This is my sister.' he said. I smiled.

My parents tried to adapt to a new way of life, a young family, no money. They couldn't seem to rally to my brother's needs. The support wasn't there for them or him. It fell to me, or I took it on, I'm not really sure which is true. I answered every call, day or night. My brother's struggle raged for over 20 years and finally came to an end with an accidental overdose. My parents crumbled. It was me collecting his effects, arranging the service, making the phone calls.

Our family unit carried on. Loss affects people differently. My Mom became quieter, an emotional stone. My Dad became more tolerant and open to people's differences. I continued to love them and learn that they were once younger parents trying to learn the ropes. Once I realized that they were like me, I accepted their failures and celebrated their successes. They became the epitome of Grandparents.

During my Dad's brief illness, my Mom couldn't cope and again, everything was on me. As soon as he passed it was her turn to slide. When I reflect on becoming the anchor, whether it fell to me or whether I choose to grab it, I'm thankful for the honour.

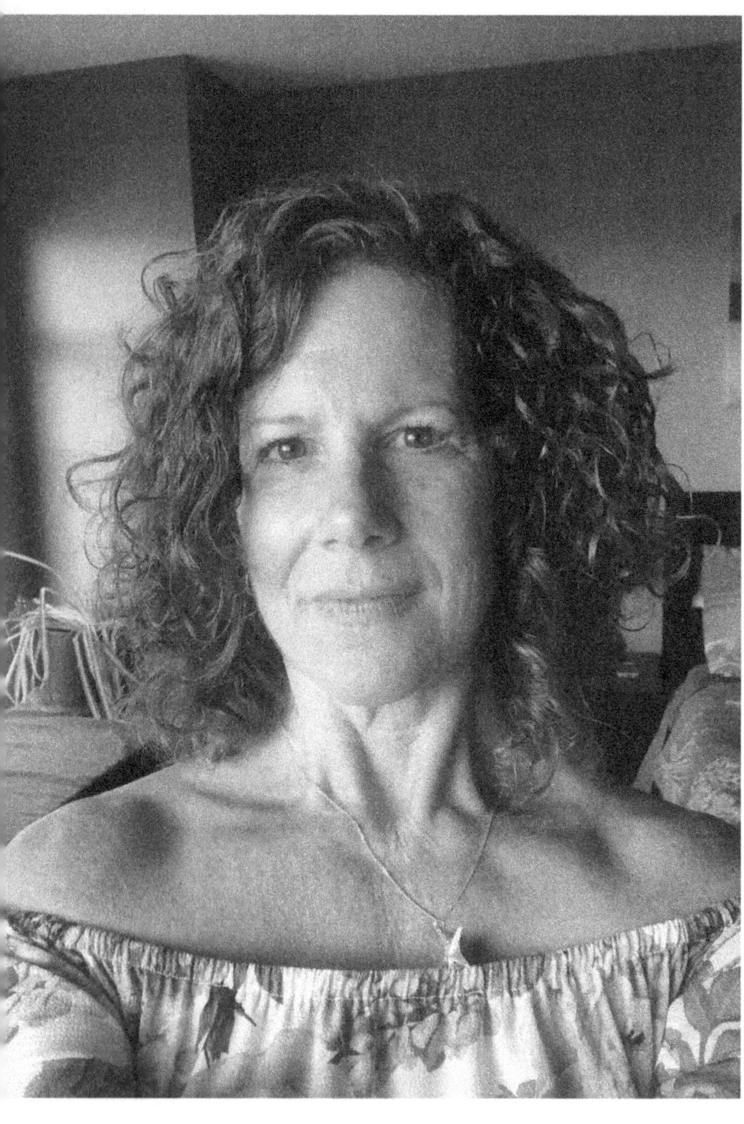

Siobhan Coates is a Stand-Up Comedian, A Storyteller, A Speaker, and a Life Coach, who has a message for her 12-year-old self.

Siobhan Coates

Dear 12-Year-Old Self,

What I want you to know is that the next few years are going to be tough, but you will get through it.
What I want you to know is that the bullying will be endless, and you will not feel safe at school or home for the next 7 years.
What I want you to know is that you are not going crazy. You feel alone and lonely, but all that writing and play-acting you are doing in your room will pay off.
What I want you to know is that you are not going through this in vain.
What I want you to know is that it may take me a few years to find your voice and your talent and embrace it, but once I do, watch out world.
What I want you to know is that after mom dies when you are 19, there will be freedom and grief wrapped up together that will confuse you for years.
What I want you to know is that it's okay not to grieve for a parent who abused and used you. What I want you to know is after she dies, she becomes your guardian angel.
What I want you to know is that she is a better mother on the other side than she ever was in flesh and blood.
What I want you to know is that this mom will take you on journeys you never thought you were capable of and keep you safe.
What I want you to know is that you move across the country when people thought you were crazy.
What I want you to know is that you jump out of planes, travel different countries, embark on many career journeys, ride a motorcycle and live life on your terms.
What I want you to know is that today I am a Stand-Up Comedian, A Storyteller, A Speaker, and a Life Coach.
What I want you to know is that Laughter is Miracle Drug, and you, my child, are the doctor giving out the doses.

What I want you to know is I am grateful to you and for you.

Paddy Meade is an artist, and a mentor who chooses to be visible and empowers others to do the same.

Paddy Meade

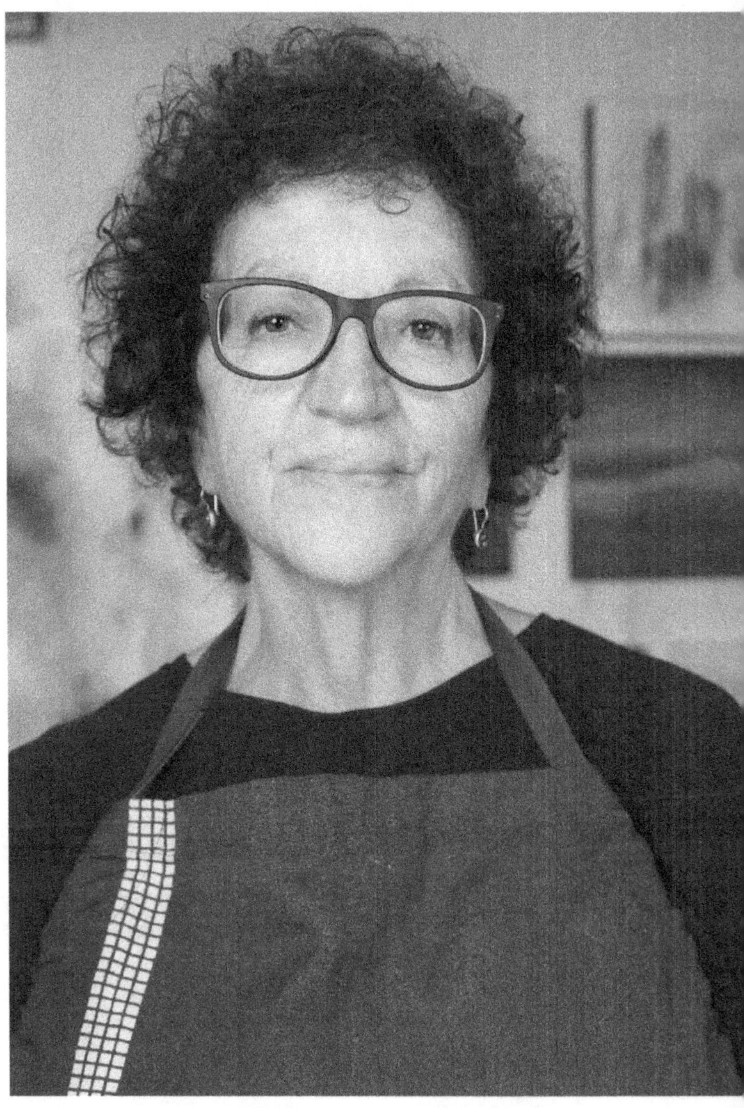

From afar, I appear strong, independent, successful. And that is true. I have had a wonderful life and career adventures, including raising a family and holding prominent leadership roles with titles of Executive director, CEO, and Deputy Minister. I have had an eclectic career, and now, as an artist, I am eclectic in medium and subject. I have tasted success, and overcome personal and professional failures and challenges, yet remain cognizant and amazed at the rich beauty and potential of the world, humanity, and life. I have also been invisible. Invisible in a chauvinistic household of male siblings, invisible as a young female in my generation, invisible to those who are important to me, and often invisible to myself.

As an older woman, I now see the world trying to cloak me in invisibility again, and yet I am comfortable, confident, and not willing to hide. There are times when I have learned to enjoy being invisible, to observe, learn, and experience through the success of others, and at times to avoid chaos and grief. I have used invisibility to absorb the world around me, as a silent leader, supporting and leading from behind.

Being invisible can feel like "less than." I have had to learn to challenge myself, push myself to feel worthy, and to know I can accomplish. Being invisible is not always less than, not always powerless, and is important in leadership. I have learned that I can choose to be invisible and choose to prominent, and there are times for ether and both.

I still struggle with self-doubt and fear to try things, be things, and overcome self-doubt and inner criticism. I have also learned to silence the fears, take the risk, step forward and walk untrodden paths. I have tried to carry the mentor role forward, giving the opportunity to other women and men during my working life. Now, I call myself an artist, a path where being invisible and yet stepping forward is critical; where having learned to overcome my self-doubt is important. I choose now to be visible in different ways. I choose to continue to mentor where I can. I choose to share through my art. And I look to support others who feel invisible.

We all should.

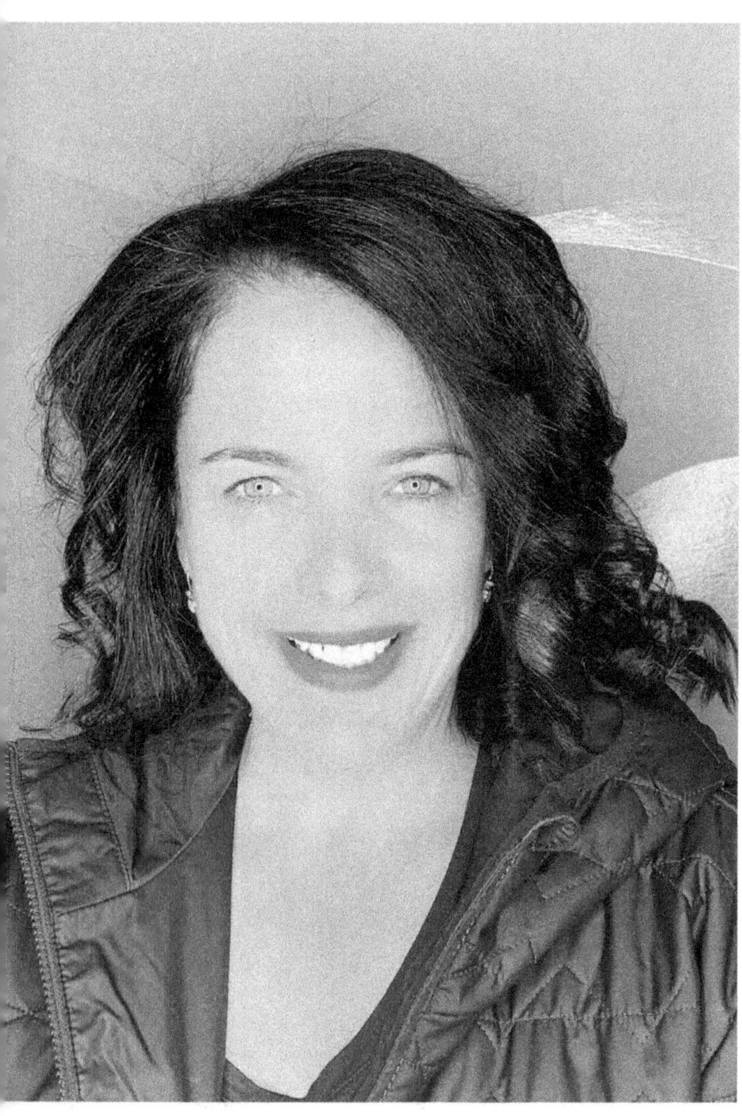

Tina Richardson is a fifty-four-year-old mother of three and a champion of causes that raise awareness for Pediatric cancers, toy shopper extraordinaire, and death doula.

Tina Richardson

In 1989, I moved from Montreal to Vancouver. In 1990, I landed my dream job, onboard the "Rocky Mountaineer." In 1992, I was thrilled to find out I was pregnant with my first child. His father and I married because I was pregnant, and I thought it was best for our son to have two parents living under the same roof. In 1996, our daughter was born, and in 2008, we welcomed a healthy son.

Fast forward to June 2011; all train hosts were locked out and ended up on the picket line, fighting for our jobs. As I was our family's breadwinner, and unemployed, we were evicted and left to reside in a trailer in my sister's driveway. In October 2011, my youngest son was diagnosed with leukemia. Sean spent four years fighting for his life and sadly passed on his sister's nineteenth birthday.

There are no magic words when it comes to dealing with grief. It's so important not to conceal our emotions, as most of us have been conditioned to do. During my grief journey, I've learned that we will never get over the loss of our children, but with time, we find ways of getting through it. Grief comes in waves, as unpredictable as the waves of an ocean. The biggest fear of a bereaved parent is that our children will be forgotten. All we have left are memories and photos.

Soon after Sean passed, I set out to find a way to honour his memory and ensure that his passing was not in vain. As Sean was born on the 24th of September and passed on November 24th, each month, I ask that people do a random act of kindness in memory of his loving, generous spirit.

For twenty-two years, my glamorous job on the luxury train was how I identified myself. When Sean was diagnosed, my perspective completely changed. I witnessed firsthand precious children fighting for their lives - just wanting to be normal kids, enduring horrific pain, life-altering surgeries, with many not surviving. It was a huge life change for me on so many levels.

I know now that my life has a greater purpose. I don't know if I would have ever learned what that purpose was if my son hadn't died. Sean's seven years with us was a true gift, as were the life lessons he continues to teach us all.

Michaelee is a proud Kanien'kehá:ka (Mohawk) from Akwesáhsne and Northern Paiute from Nevada. Her passion for creating beautiful soaps and beauty products drove her to quit her job as an engineer and start her company, Sequoia.

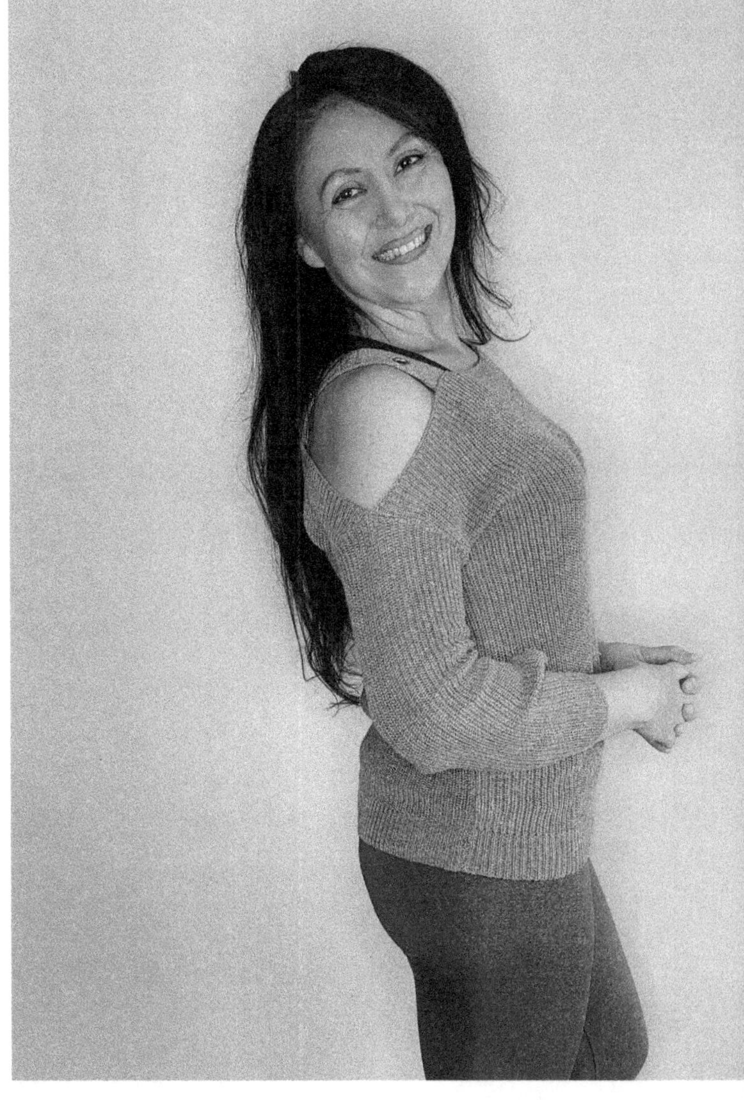

Michaelee Lazore

When I told my dad that I was going to quit my engineering job and start my soap/skincare company, his response was, "maybe you should go back to school to be a lawyer." I don't even know if he remembers that, but I understand his response. I got my degree in mechanical engineering and had started a career in the civil engineering field. That was already ten years of my life. It was a great job, and my parents were proud, but I wasn't passionate about it every day.

In order to be happy, I felt that I needed to follow my dream of creating something of my very own. Something I was passionate about where the sky was the limit. I didn't want to regret not trying. This leap of faith almost twenty years ago was when I created "Sequoia." On the surface, Sequoia may seem like a purely artisanal brand. While it's true there is a huge artistic aspect of creating beautiful soaps, blending different fragrances and essential oils to create unique smells, it is also highly technical.

I'm someone who has both a strong artistic and technical side and craved both of these elements. The hardest part was finding something that had both sides. This wasn't something I was actively looking for, and I believe that is how I found it. One day it just presented itself. I thought, why are there not any bath and body care products that are Indigenous-inspired? I looked into formulating products, and that is when the seed was planted, and it all began. I became obsessed and worked and thought about it every day. This was how I knew I found my passion.

As a proud Indigenous woman, it was very important for me to be an example to other Indigenous youth. I didn't find my passion in life until I was finished university and had already started a "solid" career. There were a lot of ups and downs but that is to be expected about any path in life. Life throws us curve balls and switching gears is something I don't regret for a second. And as it turns out, today, my parents are my biggest fans.

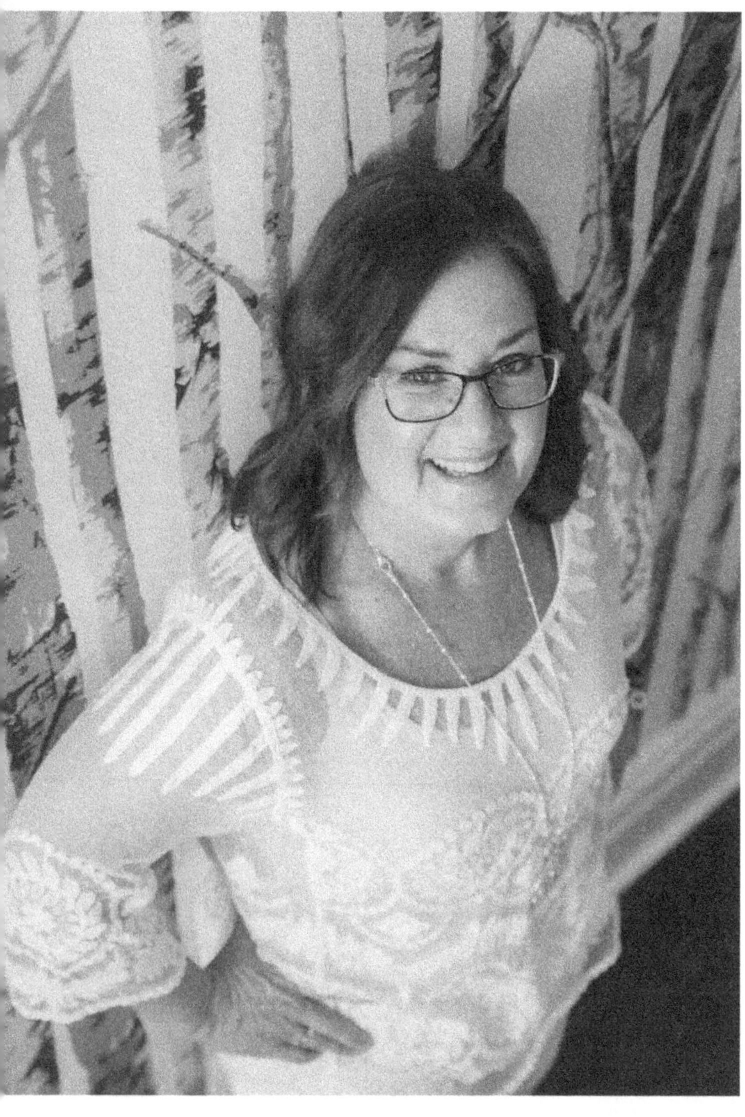

Susan is the creator of a life filled with healing and forgiveness, replacing sadness with joy.

Susan McCart

Life at age fifteen isn't very complicated; at least it's not meant to be. Little did I know that my pretty uncomplicated, safe world at fifteen would change its course bringing me to my knees, questioning my faith on every level. Why would God allow two men to get into my brother's taxi, take him to a farmer's field, and beat him to death? This was beyond my comprehension and left me with an excruciating pain I didn't know existed. Was this what life was going to be like, one of sadness and heartache that would never go away?

Oddly at this young age, I strongly believed that we are products of our upbringing. After the funeral, I returned to school and learned that the mother of one of my brother's killers was working in the high school cafeteria, and I wondered, was this some sick, cruel joke? It was no joke, but actually what saved me from living a life filled with anger and resentment. After learning she gave birth to him in prison, I thought, what chance did he have? At that moment, I was able to forgive and find peace. That may sound impossible, but that's what I needed to survive and go on to create a life that wasn't defined by this horrible tragedy; merely a bridge to help me grow and evolve.

Through healing, synchronicities, and witnessing life's small miracles, I have learned that I have the power to create a truly beautiful life. I look for the gold nugget in each and every experience and trust the process. We aren't meant to live a life of suffering. What would be the point of it all? My soul is on a journey, and I make choices along the way that are in line with my life's purpose and work hard to keep my heart open, to be kind and compassionate. I am a product of my life's experiences, which have deepened my faith and allowed me to grow, and it started when that fifteen-year-old little girl was able to find forgiveness.

Melissa Deally is a wife, mom, world traveller, educator, and Integrative Health Practitioner, and is here to guide you on your health journey.

Melissa Deally

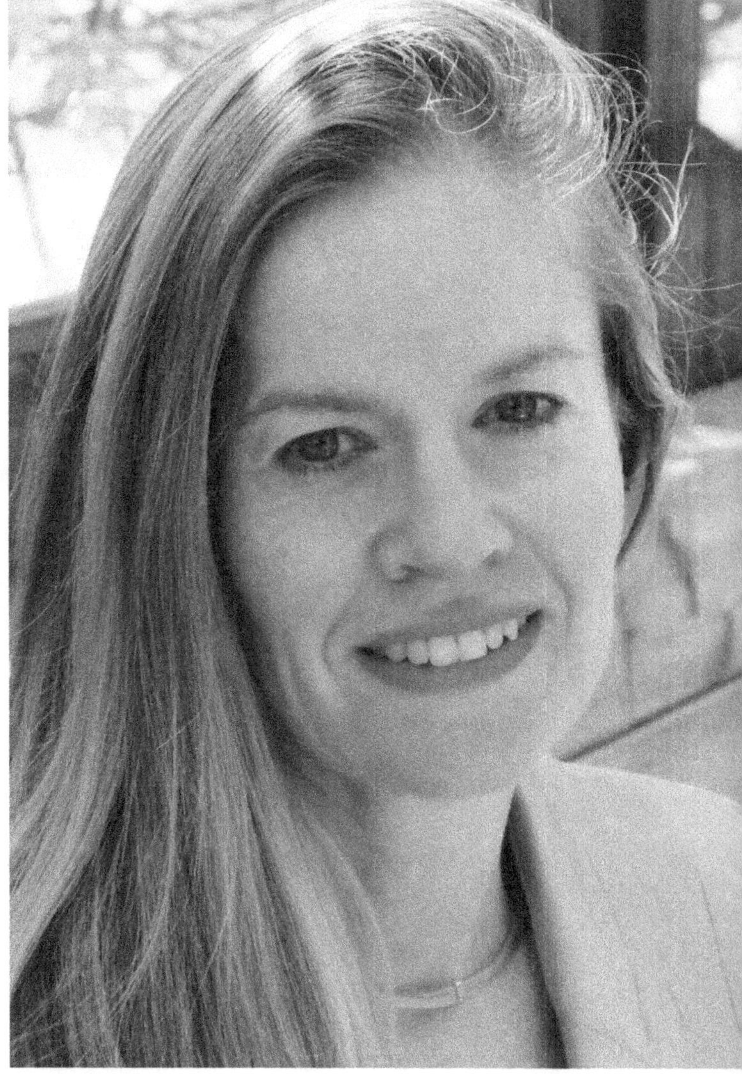

Are your trashcans overflowing? I don't mean the ones you put out on the street, I mean your liver and kidneys! After a lifetime of eating, drinking, and having toxins get inside our bodies, our liver and kidneys are getting bogged down and are no longer able to get the toxins out as well as they used to. Like garbage left out on the street too long, starting to smell and rot, the toxins are causing your body to rot. The world is the sickest ever, with near epidemic levels of chronic illness, and no one is asking "Why?".

My name is Melissa Deally, and I'm an Integrative Health Practitioner and Registered Health Coach. It is my purpose and passion to help people heal and disrupt our current thoughts on our health. Something we take for granted until we don't have it anymore...
90-95% of all diseases are triggered by the environment we create inside our body. No one goes to bed and wakes up with a disease! It grows inside us over time. What if we didn't wait to get sick? What if we knew how to optimize our health?

This is what I want to offer you!
I shift women from a life of dis-ease to a life of vitality.

This brings me back to those trashcans! I help you discover your toxic load and guide you through a program to have you empty your trashcans and re-set your health. Plus, I use the power of functional medicine lab tests to "see" inside your body to understand where imbalances lie and then use natural remedies to bring your body back into balance, at which point it can heal itself like it does a cut finger or broken arm.

A body in balance doesn't get sick, harbor disease, or hold onto excess weight.

My business is 100% virtual, the lab tests are sent to your home! I offer a guided program, meeting with you at least four times during your healing journey, providing all the support you need, including recipes, meal plans, and shopping lists for improved nutrition and health education throughout your program.

This is true health, and health is your true wealth.

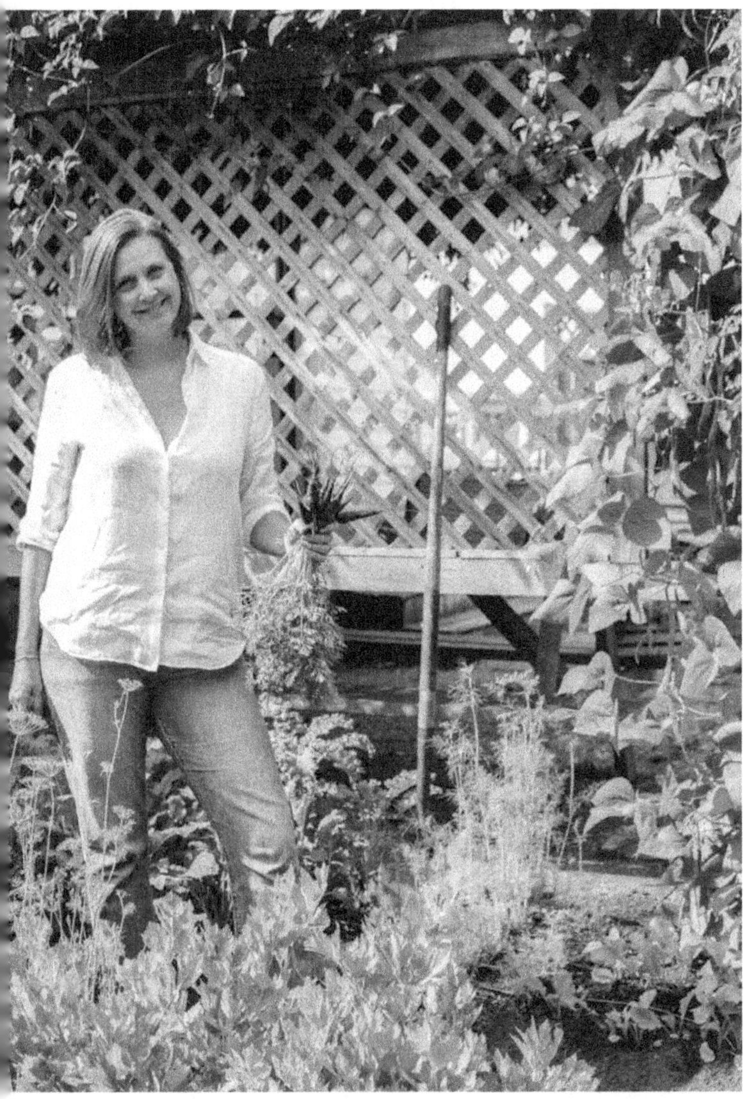

Toni Desrosiers is the founder of Abeego and inventor of beeswax food wrap.

Toni Desrosiers

In 2008, I was working as a nutritionist and started to question why we were wrapping our fresh living food in airtight plastic wrap. There's no such thing as an airtight and transparent peel in nature. Instead, you'll find lemon peels, cheese rinds, and onion skin, all of which are breathable and opaque. This is when I set out to invent the future of food wrap. Abeego mimics these intrinsic qualities of natural skins, peels, and rinds and keeps food fresher for longer than ever imagined.

Thirteen years later, beeswax food wrap is popping up across the globe! I knew my invention was going to change the world, so it's incredible to watch it lead the way as a global trend and movement; helping kitchens around the globe reduce food waste every day.

It's been a wild journey, and I find solace and creative freedom in my garden. I never listen to anything while I garden. I let my mind wander while I silently work with my hands. Some of my most developed ideas come out of my vegetable patch.

It's my front yard garden that has provided even more than nutritious food and alone time. It stops those passing by and supplies food for conversation and connection. There's nothing quite like picking a fresh cucumber and handing it to your neighbor as they stroll along, offering an opportunity to pause the hustle of our minds and let us appreciate the simplicity of food and community.

It's moments like this that contribute to my mission to Keep Food Alive and hold space for those hungry to rekindle food wisdom inherent to humankind. For me, Keep Food Alive is about every moment you're connected to food in a lively, present, or conscious manner. It's a holistic approach to eating that encompasses positive shared experiences around food that nourish our spirit. It's about the stories that reconnect us to each other and our natural world.

I am driven by the desire to capture these stories to preserve and expand what it means to Keep Food Alive.

Katayoon is an Iranian, queer woman, a mom, an artist, a successful Realtor, and a business owner.

Katayoon Webb

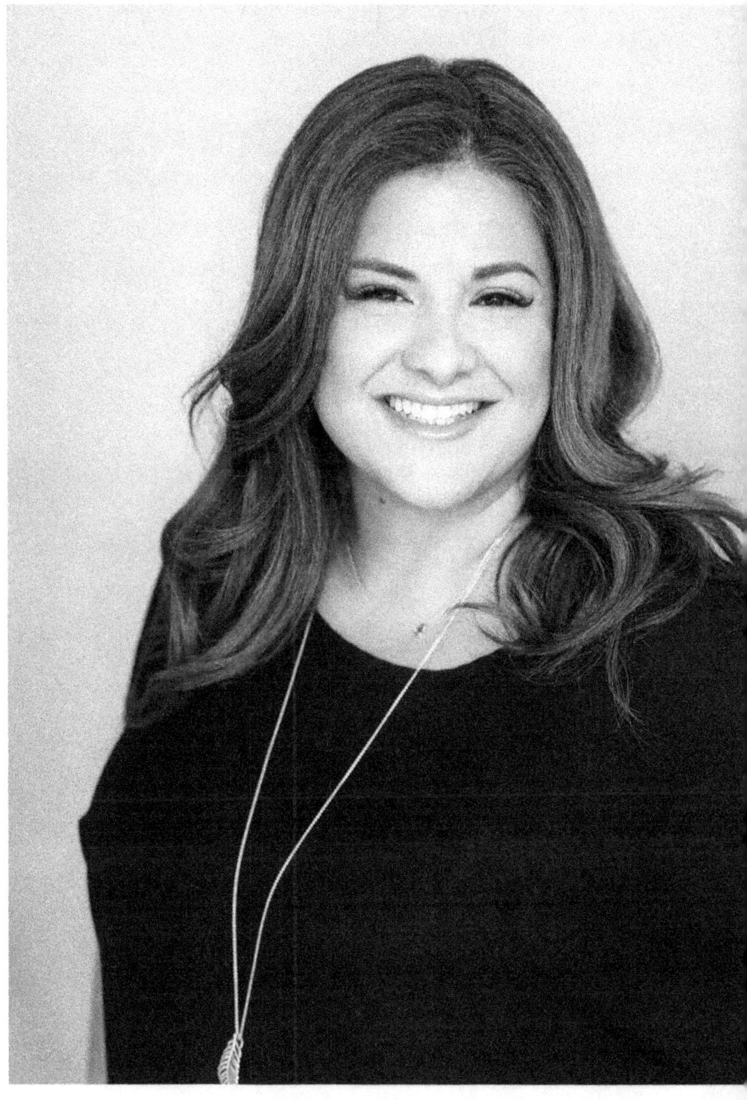

What if the life you were born into was nothing like the life you dreamed of? Imagine growing up in an Islamic country during a revolution, being young, female, queer, and having the heart of an artist. Being a woman in love with another woman is not talked about in that culture, and certainly not at that time. Being an artist, I constantly pushed the boundaries through my art and was reprimanded for it. I learned to quiet who I was, in favour of doing what was expected of me. That expectation stayed with me, through immigration to Canada, through completing my fine art degree, and through fulfilling my parents' dream of finding a husband and having children.

I had everything, or so it seemed. I fiercely loved my children, and had an amazing friendship with my husband, a fulfilling career, and felt very secure with who I was as an artist. But I was not happy. I had built my life on providing happiness for other people. I could no longer quiet the part of me who wanted to love a woman, and now living in Canada, I knew it was possible, accepted, and even celebrated.

My challenge now was to find a way of keeping my family together, but also fulfill who I am. There was no rulebook on how to do this successfully, and most people in similar situations found themselves dealing with custody battles and divorce. This was not an option for us, as neither my husband nor I wanted that – we worked together, lived together, co-parented together.

Today, I wish I could show the sixteen-year-old girl in oppressive Iran, a glimpse of what was to come for her. I am celebrating my third year in a loving and fulfilling relationship with a woman! We own side by side homes; my children see both of their parents every day. Their father and I work together and co-parent. As in every family, we have our challenges, but we face them together with love and trust, instead of hate, jealousy, or division. I hope to inspire my little girl to live a life that makes her happy, and not just what is expected of her by her family or society.

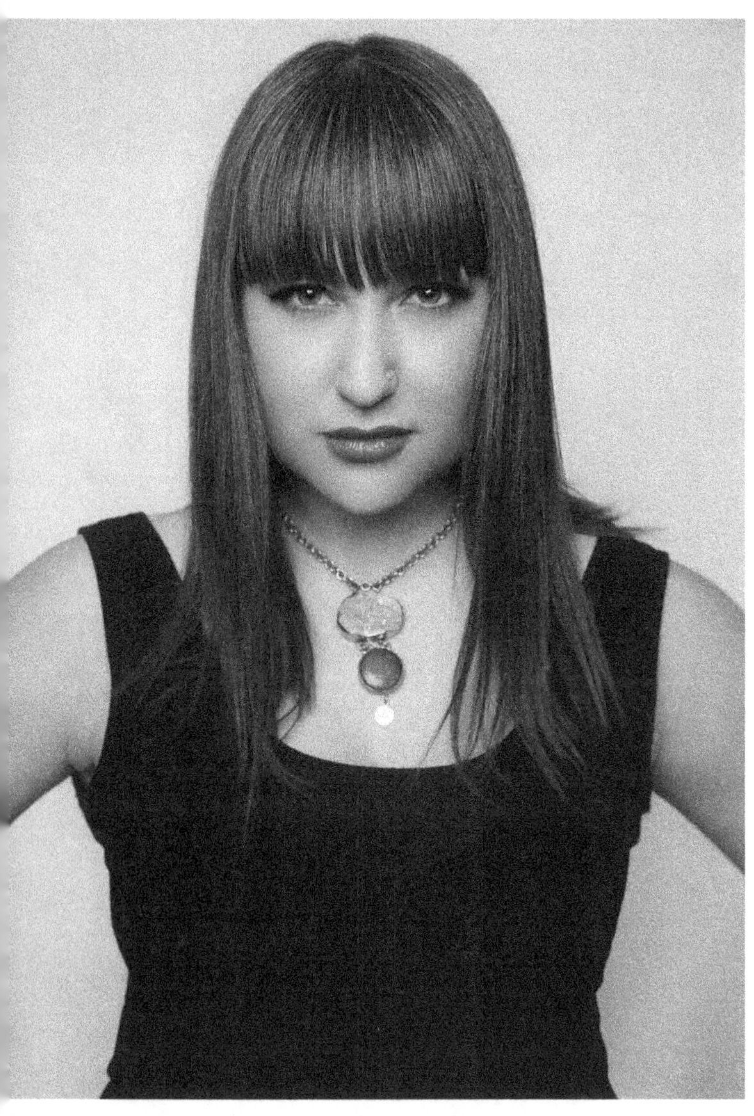

Missy MacKintosh is an internationally acclaimed professional makeup artist, and the founder and CEO of MisMacK Clean Cosmetics Inc.

Missy MacKintosh

Empowering through makeup is my passion. My personal tagline is, "Makeup Does Not Define You but is Merely a Tool of Empowerment." I believe that makeup is designed to bring out your most beautiful natural features, it isn't to cover them up or change them. Makeup has always fascinated me because of this. When I was young, my mom didn't use makeup, so I was the kid found snooping through others' makeup bags, testing products on my hand. I was obsessed.

When I was fourteen, my mom became a Mary Kay makeup consultant, and I thought I'd died and gone to heaven. When I discovered there were careers in makeup application, I enrolled at Blanche McDonald and moved to the big city, where I established a flourishing career.

Things pivoted after my husband and I suffered a silent miscarriage. We decided to return to our roots in the small town of Salmon Arm in order to start our family. I believed life there meant giving up my dream in makeup, so I worked in travel for a while, but makeup followed me. After side hustling for six years, I returned to the world of makeup in 2014. While working with Portia-Ella, I fell in love with the integrity behind clean beauty. It was then I realized, I didn't just want to apply makeup, I wanted to create makeup - but who does that? If it were easy, everyone would. After much research, I discovered there was not a Professional Performing Clean Makeup line on the market. I took matters into my own hands and created MisMacK Clean Cosmetics Inc., the first Professional Performing Clean Makeup line.

My two entrepreneurial parents provided a solid example of what was possible. There have been failures along the way, but I have learned to sit in my failure and learn from it. It is where growth takes place. I don't have all the answers, but I'm learning as I go. My mantra is; be bold, be brave and take action! I lean on my support system and use my critics to fuel me. Every day in my small town of Canoe, BC, I am busy proving myself wrong!

Dayo Alabi is an immigrant, a storyteller, an entrepreneur, PR and Communications professional, an outgoing fashion enthusiast, and a dedicated mom in pursuit of excellence.

Dayo Alabi

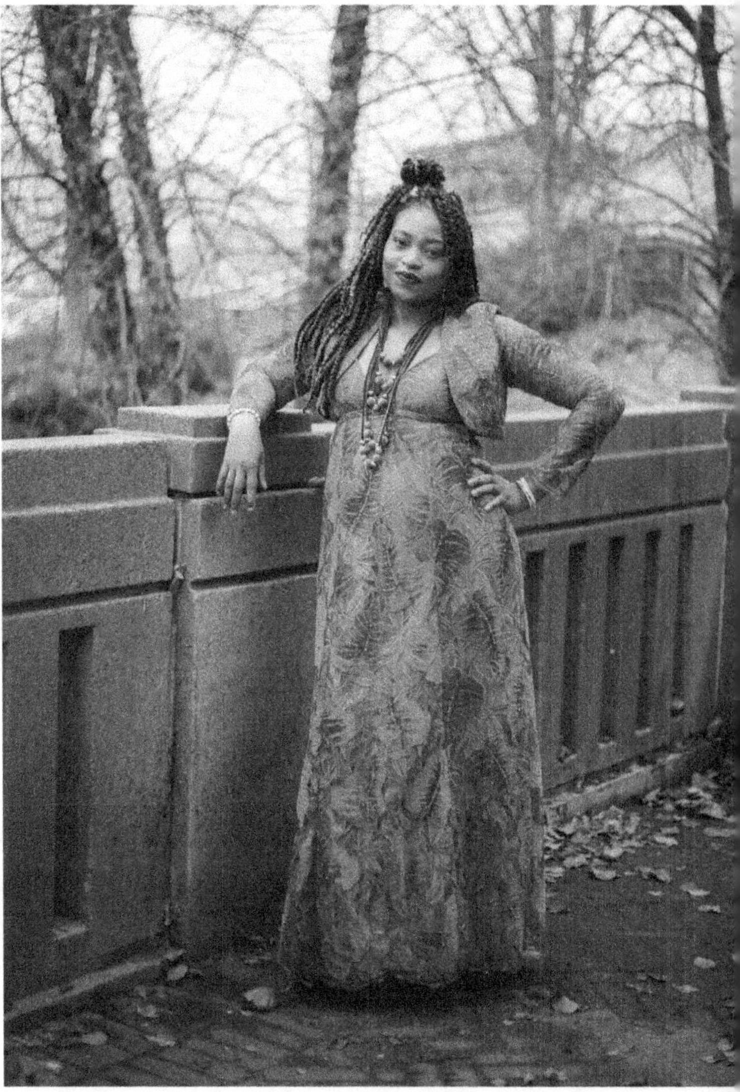

I RISE!

Happiness is my number one goal in life, enjoying every moment, spreading joy, and never taking one day for granted. My potential is endless and limiting myself is not an option. I am ambitious, positive, imaginative, and add a dash of happiness to all I want to accomplish.

I envision my life right now, and what I wanted as a child has all come to pass. I knew I would see myself behind the cameras, in front of the cameras, holding a microphone, anchoring, speaking, or motivating, inspiring people to achieve great things.

The twists and turns, pain, loss, grief, and sadness experienced in my life after a divorce was a moment in time. But then, I had to reset, reclaim my life back, and I found peace with prayer. I felt free, and now I RISE!

A major setback in your life can take you down memory lane, and then you constantly ask yourself why? Will I come out stronger, or has this setback defined me? The "why me" question began to change to YES ME. I began to say to myself, YES ME!

Failure sets you up for greatness. It molds you to keep fighting. It keeps you grounded and reminds you to never look back, but to forge ahead time and again, setting forth in pursuit of a new life, the tiny little voice saying, "You will RISE."

My Nigerian heritage is important to me, trying to balance our culture, fashion, and food for my three beautiful Canadian children. There are so many opportunities that I am involved in, bringing about change in my community. I am part of a team of educators who will be creating and putting together a curriculum for Canadian Black History. I have also been invited to participate in the revival of the JR Black Achievements Awards.

My voice is my strength; to uplift, advocate for social issues, equality, inclusion, representation, and women empowerment. Advocating for my community, supporting causes, shedding light on discrimination and racism. As a beautiful, Black, Canadian woman, I am evolving by the day. I see everything I am becoming and all that I will become, and so today, I RISE!

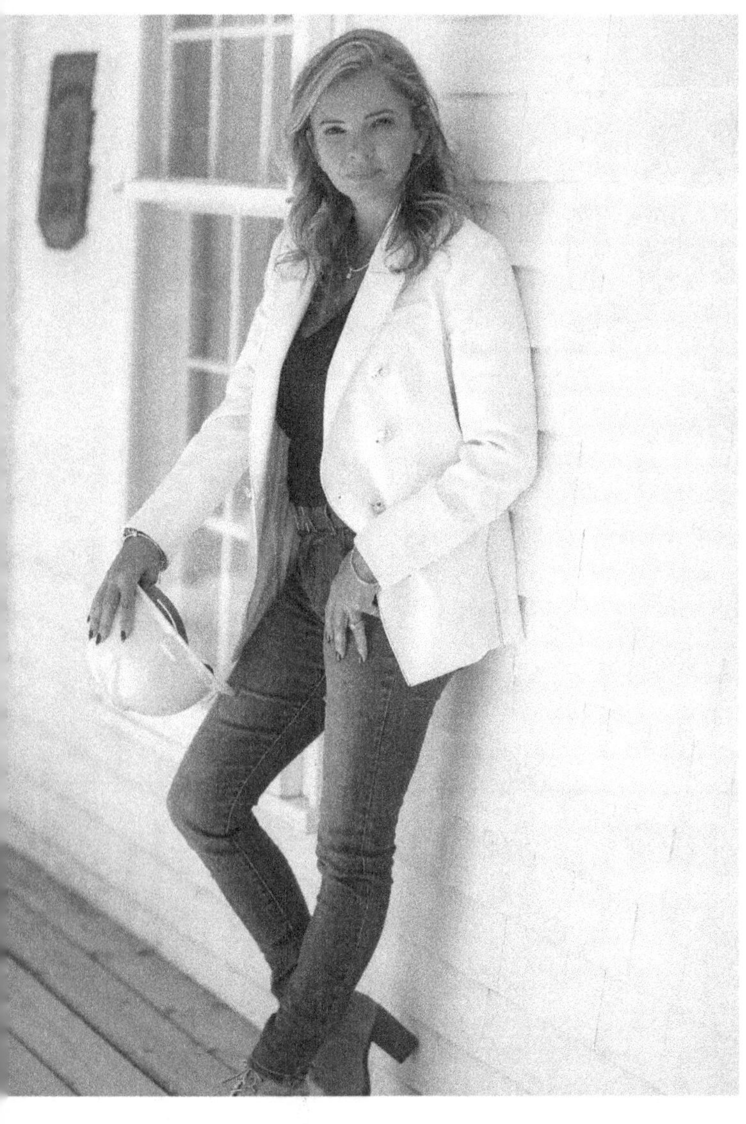

Tamara Barker Watson is an entrepreneur, an award-winning builder, Realtor, and Harley riding mother of two.

Tamara Barker Watson

I do not let other's perceptions of me, define me. Belief in myself and my abilities have made me who I am today. Honesty, keeping my word, displaying a strong work ethic, and communicating clearly are the foundations of my success.

It has long been said that the Newfoundlanders are a hardy breed but being a young girl with a scoliosis diagnosis and a body cast, had me questioning that belief. I found strength and inspiration in observing the no-nonsense business spirit of my mother and in the solid belief held by my father that his three girls were as capable as any man. My parent's faith in me created a strong belief in myself and my abilities. Leaving Newfoundland to attend university, my parents were still the first people I thought to call when I wanted to share an achievement or when I encountered a seemingly insurmountable problem. They were there to ask the right questions, offer support, and guide me to my own conclusions.

While in university, I developed an interest in housing, becoming a realtor. Now I do everything from landing acquisitions to overseeing construction projects, negotiating contracts, scheduling, and budgeting. Passionate about eco-friendly and energy-efficient living, I created Whitestone Building and Renovations, with my Partner Andrew Watson, one of the first green companies on the local construction scene. We have been building and designing homes in Halifax, since 1995. Our success with Whitestone spunoff into 6 other companies including two landholding companies, a commercial Rental company, and a storage facility.

Each day I get up and jump out of bed because I can't wait to get to the job site to watch the process of a homecoming to life and feel the excitement of my clients. I am not just building houses; I create homes for friends. I don't believe in work-life balance because as an entrepreneur, when you find more free time, you fill it with work because you #lovewhatyoudo and see it as a lifestyle, not a job.

Today, ranking as one of Canada's Top Female Entrepreneurs, I hope to inspire other ladies to look at entrepreneurialism as more than just a dream." It can be a way of life if you just believe."

LeiLani Kopp brings her experience as a Paramedical Corrective Makeup and Scar-Re-Pigmentation Specialist, as well as thirty years in film and TV to her own cosmetics line, Sweet LeiLani Cosmetics.

LeiLani Kopp

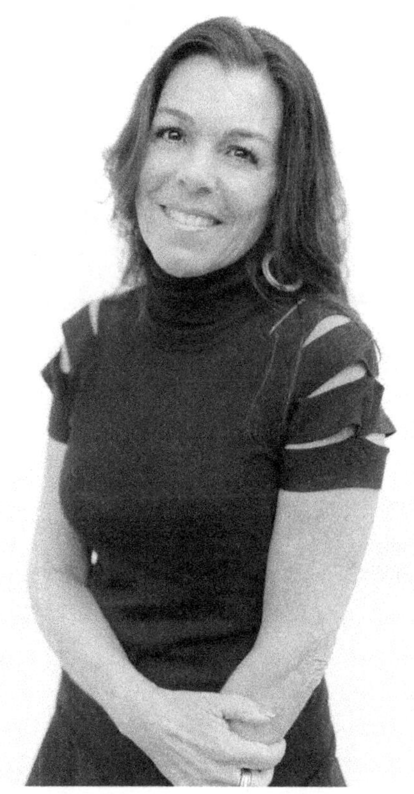

Since the age of twelve, I dreamt of becoming a special effects Makeup Artist for film and TV. Becoming a Hairstylist right out of high school allowed me to save money, and at the age of nineteen, my journey started, and I moved to LA for FX/Makeup school in Hollywood. I was very fortunate to do work experience in some film studios and met a lot of famous actors early in my career. My first real job, I was hired by a Cosmetic Company to go to Zsa Zsa Gabor's house to demonstrate their Joe Blasco Film Makeup.

It was at Christmas, and I remember walking into her home, and there was a tree in the foyer that went up three levels. At my young age, I'm not sure if I was more impressed by Zsa Zsa, or her home up in Beverly Hills.

Upon returning home to Vancouver, my gramma passed away, and sitting with my mom at the funeral home, I blurted out that I would be doing her hair and makeup. My mom almost fell off her chair, but hey, I was always the one that did her hair, why would I have anyone else do it. Crazy, how this led to me teaching embalmers how to do makeup at funeral homes.

I did go on to living my dream of doing FX Makeup for Film, as well as every cheesy Hallmark movie. Ironically now, I volunteer with plastic surgeons to teach clients how to cover injuries I once created, which led to creating Sweet LeiLani Cosmetics.

I never set out to have a Company; I wasn't book smart; I couldn't pass a math test if I tried. I always told my kids grades aren't everything. My advice was to stay focused, stay in your own lane. It's about reaching, striving, dreaming, and using your talents to help others. When my daughter hears me swearing when something is going wrong, she says, say thank you, the universe is pushing you in a better direction. My mom's advice is to enjoy the journey. She gave me a mug when I left for LA that says those who reach, touch the stars. I still have the mug, and I'm still reaching!

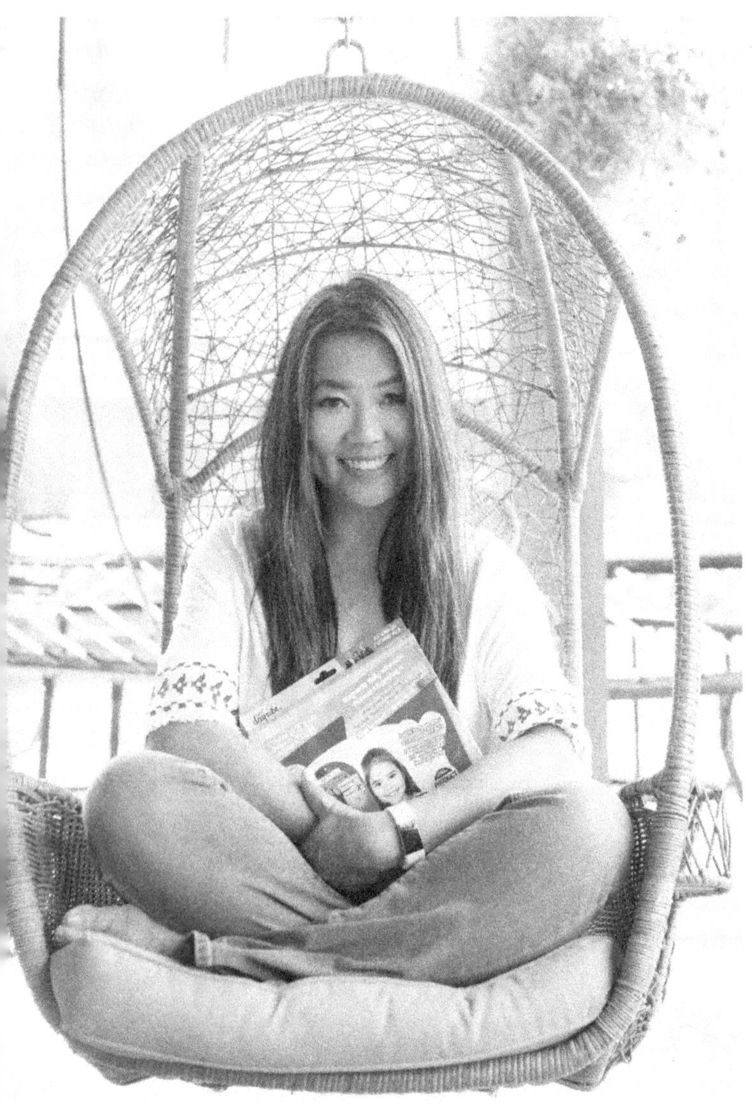

Elaine Tan Comeau knows the ups and downs of being a mom entrepreneur, from launching her award-winning product line, Easy Daysies, off her kitchen table to inciting a bidding war on Dragons' Den. She seeks to help women entrepreneurs thrive on her podcast "Create Better", and in her book "Sell Your Passion".

Elaine Tan Comeau

Please touch your nose with your left pointing finger. Do I have your attention?

I attempted this simple task every day in May 2018, with utter gratitude. My life had been abruptly interrupted on April 25 when I had a stroke. I made poor choices all day, starting when I awoke with half my body not functioning. Instead of asking for help, I chose to ignore all the signs because I had three children and three small businesses to run that day.

How often do we feel we need to do it all and be everywhere, when in fact, very little is urgent and important?

I remember in the hospital thinking, "This stroke is completely inconvenient". I had speaking events, plane tickets booked, a test order of my product Easy Daysies shipping to a U.S. mass retailer, and I was launching a book. I did not want to let people down, but I had a three-month flight and driving ban.

I pleaded with my cardiologist to attend my daughter's upcoming Nationals volleyball tournament in Edmonton. After three days, he finally said, "Elaine, you can go to your daughter's tournament, or you can go to her wedding." Mic drop. He then increased my flight ban to 6 months!

I learned that I want to be the person who says, "I choose to" rather than, "I have to," to live a life by design rather than by default. And this begins with making small, sometimes difficult choices every day to put my time and energy where my heart is. Life should not be about getting as much done as possible, but about getting the right things done.

I am learning something new – I call it "single-tasking" – focusing on one task or person at a time. It works in relationships, business, and parenting. It produces better results, and my body thanks me!

Our children, spouse, and clients will not remember our multi-tasking moments. But they will remember the single-tasking times spent with them. Go forth and embrace your single-tasking moments. Own them, because, through them, you will make an impactful difference.

Tina Llewellyn is on a mission to create a life that fuels her body, mind, and soul. Tina is a lover of plants, horses, magic, and art, it is through all of these facets that she has built a place where women and children can come to heal.

Tina Llewellyn

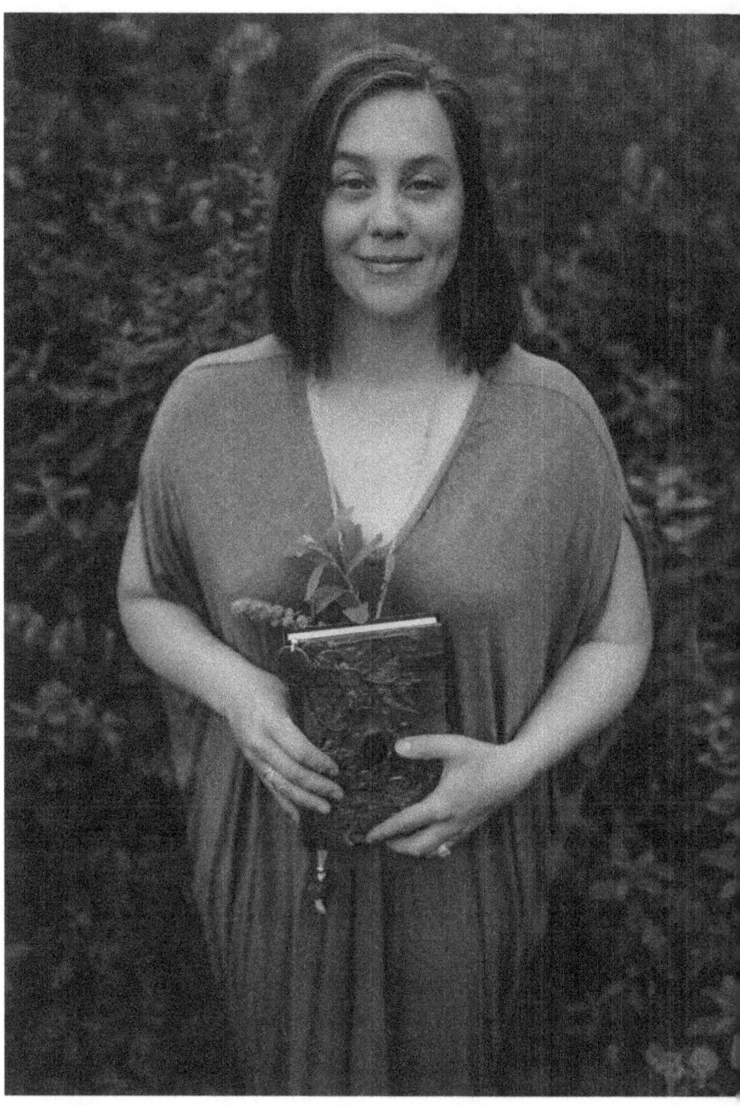

Have you heard the term; life is circular? In my experience it truly is. As I look back on my life, I realize I dreamt the life I am living now into being. As a little girl, I would dream of horses and would wake up in the wee hours of the morning, go downstairs, and draw what I dreamt. I would spend summers in nature, singing and being free.

Horses have been a constant in my life, especially my heart horse Lucinda. Lucinda was with me as a crazy teen and throughout my career as a Farrier, a male-dominated trade, where even women believe women shouldn't do it.

Have you ever been told you can't do something, and what did you do about it?
I was, and I showed myself what I was capable of by becoming the 5th female Journeyman Farrier in Canada. Although I loved my job and the horses, it was not life-sustaining. The same year I transitioned to a new path I also said goodbye to my heart horse, Lucinda. It was time to follow the way of my soul.

Being a curious one, and always wanting to grow, I took course after course, and all have become facets of myself.
I became an Herbalist and fell in love with the way we live in reciprocity with the plant world. We know each other on a cellular level; learning ancient traditions of when women use to be in circle together, during a Priestess apprenticeship. This is when I found my voice, and something in me was changed forever. I wanted to discover more of myself. Rediscovering art and a new way of working with horses that are both so healing to myself and those I work with.

So, when you're scared you've lost something, remember it can show up again when you least expect it and bring you immense joy. Just like the earth goes through cycles and the snake sheds its skin, it is OK to start fresh!

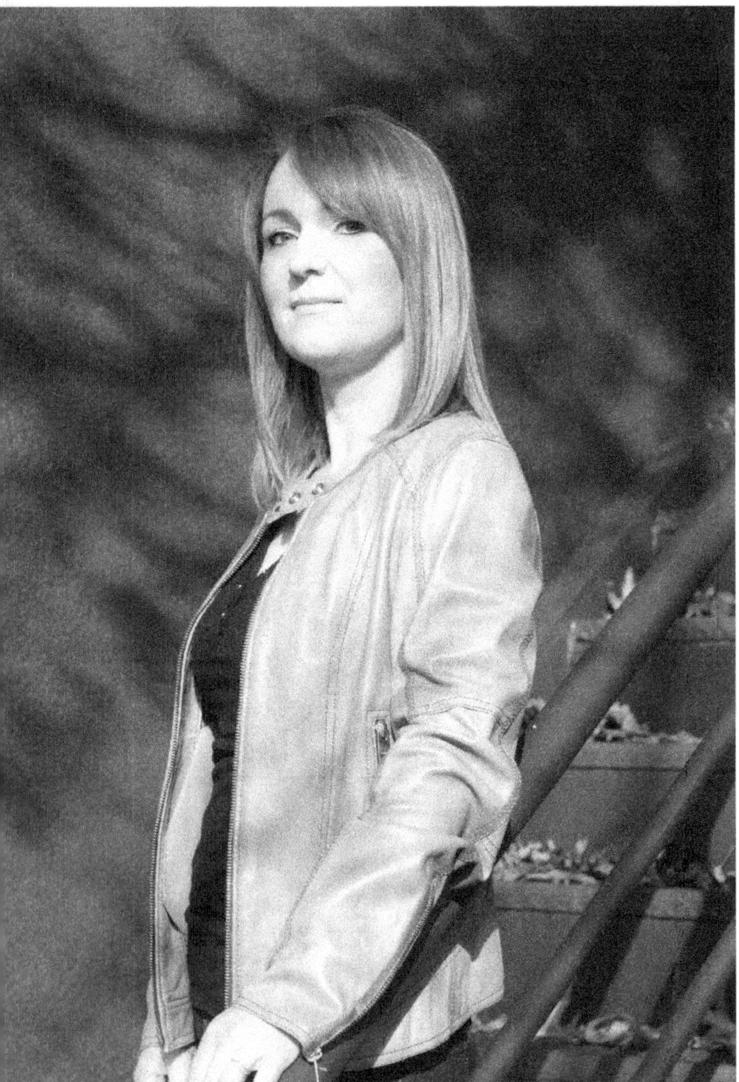
Photo Credit: Trina Schlingmann

Marzena Skowronski is a single mom, a successful make-up artist in the film and television industry, a skincare specialist, an avid traveler, a resourceful soulpreneur, and an amateur astronomer.

Marzena Skowronski

Life seldom takes us where we plan to go, but we always end up where we need to be.

Very early in her career in the cosmetics industry, Marzena Skowronski took an interest in the ingredients that beauty products contain. She was surprised to find that most commercial brands use chemicals that are toxic to human bodies and the environment. It seemed obvious to her that you shouldn't have to compromise your health while trying to look your best, and thus the idea for her own line, Green Envy Cosmetics, was born.

It was easy to find excuses for putting off getting started. How would she finance it? What would packaging look like, and where would she get it? How do you build a website? How does e-commerce work? And then she took a leap of faith and just did it. She had confidence that the universe would provide, and she wasn't disappointed. In short order, people who could help her navigate all of these questions had made their way into her life.

She worked hard and listened to her customers. They loved the cosmetics she had designed, but many of them were also looking for something else, something to nourish their spirits. Marzena designed a line of all-natural aromatherapy products using organic ingredients and high-quality essential oils. In short order, her massage oil became the bestseller in its category of more than seven thousand similar products on leading e-commerce website Etsy.

Marzena believes deeply in the power of self-love and positive thinking. She infuses her products with them and attributes much of her success to doing so. She loves hearing about the successes her customers have experienced in their own personal journeys of soul healing using her products.

True success is living a life that is authentic to who you are. Don't let doubt and fear hold you back.

Shelby Kargl is an entrepreneur and mother of two, who has been inspiring children to learn and experience the joy of dance for over twenty-five years.

Shelby Kargl

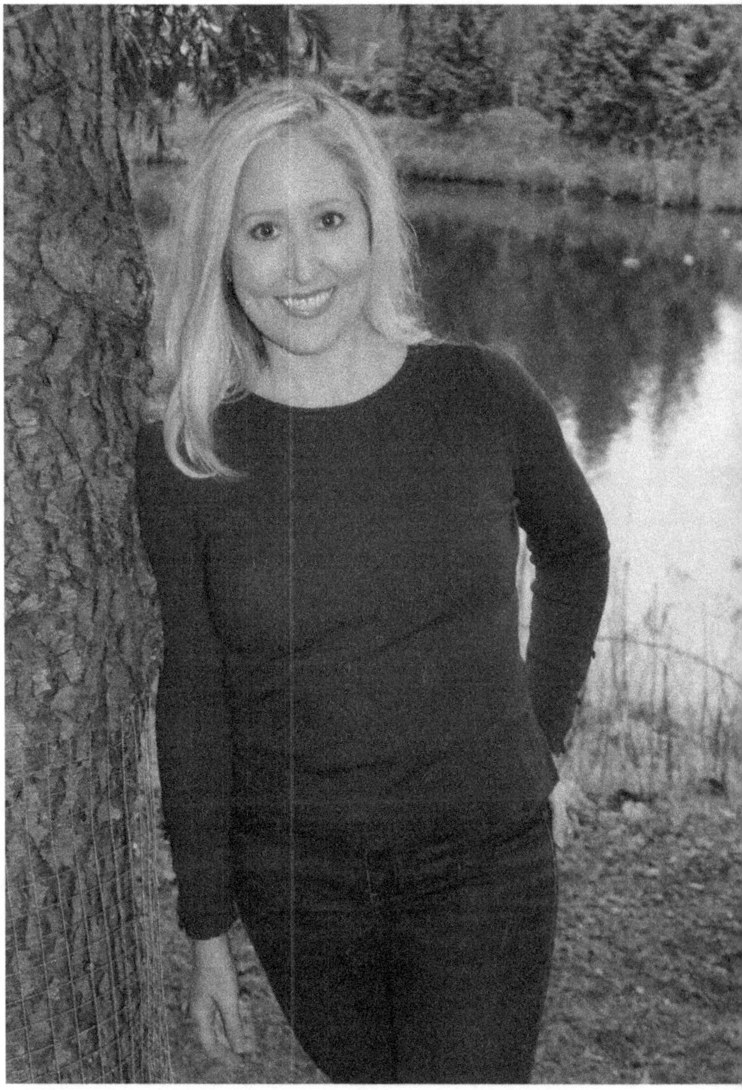

I trained in classical ballet with the Royal Academy of Dance my whole life. I became a fully certified, registered teacher at 19 years old. Through that accreditation, I took university courses with the University of Waterloo in kinesiology & child psychology and began to teach. Ballet is hard work, but life is harder. I tend to escape in the studio. Being a teacher and inspiring the next generation of dancers makes me very happy. I find working with younger children especially wonderful, which is why I established Wee Dance to teach children the joy of dance and movement. It's through their eyes, wonder, and full expression that I truly feel joy.

I never thought of myself as wanting to be an inspiration, but the truly dark times in my life have taught me that God leads you to people who can help you on your remarkable journey. That, in fact, is one of the reasons why I'm licensing my Wee Dance business model. I'd like to help others who have a passion and appreciation for educating children in the arts but are not sure where to start and need a helping hand. After being through my own personal and professional trials, and learning from them, I am coming to the realization that I can lead and help others. To other women entrepreneurs who are chasing their dreams, I would like to simply say, keep going. To those feeling blinding anger, acknowledge it, and let it go. It hurts you and those you love, more than anyone else. To those dealing with loss, the pain will recede, it will become an old friend and will make you both stronger and softer at the same time.

It is when things seem darkest, we have to remember that we are blessed in that darkness. It is in that time before growth, and the time in which we should be reflecting and choosing our way, that sometimes we feel like we're buried. We feel buried in busy-ness, anger, regret, or sorrow.

The next time you feel buried, think of this: Perhaps you've been planted and now is the time you should grow, and bloom, and start to dance.

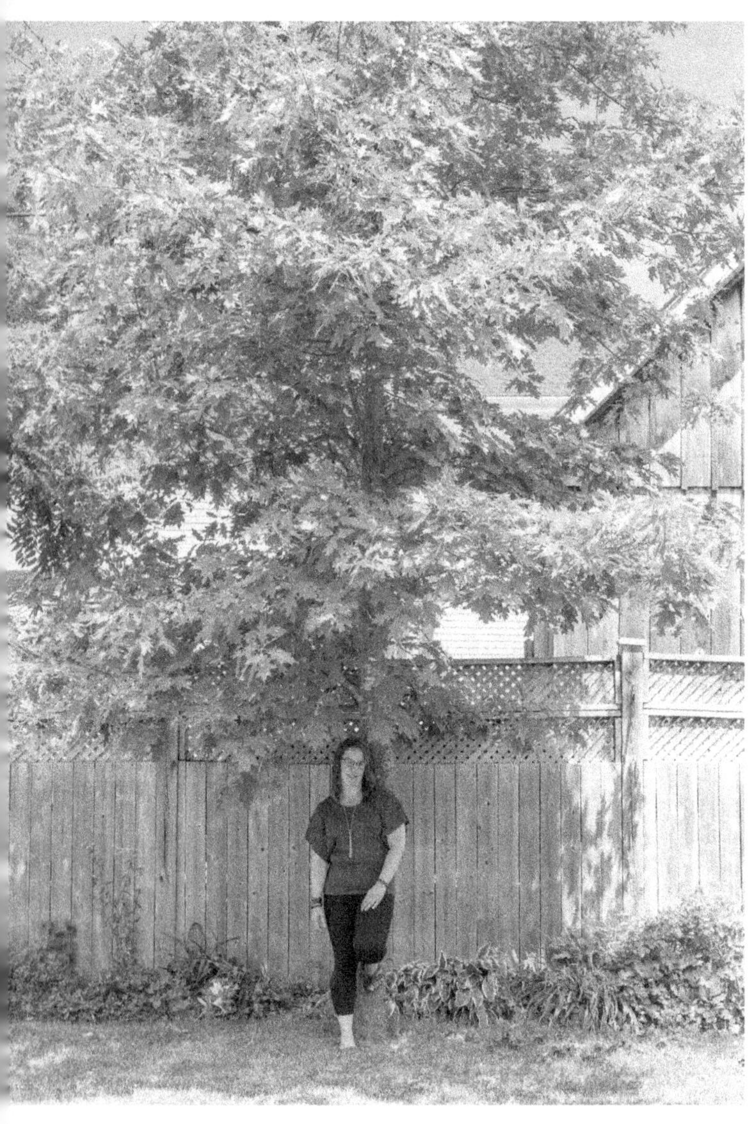

Melissa Wormington is the mother of two amazing teenagers and the Facility Leader at NV Fitness Goderich Fit Body Bootcamp where she works to empower women (and men!) every day to realize their potential for greatness. She has always loved to write, and this is her second time being published!

Melissa Wormington

If I was to choose one word to sum up my 2020, it would be "RELENTLESS".

The hits just kept on coming. I could not allow myself to sink. I had to find creative ways to swim, over and over and over again. I worked hard to keep my head above water. In March I worked to help transition a fitness business online while continuing the transition from "married mother of two" to "separated, co-parenting mother of two." While attempting to avoid layoffs of my team or myself, I was also navigating the waters of homeschooling in a global pandemic.

In the Spring while under lockdown we listed and sold our home that had been rebuilt nine years earlier after being destroyed by a tornado, my children and I moved across town. In July we re-opened our facility doors while also maintaining our existing successful online program. I led my team through strict pandemic protocols in an effort to keep us safe and employed. In July, for the first time since 1998, I also went on a "first date."

While I worked hard at healing my heart, I fed the uncertainty, anger, sadness, guilt, worry, anxiety, hurt, shame, success, winning, and happiness, with food. The choices I made didn't reflect on the outside, all of the hard work I had done on the inside. I had let myself down.

In the winter of 2019/2020, I lost 20 lbs in six to eight weeks because I barely ate. Later, in the spring and summer of 2020, I gained 30 lbs through emotional eating.

Now, my word for 2021 is REDEMPTION. I commit to becoming the best I can be. To gaining my confidence back. To being comfortable in my own skin and my clothes. To being the best role model to you, to my community, and most of all, to my two teenagers. To leading from the front and being the woman of influence, I have the potential to be and you all deserve.

2019 nearly broke me. 2020 opened my eyes. 2021: I'm coming back.

Want to come along for the journey? I'd love some company.

Heather Haslam, CHt is the owner of True Spirit Healing Arts in Vancouver B.C., and enjoys sharing her gifts of Clinical Hypnotherapy, Life Fulfillment Coaching, Reiki Energy Healing, and Skin and Body Therapy with those in need. Heather believes in healing from the inside out and is passionate about helping people in meaningful ways, connecting to their true selves, and helping them express that in their daily lives.

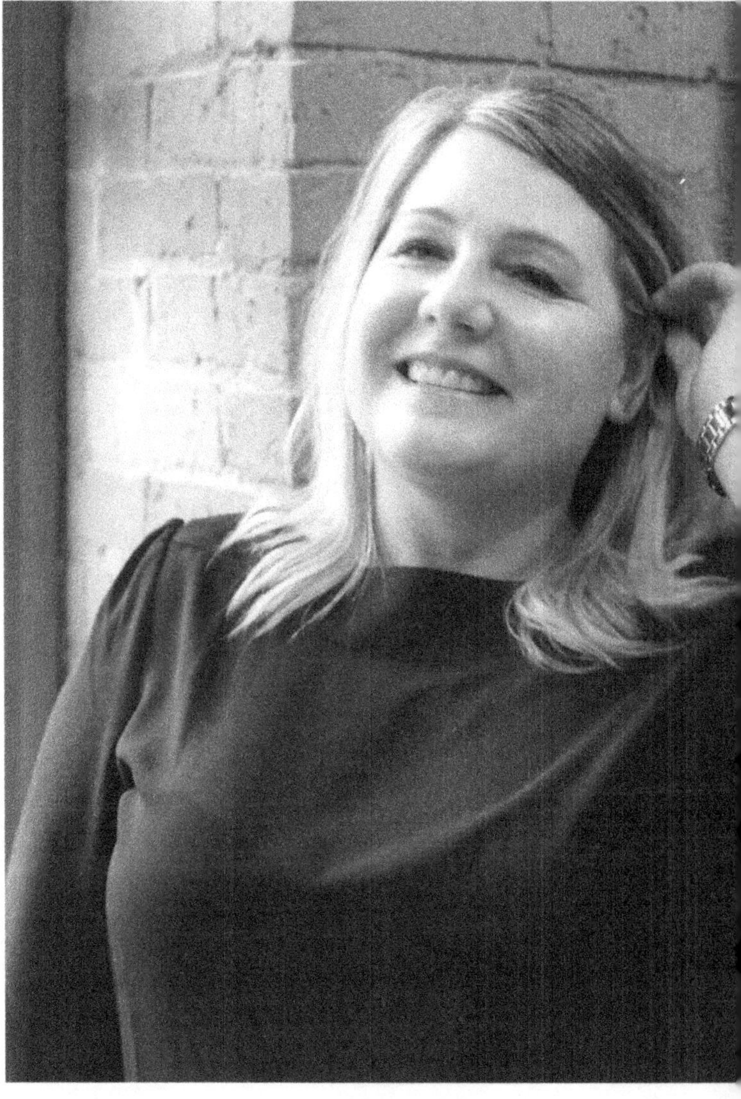

Heather Haslam

I have always been a firm believer in walking to the beat of my own drum, even at an early age. For me, that meant leaving home at twenty, packing my dad's hockey bag, and moving across the country to explore and see more of Canada on my own and create my own life from scratch.

At forty-eight, when I reflect on my life/career, where I went completely right was following my intuition in my decisions regarding what I chose to spend my time on, and what needed to change in order to make me feel my best, and to always speak my truth. My career has changed and morphed in a way throughout the years that has allowed immense growth and learning opportunities for me, from starting out as a Beauty Therapist, moving into Instructor and Directing positions at various schools, helping students create their own business after graduating and finally adding Clinical Hypnotherapy and Coaching in 2015 to the list to help empower women to follow their inner voice.

One of my favorite quotes is "Be the Designer of your own Destiny," and I believe this to be true more now than ever, especially for women. Don't be afraid of growth, change, failure, or breaks in your pursuit of happiness. This is life and all part of the learning process.

My greatest recent accomplishment was travelling to Mexico to empower girls with the skills needed to provide for themselves in the beauty industry. It impacted me in that we all have so much to offer in sharing with other women; the more you share and empower, the more you see others shine. This was a silver lining so far, and I'm looking forward to more opportunities like these in my future!

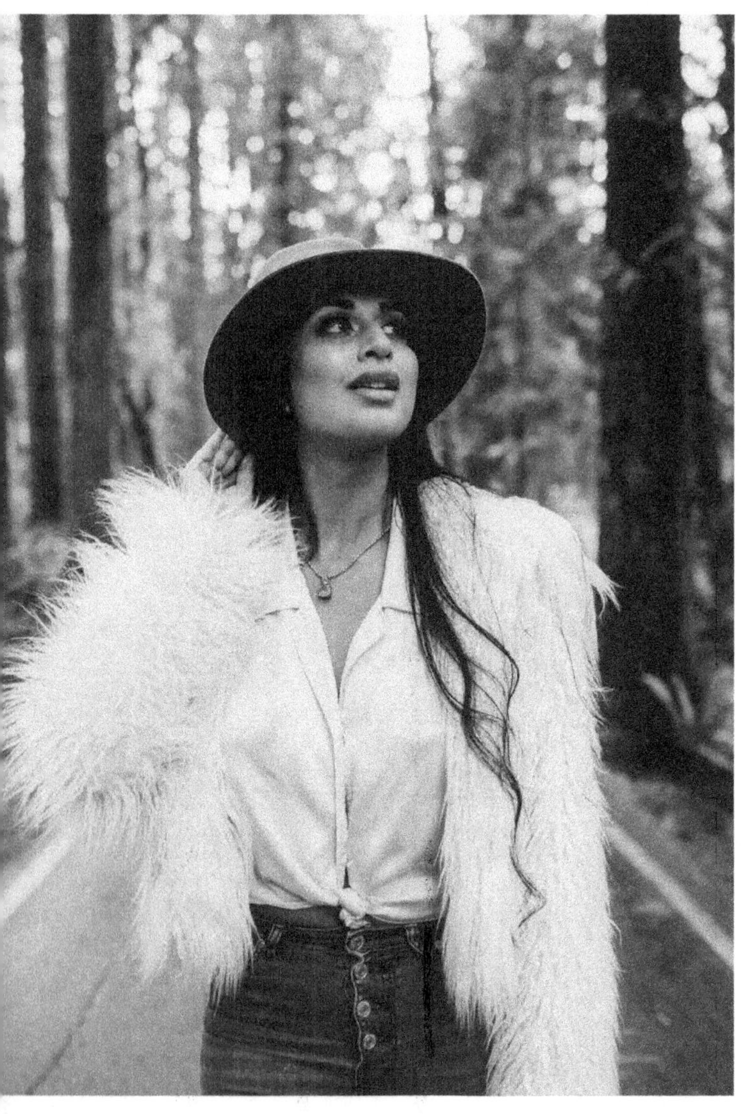

Natasha Raey is a serial entrepreneur and philanthropist who focuses on healthcare, women's empowerment, and medical marijuana. Natasha Raey is also – too much.

Natasha Raey

I know there are people who think I'm too much. I dress up too much. I'm too opinionated. I do too much; and I think there are a lot of women who feel the same way as me. Luckily, many of you also happen to be friends with me or have a friend like me that takes up a vibrant space in your world.

As women, we need to push back. We always have the choice to go with the flow, be more regular, dress like everyone else, live your life trajectory like everyone else; but is that really what you want? I'm in my late 30s, and I've had my fair share of failed relationships that brought me now to my forever person. I have entered and exited a number of career paths [lobbyist, model, Executive Director, researcher, fund developer, event planner, journalist – you get the idea] and now feel most fulfilled as a serial entrepreneur who creates and executes on business ideas. Some fail miserably, and some do really well... but that's where having an appetite to take big risks comes in.

I didn't follow a conventional path in my life. I said no to every man who proposed to me and decided fairly young that I didn't want children. I refused to settle down into a regular job, and every time the opportunity to move or visit another city or country was presented to me, I took it.

I believe so much in the power of manifestation. I don't believe in acting small because others get uncomfortable when your light shines bright. I believe in helping other people brighten their light, and I'll shine mine on yours for as long as you need it.

So the next time someone tells you you're "too much," just smile and say, "Thank you." Because it's okay to be too much. We need more women to be too much.

Jane Stoller is a Swiss-Canadian life-biz organizer whose passion is in decluttering spaces and organizing business processes. She draws inspiration from Benjamin Franklin's words, "For every minute spent organizing, an hour is earned" as she shares her passion with her clients and community.

Jane Stoller

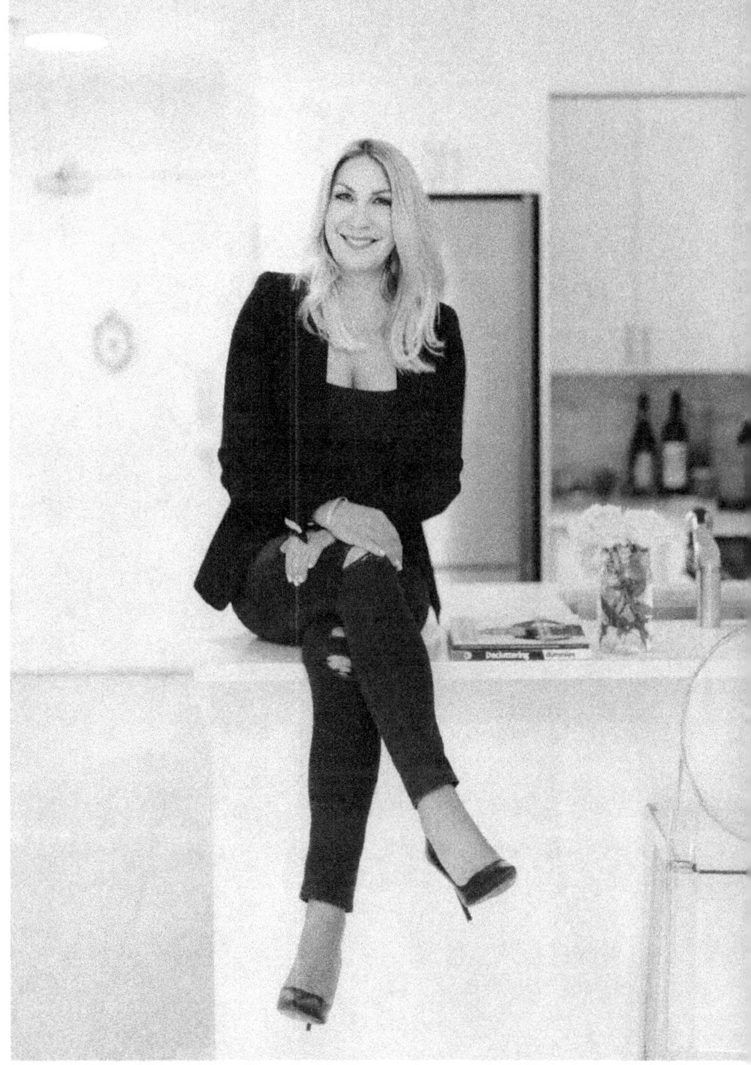

Not only am I a compulsive organizer, but I truly believe the more productive and focused we are, the more time we have to make the world a better place.

Raised on a farm in a small town in Ontario, I manifested tiny, tidy tendencies: lining up my pet cats in order of size, stacking my books by publication date, and creating a colorful bed-top spectrum out of my stuffed animals. As I continued developing my organizing passion through school, I was stuck on what society's image of success looked like. I was terrified to market myself as an organizer. I went on to work in the corporate world of the construction industry, and during this time I did attempt to start my organizing business, the very same business I have now, but failed.

It was 2007, before the lifestyle blogger era. I got advice from people I thought were great corporate mentors, but they told me the only reason I should do this business was if I wanted a husband, or if I was fired. Worst advice ever. Looking back now, I cringe — if I had the support that is available today, I would not have failed, and my business would be ten years old and ten times bigger!

I am grateful for the experience I got in the corporate world, but my true passion is helping women get organized and scale their own businesses. A few years ago, I finally took the leap of faith and started my business, Organized Jane, full-time. I share this openly, hoping that others will learn from my mistakes. And that is my biggest lesson from failure; share authentically so others can learn, and I can learn from others who do the same.

Take it from me: Whether your passion is a side hustle, a full-time business, an idea for a business, or even a hobby, never discount its value, or think it isn't worthwhile.

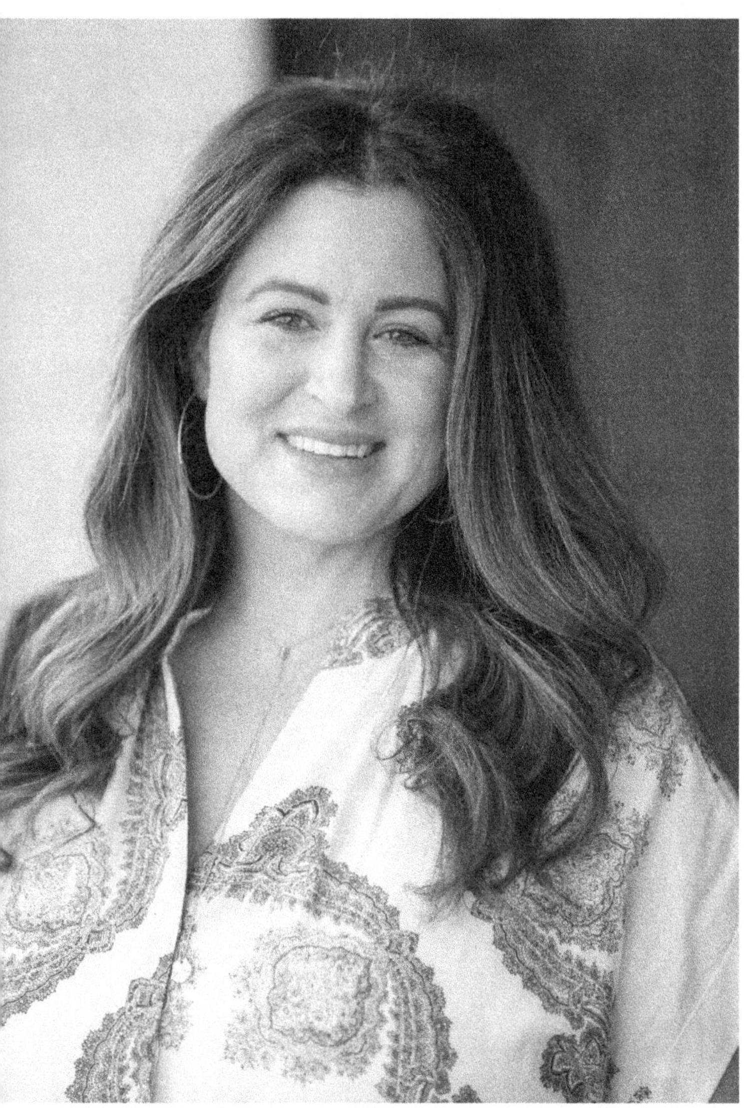
Photo Credit: CBR photography

Jessica Marola-Hugh is a bi-lingual Christian entrepreneur with a passion for holistic marketing, nature's science, and eco-tourism.

Jessica Marola-Hugh

I was born in South Africa. Growing up, my parents' values were established through loving biblical principles that I cherish. I was always a determined child. I absolutely loved to explore, the opportunity to test boundaries without fear of the consequences was a passion of mine. I honestly HATED any box; the idea that I needed to fit a mold elicited total rebellion. In school, I found it hard to adjust, often the class clown or the wild independent thinker, my classmates either teased or avoided me due to my peculiarities. I wasn't part of any winning team, aside from my own, and without the right mentors, I pursued career choices that weren't in line with my gifts or interests.

Leaving school feeling quite defeated, I took a few college courses, then dropped out to get a "real job," or so they said. The glorified nine-to-five was such a bore. I felt each moment spent behind a cash register was a loss to my soul. Something wasn't quite right, and I began a spiral into depression. After a few poor relationship choices, and surprise of motherhood at twenty, things turned. I realized that my son was going to be a massive responsibility and would require a great deal of tenacity. I also knew absolutely nothing about life. My husband and I were eventually married, and over the next ten years, I held a series of corporate roles and welcomed two more children. Then I was offered a marketing internship. I dove right in.

I've never looked back. I continued to work full-time, building out my marketing skills, taking online courses, learning from industry leaders, while also raising three boys with a disabled spouse. I was never more exhausted or worried about what tomorrow would look like, but I believed I could. And I did.

I recently welcomed a little girl, who just turned one this past December, and she is the absolute completion of our little family. I owe this journey to my faith. It has taught me some valuable lessons in perseverance, compassion, forgiveness, grace, priorities, wisdom, and so much more. I'm so very grateful I've had it to lean on with every win and every failure. It's honestly helped me to be a better person, mother, and spouse.

Elisa Kurylowicz is a body image and self-love coach, an awareness mindset specialist, a podcast host, and a former Canadian National Team Athlete (2x National Champion + World Cup Gold medalist) in the sport of freestyle mogul skiing.

Elisa Kurylowicz

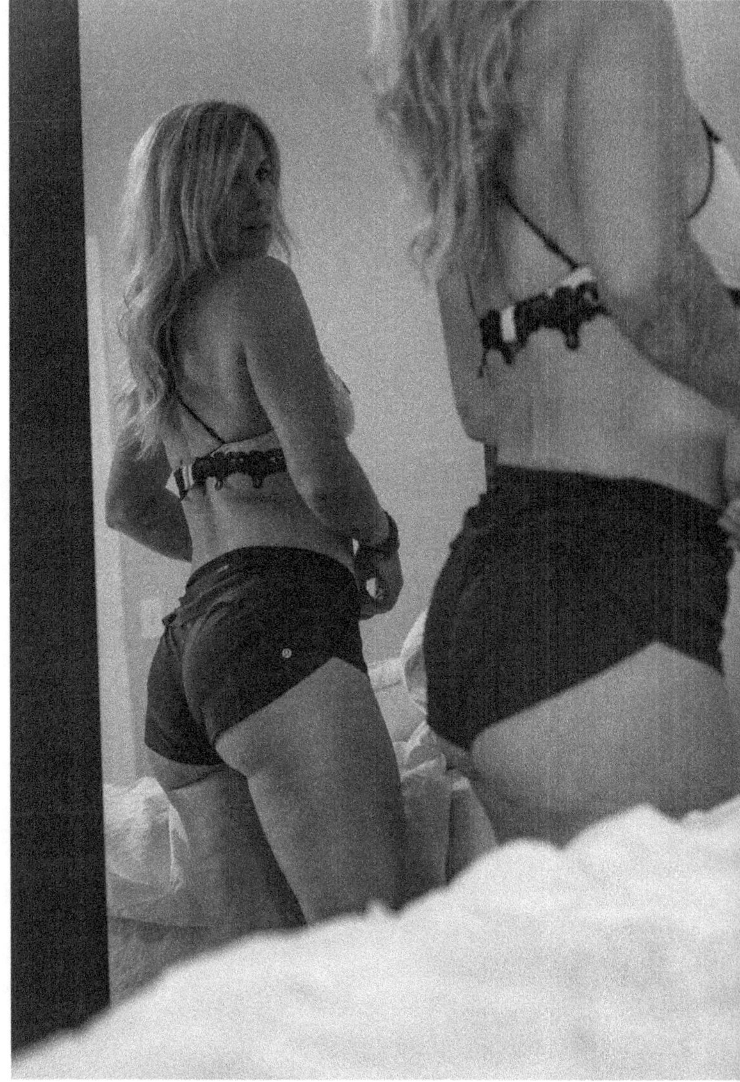
Photo Credit: Els Durnford

Throughout my adult life, I have said thousands of mean, degrading, and inappropriate insults to myself about my body. My thoughts about how I should look were dominant and came to me as routinely as brushing my teeth. I have lived in a 145lbs, World Cup athlete's body, a 235lb, unhealthy, depressed body, and many versions in between. No matter what version, I was never enough. Not only that, but most of my accomplishments also lived in the shadows of these beliefs and were never fully celebrated.

I divorced a toxic man.
I started my own business.
I ran 7 marathons.
I travelled the world alone.
I learned to cook...

All of these things I undervalued because of the way I looked with thoughts such as, *"this would be so much better if I was thinner,"* or, *"I would be so much happier if I weighed less."* You see, I didn't know that I was under the spell of diet culture conditioning. I didn't know how deep its roots were intertwined in practically all of my beliefs. I didn't know. That was until I woke up. Now I know.

Now I know how much pressure I put on myself thinking a size six would make me better. I'm a size ten, and I'm gorgeous. Period. Now I know how many times I saw my cellulite, rolls, loose skin, hairy legs, toes, and upper lip as imperfections. The world does not have the right to tell me what is perfect. My body is none of your business. Now I know the impact of dropping my food, fitness, and fatphobic obsessions and how this has allowed me to step up and show up for who I truly am. And now I know who I am. Now I know the world doesn't have the right to tell me who I am. My body is not a measurement of my worth. Not now. Not ever. This is my pursuit of happiness.

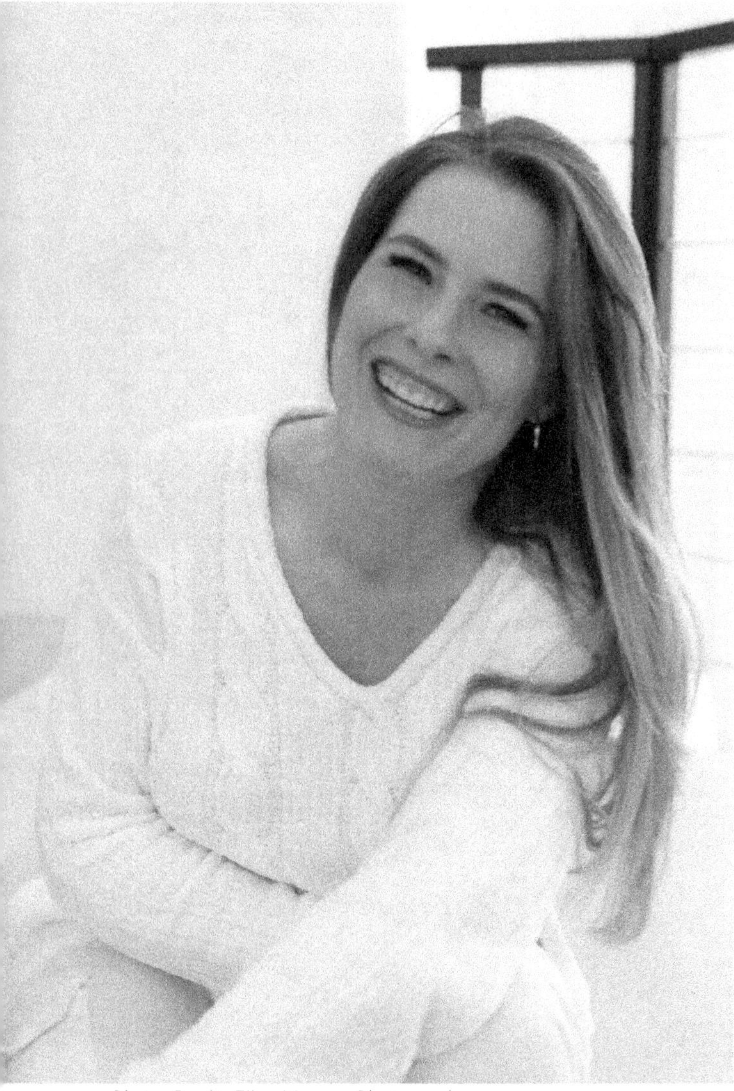

Photo Credit: Ellen Nguyen Photography

Good God! I'm Gay!
Saying It Out Loud To The Biggest Influence In My Life

Holly Skyy

You would be surprised to discover that past Holly's bright blue eyes, humour, and easy-going, warm, compassionate demeanour, her journey has been filled with unexpected twists. Vibrant and engaging, Holly has had an interesting career in the Film and Television industry, including serving as an Adjudicator for Miss World Canada and the Inspiring Youth Awards for EveRIAthing Wall of Stars awards, which was presented to youth across Canada. As a humanitarian, she is filled with passion in all she does and who she comes into contact with but is always ready to take a step back for her loved ones.

After nineteen years of marriage, on my own as a single mom, in January of 2015, I would find myself in Portland, Oregon at the Gay Christian Network Conference to connect with other individuals that had walked a similar journey in reconciling their faith with their sexuality.

Never expecting to be face to face with people who would spew out words of condemnation and hate telling my family of LGBTQ+ that God hated us. The infamous Westboro Church. Suddenly in a surreal position that would either make me run in fear or stand strong in my faith, it would be from experiences such as this that I would learn, and I would grow and think back to the story of David and Goliath. This would prompt me to start the writings of my memoir, "Good God! I'm Gay!" with an expected completion of 2021.

Finding myself in the dating world, travelling halfway across the world to Japan, trekking through the jungles of the Philippines, and peering down into the craters of volcanoes, my life would take another unexpected turn; a motor vehicle accident and dealing with a post-concussion brain injury and internal injuries, as well as being a COVID survivor. I believe in living life with authenticity, a generous heart of love, courage, joy, integrity, kindness, and faith.

"I learned that courage was not the absence of fear, but the triumph over it. The brave man is not he who does not feel afraid, but he who conquers that fear" - Nelson Mandela

Mariana is a designer from Rio de Janeiro, Brazil, living in Vancouver since 2016. Before finding her love for jewelry, she experienced many ways to express herself visually. She worked as a visual artist, painter, graphic designer & clothing designer.

Mariana Carneiro

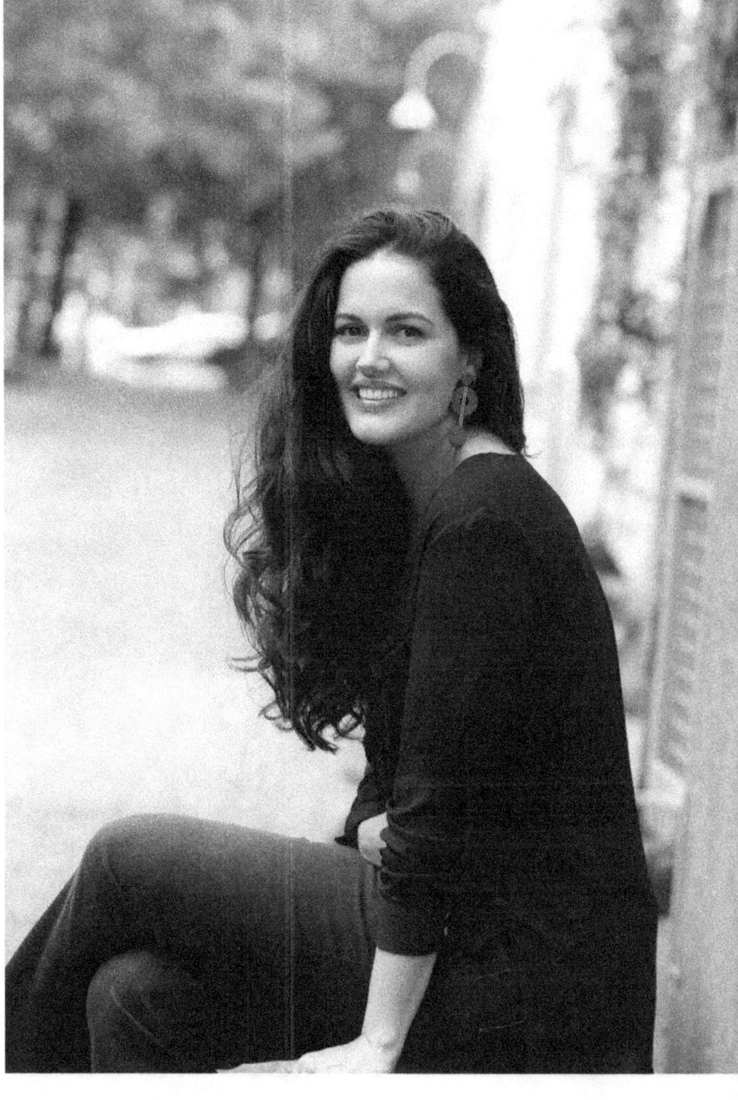

Since a really young age, I have been curious about art, shapes, colours, poems, music, anything that would capture my attention, anything that would make me feel alive. I had so much inside of me to put into the world but didn't know how. Art was my way to go!

At thirteen, I started to paint and was lucky to find an amazing mentor that changed my life!

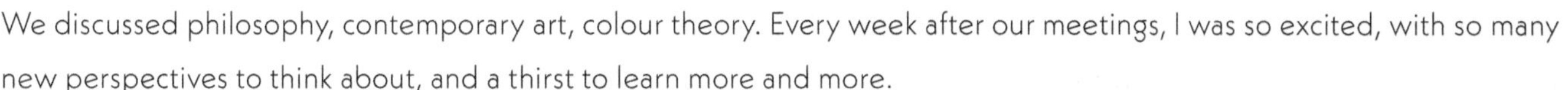

We discussed philosophy, contemporary art, colour theory. Every week after our meetings, I was so excited, with so many new perspectives to think about, and a thirst to learn more and more.

Since then, I knew I needed to be creating! The challenge to learn how to work with new materials and techniques in different areas was, and still is, my fuel. It is what keeps me going every day. To be out of my comfort zone is to know that I am moving forward and learning.

Today, my passion is to bring joy and confidence in the form of jewelry. I would like to think that with my work I can incentivize women to see themselves with different lenses, see themselves powerful, beautiful, bold, and brave.

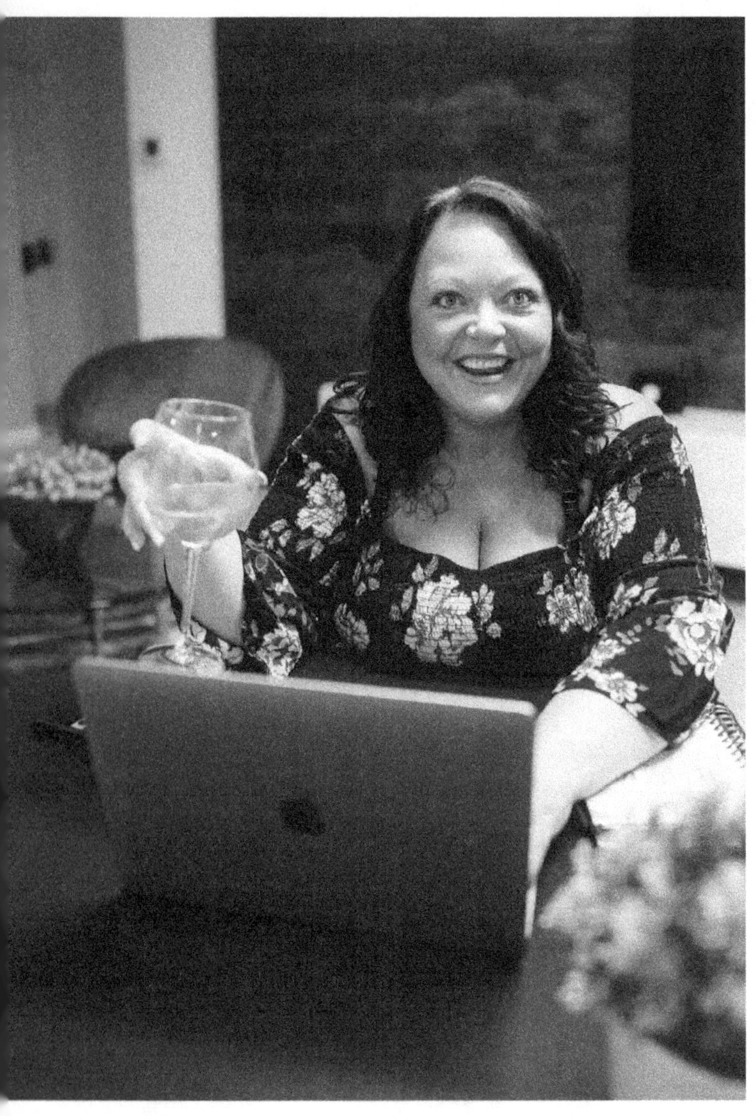

Donica Canova is a network marketing professional who focuses on empowering the people around her through a culture of teamwork.

Donica Canova

I have spent the last five years mentoring and leading a team across Canada, the USA, and Europe. I promote an empowering team culture that inspires women to live their best lives. By encouraging them to seek out and understand their core values, passion, and purpose in life through self-development, self-care, and goal-setting techniques, they experience a shift in their mindset and gain an understanding of the power of positive thinking. Once someone has the right mindset, they will see that they are capable of living life on their own terms and that anything is possible.

It was through taking a good look at myself that I realized it wasn't time freedom or financial freedom that made me truly happy. Those were things that people told me would make me happy, and although it provided me with an exceptional income and time freedom, I was still lacking my true purpose in life.

It is my mission to impact and inspire us all to give more and practice gratitude in our daily lives. The goal is to have us come together and be part of something bigger, where together we can truly change the world and make an impact while we are here.

Change is possible, and every day we have the ability to create change within ourselves. It starts with knowing who you are, why you were born and knowing what your goals and dreams are, and then taking action. Knowing what you need to do and taking the action steps to create success, happiness, and live within your true purpose.

My greatest joy has always been in helping others. One change challenge came about when I realized that people truly want to help where they can, but they can't always see the big picture of how their contribution is having an impact on the world. When you become part of something bigger than you ever dreamed of and realize that you can make an impact, you start to realize the power of working together, and the impact that we can achieve together.

Listen to your heart, follow your dreams, there is greatness inside of you, and you are just one change away from living the life of your dreams.

Tori Dolmans is a passionate advocate and licensed Independent Mortgage Broker with Mortgage Architects as Mortgage By Tori

Tori Dolmans

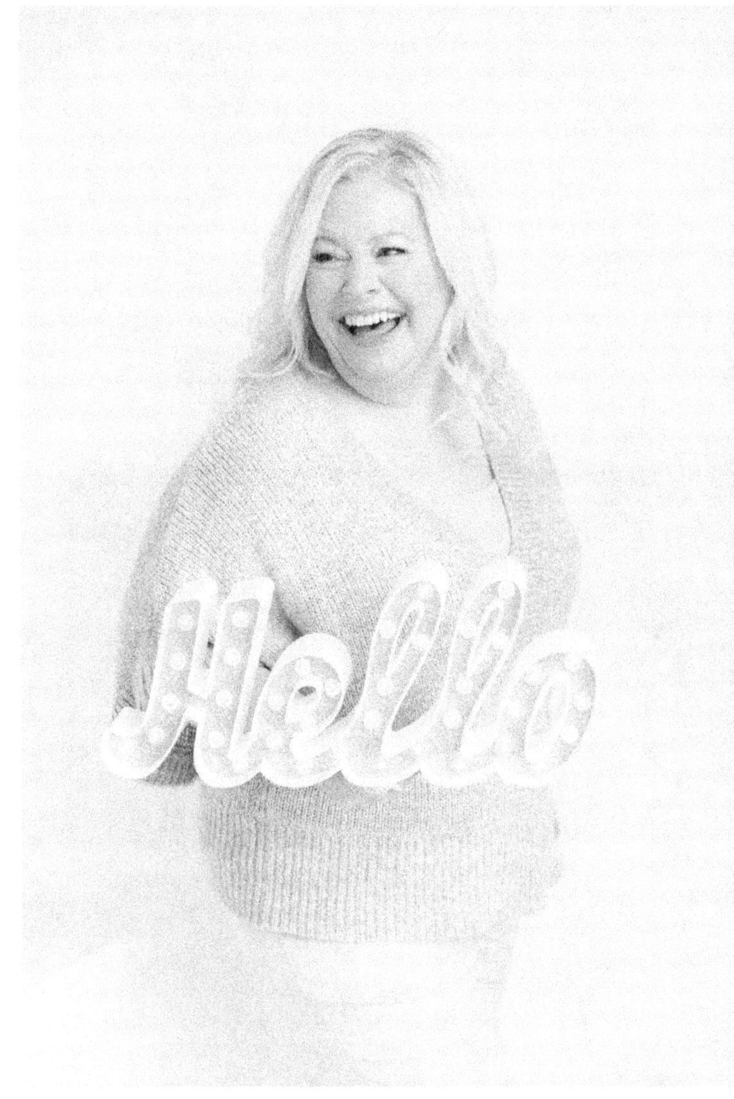

All I've ever wanted to do is help people. And after spending fifteen years in banking, where our job is to put people in boxes and treat them a certain way due to a few numbers on paper, I got frustrated that I couldn't do more to help.

No two people or situations are the same, and as someone who's never been "cookie-cutter" herself, I saw the need to go out on my own where I'd be able to get to know my clients as humans with a story to tell. This means I can give them options that fit their lifestyle and shine a light on the truth which ultimately leads to helping bring their dreams to life - cheesy but true!

I learned all the important lessons in life from my mom, my hero. Strength, self-worth, self-love, and resilience... and one of the most important: intuition.

When I reflect on my career, where I went completely right was in learning to trust my gut and leaning into what my intuition was telling me was the right path. Jumping ship from a salaried job when my kids were one and three was obviously a risky move, but I knew what I had to do. I craved connection in my work and to feel like I was actually making a difference.

Today, everything I do is guided by my PINK Principle...

Proactive - I'm always thinking ahead for you on how we can reach all your goals, not just the immediate ones. I'm in this for the long-haul and there's always more for you on this journey with me when you want it.

Investment - I'm investing my time, energy, and expertise into our relationship but most importantly, investing in your dreams. Your dreams are now my dreams.

No Judgement - I'm your advocate, your cheerleader, your supporter, and your friend. You'll always be made to feel safe, comfortable, and unpressured. Show up as you are.

Knowledge - I want to make mortgages easy for people. I seek to educate, share my expertise, and add as much value to your life as I possibly can.

I use this to guide my work, empower my clients and create a lasting legacy.

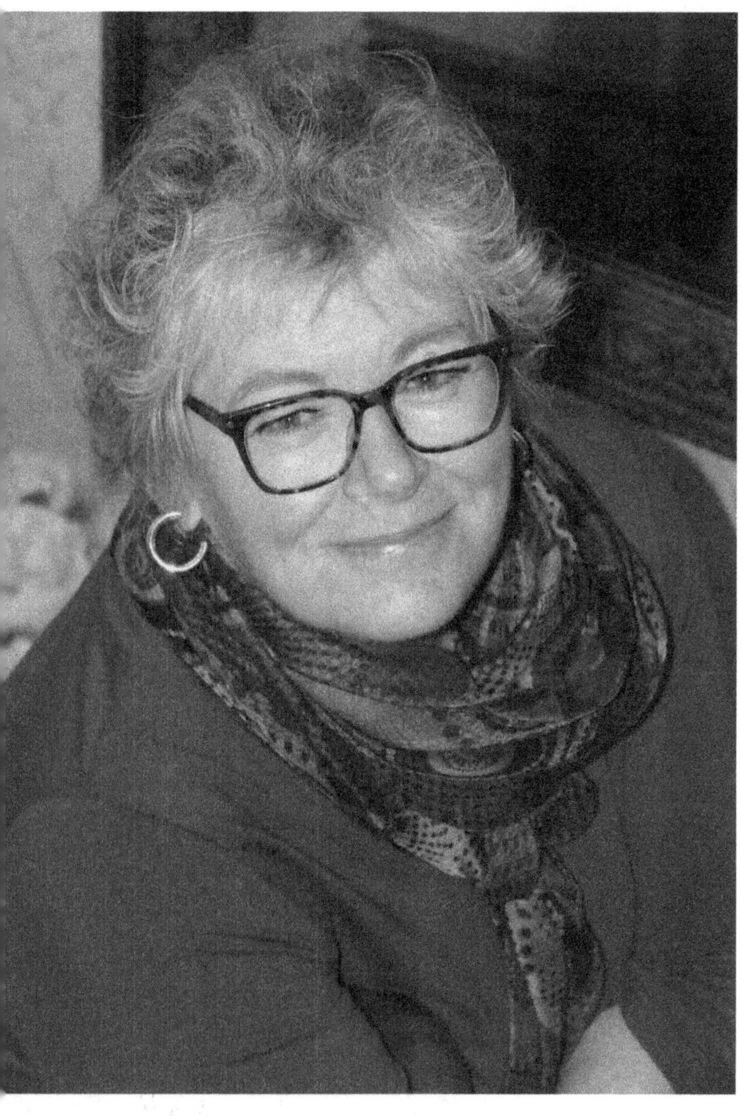

Kimberley Payne is a thought leader, a volunteer, and loves to lift others up.

Kimberley Payne

'This too shall pass.' 'Whatever doesn't kill you makes you stronger.' 'God never gives you more than you can handle.' These are phrases that shaped my life. They were the structure, the glue that seemed to hold it all together. A good friend once told me that she had never known anyone who had reinvented herself so many times, managing to rise above the adversities of life. The one phrase I use when life is challenging: there is always another way. Oh, and proceed until apprehended!

I grew up in a very violent home, a place with little love or affection. Punches or lashes with the belt were commonplace; hugs were things I shared with the dog. I promised myself my children would always know they were loved. The one thing I wanted from life was to not be like my mother. She never protected us; she always put her needs first. I knew there was another way. I watched Little House on the Prairie, and I saw love and hope, and I was determined to have that in my life.

Two failed marriages gave me five incredible kids. They also gave me resilience and determination. I discovered there was always another way through, and I relentlessly forged my way through one disaster after another. I have used food banks, had my hydro and telephone cut off. Raising a large family primarily on my own was hard, busy, and primarily, rewarding.

Volunteering and community became essential to me. The more I gave, the more I received, literally. District Commissioner with Girl Guides, secretary for two minor soccer leagues, chair of the local cooperative nursery school, all because I wanted to be engaged in my children's lives, and that led to a love for community that identifies me to this day. I was not my mother; I found another way.

I love lifting people up, especially women. I have been the leader of organizations that invest in the local community for over thirty years both professionally and as a volunteer. I actively seek ways to improve lives, to build a safer, more caring community. As difficult as things may seem, there always is another way.

Katie Fuller is an entrepreneur and the owner of the Fox and Hound Canine Retreat.

Katie Fuller

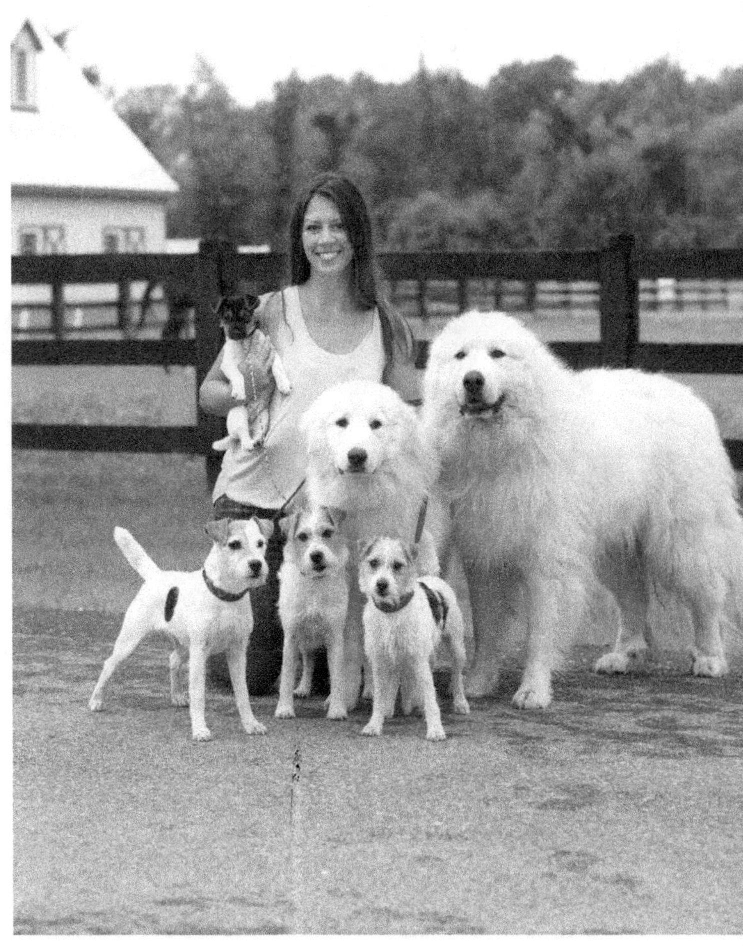

Do what you love, and the rest will follow! As an entrepreneur, mother of two, dog mom of nine, employer, and owner of the Fox & Hound Canine Retreat, I grew up surrounded by dad's foxhounds and Jack Russell terriers. My involvement with Dad's kennel, dogs, and trials established my life's dream of working with dogs. Combining my knowledge of dogs with a passion for their well-being allowed me to create a healthy and authentic lifestyle, abundant in meaningful work and joy!

At nineteen, I opened my first grooming salon in my hometown of Arkona, Ontario. In 2003, I began a career in pet nutrition with an international company, travelling throughout North America. During those years, I worked with industry leaders, veterinarians, breeders, world-class trainers, and even sled dog mushers. Travelling allowed me to visit hundreds of boarding facilities. In 2011, life changed with the arrival of my daughter and then my son in 2012. With two small children at home, travelling came to an end, so I began to design my own facility, putting lifelong dreams into motion. The Fox and Hound, named as a compliment to my dad, became a reality that allowed me to work from home and be with my children.

Opening January 2015, The Fox and Hound was a facility that provided overnight accommodations, daycare, grooming, training, and retail. Putting myself in the mindset of nervous dog parents aided me in creating something dog parents would feel good about.

During the first three years, growth was quick and challenging. By 2017, assistance was required, and the hunt for a manager began. With guidance from Fraser Perry of the Sarnia-Lambton Economic Partnership, Kelly, the most perfect manager, was installed at the F&H. She recognized a need for team management and began to delegate roles, creating success and a positive culture. Lessons learned include, find people you can trust, who have faith in your ideas, and can help bring them to fruition. Hire slowly, adding new staff to the team while supporting the current team members until balance is achieved.

I have built a life doing what I love and hope to share this with others.

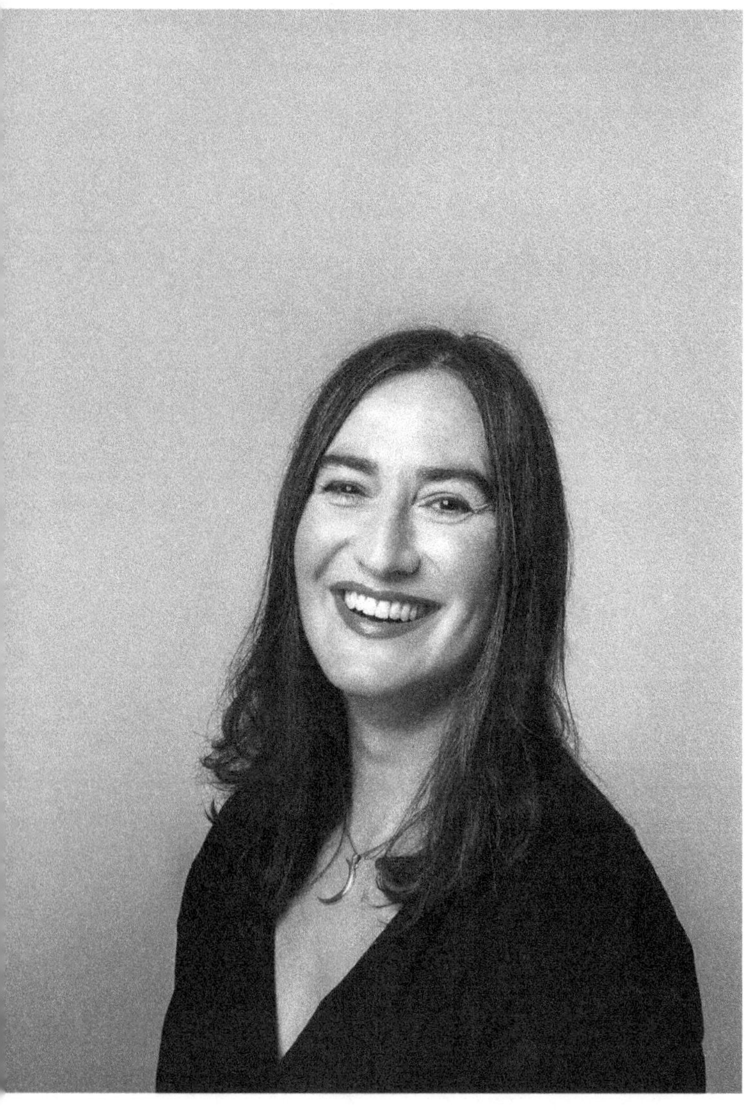

Chrissie Bettencourt is a Digital Business Strategist, writer, and changemaker.

Chrissie Bettencourt

If there is one sentence that people often use to describe me it is, "a force for change," both personally and professionally. I believe that change is a key driver for helping us step into our highest potential, and this belief is something that I use to create an authentic life.

Eighteen years ago, I had one of those "dark nights of the soul" when I realized I had built a life around others' expectations of me rather than one based on who I truly was. It was a turning point and the beginning of a long journey back to myself. I ended up leaving that life and began building a new one, beginning a deep inner journey that helped me heal and become more connected with my inner self. Then one day, I realized my inner world no longer reflected my outer world. A change was required. So, I quit my unfulfilling job, sold all my belongings, and bought a one-way ticket to South America. I had no idea what I would do when I got there and knew absolutely no one, yet it was one of the best decisions I have ever made. What I thought would probably be a few months turned into twelve years with zero regrets.

This experience taught me the importance of being true to oneself and making decisions that reflect that. I still see so much fear around stepping outside of the box and the life "blueprints" others expect us to follow. Especially as women, the expectations layered on us are immense. Yet, the risk of not stepping outside that box, to me, is even greater. If we don't, we will never discover our potential, what is true for us, and who we were meant to be.

I am now using my "changemaker" skills to teach organizations how digital and agile concepts can create a positive impact both externally and internally, as well as a thriving environment for its people. I am also writing a book to help individuals move through their own journeys of change, transformation, and empowerment.

What is the biggest impact I think we can all make? Stop fearing our power and embrace it.

Cheryl Bodnar's art is her therapy and passion.

Cheryl Bodnar

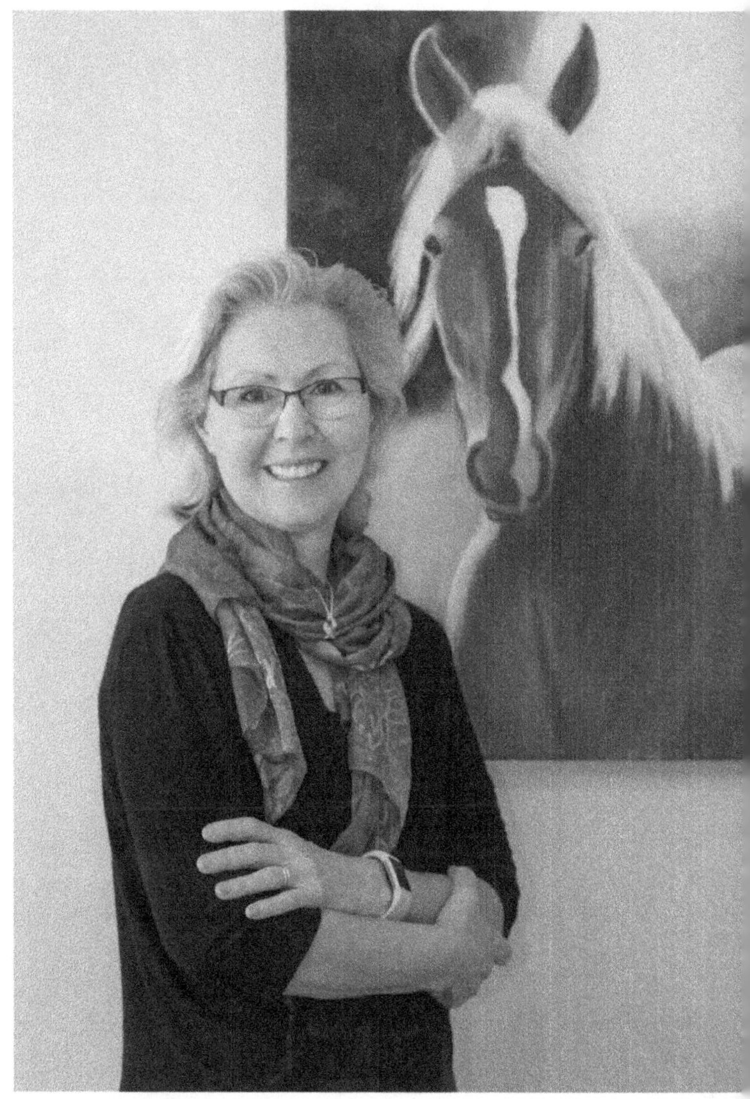

I am an Artist. I live with my husband and together we have two grown children. My family are my cheerleaders, and the most important people in my life and I am the cheerleader in their lives.

I am a culmination of my mistakes, my experiences, and my achievements. My life has had its ups and downs like everyone else's. As a child I was very shy and uncertain of myself. I have had low periods of time in my life and had suffered some trauma and depression. Being an Educated Professional for 40years gave me great confidence. As an Intensive Care Unit Nurse, I worked with tragedy, sorrow, and pain.

There was also great joy when our clients returned to health, but not all people got well. Bearing witness to that carried a heavy emotional burden and a particular kind of stress. With deliberate and mindful changes, I began a Spiritual Journey for the past 30 years.

Lifelong learning is paramount to my happiness. It is through continual learning, self-awareness and personal change that I was able to heal and grow. I am a serious soul –perhaps an old soul. Becoming who we want to be requires good choices.

My art has provided me with serenity and healing throughout my years. There is a peace and tranquility when I am in my studio. Art is therapy for maintaining inner calm. When I worked on the painting Teagan, the horse pictured here, I felt like I became one with her, like she was standing right in front of me. I could smell her and feel her calm. Time becomes suspended! Emotions become balanced through creativity. I am incredibly grateful that I have pursued my craft and worked hard at reaching my goals.

Trust in the process .... in art ...as in life. We all have our own unique creativity. Nothing happens or improves overnight—it all takes time, effort, and intentional deep inner soul searching and work.
I wish that you find your passions – find your happy, your joy, your love, your creativity, and a bit of good madness.

I support these Societies: ALS Society, Covenant House, and the LGBTQ Community.

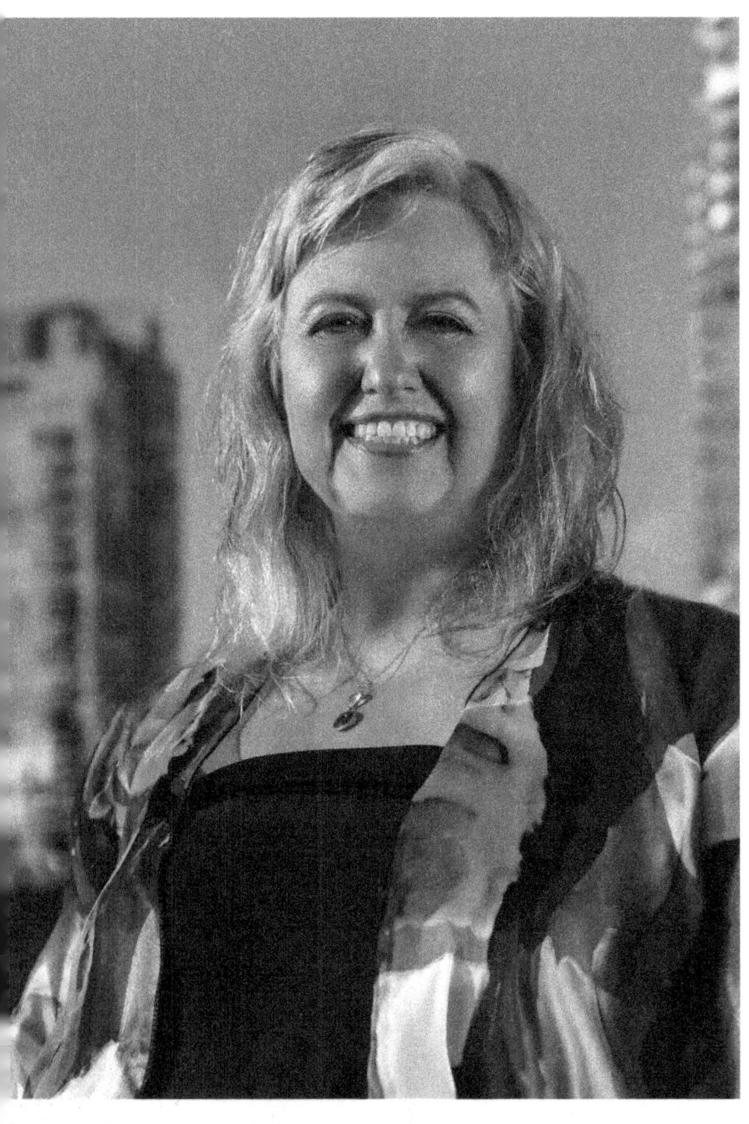

Lauren Labas is an opportunity-creator, a marketing savant, and is a perpetual ray of sunshine.

Lauren Labas

After fifteen years of marketing large corporate investment projects, in late 2019, it was time to source a new project, and I wanted it to be exciting. I could feel my life taking a shift. Yearning to market something I was passionate about - something adventurous and fun.

Having grown up in the touristic Okanagan region of BC, I fell in love with its beauty all over again visiting Penticton the last few summers with my girlfriends. Scenic, sandy beaches, a winery every 400 feet with stunning patio lake vistas, were what attracted us to this region. The problem was, we never had enough time to visit where we wanted to go and did not even touch what this region had to offer. The more we saw, the more we knew we had to experience.

Knowing it's about making connections and relationships; I organized a large tradeshow to bring the Okanagan to Vancouver! A place of connection, joy, and festival. To bond with the exhibitors, I bought, outfitted, and set out with my new RV digital remote office hub! I wanted to create, experience, and define a vision for my audience.

Then a pandemic! My Vancouver wine festival could not happen in 2020, but my website established me on the ground in the Okanagan with Vancouver VIPs having questions on how to connect with the Okanagan and the Island – time to push forward and develop something new. This challenge excited me.

On my first trip out with my RV, I decided to enjoy the summer on beautiful Skaha Lake, BC. It was one of the best summers I have had in a long time. Stepped back from the city, I bought a smart hub for wireless, and developed websites from the lake!

I recast my vision to be www.bcwineworld.com, and hired a wonderful new friend and International Champagne Judge to help work with wineries and hopefully become a new business partner.

In this shift I found myself selling my rental property and buying a lot on Naramata Bench, BC.
Wanting to share my vision, I am creating a three-bedroom suite for short-term rentals as an adventure vacation in wine country, designed in a Tuscany style and a swim spa to relax watching the sunsets over the lake. If you love wine, join our VIP club and experience wine with us.

Tanya Slingsby is a daughter, an artist, a woman, and a mother.

Tanya Slingsby

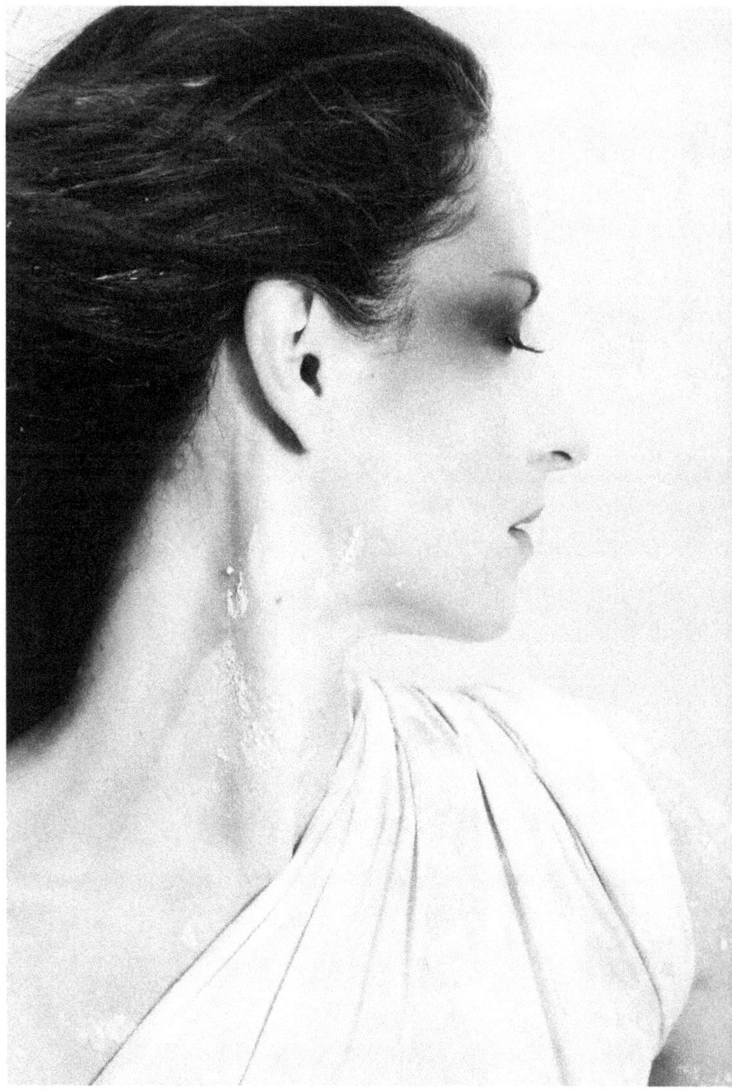
Photo Credit: Darko Sikman, Film Still from SHORU exhibit Vancouver, BC.

My identity shifts — daughter, artist, woman, mother — each inform the other, pushing my exploration of nature and the sublime to glean experiences of our collective identity. I'm all too aware that time won't wait for me. With intense post-secondary and graduate studies abroad, my academic training acted as a barrier to my early art practice. As a result, I painted only occasionally until my mid-twenties.

When my mother died from cancer in her late forties, I was shocked into realizing that I had to live my truth while I could. One night I woke in the small hours and painted a bold abstract canvas.

I walked straight into my fear and remorse, into the catharsis of loss, letting my emotions spill freely into the work. It was this painting that launched my art career.

I title my work in foundational languages such as Sanskrit, Latin, and Arabic because they speak to the universality of human existence and the deep allure of the sacred feminine. My parents raised me in the pristine beauty of Salt Spring Island, BC. They nurtured my fascination with natural spaces and the way light shapes our perspectives. It took losing my mother for me to set aside my formal studies and reconnect to that childhood power of surrendering to natural beauty. Even now, seeing the morning mist clinging to a branch or a blanket of frost-tipped leaves on the ground returns me to that childlike sight, where I can paint unfettered.

Becoming a mother myself challenged my identity as an artist, but it also forced me to change my desire for constant novelty into one for balance, and from there, to connect to my greatest commitments and experiences. The patience and acceptance I've cultivated in my artistic process help me connect with my son. He now teaches me new ways to see.

Within all of this beautiful interplay, I can re-experience the moments my mother gave me. Until motherhood, I could only express these on the canvas. Motherhood embeds, humbles, and inspires me, and so affects my creativity and experiences irrevocably. This identity is the greatest gift.

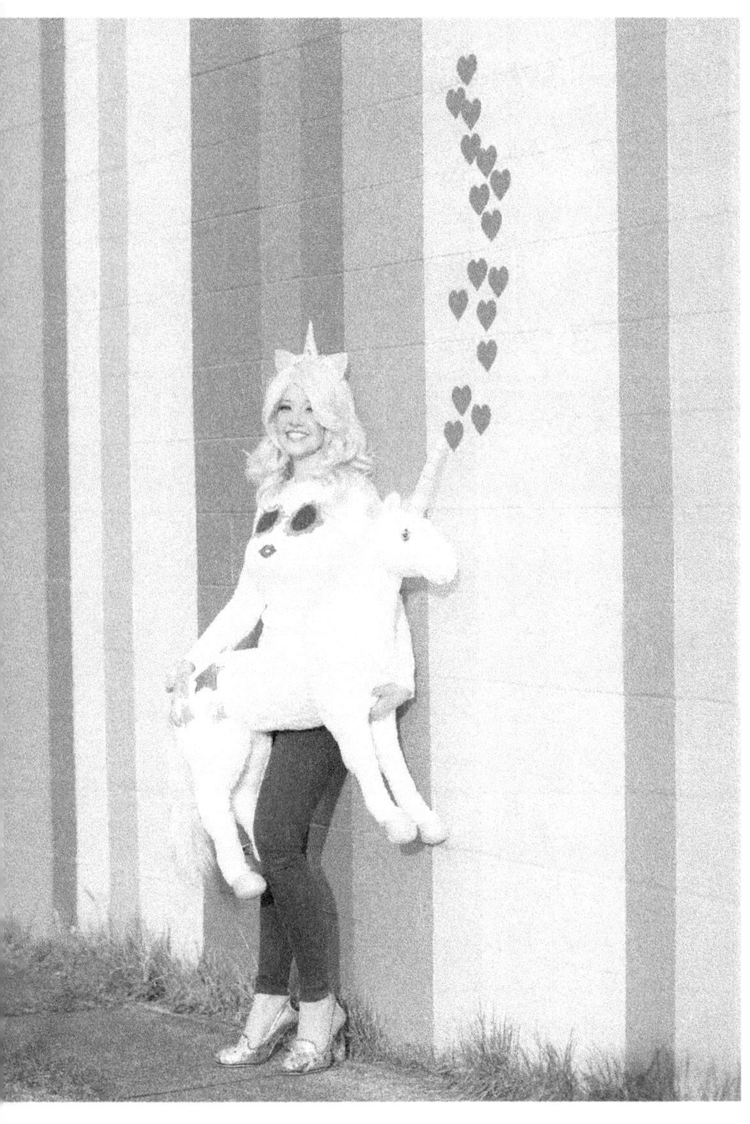

Kyra Wong is a true original and sparkly force of nature on a magical mission to promote unity, equality, and greater humanity. Kyra believes- we are ONE.

Kyra Wong

In my pursuit of happiness and success, my greatest lesson has been to stay true to myself and never let anyone try and tame me. I came into this world a creative free spirit, rambunctious and playful, with no interest in living by the rules. I was the kind of girl with a perpetual twinkle in her eye, who loved to add glitter and charming outrageousness to the lives of the more conventional. Looking back on it now, it's obvious to me I was born with a unicorn nature; untamed, imaginative, and forever seeking a rainbow-coloured escape route towards a life less ordinary.

Unfortunately, growing up, I was raised in an environment where kids obeyed their parents, with no questions asked and even more so if you were female. I was expected to be an obedient member of the herd and dim the sparkle from my unicorn hide to fit in. But I knew I would never find my fairy-tale ending if I settled for a cookie-cutter version of myself to try and please others. So instead, I chose to break the mold and follow my untamed heart with faith, trust, and a little pixie dust. By accepting my uniqueness as a gift and refusing to bend to societal pressures, I've tapped into my superpowers and created a life by design on my own terms.

Today, I'm challenging the status quo as a passionate crusader for unity, equality, and justice, to be a positive force for change in the world. I'm on a mission to help inspire and empower women and other society underdogs so they can reach for the stars and achieve their full potential. I envision a future where we recognize the "oneness" of our humanity, and show up for each other with greater consciousness. As someone who fearlessly glitters outside the lines of convention, I know that anything is possible, and magic happens when we're bold enough to stand in our truth, use our voice, and let our light shine. We can do extraordinary things when we're brave and free, so embrace the person you were born to be... your dreams are counting on you.

Beverley Boone is an award-winning Realtor with an enthusiasm for building community and supporting others.

Beverley Boone

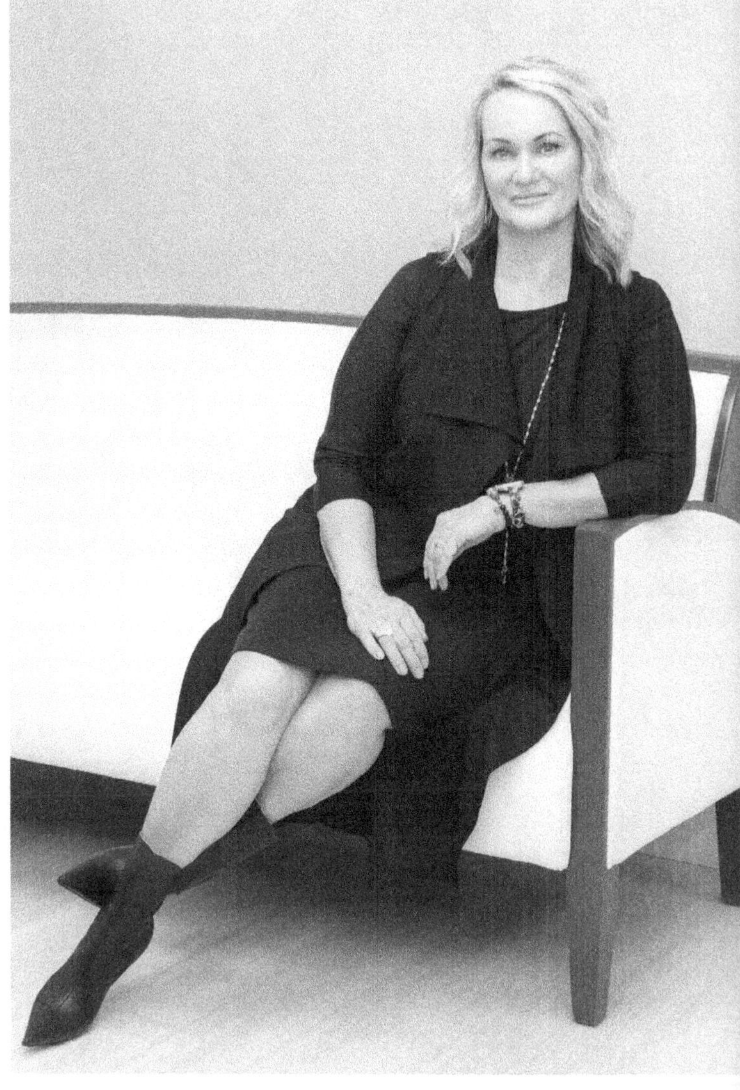

BREATHE – You've got this, Bevie. Just breathe!! That was the daily mantra I repeated while staring out at the lake after moving to Sarnia. Having been married, a mom, divorcing, remarrying, nursing my ill husband, and losing him, I was no stranger to change. I married him knowing he had a life-threatening illness but didn't think I would lose him. I trust I arrived in the right place at the right time to help him prepare to leave this world. Things unfold as they should, even if we are not always aware enough to see them. After his death, starting over again and remaining optimistic seemed overwhelming. Taking that daily moment to just inhale and slowly exhale allowed me to refocus and readjust. Transformation isn't easy, but putting in my best effort during the difficult moments prepared me for all the moments to follow. Tribulations are the real treasures that help us to shape how we face the future.

Having experienced much in fifty-six years, causes me to joke that 'I'm every woman'; the daughter, the mother, the divorcée, the caregiver, the widow, the professional, the friend, and now the fiancée. When someone gifts me with their story, I connect with them in such a personal way because my many experiences coincide with their own. Hence, 'I'm every woman'. My success is based on my ability to relate to others. I aspire to treat everyone I meet with kindness. I am passionate about helping others recognize their talents and apply them.

Four years ago, I established BREATHE, an online sisterhood that was born from my desire to build a positive and supportive community for Sarnia-Lambton women; a place where women can connect, share, motivate each other, and support one another through joy and strife. Currently, the group at one-thousand-plus members strong brings together women from every walk of life. Living my best life means being passionate about others, giving back, and building community. Being a full-time realtor, a makeup artist, and the founder of an online community, I sometimes must remind myself to just BREATHE.

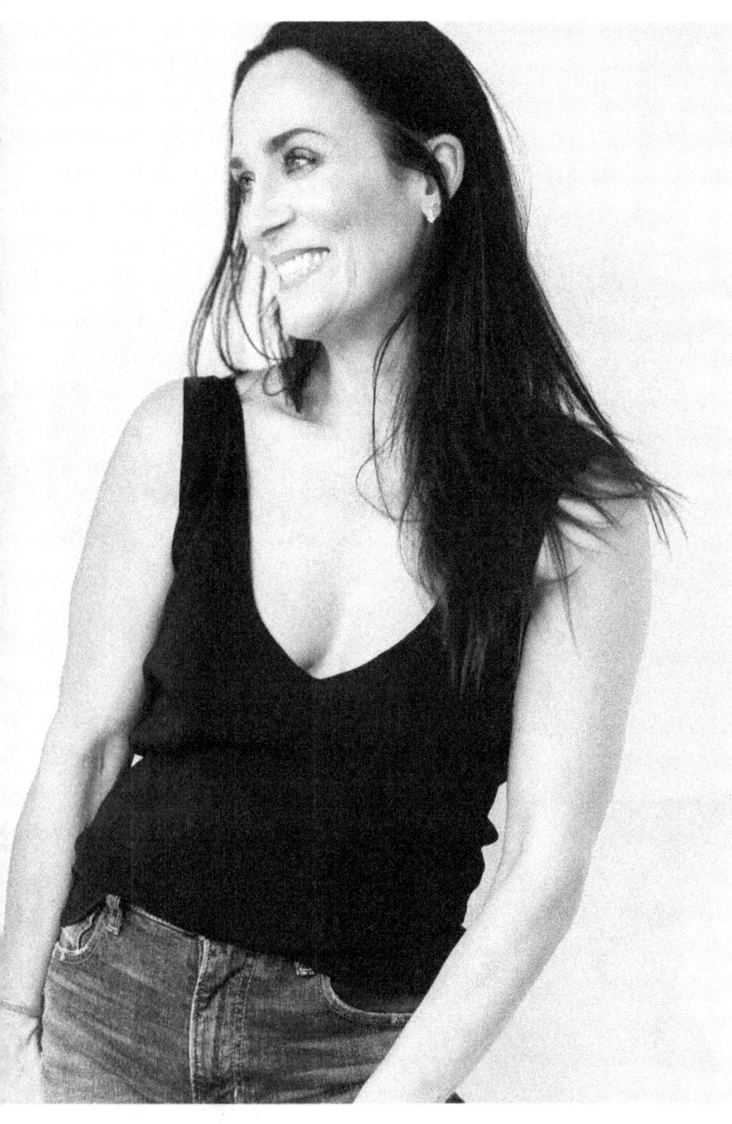

Corinne DiPietro is an artist who celebrates uniqueness, imperfection, and "enough-ness."

Corinne DiPietro

Am I enough? ... I've been haunted by that simple question for as long as I can recall. Once a playful girl who loved to draw, create and animate, I grew into a young woman who somewhere lost this ease, imagination, and freedom. I traded youthful abandon and became trapped by self-consciousness, more concerned with what others' experience of me was over my own. Insecurity turned my appreciation of beauty against me. Was I thin enough, pretty enough, cool enough? I went beyond the typical striving to fit, desire to assimilate, brutalized my body image, and over-accommodated for acceptance. Early coping methods involving food and drink took root and became problems themselves.

On the surface, I was seemingly all together, bold even, but I had buried doubt and lived life avoiding the hole. Opportunely, my facade and skills found a career in makeup artistry. It blended the love of beautification and transformation. I loved it, though, at the end of the day, I still questioned; was I successful and creative enough, let alone intellectual enough? Airs and fears undermined my joy and pursuits. Especially in relationships, I held back, fearing rejection of the real me.

Bravely addressing these emotional questions with self-reflection and personal work, I gained perspective, enough to regain trust in myself. Following my heart, I left my career and country. However, as my rewards got better, my tests felt harder. In a new marriage, blended family, social scene, and role, I considered; am I wife enough, yet still me enough? No longer in the film industry, but fine art, how do I measure success now? As a woman in my fifties, simply aging undermines the "enough-ness"!

It's not easy feeling complete in a world selling expectations and illusions, especially as we exist online with filtered faces and curated feeds. Society's feedback, fabulous or not, isn't as crucial as that of our inner voice. We are all unique, perfectly imperfect, and on our own journey. Coach yourself gently, but confidently. Ultimately, you are the one that says whether you are enough.

Propitiously, when grounded in the feeling that I'm enough, I'm able to be so much more.

Adera Angelucci is a creative entrepreneur who works with women to step out of their comfort zone and lead with confidence.

Adera Angelucci

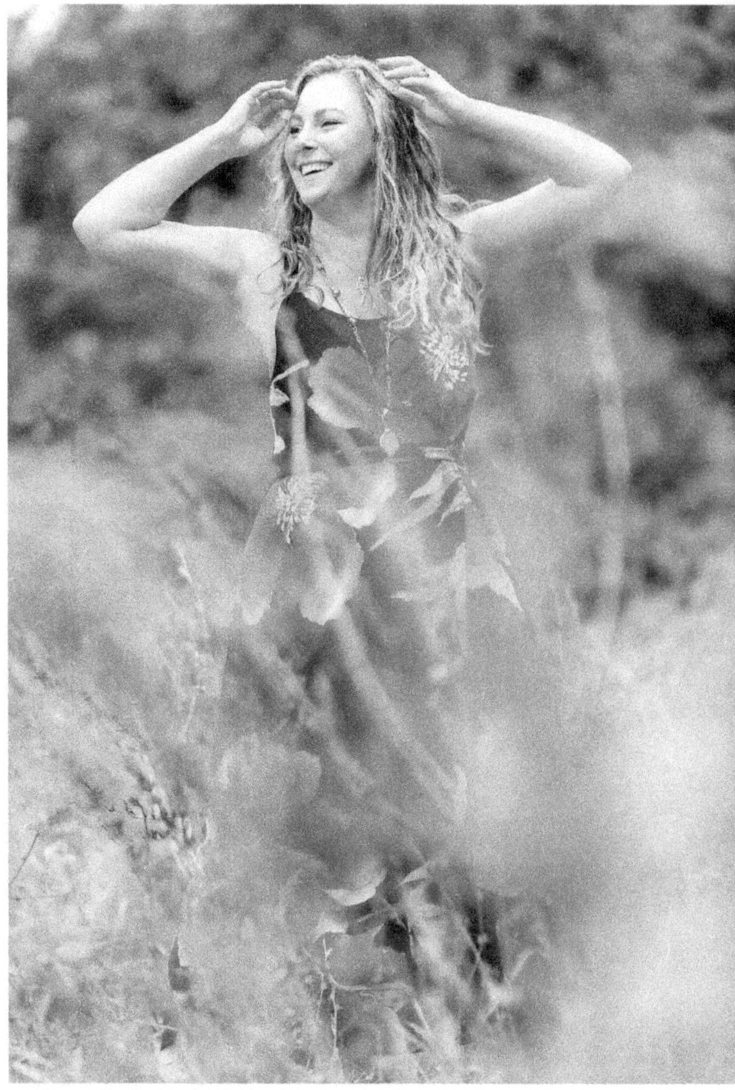

Photo Credit: Linda Mackie Creative

The first time things went horribly sideways for me on stage. I was nineteen, performing with the Vancouver Theatre Sports League. In the heat of the improv, I "gunned" down the other players on stage, leaving me all alone.

Not a smart move when the goal of improv is to play off each other. The lights mercifully went out, and the crowd cheered. I did great! I did not. Backstage, I was told I had destroyed the whole thing.

There were many more disasters.

When I was twenty-seven, I co-hosted the annual talent competition at the PNE fairgrounds with the iconic Red Robinson. The wind kicked up out of nowhere, and my dress flew up around my chest, exposing my underwear to thousands of spectators in the crowd. I must have had an out-of-body experience because I can't remember saying this, but my Mom told me I gracefully flattened my dress back down and said, "Well, I guess you got to see more of me than expected," before swiftly introducing the next act.

With each blunder, I carried on with more and more grace. They taught me I couldn't attach my self-worth to any particular instance. Instead, I saw them as gifts along my journey to find my flavour of happiness and success.

They built my self-trust and confidence.

By taking action (even less than graceful ones) without concern for the results, I lead myself to understand who I was and what I wanted. I gained clarity on my guiding values: freedom and creative expression. I kept altering my course by making new choices guided by this compass. My inner happiness and definition of success have been seeped in muck ups, wrong turns, and failures, each bringing me closer to where I wanted to go.

So, if you are ever in a circumstance that is less than what you imagined, remember your confidence, self-worth and trust are built on mistakes. You don't always stride into success, whatever that may be. Sometimes, you stumble and find a better path.

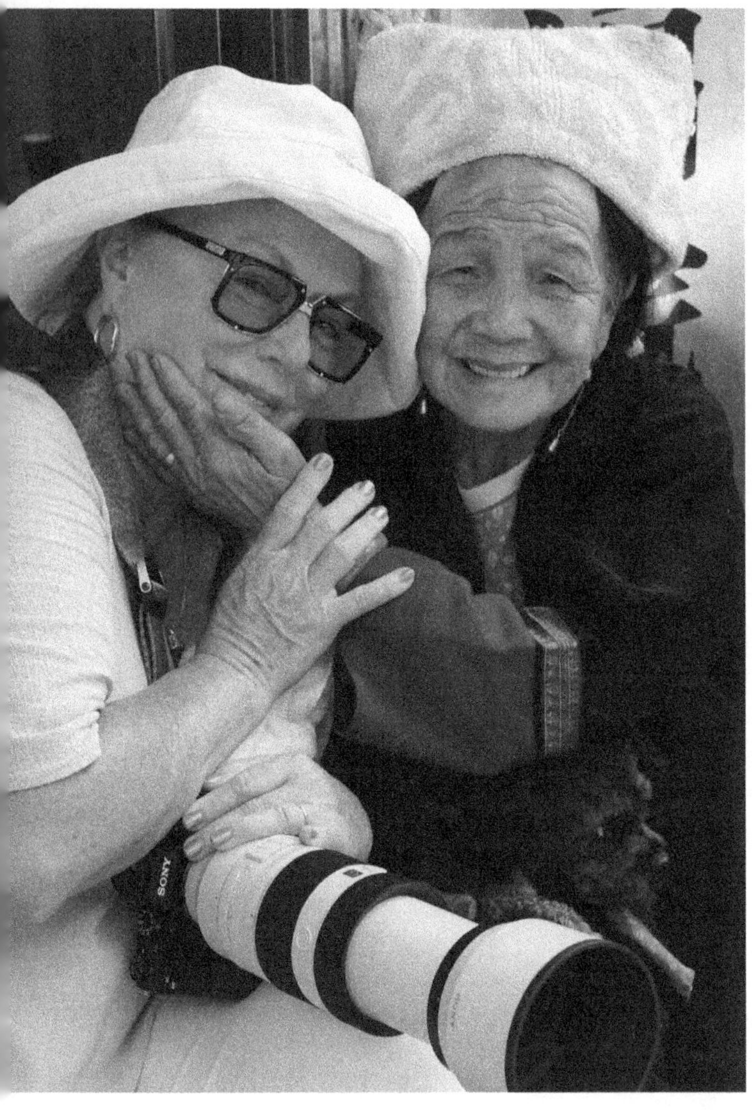

Mary Lynn Fluter is a photographer, a leader, and an artist.

Mary Lynn Fluter

My life has been a kaleidoscope of fractured glass. In my seventy years, there are many shattered pieces, but with every break, the colours of my life have become brighter.

I am the youngest of four with three brothers. When I was born, the angels were either singing 'alleluia' or crossing themselves. My mother was a woman beyond her time, a beacon of inspiration and hope, not only to me but to her community. My gentle father trusted her every move.

Memories, I have aplenty. In my late teens, I was blessed to travel with a singing group called 'UP WITH PEOPLE' throughout Canada, the US, and Mexico. Fanshawe College followed, where I achieved a diploma in Communication. At twenty-two, I was married and started my photography business. The truest pursuit of my personal happiness arrived with the birth of my two amazing sons.

With divorce, the glass fractured. Raising my sons, I kept them close, carrying my camera gear, and away from mischief. With a production company and established presence in Toronto and Los Angeles, they are both a tribute to me and the family. Their TV productions warm the heart of my kaleidoscope of memories.

My own work has been featured in numerous fashion and bridal magazines and displayed in galleries in Toronto and New York. My studio employed five to seven photographers. Returning to Fanshawe to teach advanced portraiture, I mentored numerous photographers who are now established throughout Southwestern Ontario.

Leaving London for Grand Bend, my work evolved into symbolic and transformational art. My photographs found their home in a Gallery in Grand Bend. I am now focusing on large format photographs to be displayed as art in offices and homes. Travelling the world with my husband, I keep him close to me, as he now carries my gear. He is great and loyal support.

My pursuit of happiness has taken me through the happiest and hardest of times: divorce, betrayal, and death. But here's the thing, every time I look through the lens of my camera, I see the beautiful kaleidoscope of my life refracted in the brightest of possible colours. And that is what my pursuit of happiness is all about.

Cheryl Ann Brewster, B.Msc., is a business intuitive, mindset coach, author, speaker, and ordained Minister of Metaphysics, living in West Vancouver, BC, Canada, serving globally.

Cheryl Ann Brewster

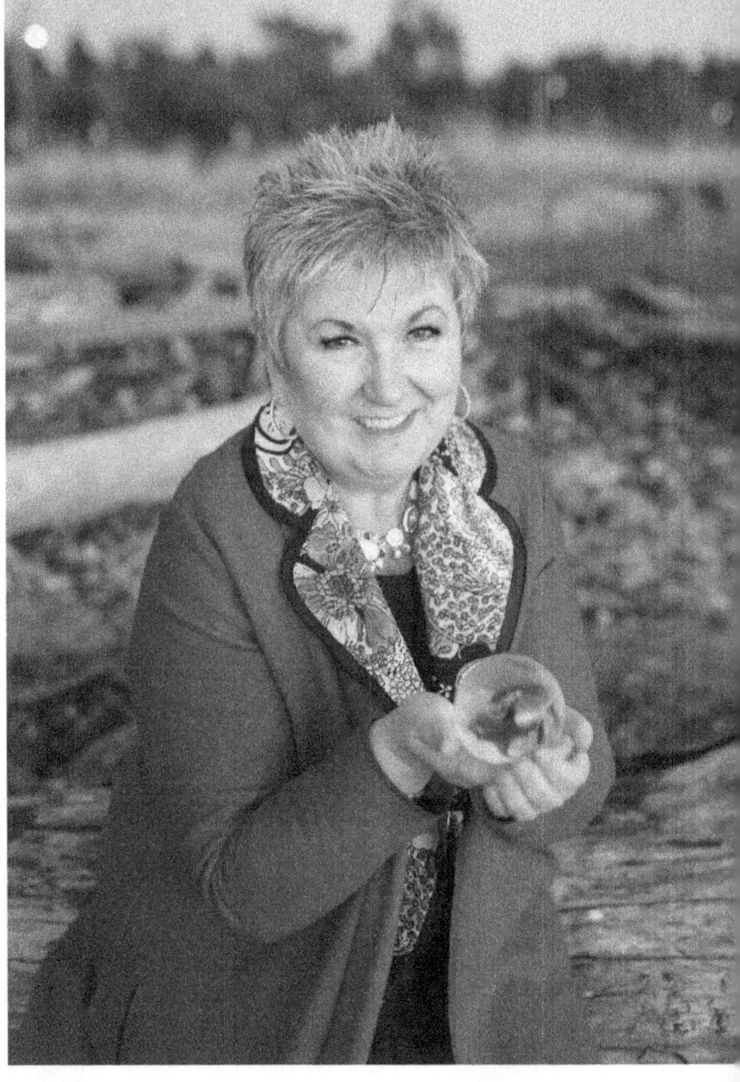

How did you decide your career path?

I didn't - it chose me! My story is one of extraordinary trust. In 2004, I experienced "a calling" to leave a successful position in the corporate world to found The Intuitive Life; a soul-centred business dedicated to developing the ability of both leaders and individuals to be self-directed, and to confidently shape a better future, especially when faced with challenge and uncertainty.

My work with clients heightens their capacity to act swiftly and feel better NOW. The emotional relief of increased clarity nurtures confident decision making, more effective communication, speedy resolution of challenges, and the joy of success that feeds peace, prosperity, and fulfillment.

My services are tailored to each unique client or situation and can include intuitive consultations, coaching, educational programs, and masterminds. I have a passion for joy and celebration and as an ordained Minister of Metaphysics, am licensed to provide spiritual mentoring and officiate weddings, celebrations of life, and other meaningful events.

My work has been shaped by the profound stories of courage and fulfillment that my clients recount from our work together, my own dark nights of the soul, and the many mystical and out of body experiences that are a testament to the exciting possibilities ahead of us. In my soon to be published book "Limitless, the Call to Joy in Life and Business," I describe how "living your joy is the most courageous, important, radical thing you will ever do. It is your gift of service to humanity, the ultimate act of leadership, love, and legacy that births a greater reality and assures a life of no regrets."

We are in the midst of an historic shift in global consciousness, a critical juncture in our personal and collective evolution. Creativity, self-directed leadership and soul-centred community at its deepest, most courageous, compassionate, and authentic level is required. I invite you to a deeper conversation to explore and activate the emerging potentials within. Synchronicity guides and action transforms.

Photo Credit: Kristy Powers Photography

Tracy Donald is an entrepreneur and business owner, helping women find their power.

Tracy Donald

Staring at a pregnancy test stick in a bathroom stall of the local drugstore, I couldn't believe my eyes. At eighteen years of age, I was pregnant for the second time. I had just ended my relationship with the father of my son and had moved in with my grandmother in hopes of finishing my schooling. I was already struggling to finish school with a baby at home. How was I going to finish with two babies? Where there is a will, there is a way. The day that I walked across that graduation stage, diploma in hand, my entire family was able to see what being tenacious can accomplish. At that time, I still worried about how I would support my beautiful babies and give them a life they deserved, and then someone introduced me to the world of direct sales.

Direct sales changed my life. This was a career perfect for a young single mother. I was available for the kids during the hours they needed me, and I could work as hard as I needed to, while they were sleeping or in school. When the kids were small, I hoped I would meet a man, who loved my children as much as I did, but work and two babies kept me busy. While out one evening, I met a wonderful man. Twenty years ago, I married him, and we added a third child to our brood. I felt so blessed. Over the years, I have had four different direct sales businesses. It has sometimes been a feast and sometimes famine, but in my case, mostly a feast.

Belief, our greatest asset, can sometimes wane, so if yours is lacking, borrow someone else's faith. I borrow my husband's belief. I love doing what I do because I relish helping women find their power. As a collaborative leader, I show others how to move forward. I help them find their potential and encourage them to chase their dreams. People often say that I am lucky. I say, "I make my own luck through hard work and helping others help themselves." A confident woman is unstoppable!

Jenn Harper is Anishinaabe-Canadian and the founder of Cheekbone Beauty, helping Indigenous youth see themselves in a beauty brand while crafting sustainable cosmetics.

Jennifer Harper

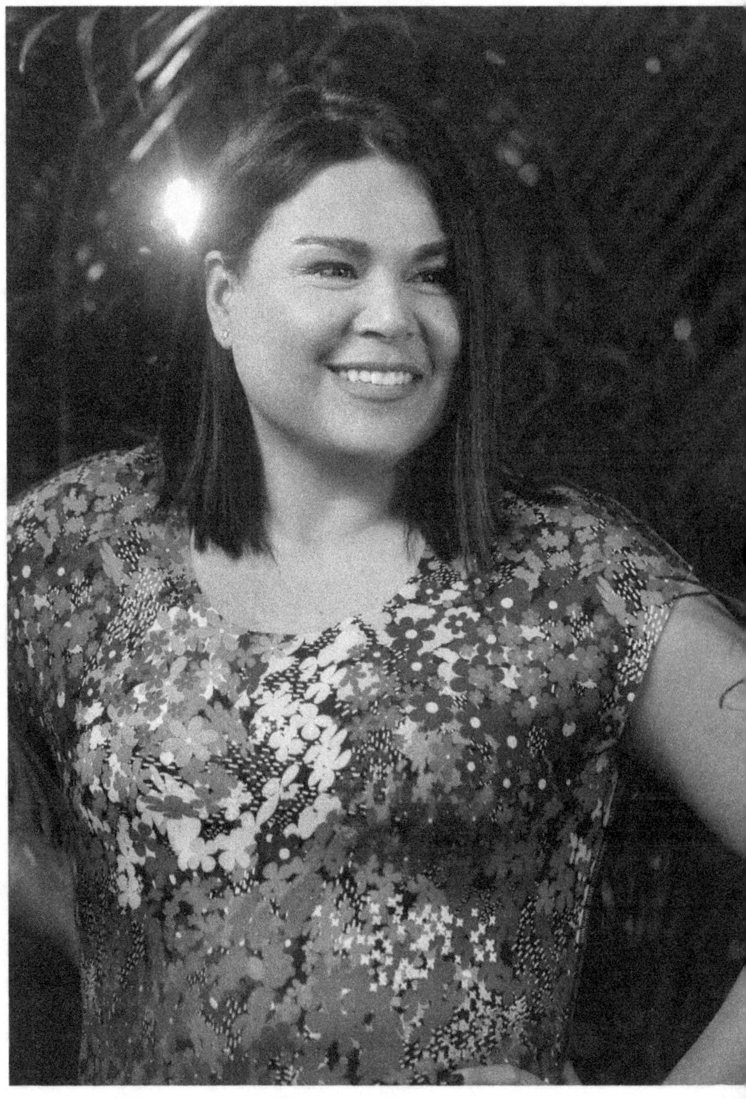

Let's rethink our relationship with the environment and our community. We live in a world where individual benefit is more important than the well-being of our community and our environment. In Western culture, competition and accumulation are among highly celebrated drivers in Western behaviour. On the contrary, sustaining our people and sustaining our environment have been key drivers within our Indigenous communities for thousands of years. The main ingredient in Indigenous leadership is humility: it is horizontal and egalitarian, not hierarchical, and the term used by Indigenous people practicing well-being for our community is collectivism. With the realities of our climate emergency, a step in the right direction in order to help our partnership with nature is to practice this in the workplace. But first, it begins by changing our mindset.

To protect our planet and Indigenous knowledge, we can prioritize collective goals instead of focusing on our individual ones. Integrating Indigenous wisdom in our business models should be as relevant as the scientific facts and data that exist in everyday objectives and business decisions. Now, we can do our part to incorporate Indigenous wisdom in our current Western economic thinking, create a value system to benefit our community and the environment, switch our mindset and business models to ecological mode. Through the practice of integrating ancient design into our modern world, we can re-learn how to consume responsibly in order to leave enough for those who will come after.

Indigenous people are responsible for a quarter of the world's land conservation and 80% of global diversity, yet only makeup about 5% of the population. As a Native beauty brand, while we can't mimic nature completely, we can try our best. From our roots to your lips, and from our innate connection to land and water, we can re-emerge kindness, community, and compassion in our world!

Only take what you need.

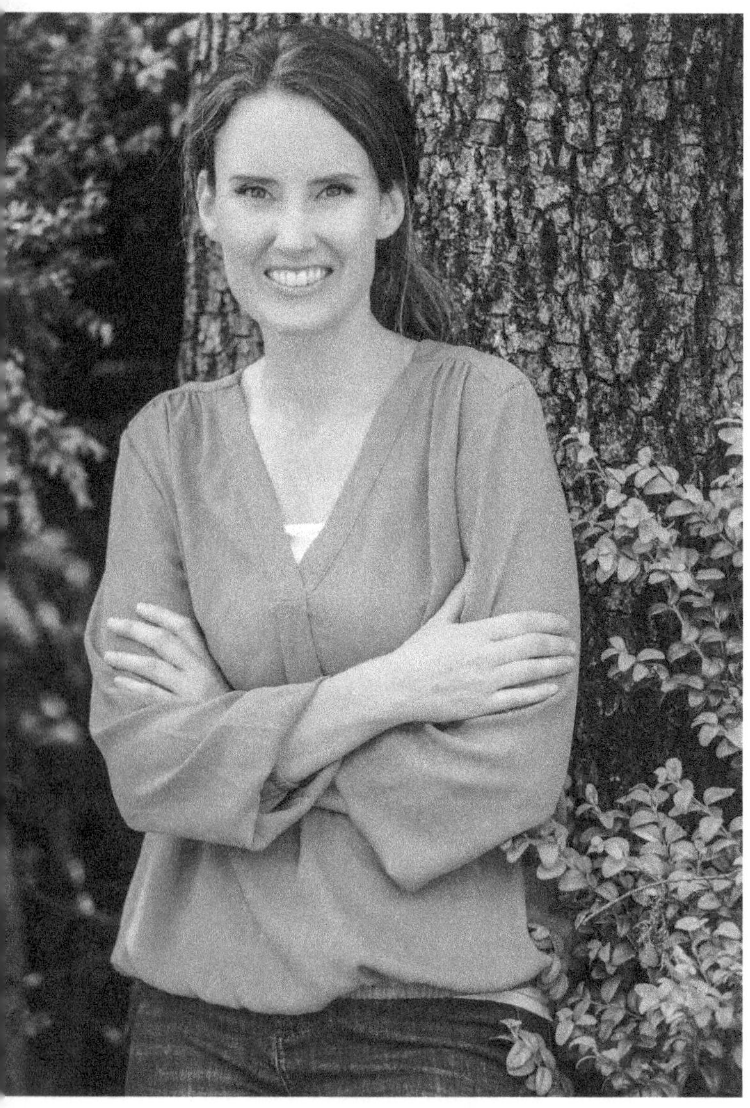

Tawnya Ritco is a mom, partner, daughter, sister, friend, and teammate with more than twenty years in the natural health industry. Tawnya is a registered holistic nutritionist and dedicated relationship-builder.

Tawnya Ritco

My amazing parents tell me that two of my first words were "me do!". They reflected how much I seemed wired for independence. I often smile at the thought of "me do" and how our character starts to develop so early in life, shaped by our experiences along the way.

I've never lost that sense of independence. Like everyone, I've faced challenges and opportunities, had failures and successes, and have felt both profound heartache and incredible joy. Like many, I've learned the most from the difficult moments; the ones that pushed me entirely outside of my comfort zone. Those moments helped me realize not only how fragile we are, but how resilient we can be in the pursuit of life.

One came at the age of sixteen when I survived a terrifying drowning accident. It happened when I was tubing down Skutz Falls on a hot summer day on the Cowichan River on Vancouver Island. I suddenly lost my innertube, was sucked under the rapids, and became lodged underwater between two rocks. Thankfully, I was pulled out of the rushing water, unconscious but alive. I survived that near-death experience solely because of the relentless efforts of my friend and a complete stranger, who both risked themselves to save me.

That accident changed me forever. It taught me the importance of selfless acts and that this one had saved my life. I also learned that I couldn't do everything myself and that we often need help, especially in urgent times. The strength of my independence became the power I've found in interdependence. "Me do" became "we do".

I'm eternally grateful for what that perilous moment taught me and for the inspiration and strength I've drawn from it and other key moments. I've found that the more we allow ourselves to be inspired, the more we inspire others. I've realized that each day is a fresh start – a new beginning -- and that we're constantly learning, adapting, and evolving as we strive to be the best that we can be.

Jodi Takhar is a mom, a counsellor, a person in long-term recovery, and a cheerleader for many. She has been told by family, clients, and friends she gives people a safe place to land.

Jodi Takhar

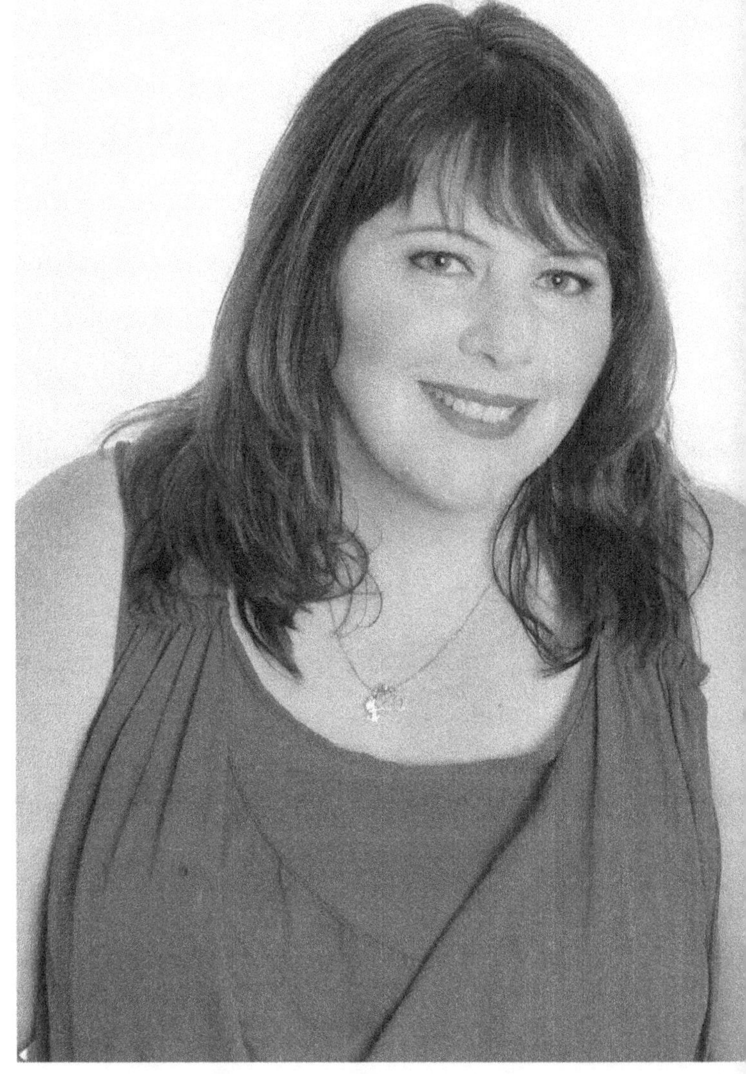

My personal slogan for many years has been, "and, that's okay!" Since childhood, I have felt the need to justify, explain and defend my beliefs, values, opinions, and behaviour - pretty much my whole self. I spent a massive amount of time and breath apologizing for myself. And then, at twenty-four, I got sober.

What I have learned between twenty-four and forty-nine, on this fantastic journey in recovery, is everything happens for a reason. People do what they do and say what they say because of an event, belief, or teaching. Situations happen and things are said or done, and there is always a lesson or a purpose. Whatever the circumstance might be, I believe, it will always work out exactly how it is meant to, "and that's okay."

This does not mean I haven't hurt, been sad, angry, or disappointed. My divorce was no picnic, and neither was that car accident. Having arthritis hasn't been easy either. What has happened in all the ugly and gross situations, often more than the wonderful happenings of life, is that I have grown, learned, changed my perspective, and accepted.

I have given myself and many others permission to make that mistake and learn from it, have that feeling and really feel it or share that experience and grow from it. It is okay to be you exactly as you are with all you have learned and all you don't know yet.

I believe we grow from the inside out, so the next time you make a mess of something or have a horribly painful experience, see if you can find that place in you where "it's okay," and give yourself permission to feel, grow, heal or change your perspective.

It really is okay to be you because you are perfectly perfect in every way.

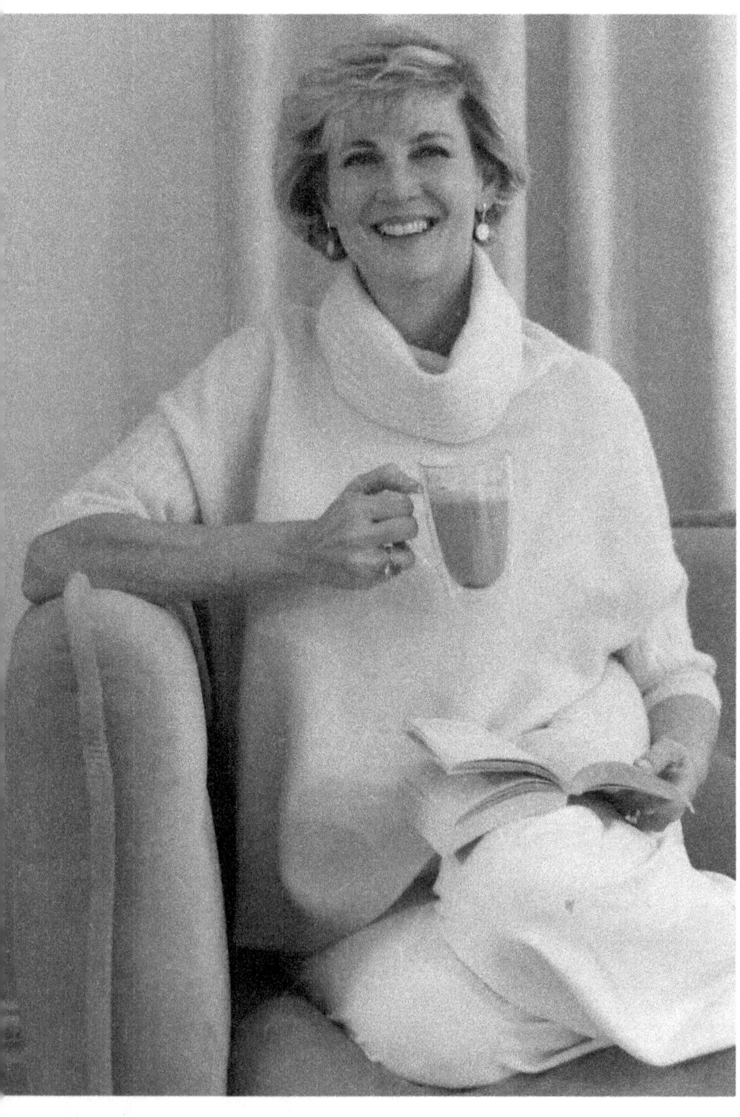

Nicola Arndt is an educator, administrator, and lifelong learner with undeniable enthusiasm for life.

Nicola Arndt

I believe that learning is a lifelong process. Every time we open our eyes, the process begins, and it doesn't stop until we close them again to sleep. Learning is the human purpose. It is the reason we strive for excellence, and it is the reason we achieve it.

A yearning curiosity is our springboard into an ocean of learning and wonder. Everything that has ever been thought of is written down for a student to discover. As an educator and administrator, my role is to act as a guide to each and every student. I am present to point out possibilities, push a little further, and encourage their process to continue.

Each time knowledge is rediscovered, it is new because the discoverer brings their own thoughts and experiences to the discovery. Every time I take part in a journey, it is different, yet exciting, because I can see it through the eyes of someone new. I hope I can inspire the students and staff whose lives I touch to relish the adventure of learning as much as I do.

My own educational enlightenment continues. After the recent loss of my husband and a throat cancer diagnosis, I find myself reflecting on the importance of resilience and optimism. Resilience has allowed me to move forward. I do not, however, move forward alone. I take those that have gone before with me because they have shaped who I am and who I will become. Optimism: a hopefulness and confidence about the future allows me to recognize life and learning as the possibilities that they are. I am passionate about possibilities, wonder, and a love of the search for wisdom. Some of my journey's moments have been devastating and some dazzling, but I believe it is how we rise to meet those moments that will define us. I tell my daughters that happiness is a by-product of living a life that matters. Pursue your passions, seek human connection, elevate others, and above all, be kind! I choose to wake up every day and live a life that matters. My passions are now directed toward the completion of my Conflict Management Certificate and my arbitrator's qualifications. After all, learning is for life!

Caitlyn Vanderhaeghe is a mother of three daughters, a Frozen and Peppa Pig expert, author of a children's book, wife to a supportive husband, the youngest of four children. Caitlyn is a Co-Founder and the President and CEO of KidStar Nutrients.

Caitlyn Vanderhaeghe

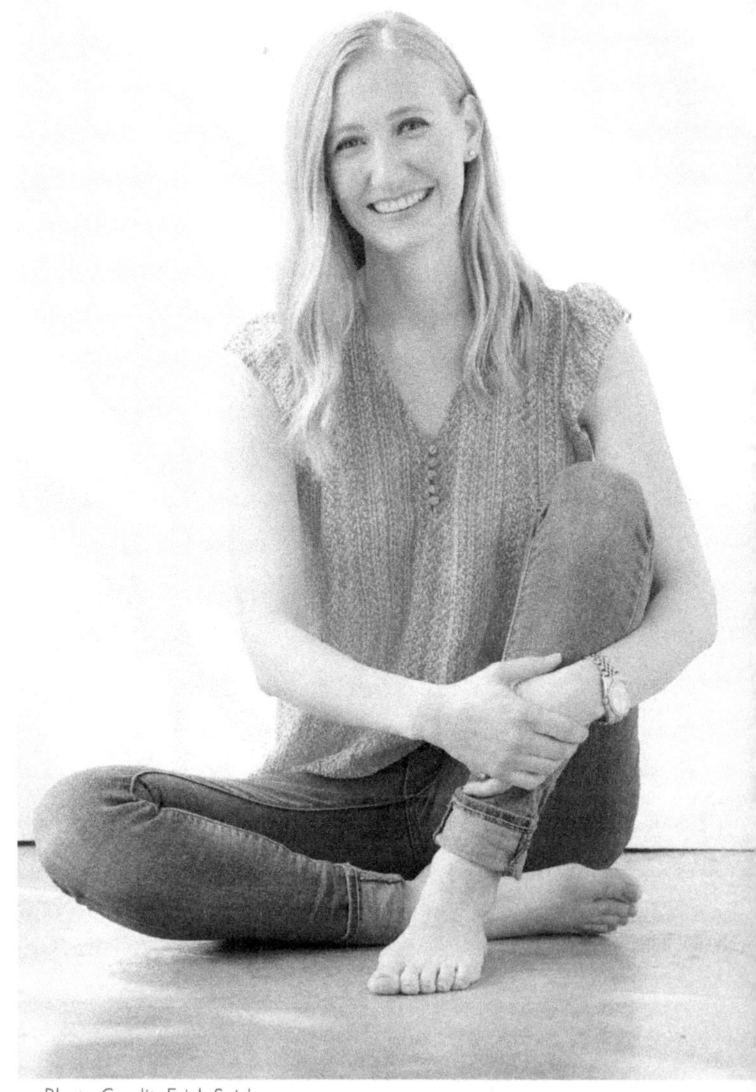
Photo Credit: Erich Saide

I grew up immersed in the natural health industry. Raised by my nutritional health expert mom, Lorna Vanderhaeghe, I was encouraged to ask questions and seek alternative solutions when possible. I come from a long line of passionate women, who have taught me to step out of the box and live my dreams. Even though I became an elementary school teacher, I kept being pulled back to my nutrition roots. For over ten years I ran the supply chain for my mom's company, so I knew how nutritional supplements were made.

When one of my daughters needed help for a serious iron-deficiency issue, I searched for decent products to help her, and none were to be found. That need led me to think about creating a nutritional supplement company with products parents could trust and kids would love. With the support of my family, I co-founded KidStar Nutrients with my youngest brother. My role as CEO and President takes me way out of my comfort zone. No longer was I behind the scenes but now out front and center helping people. From learning how to be a social media maven, developing products, writing educational materials, and sometimes putting on my steel toe boots to work in the warehouse, I am so grateful that I get to do what I love — advocating for kids' health and giving parents the tools to help them raise healthier kids.

Bravery, resilience, and determination come to mind when I think about how I am going to succeed. My company is like my fourth baby, and no amount of sleepless nights will stop me from seeing it grow into the business I know it can be. I want my children to see my passion, and grab hold of what they love in life, and know they can achieve anything with focus, commitment, and hard work. Ultimately, educating moms and dads on nutrition for their children will have lasting effects. I believe if you see where you are going you can make it happen — all it takes is a strong desire, lots of gratitude, and never giving up.

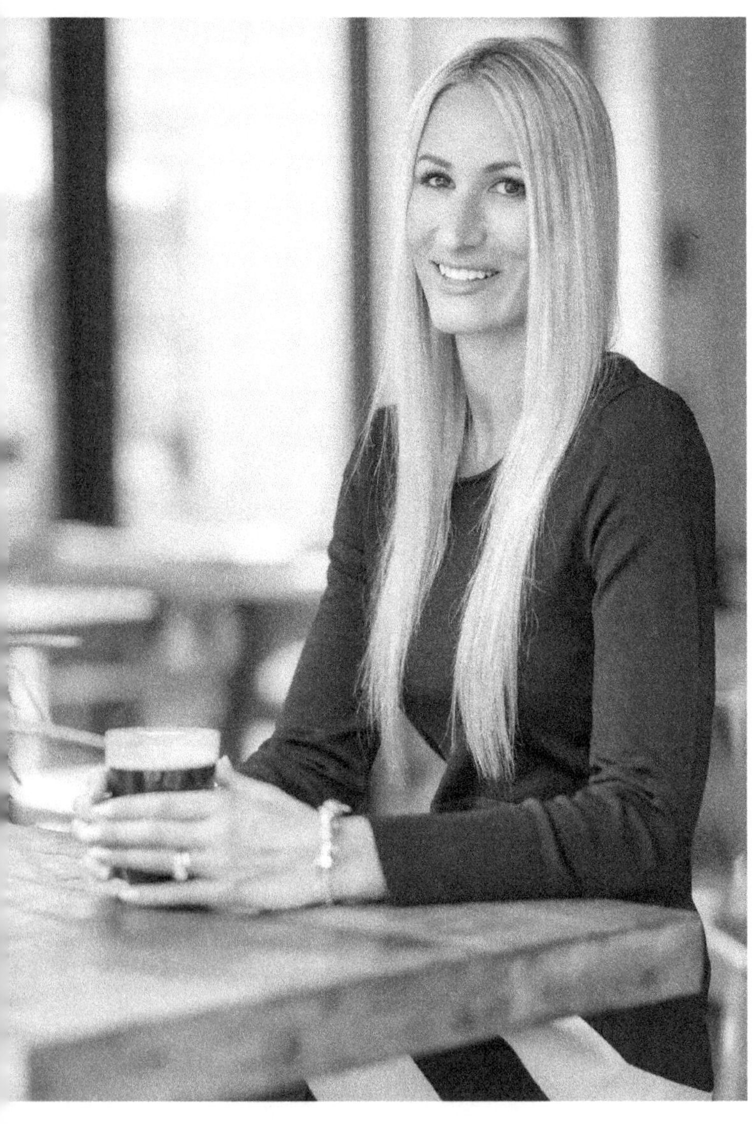

Kristin Hazzard is a self-described high achiever who has learned that the greatest rewards don't just come from accomplishments – they come from the heart, and the courage to harness your inner power.

Kristin Hazzard

Born into a family of high achievers who broke world records and glass ceilings, it's easy to understand why I'm driven. It's in my DNA. From a young age, I thought that in order to stand out I had to be the best.

I played national-level hockey, was named an Academic All Canadian in university and competed internationally in fitness competitions. I earned my Master's in Education specializing in motivation; taught, coached and founded a fitness company - focusing on elite athletics - to empower people physically and mentally. Despite awards, trophies and championships; endorsement deals and recognition – it was never enough. I had learned to equate success to self-worth and love, and the self-imposed pressure to be the best came at a high cost.
Then, the life I knew suddenly ended after a car accident devastated this persona. My super-hero spirit was crushed. I felt like a shell of my former self.

Recovery was slow, and not just physical. I finally understood I could no longer pay the high cost of the pressure to be the best and realized that the power to step back into my light came in finding lasting, internal belief rather than the fleeting gratification of external perfection. Inspired by my mentors and coaches who had helped me, I saw that I could take everything I'd learned and experienced to further help others.

With my purpose clear, and fueled by my love for learning, I studied to become an Executive Coach, choosing the world of elite business leadership because I could relate to the pressures of the drive to succeed. I knew I could help leaders shift their perspectives by leveraging their purpose to improve their overall performance.

I am now aligned with what I am really here to do – and am happy to say that not everything has changed. I'm still a fierce competitor who loves to win and loves epic adventures – but now I play for myself, with my golden heart shining bright and leading the way.

Jennifer Italiano is a single mom, a passionate businesswoman, and co-owner of Live Organic Food (Live).

Jennifer Italiano

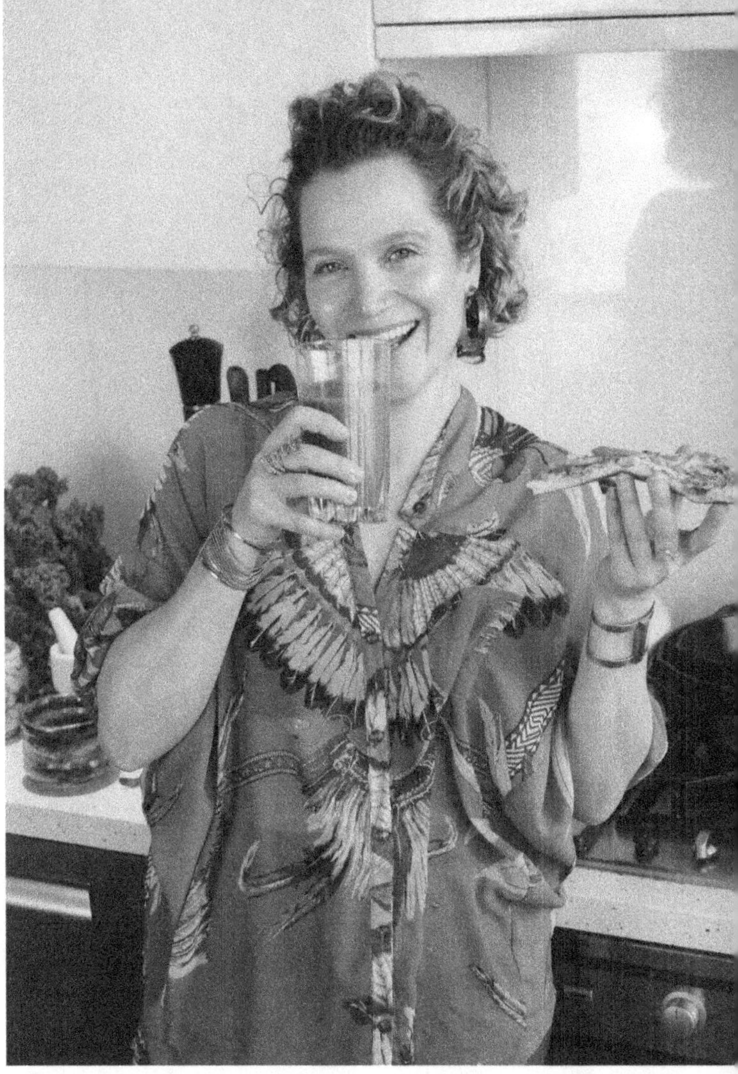

Live is an organic, plant-based, food manufacturing facility producing products for hundreds of Canadian retailers. My humble beginnings started in 2002 with a four-seater, organic juice bar. My vision was to make healthy products universally accessible in a nascent industry that wasn't yet fashionable. I think that for the most part, I have delivered, and I continue to expand on that vision every day as my life, work, and the market evolve tremendously.

My success boils down to never having a fear of my ambitions. The happiest and most successful times for me have been when I was able to let go of conventional mindsets and do things my own way. Things were tougher in the beginning due to my tendency to take things personally. There were times when I wondered if any of it was worth it. In time, I realized and accepted that there is no success without failures and that I would never have a nine to five career.

Today I feel lucky! I'm in a place where I'm living my passion. It's something I have to keep reminding myself of, and it gets easier with each coming year. I've realized that our food is making a difference in people's lives and that I am, in fact, making healthier food universally accessible.

Fortunately, my passion for what we've created here at Live has not stopped me from enjoying a 'balanced' lifestyle. I'm a mom, a sister, a daughter, a friend, and a partner to those around me. I've learned when it's time to turn off the businesswomen in order to enjoy time with my loved ones. Sometimes, when I'm able, I enjoy kicking back, relaxing, and doing absolutely nothing. You will find me on any given day drinking my green juice, but I enjoy my pizza too.

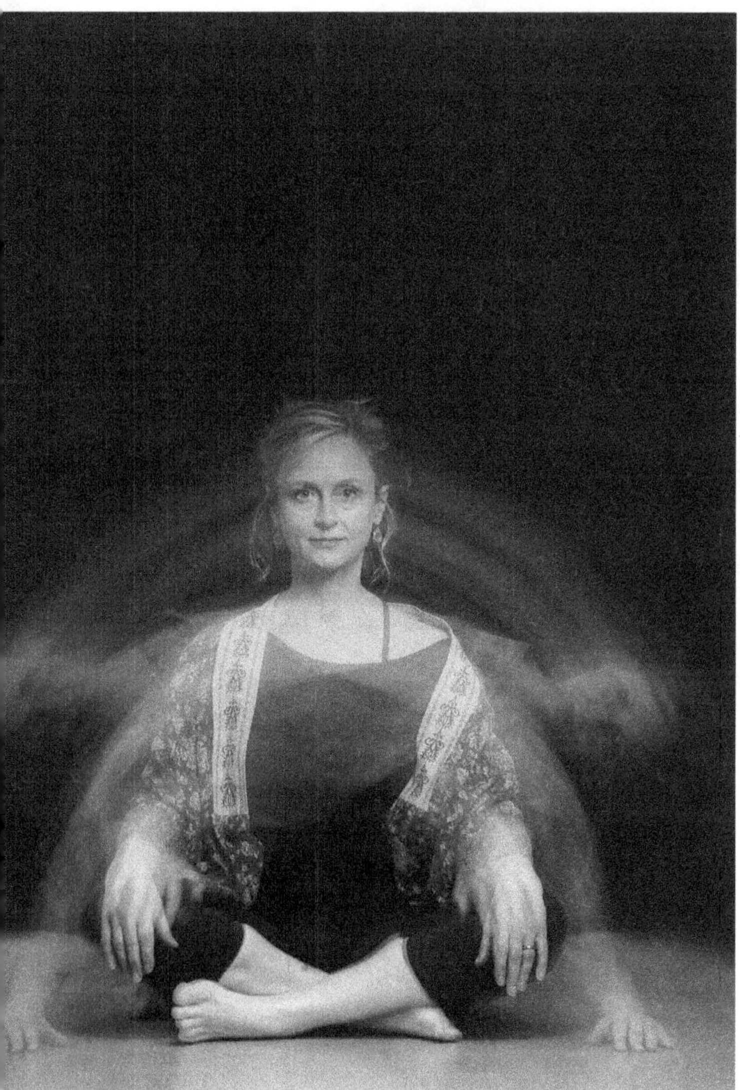

Photo Credit: Radina Photography

Laura Burns is the Flexible Life Coach, helping individuals to reconnect their body and mind.

Laura Burns

Building a foundation for my dream life: the partner, the dog, the house, and the career, when, two freak car accidents later I find myself laying on my couch, for three years, with no one calling or coming to visit. Even the dog ignored me. What did I do wrong?

In that moment, I realized I'd been engaged in my life like it was a buffet, not a museum. I never trusted anyone to truly connect, invest time, to curate real connections.

Instead, I would skirt around the edges, nibbling, enjoying the flavours, and then disappearing into the night. I was disconnected from my body pain and the people around me. I knew something needed to change. I started with meditation, which was like trying to tame a tiger. Alarm clocks were destroyed through the process. Then, I learned to stretch with an elite athlete and became pain-free. I returned to learn how to share this method to eliminate muscle tension in the body which helps most conditions of the musculoskeletal system.

Once certified, I discovered through all my experiences that this creates a unique program when I use the stretching with coaching inquiries. I now help others see the messages in their body and become pain-free, more mobile, and use this freedom to pursue a limitless future.

I learned that my future would only shift when I devoted myself to reconnecting to my body and mind. Then I would be able to reconnect to others and build a happier life.

My wish is to live my life through small acts of greatness curated over time and that it will make the difference to reconnect the world.

Crystal Carson is a trailblazer, a connector, and a businesswoman, but regardless of the industry one will always find Crystal at the forefront of innovation and change. Operating at the intersection of creativity and commerce she is often referred to as a modern-day renaissance woman.

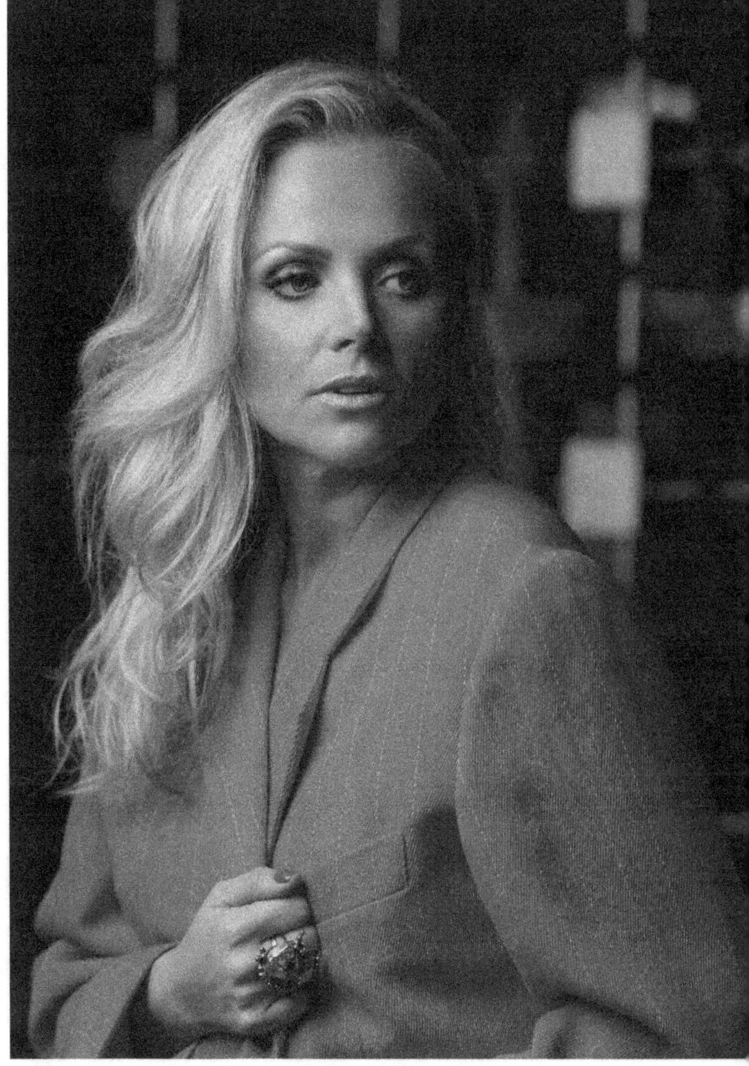

Crystal Carson

Crystal is a small-town Canadian girl with big dreams. Think "Sex in The City," and she's Carrie and Samantha combined - an adventurous alpha female with a bohemian soul and champagne taste. Crystal hustles through life, learning failures are simply the channels to success, her insatiable curiosity is the inspiration of pioneering a unique path in the journey to life's purpose.

Crystal believes trauma can truly be a powerful experience if one lives in their truth because of it. Her ability to overcome her greatest challenges in business has come through the strength and knowledge gained through challenging personal experiences.

An influencer and storyteller, Crystal's passions naturally led her to a career in media. In 2006 she began her career in the traditional media world as an editor and contributor to multiple publications such as Elle Canada, Vancouver Sun, and Fresh Magazine. A few years and many tear sheets later she entered the world of television, working in front of and behind the camera for CTV, ET Canada, and Global News. At the core of everything is Crystal's relationships. Energized by others she has cultivated a global point of view with circles of international tastemakers and friends.

Crystal is about the WHY, continually inspired by the innovation of leaders in their industries, she loves connecting the brightest minds to create something new. Working with high profile entrepreneurs, global brands, and media outlets, she has built a vast network of unwavering trust, A personalized 'search engine' for entrepreneurs, investors, and innovators with her ability to spot patterns that facilitate new opportunities.

Through risk and renewal, Crystal has transformed herself throughout her life, entering new arenas without fear. She recognizes each transformation as revolutionary, as from each she draws the knowledge and experience to succeed. There is a fine sense of harmony and contagious energy in everything that she does whether facilitating change, connecting the right people, leading a team, or building a brand.

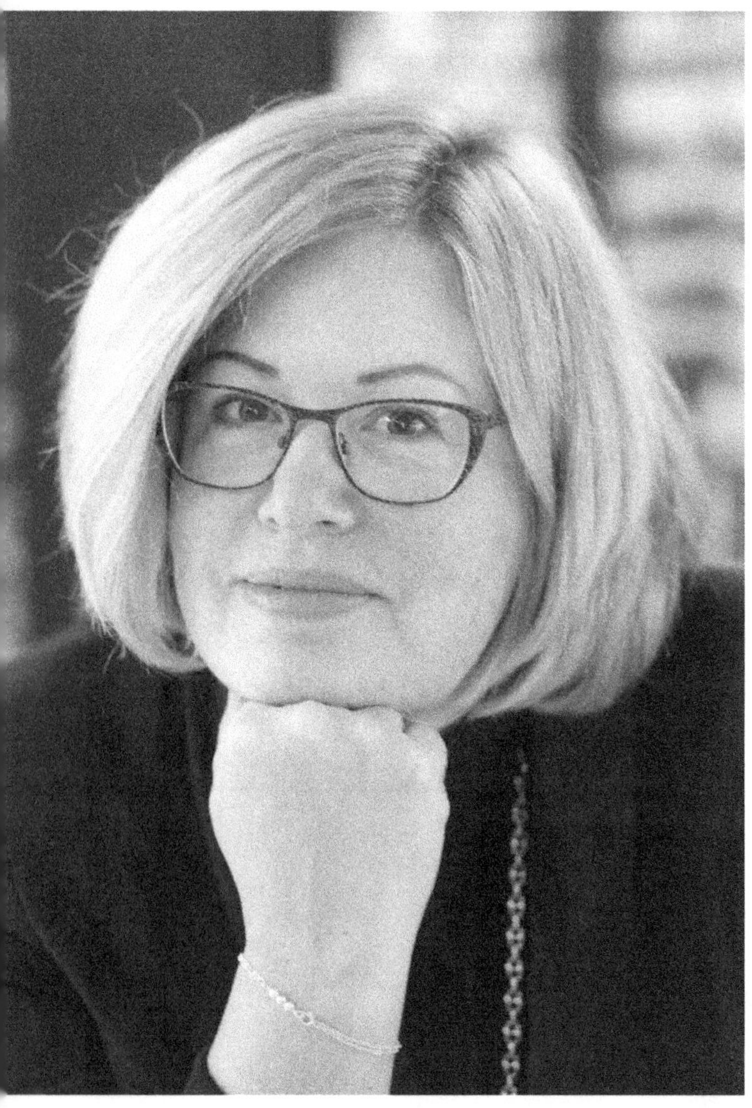

Shelly Smee is a Realtor, Managing Broker, World Class Athlete, Artist, and Poet.

Shelly Smee

Writing about oneself is daunting, and like most important assignments in my life, I've spent a great deal of time thinking first, knowing a deadline tends to crystalize my thoughts at the last moment. I am of the opinion that creative procrastination is an essential element of the writer's craft.
Life has deadlines, hard and soft, limits that are of our own making, and boundaries we don't know exist until they are crossed. From these 365 words on the page, you will get the essence of me; that is my intention.

You will come to understand I do not suffer fools and have worked very hard to find more graceful ways to express my indignation. This is the gift of the fifties.

A Gen X renaissance woman, I am a firm believer that hard work is rewarded by magic and that human potential is limited only by hate. I know we are created equal, yet we do not always have equal access to the same resources, be it financial, emotional, or the circumstances of our birthplace. I know that love, hope, and time are the trifecta.

My two favourite words are "I know". This simple statement said with confidence and conviction can end conflict and create collaboration. I do not use words frivolously. One of the great lessons of leadership is the understanding that it is also ok to not know. Being wise is knowing when I know that I don't know. Being in possession of unbounded curiosity to seek the truth is my greatest resource.

Maturity is understanding that inertia is a decision. Leadership is the ability to foresee consequences and choose the best course of action. What does all this have to do with Real Estate? Everything. My accomplishments as Realtor, Managing Broker, World Class Athlete, Artist and Poet, all have their place in my psyche. What drives me is being in relationships with my fellow humans. Striving for authenticity in all interactions with integrity and kindness. My twenty-five-year career in Real Estate has provided a platform to serve and time after time proven that trusting the universe means trusting myself first.

I create lifestyle solutions. How cool is that?

Sherry Klassen is an artist and painter with pieces displayed in Roam Gallery in Vancouver.

Sherry Klassen

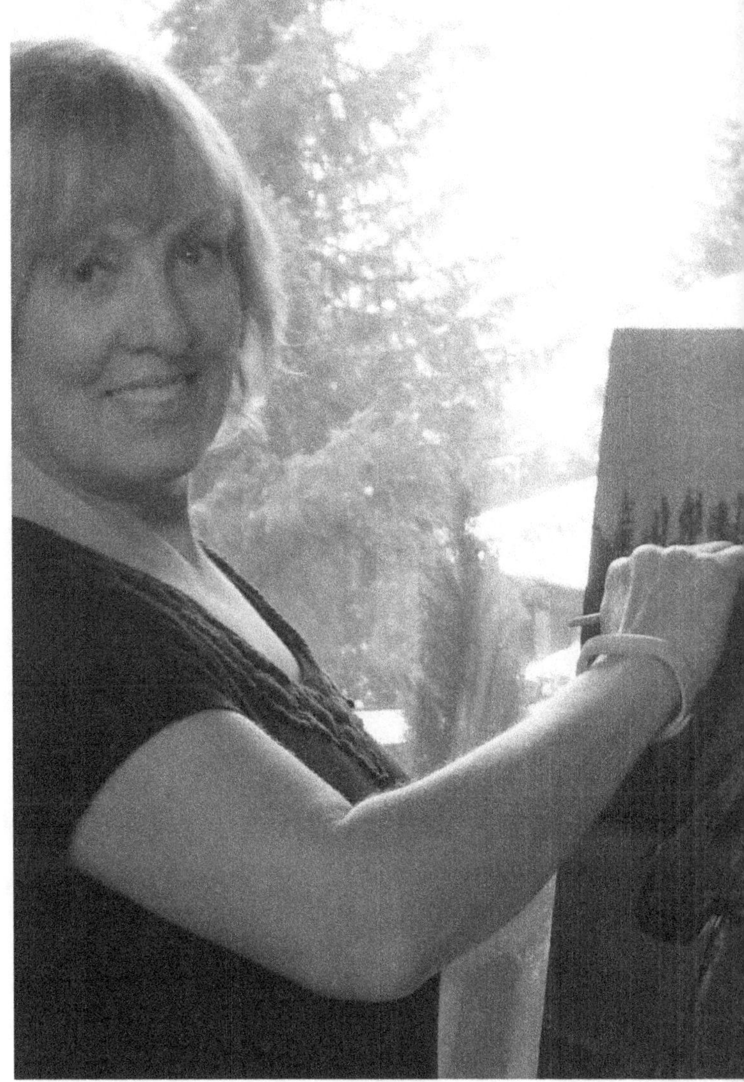

I have always set goals for myself in all areas of my life. I make sure they are specific, break them into small steps, and set out an order of approach. I strive not to work on too many at the same time to ensure successful completion. Although, as an optimist, it is sometimes difficult for me to limit myself.

I am a "can do" kind of person. I have been blessed with a positive attitude and a lot of energy. An employer once said to me, "you can teach skills, but you can't teach attitude," and that stuck with me. I believe that if you have a positive mindset and a strong work ethic, you can build a great life.

As a young woman, I met Jim on a ski trip. He had graduated from UBC and recently landed his first engineering job. We quickly fell in love and decided we wanted to share our lives however, we had a major obstacle to overcome. In his first year of university, Jim had a horrific accident and was unable to work. He had incurred a lot of debt.

When I realized how much Jim owed - more than twice his annual net income, I knew we were going to have to do something drastic. We had to find a way to live rent-free, so we could dedicate Jim's salary to debt reduction. We were able to find a position managing two apartment buildings in exchange for a suite to live in. I was working as a retail store manager at the time and took on an extra job assisting in the showroom at a newly built condominium complex. Additionally, we earned extra money by painting the suites when people moved out.
Within two years, we had paid off the debt and saved enough for a down payment on our own apartment. Although it was daunting to face such massive debt, it taught us to work together through adversity and set a tone of unity for our thirty-plus year marriage. At the time it seemed so difficult, however, I realized that it taught me so much about possibilities, grit, strength, and determination.

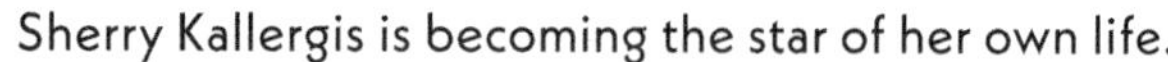

Sherry Kallergis is becoming the star of her own life.

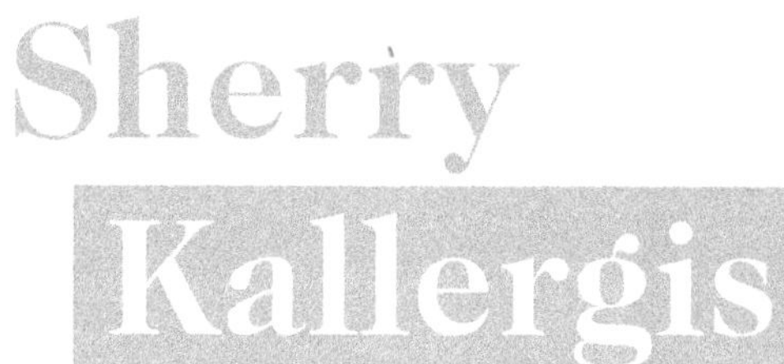

Sherry Kallergis

"Your life is a story, so sell the movie rights girl!" was a catalyst to change. The imagery of me being a star made it easy to adopt the empowering perspective daily. Are you the star of your life, and are you intentionally making every moment movie-worthy?

I am the oldest child and girl of five children however my family was always taking in others. Foster children, extended family members, neighbors, anyone needing a hand up, even strays from the bus station moved through our house. I was expected and trained from an early age to put others first. I didn't get the opportunity to learn how to put myself first, and it followed me through my adult life.

Repeating what I knew, at times, I ran a household of thirteen with eight under the age of twelve (not all mine). I was so busy just trying to get through life, to the next paycheck, the next promotion, through the next school day, the next project, I forgot about enjoying it. How could I, when "me" was on the perpetual shelf?

A rogue question from my daughter in my fifties stopped me dead in my tracks. I had no idea what my favorite color was. Like, who doesn't know that? It dawned on me that I was just existing, not living. Shortly after someone recommended "The Power of Now" by Eckhart Tolle. The trifecta of reading the book, embracing my life as a movie with me as the "star," and reconnecting with the fabulous me brought color into my life and a joy I never imagined. Putting myself first caused me to take stock of what I wanted, liked, and what was missing. Disrupting the status quo became my new approach.

That is how my magazine At Forty-Five came to be. It is a vehicle for connecting me with women who are dabbling in new things and discovering facets of life they totally missed. Helping others might be in our DNA as women however, putting ourselves first has got a bad rap. It is not being selfish but a pre-requisite to living your life in technicolor.

Who knew taking out the trash could be a starring role?

Lynda Turner is a vegan biologist and the founder of Fauxmagerie Zengarry all natural vegan cheese company.

Lynda Turner

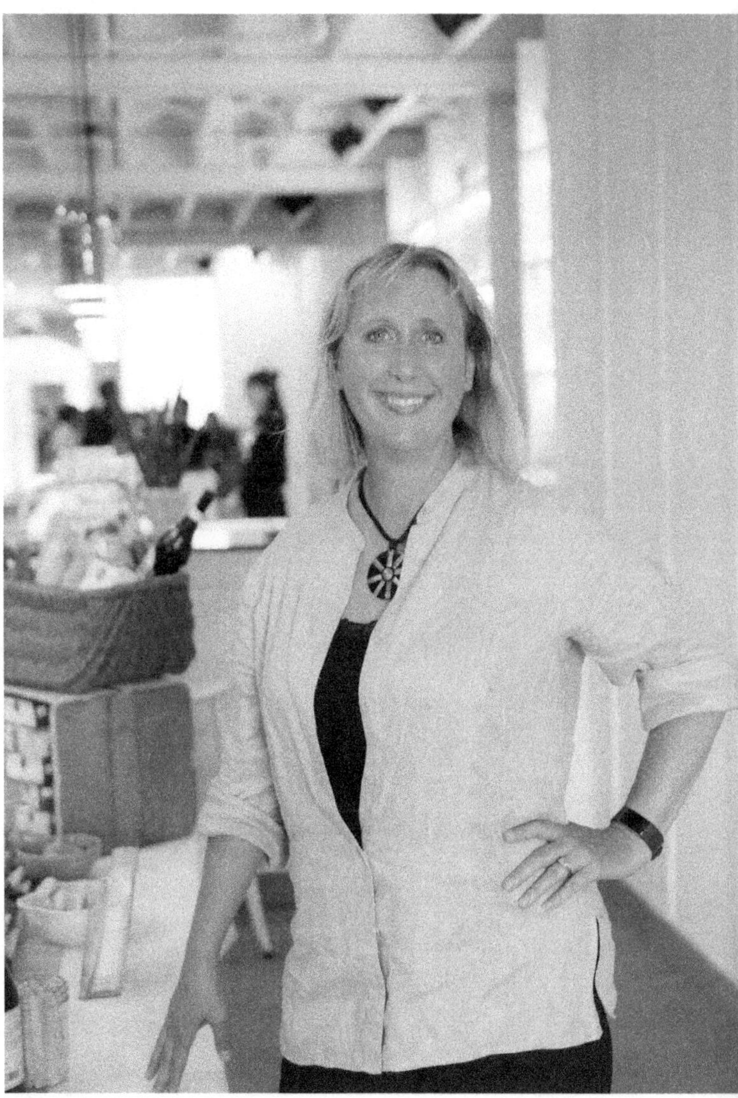

Growing up, like most girls my age, I dreamed of living happily ever after. I thought life was a straight line, that hard work and perseverance would inevitably lead to the proverbial pot of gold. But that's not how life works, does it? You can have the best plan, put in the extra hours, and make all the right moves, but sometimes life throws you a curve, and you have to re-evaluate your goals.

After studying biology and ecotoxicology, I landed a dream job at Health Canada, where I worked for almost twenty years. I expected to be happy working there until retirement, until I read a ground-breaking research study: The China Study. A comprehensive study on the incredible benefits of a plant-based diet. After doing my own research, I decided to put my learnings into practice and adopt a plant-based lifestyle.

In 2010, vegan options and restaurants were rare. Out of necessity, I developed a keen interest in cooking and became rather good at it. But the one thing I missed most was cheese. Back then, vegan cheese wasn't great, so I experimented with making my own. The feedback from friends and family was overwhelmingly enthusiastic, so I decided to rent a booth at the Ottawa Veg Fest to see what other people thought of my cheese.

This decision set in motion a chain of events that altered the course of my career, and my life.
I started producing vegan cheese in my kitchen on nights and weekends until it was clear that my passion project could be a viable business. Eventually, I left my government job and embraced the busy life of an entrepreneur.

Today, my business creates ethical products that are good for people and the planet, creates employment in my rural community, and gives my life purpose. I could never have predicted the direction my life would take and all the lessons I would learn along the way. One thing that has guided every major decision I've made is to trust my instincts. You never really know where life will take you, but if you listen to your heart, the journey is so much more satisfying.

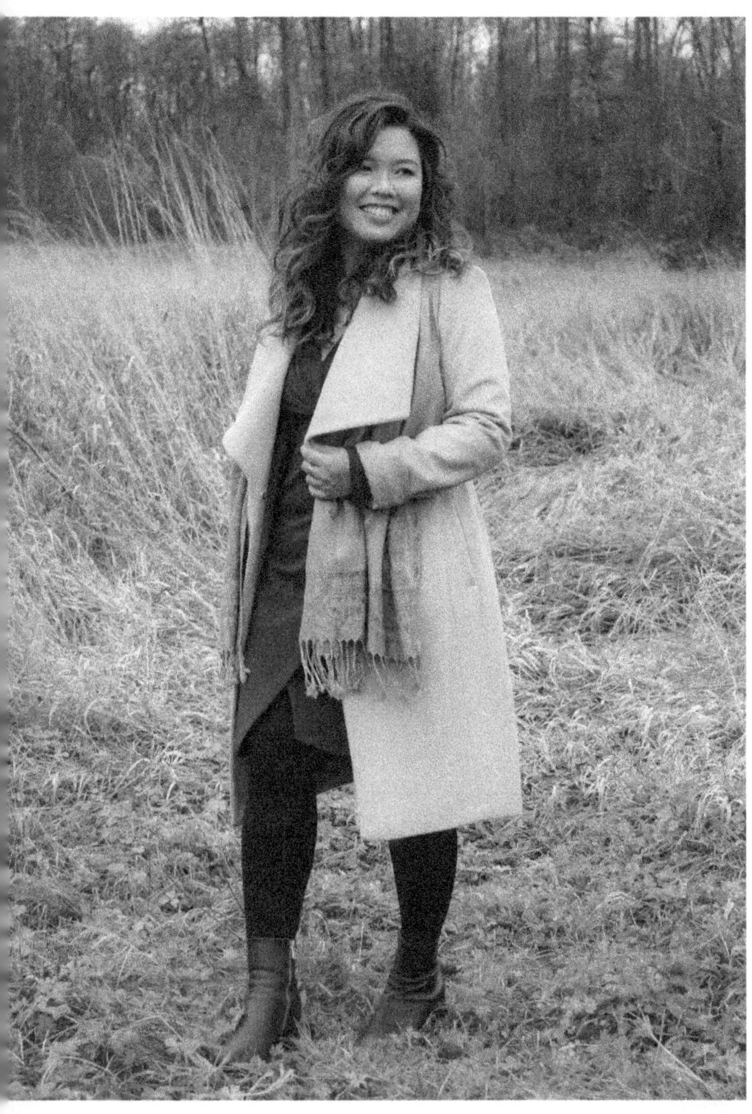

Jiali Kimoto is a mother of two, a corporate creative turned wellness advocate, and an essential oils specialist.

Jiali Kimoto

I remember vividly when I was about to graduate high school, prompting my dad, 'What am I here to do?' Seeing people graduate from university, finding a partner, having children, is that what I'm supposed to do, too? But... is that it?

Shortly after asking those questions, I found myself on an airplane from Kuala Lumpur, Malaysia to Vancouver, BC, by myself, at the fearless age of nineteen, with two suitcases and nothing else. I went to school for Interactive Digital Design and Graphic Design.

I got a job, then another, climbing the corporate ladder, and before you know it, I was travelling the world, seeing places and meeting people, and making more money than my parents ever did.

I also met the guy of my dreams, we fell in love, got married, and then got pregnant. Checking all the boxes. And yet, this question I had asked back then kept haunting me. "Becoming a mother is the greatest job in the world," they say. So, I devoted myself to my baby with every ounce of me. I didn't think much about anything else, until I was forced to pay attention when I developed a debilitating skin condition during my second pregnancy.

It was the most trying time of my whole life, not knowing answers, and suffering, with no end in sight. Tears of disappointment and hopelessness followed after medical appointments and doctor visits. It was during this bleak time where I felt the loneliest, even when holding my precious newborn in my arms. I was broken wide open and was pushed to face the rawness of it all, quite literally.

Through unapologetic self-love, self-trust, and self-empowerment using nature's medicine, I found answers. All my life, I was always chasing for what's next, what was expected of me, and perpetually looking outwards for guidance. Working with nature has taught me to remember who I am, to stay curious, to be relentless, and follow my inner-knowing to find what I'm looking for. After all, life isn't about how many checked boxes; it's about surrendering to the ever-expansive beauty that surrounds us daily.

Angela is a multi-award-winning Mortgage Expert, Author, Speaker, host of The Mortgage Show, and philanthropist striving to enrich the lives of everyone around her.

Angela Calla

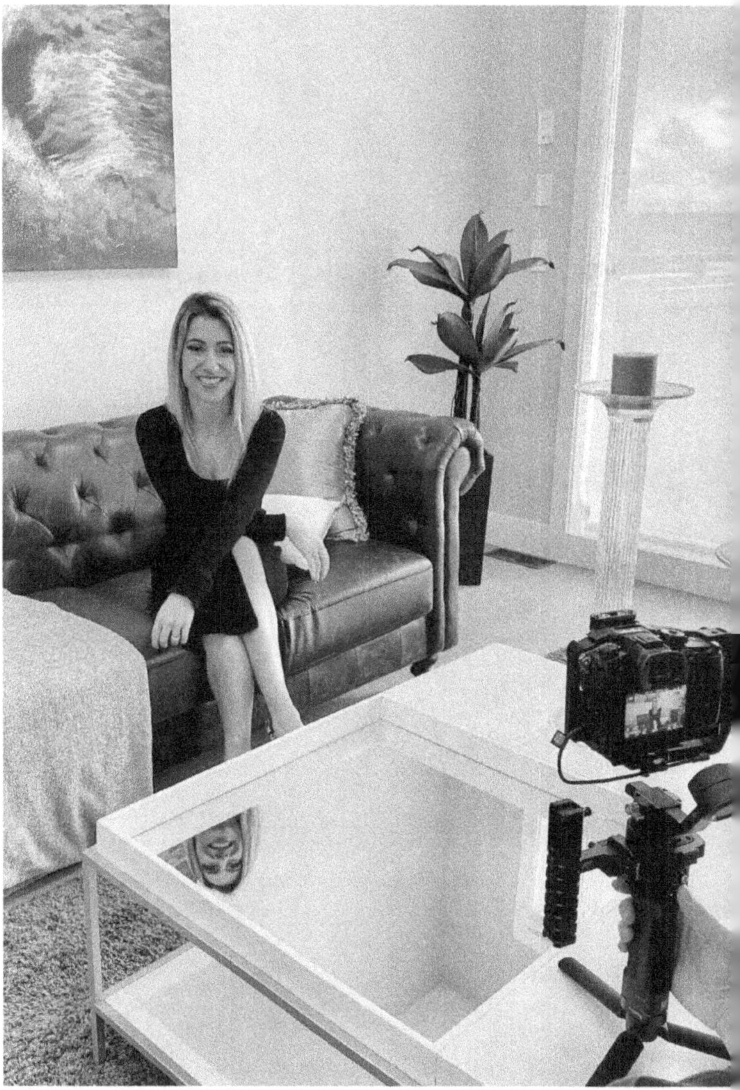

When your passion meets your purpose, you will stop at nothing to find every way possible to share it with the world. Once you learn what your unique gift is, you will continually draw people and opportunities to you.

I was fortunate enough to learn at a young age how to use financial knowledge to get ahead. There's a huge weight on your shoulders that comes with the desire to do the best you can for everyone around you. This drove me to put myself in the public eye and with this came a significant amount of responsibility.

For me, being in the media wasn't about scaling my business, but rather who I was going to take with me on that journey. Finding those whose core values align with mine so I could enhance their lives and bring that experience to others.

Having the confidence to be on the news, write books and articles for magazines, host a radio show, and sing the national anthem in front of thousands, only hold value because of those I get to help along the way.

There will always be people that will oppose you just to oppose you, or that don't understand the hard work and difficult choices you had to make to grow your business and educate others. Of course, those things are scary, and the comments will have an emotional impact on you, but it's the benefit of helping people that makes it all worth it.

When your passion to help others is so profound, your fears dissolve. You become fueled by seeing the results of people living their wealthiest and most enriched lives. So, take that fear of NOT being able to help as many people as humanly possible because that exceeds any doubt.

The real beauty in life is that most things aren't perfect. When you reach a point where you're comfortable with about 80% perfection you'll overcome that – freezing in decision moment – that will end up costing you the opportunity. When opportunity arises, have the confidence to jump and take the lead.

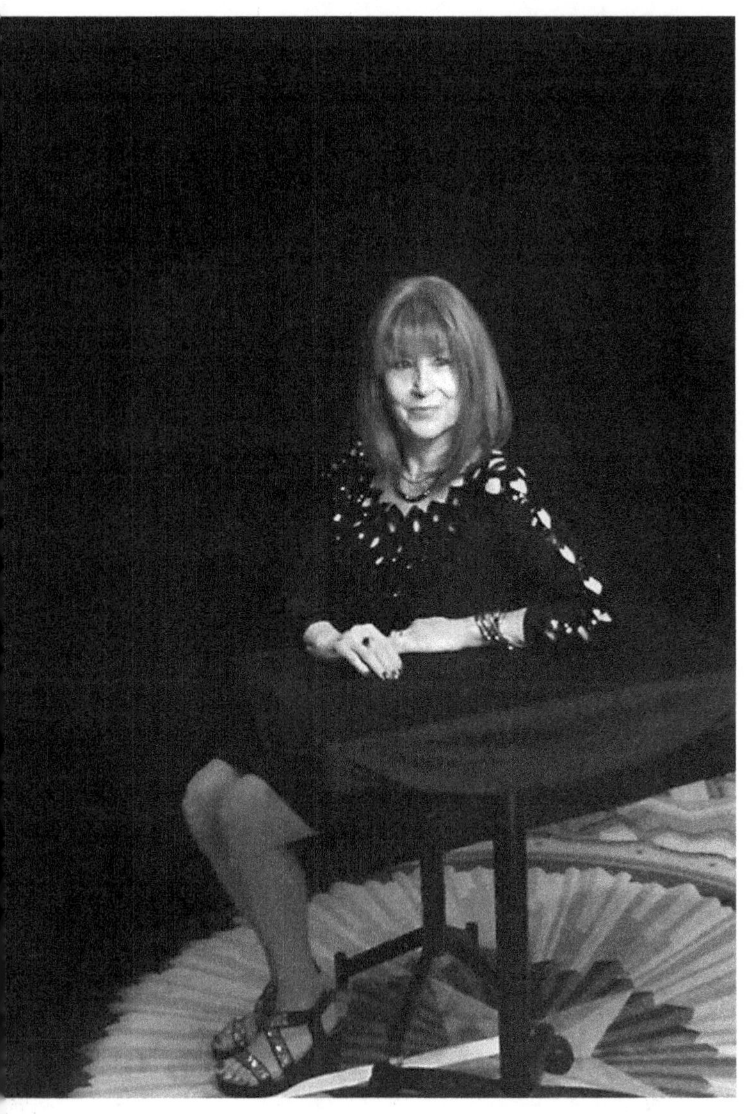

The common thread that is woven throughout my life is my love for people, my great appreciation of life, and for all I have.

Esther Topaz

I am a child survivor of the Holocaust. Born in a concentration camp in Gurs France, and then raised in my homeland Israel. For the past fourteen years, two professors from Keene state college in the United States have been documenting my story and creating a film about my life and my art. They have travelled with me to visit the concentration camp where I was born. I have always been adventurous, which led me to live in Germany and Switzerland, where I worked as a kindergarten teacher in a Jewish school. My next adventure brought me to Montreal during Expo 67 where I was teaching once again.

I then returned to Israel after four years and travelled the world as a stewardess with El-Al airlines. Fate brought me back to Montreal where I became a Canadian citizen and mother to two amazing children and eventually grandmother to five beautiful grandchildren. I started working with stone in 1972.

Motherhood had a great impact on my life as a woman and as a stone sculptor. Stone was a great medium and a challenge for me to express all that was in my heart and soul. The essence of life and the human connection. It was thrilling to use a cold and hard material and create such powerful emotions like the passion of lovers, carrying a child, and always the message calling to protect our children in this world. My Sculpture "Reach for the Star's" was on display at the NASA space centre for many years.

Over the years I became a professional Sculptor and teacher. Teaching gives me great satisfaction and the opportunity to share my knowledge. It gives me great joy to see my students work in Stone and find their own way.

And then came 2020...
So, what is there for a sculptor to do? Sculpt!
And that's exactly what I have been doing.
Wishing for the world to heal.

Teresa Phillips is an artist and a citizen of the world.

Teresa Phillips

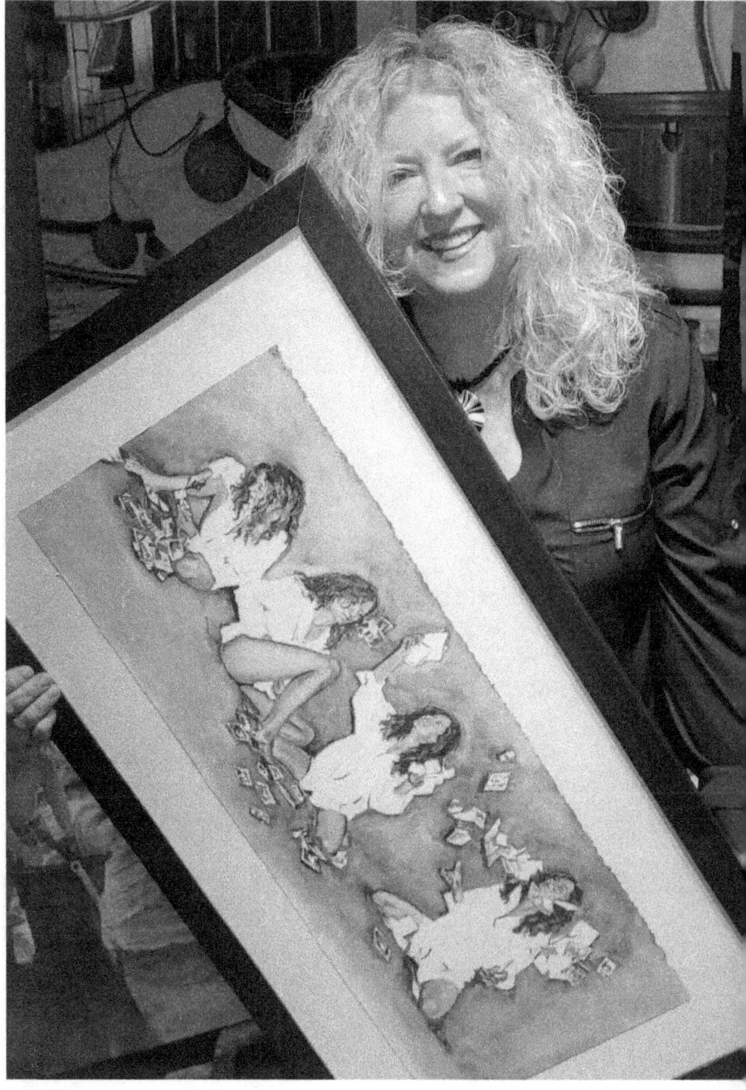

For me, it's always been about letting go; childhood memories, difficult families, illness. I was raised with love, but there was too much drink and too much drama. Two fathers raised me, neither biologically mine. My birth father? That meeting would come when I was twenty-one. Imagine an instant, deep connection, like looking in the mirror and seeing right to your soul. All these men have long since passed away, the first when I was only thirteen.

I was fifteen and a half when I left home. I had skirted around the dark side, waitressing in strip clubs and bars; I experienced a number of drugs. At nineteen, I found myself in a small town and pregnant. I tried to do the right thing. "I'd made my bed and I should lay in it," I was told. I stayed for eleven years and two more children. I wasn't abused, but we were broke and miserable. I knew I could do better on my own. And I did. Hard does not scare me. Telling me I can't do something is a challenge I love to rise to.

I didn't know who I was anymore. It wasn't until I picked up a pen to draw a picture of a plane for my then father-in-law that everything changed. My world opened up beyond my wildest imagination. It took a few Monday nights: two hours painting with a group of talented artists, then off to the pub.

These were people I could relate to: I could be this free version of myself. My creativity became my new superpower. I started selling commissioned paintings and opened a gallery with six other artists. Wow, what a ride!
Now my life is filled with a wonderful husband, children, grandchildren, friends, and the community in which we live. The opportunity for worldwide travel has opened up our lives. I love being a global citizen. It makes me smile when I can make other people smile.

The painting in this photo is called "Letting go" - my self-portrait, and also my mantra: a reminder to take a good look at your life, accept what you cannot change, cut out the s*** and live your best life.

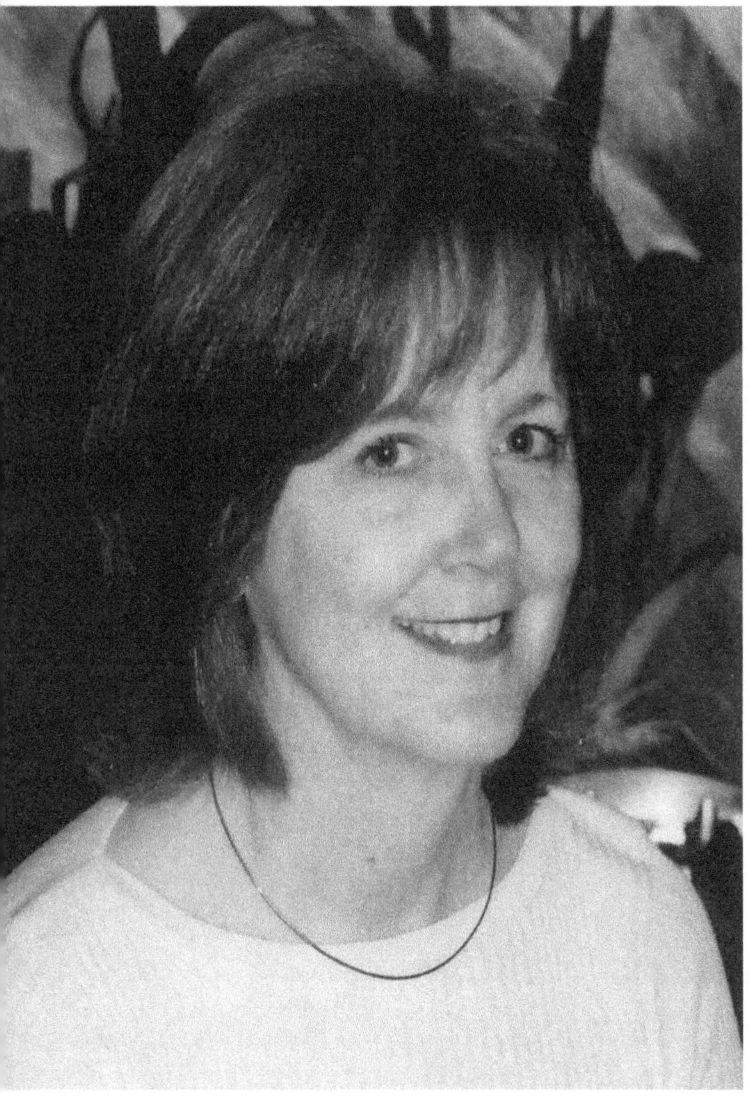

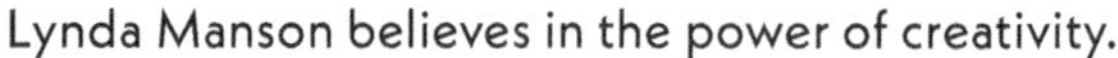

Lynda Manson believes in the power of creativity.

Lynda Manson

These are chaotic, stressful, and uncertain times in which we live.
Much is demanded of us all: patience, love, kindness, compassion, grace, resourcefulness, resilience, tenacity, and more. Previous generations met the challenges of the Great Depression and WWII with strength, stoicism, and **creativity.** Bennett Buggies and eggless cakes are two examples of overcoming adversity. What can we learn from them?

"You can't use up your creativity. The more you use it, the more you have" - Maya Angelou.

When I was very young, I discovered the joy of creating and amused myself through drawing, colouring, and sewing doll's clothes. In my teens, I learned to knit, design, and sew my clothes. After earning a degree in Clothing, Textiles, and Design, I taught and created a fashion design business. In 2011 I switched gears and started painting seriously.
My husband and I raised three sons. Our lives were busy, and our journey as a family was occasionally littered with boulders, potholes, left turns, narrow shoulders, and many trips to the hospital for treatment of anaphylaxis, stitches, and broken bones. One son was hit by a car and spent three months in hospital. Within one year, my husband and one son were diagnosed with cancer. Two sons were viciously swarmed and assaulted. One son and I contracted a virus that left us with invisible diseases, CFS and Fibromyalgia. Coping with a debilitating chronic disease, and at times reeling with fear and uncertainty, the antidote for me is my creativity. When I could barely sit in a chair, I knit. When in pain, physical or emotional, immersing myself in painting is a distraction and a relief.

How does one find creativity? It is nurtured through one's passion, determination, uniqueness, positive attitude, lack of fear, willingness to make mistakes, ingenuity, and curiosity. Where does one utilize one's creativity? The arts, music, and writing are obvious, but consider other endeavours: business, education, innovation, science, relationships.
Why find your creative outlet? It can bring joy, satisfaction, a sense of accomplishment, improved mental health, and possibly prolong life. Begin your search!

Donna West turns fifty-five in 2021. Is a dual citizen Ameri-Can, a boy and dog Mom, serial entrepreneur, a true Gemini, Type A, and a woman who values friends and family above all else.

Donna West

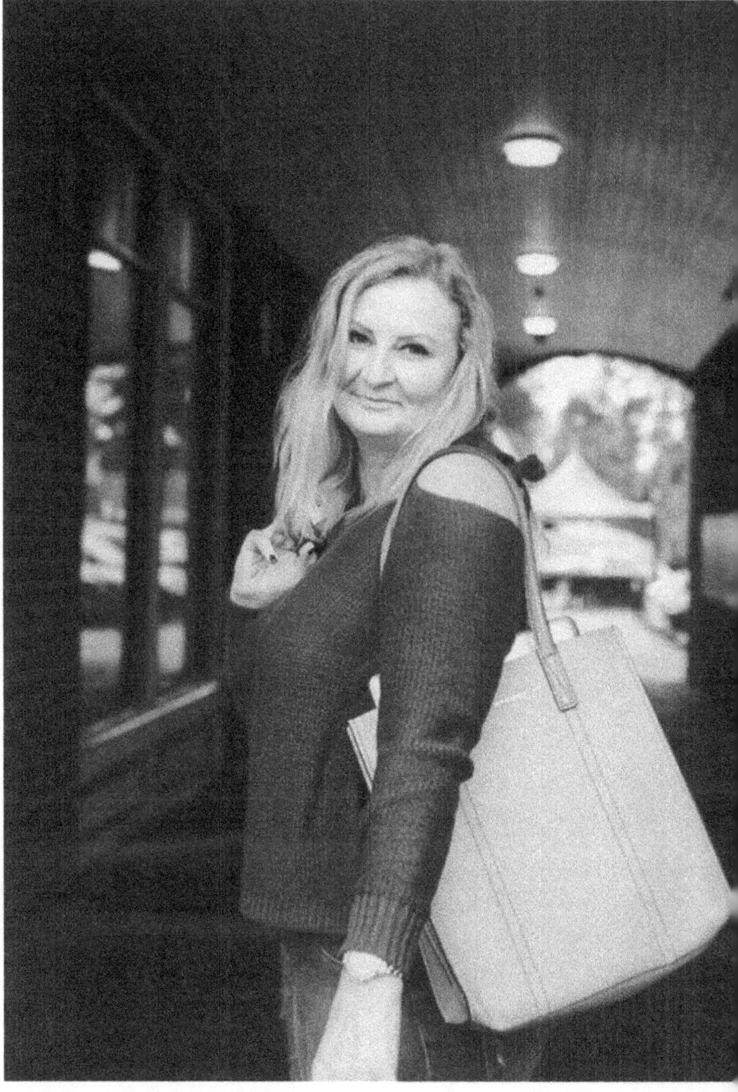

I was born and raised in a middle-class family in Wisconsin, two parents, a younger sister, a dog, and Grandparents who lived next door. I went to school through University in the state, didn't know anyone with their own business outside of a restaurant, had never travelled outside North America, didn't know anyone outside of the U.S., and never lived anywhere outside of Wisconsin.

Therefore, I never imagined or dreamt of living in another country, meeting a Canadian boy in Vegas, moving away from family and friends, having a child in my late thirties, being divorced and a single mom, being in business for myself, or having travelled to destinations like Egypt and Vietnam, yet here I am.

Truth be told, I have never really had dreams, set goals, or chosen much of my life's course. I just happen to fall into things and often feel guilty for accomplishing and succeeding in life without having to put in much thought or effort. Please don't get me wrong, I have failed miserably at many things, and my Gemini "personalities" have gotten me into trouble but the positive far outweighs the negative.

I really got to thinking recently and asked myself, "why have so many amazing people and experiences gravitated towards me, or at times, away from me?" That's when I finally came to the realization of my super-power – the super-power of thought.

From as far back as I can remember, I've always been challenged with relaxing my mind.

Therefore, I am always thinking. Whether I envision something, I think deeply about something, subliminally see or hear something, my mind is always working, and my thoughts are always present; many times, these thoughts turn into actions. Good, bad, or otherwise.

Realizing my thoughts mapped out my path in life is very powerful. Next challenge to focus and use my super-power of thought to align with who I am today and who I want to be.

Final thoughts – here's to hoping everyone finds their super-power.

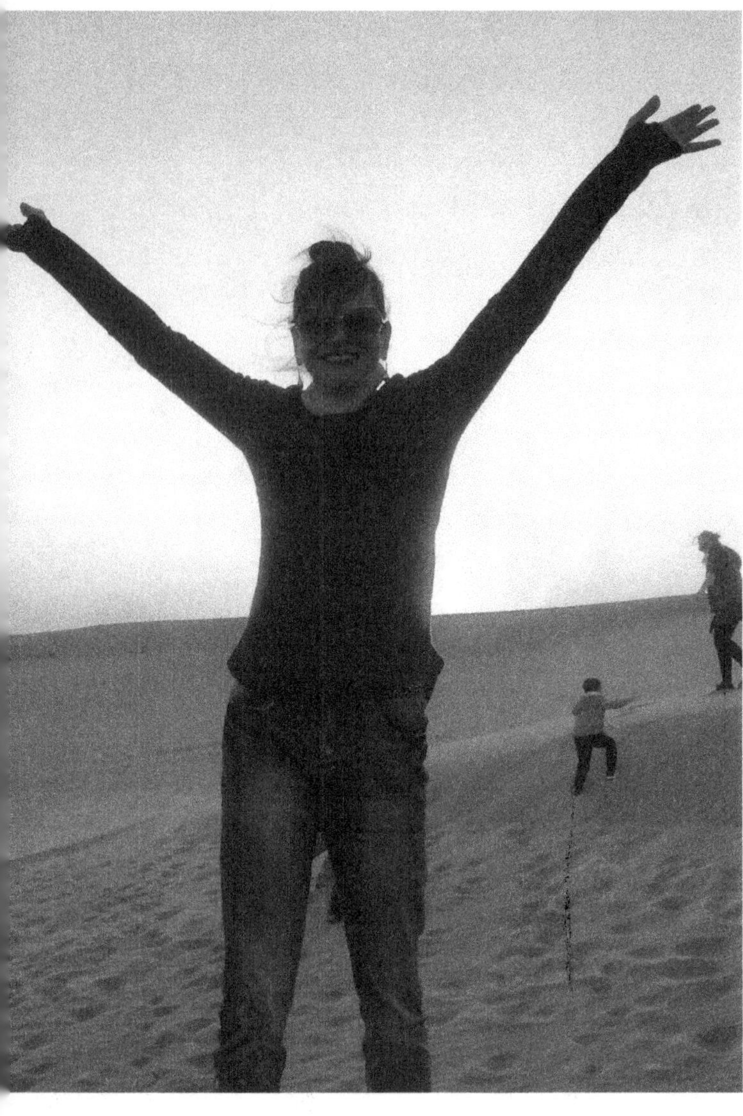

Marcela Bahar is an award-winning clay and glass artist.

Marcela Bahar

In 1968 the Warsaw Army invaded Czechoslovakia. All non-citizens were told to leave. My father, Ralph, was told to leave, as it was not safe for him to stay. Ralph travelled by train to Nuremberg, Germany. At that time, Afghans did not require a visa to enter West Germany. Dad managed to find some work and accommodation at a dorm.

My mother, still in Czechoslovakia, decided to meet my father in Germany to convince him to return. My grandfather drove my mother to the train station. The plan was for my mom, Nadia, to travel alone and bring dad back. But my grandfather knew better. He handed me to my mother and took off. The borders were closed an hour later. My grandfather knew that if mom didn't take me at that moment, she would never see me again.

My mother finally caught up with my father. Unfortunately, we could not stay at the dorm. We had entered Germany illegally now, without visas, so my mom and I were held in a detention center for five weeks. Dad would come daily, and we would speak through the barbed wire fence. Long into my adulthood, I would have dreams about seeing my father through that fence.

We were eventually allowed to travel to an embassy to weigh our options, but because my father's country, Afghanistan, was not at war, the embassy couldn't help. It was looking like my parents would have to separate because of the political situation. In a moment of brilliance, they let us make my mother the head of the household, allowing the rest of the family to come along.

We had four choices: One, stay in Germany and apply for citizenship. This could take approximately twelve years and was not guaranteed. Two, go to the USA, but we needed to be sponsored by a citizen. Three, Australia, which was three months by boat. And four, Canada. We could stay in Canada indefinitely as landed immigrants, and after three years, we could apply for citizenship.

So, off to Canada we went. We waited for the government representative to meet us when we arrived, but no one came. The terminal was closing, and the janitor noticed our family of three. The kind gentleman took us to his home. He and his wife gave us a place to sleep. And in the morning, he drove us to the immigration office.

Kimberly Dolan is a multi-passionate entrepreneur and life-long learner. She is a certified music therapist and wellness advocate who thrives on seeing and helping people live their best lives.

Kimberly Dolan

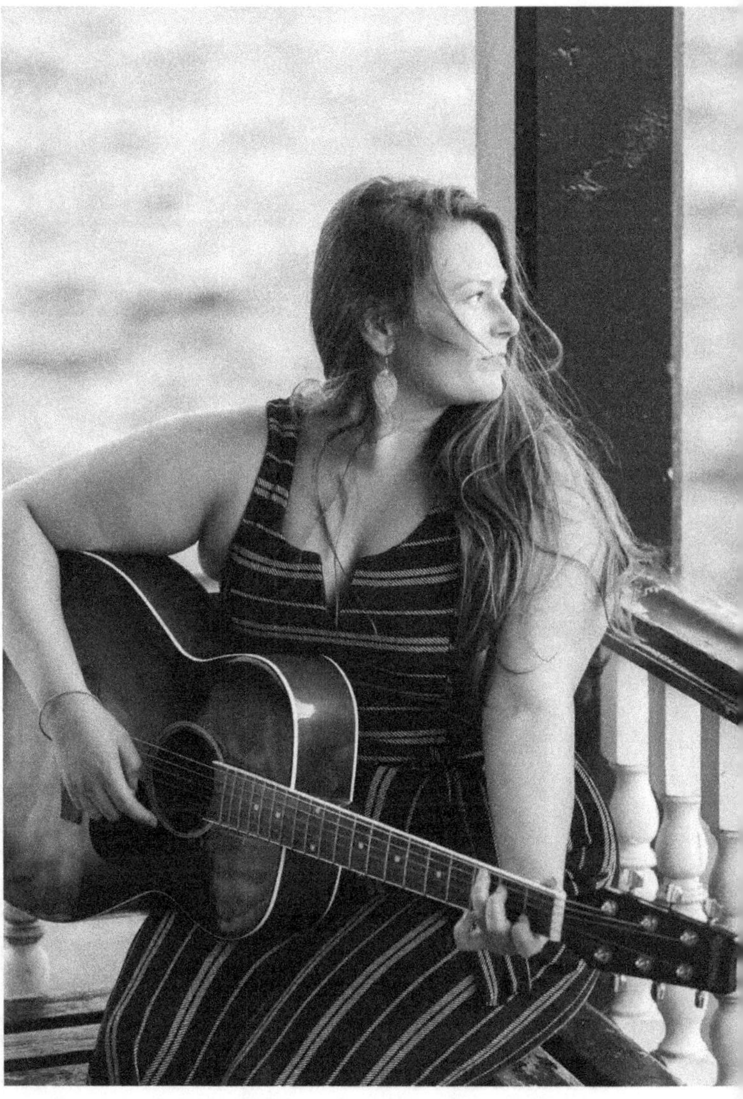

I am a woman of many passions. As a result, I am also a very busy woman - and I love it! I am a certified music therapist, singer-songwriter, theatre administrator, actor, businesswoman, dog mom, dog lover, and the list goes on.

All my life, I have maintained a busy schedule, and frankly, I feel most fulfilled when it is kept full; of course, there is always a limit. Within my first two years of my career, I was completely burnt out. I was exhausted, deflated, unmotivated, and drained of creativity. I found myself living checkpoint to checkpoint, craving the next break just to stay afloat. Then the world stopped, and I had time to breathe. It was in this breath that I realized the issue wasn't my busy schedule but rather its makeup. I was putting in more energy than I was receiving. I was not living a life that aligned fully with my wellness needs.

We are busy people. Sometimes our perfectly scheduled day is interrupted by life. Sometimes you need those extra fifteen minutes of sleep. Sometimes you need to eat that donut. Sometimes you need to bust a gut laughing with friends. Sometimes you need to feel lit up by work, or work up a sweat, or lay on the couch and cry, or pet a dog (or three).

Wellness isn't about perfection; it's about balance. It's about knowing yourself well enough to give yourself grace when you need a break, but to also call yourself out when you're slacking off on doing the work.

I believe, wholeheartedly, that life is a journey meant to be explored and enjoyed. We aren't meant to live with the "just hang on" mentality. We are meant to learn and grow and connect with the world around us.

You deserve to do things that light you up.
You deserve to feel fulfilled in every element of your life.
You deserve to thrive and live your healthiest life.
You are worthy.

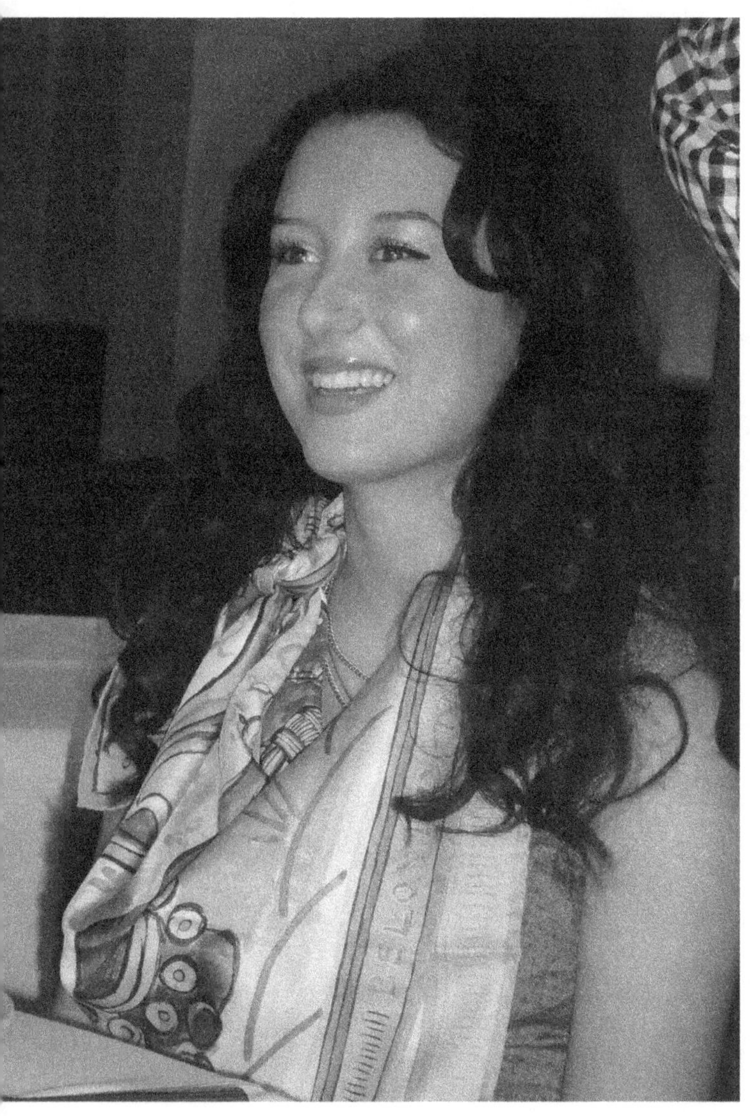

Jannette Salvador is the co-founder of Enhancing Simplicity, bringing attention to the importance of self-awareness within a self-care regimen.

Jannette Salvador

For many women, a standard day includes being a successful businesswoman, wife, sister, mother, best friend, chef, cleaner, chauffeur - standard superhero stuff - all while being emotionally sound. There are personal and professional relationships to navigate while establishing healthy boundaries, displaying constant compassion, and of course, disguising any weakness or shame.

I lost my superhero status when I suffered two concussions within two years. First, my motorcycle met a streetcar track downtown Toronto. Then less than a year later, my head hit a bridge pass on Centre Island. I quickly realized I had to re-evaluate my lifestyle. Daily tasks became arduous, and I needed support more than I had ever before. I felt I was losing my sense of self. Traumatic brain injury is called the invisible disease. I found that not many women suffer head injuries of this nature, but I also found the support of my peers and friends failing as they didn't understand why I was changing.

Working through my own anxiety and depression issues had always been difficult, but was greatly amplified by the injuries. It's described as greater peaks and lower valleys; peaks being heightened hostility (anger) and valleys being deeper sadness (depression). It's like adding 30% internal reaction to any arbitrary situation, then adding 30% to the melancholy of the reaction, even if these emotions are all inside, they quickly became overwhelming.

Enhancing Simplicity is a wellness community aimed at creating a platform for informing, educating, and sharing life stories and solutions. There is no rulebook on how to rebalance your emotions, sleep patterns, brain chemicals after trauma of any sort, not just physical, but emotional or spiritual traumas. Women have the heavier burden in most cultures and are expected to be the backbone of families, relationships, and societies. The scars we inevitably get while growing through hardships stay with us and can end up running our lives and affecting our health physically, mentally, and spiritually as well as our relationships with loved ones.

Most people don't get the wake-up call that I did when I was forced to refocus myself on creating a healthy work-life-relationship balance. Giving women the safety of community and space to understand the importance of self-compassion is what we are aiming to achieve with **Enhancing Simplicity.**

Golfo Tsakumis is a multifaceted individual who embodies many roles including artist and nurturer.

Golfo Tsakumis

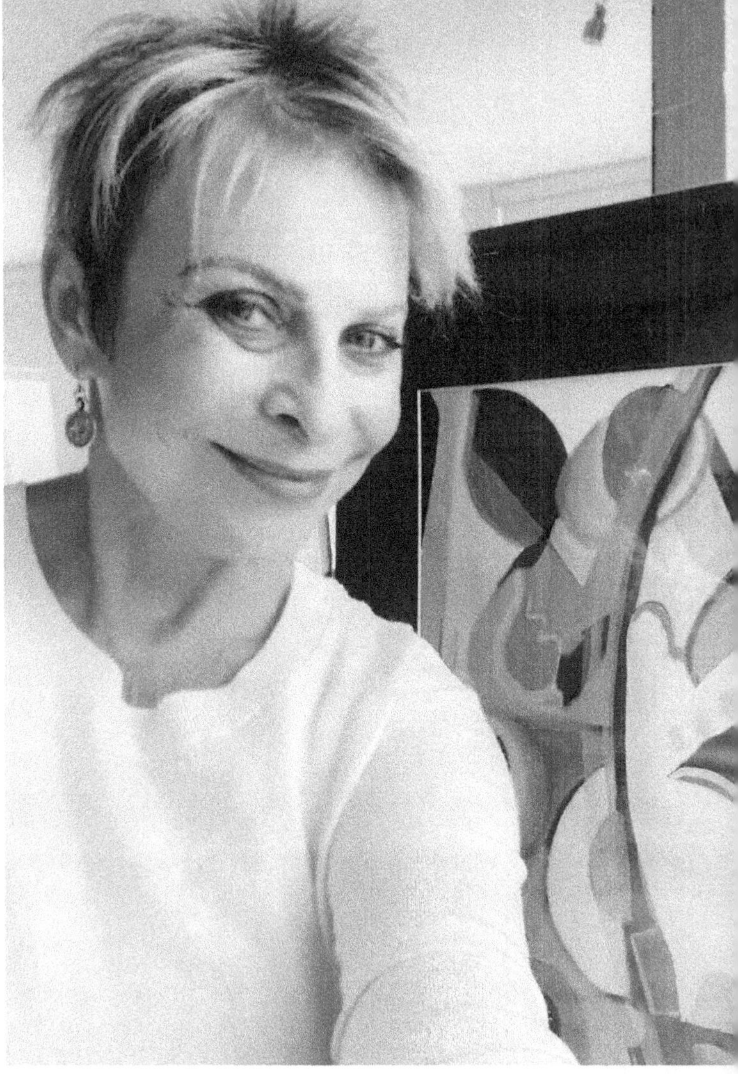

Daughter, wife, immigrant, mother, student, entrepreneur, grandmother, artist, philanthropist... these are the people I have been at various stages of my life. When I say them to myself, I think of one thing that links them all to each other: courage. I didn't always feel courageous. Often it was the opposite. When I reflect through sixty-five years of life, I realize that none of these versions of me could have existed without courage. It helped me move forward when I thought I couldn't, after experiencing debilitating loneliness upon leaving my home and country that I fiercely loved, to one that I had barely heard about.

Courage helped me realize my purpose and see my future once I became a mother. It kept me fighting through my fears and grief every day to be a caring, motivated, and strong example to my five children.

To my core, I am a nurturer. It is my 'raison d'etre'. However, it wasn't until I found the courage to nurture my own soul, as well as others, that my journey to true happiness could begin. That is when I knew that my life felt completely right. I focussed on my education, achieving my goal of obtaining my high school diploma, and applying for post-secondary studies. Eventually, I turned to creating art, and that is when the real me began to emerge.

Painting gives me courage and freedom. It is my past, present, and future coming out from my heart onto my paintbrush and then onto my canvas. I learn so much with each new piece that I create. Every person's reaction to my work is a step in my personal evolution; I become a better version of myself because of it.

Connecting with others through art has been vital in my pursuit of happiness.
Today, I am grateful for every single one of my years and optimistic about the ones ahead. I feel unstoppable. I wholeheartedly believe that each person can find their courage-it is never too late. I am proof of that. I am a completely transformed person, having stepped outside of so many old comfort zones, and I finally trust my once-absent inner voice when it courageously says, "GO FOR IT!"

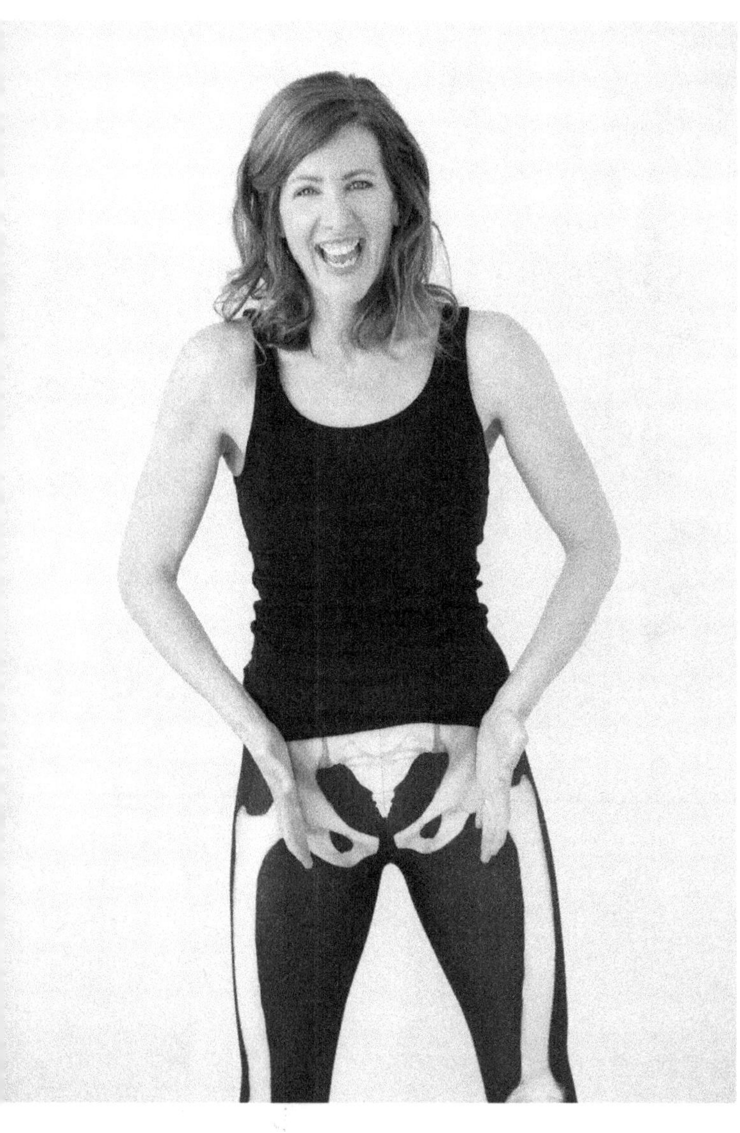

Kim Vopni is a pilot's wife and a passionate entrepreneur working in the field of women's pelvic health while doing her best to raise two boys who are comfortable with the word vagina.

Kim Vopni

Health and wellness have been a passion of mine since I was a teen. I was always buying the latest fibre rich cereal, reading every fitness magazine I could, and joining every sports team. I focused mainly on soccer and running until university and then dropped soccer. I ran to stay fit, to clear my head, and to stay fit.

I spent my twenties trying to find my way in the world. In my thirties, I started my family, and while I still prioritized my health, my fitness started to take a bit of a back seat. I had somehow lost my motivation. In my forties, I struggled. I was raising two young kids, running two businesses, and for several years doing it with no family support nearby. My body was sending signals that I knew were a form of SOS, but I had no idea where to start.

It was late in my forties that I found out I have an autoimmune condition called Hashimoto's that affects the thyroid and leads to brain fog, heavy menstrual bleeding, low energy, lack of motivation, poor recovery, constipation, anxiety, and other challenges. I took immediate steps to learn as much as I could and begin to heal my body with an aim of putting the condition into remission.

I will be fifty this year and am determined to make this my best decade yet! I have sold one of my businesses to allow me more time to prioritize my health, spend time with my family, and focus on building my women's pelvic health business. I am informed about menopause and plan to throw a white pant party once I reach it and not let it stall me.

Even though I have been a health nut for most of my life, I was still sidelined by a health condition I had never heard of. Women's health deserves more attention and it is my mission to help others navigate the various components with ease and confidence.

Cate Giannousopoulos (pronounced: John-is-hopeless) is a passionate, driven, layered woman who has worn many hats through the years, including marketing director, childbirth doula, kickboxing instructor, TV series executive producer, and serial entrepreneur (current: UntsuckCo). She attributes her personal/professional growth to her failures and most painful experiences, not her victories.

Cate Giannousopoulos

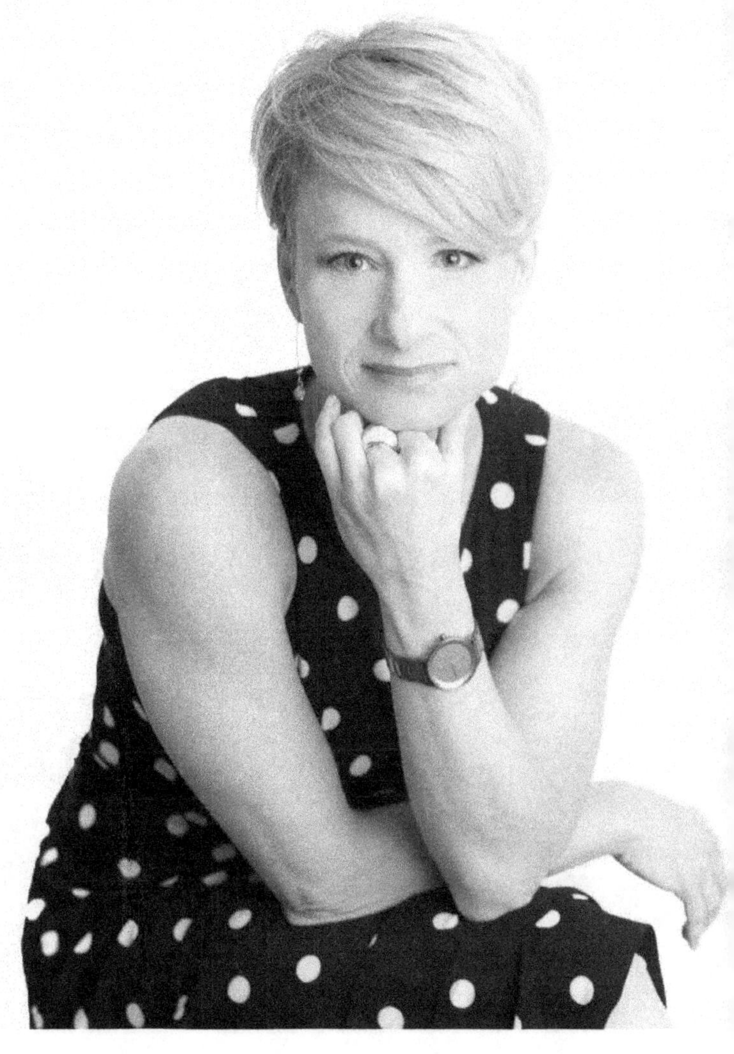

I believe in owning every inch of our stories... the messy parts, the successful parts, the magical parts, the parts we hoped would be different, and especially the parts that no longer fit because we have changed.
I believe our lives are meant to be wholly, fully lived: showing up, especially when it's painful or tough. Using our voices. Refusing to sterilize, diminish, or polish who we are or what we need so others are more comfortable with their choices.

I believe our lives are about learning and unlearning, growing, expanding, falling, getting it wrong - and then trying again. Humbly asking for forgiveness from others and forgiving ourselves. Then recovering, rebuilding, and reclaiming.
When things get messy or ugly, have the courage to look inside at what needs healing. And healing is not fixing.

For me, the most painful parts of my life have also been the most beautiful. I have learned to feel deeply, love hard, and laugh at myself. Even when it feels cringy. I have also learned to show up for myself and others. To fall, fail, hurt, grieve, and then get back up. To share my mistakes and experiences, unvarnished and truthfully. To choose closure, honesty, and courage. To recognize I will fall short of others' expectations – and to still choose to not fall short of my own. To fiercely trust, with everything I am, because what is meant for me will find me.

We all get stuck sometimes; we're supposed to. Isn't life about living and loving and feeling and growing in healthy ways? Our stories belong to us. Our stories brought us here. Now. With this soul. To do this.
Hence, UnstuckCo – my soul project, my business.

My pursuit is about becoming whole, for self and others; it's about unwavering trust in abundance, in the generosity of the universe, in the inherent goodness of myself and others, and in the whole, beautiful, layered process.

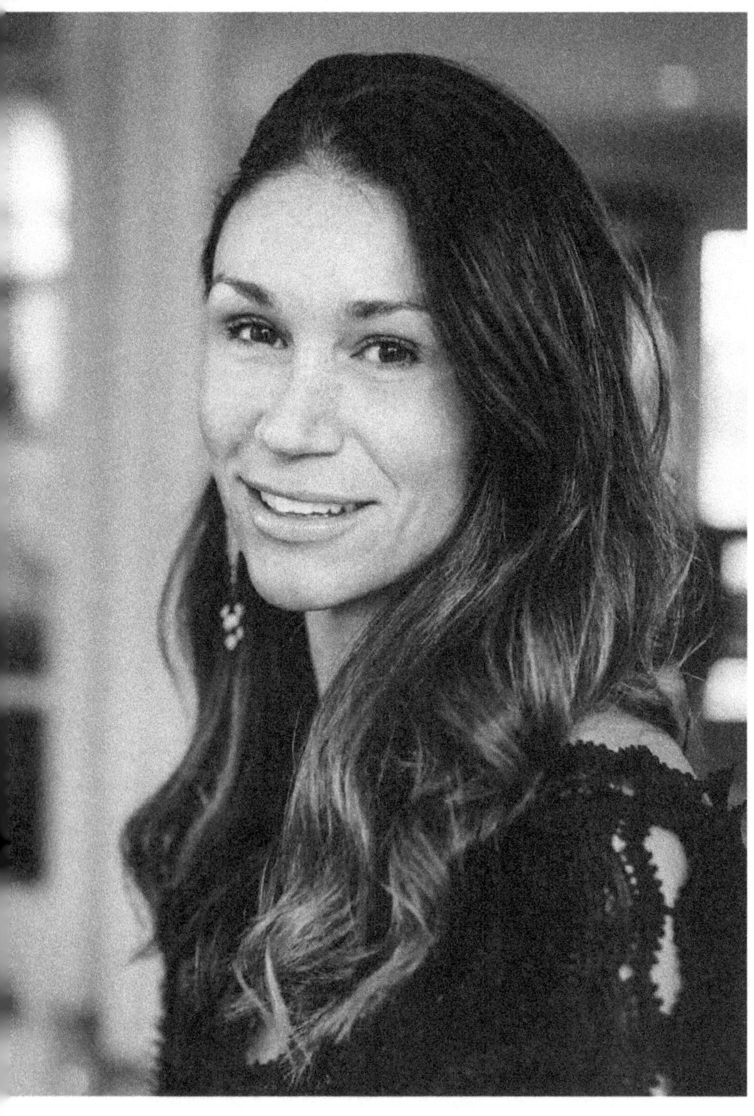

Trisha Pitura is a creative force, mother, entrepreneur, co-owner of MiNi TiPi, and she's definitely not a quitter.

Trisha Pitura

Even though some days are tough, I push through. My three children motivate me. I'm responsible for feeding their hungry minds and showing them that hard work pays off.

I'm originally from Sudbury, Ontario, and I'm a member of Nipissing First Nation. I currently live in Gatineau, Québec with my kids and husband. Growing up, I didn't have a lot of connection to my culture. Now I'm able to explore my identity as an Ojibwe woman through fabrics, creativity, and our business, MiNi TiPi. Will Smith said, "Every morning you have two choices: continue to sleep with your dreams or wake up and chase them."

Everyone has ideas and dreams, but those who take risks and make those leaps to follow their dreams will be the ones to reap the rewards.

Roadblocks happen to all of us, and when you hit one, you have to remember to take a break. Do something for yourself and find ways to make yourself whole again: physically, mentally, spiritually, and emotionally. When things get overwhelming, I have to remind myself that tomorrow can be a fresh start and that absolutely no one out there is perfect.

This work demands that I be continuously evolving and growing. Our dream is not a fixed destination. Failure has taught me that a solution can always be found with just a change in perspective. I don't view failures as failures at all, but as a lesson that needed to be learned; a gift.

My greatest lessons so far have been to be myself, to learn to say no, and to challenge myself every single day. All of these lessons have required me to find my voice and express my thoughts, feelings, and ideas with more confidence than I ever thought possible. The elder women are my mentors and have helped me find strength and inner wisdom.

My encouragement to other entrepreneurs is to try and surround yourself with a strong network of people who have experience in business, or who just believe in you. Take time for self-care and take every opportunity presented to you, even if you have to step outside your comfort zone. Never have regrets, try everything once, and always show up!

Jill Earthy's passion is accelerating the advancement of women leaders and entrepreneurs.

Jill Earthy

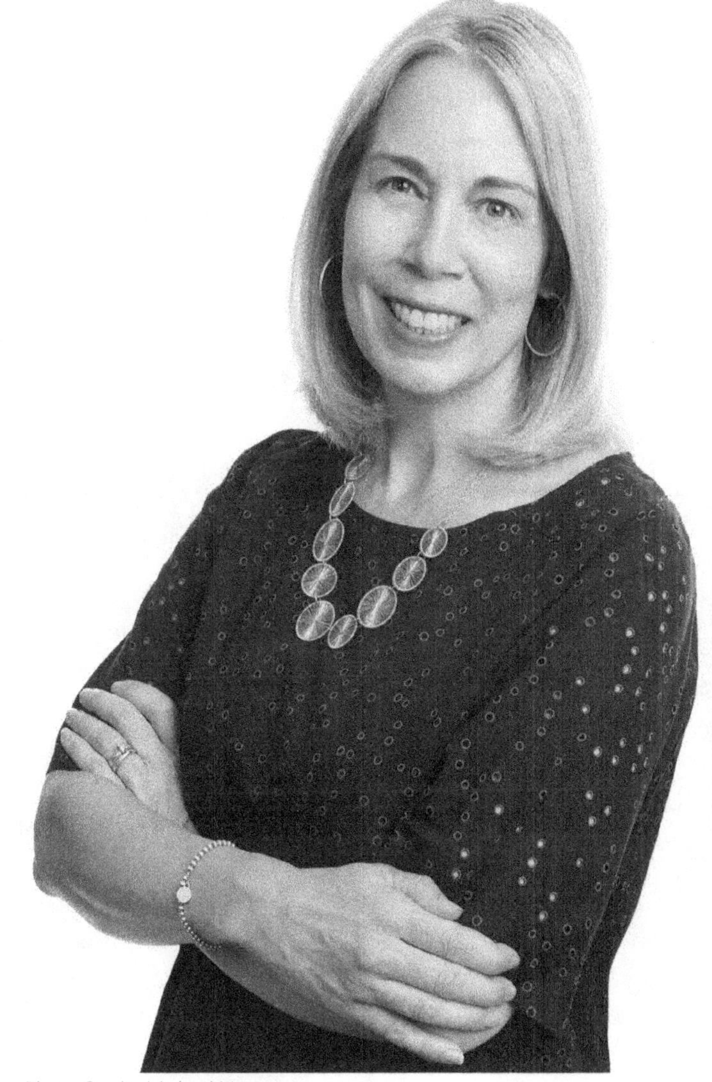
Photo Credit: Michael Hintringer

After eight years on the Board of Directors of Women's Enterprise Centre (WEC), a non-profit organization devoted to helping BC women start, lead, and grow their own business, I stepped into my current role as WEC's Chief Executive Officer, just as the global pandemic was beginning. It was an extraordinary time to take the next step on a winding career path.

Reflecting on this path, there is a clear theme of advocating for gender equity with a focus on women entrepreneurs. I have been an entrepreneur, served in leadership roles in non-profit organizations that support entrepreneurs, and held executive positions in private organizations that explore new forms of capital to increase access for diverse entrepreneurs and investors. I have been fortunate to have been given opportunities and made choices that enabled me to activate my passions and strengths of helping women identify and develop their spark, and to advocate for positive change.

At WEC, we support women entrepreneurs throughout BC with education, mentorship, advisory services, and an accessible loan program. Women represent 16% of small- and medium-sized business owners in Canada and receive less than 4% of venture capital and less than 19% of bank financing. WEC's integrated approach recognizes the unique pathways to business growth taken by women who, for many reasons, tend to start businesses that focus on impact that grow over a longer period of time. This concept challenges the traditionally acknowledged ideas of growth and success. Yet data supports this different approach and when we recognize diverse paths to business growth, more entrepreneurs thrive.

This is a time of incredible change and opportunity, with new models emerging that acknowledge the strengths of a more diverse ecosystem. As a long-time advocate for gender equity, it is powerful to see the conversation deepening to acknowledge many underrepresented voices. We need these diverse perspectives to create a more inclusive and just world. It is a challenging, yet exciting time. So, in this moment, I realize this is exactly where I am meant to be.

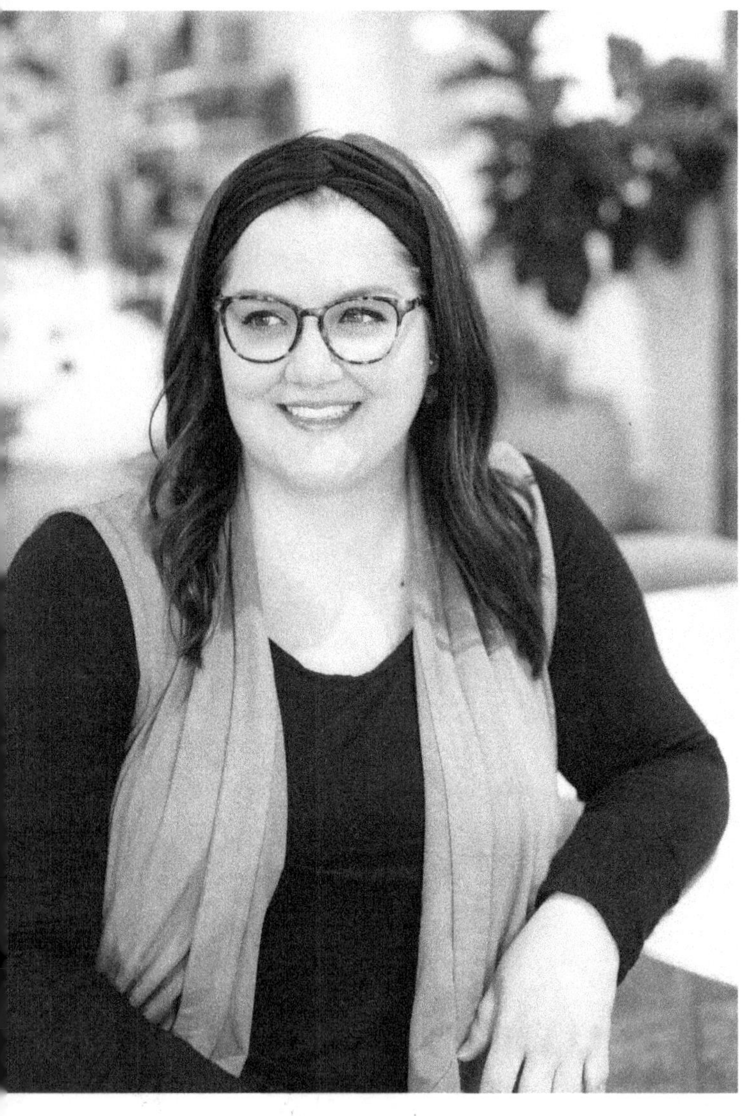

Samantha Brazeau-Wilson is a Social Media Marketer and Owner & Designer of Birch Jewellery.

Samantha Brazeau-Wilson

Growing up in small-town Northern Ontario, my backyard was a forest, and our street didn't have sidewalks. Most folks in my hometown had lived there all their lives. My grandparents lived just down the road, and much of my extended family resided five or ten minutes away. Childhood days were spent outside, using my imagination to play with foraged pinecones and sticks, building houses with leaves, and making mud pies. My way of life was idyllic, but my ambitions were far greater than the opportunities my hometown could ever provide.

Infatuated with New York City, I watched movies depicting women with flourishing careers living in the urban jungle. So, at the bright age of eighteen, I packed up my things and moved to the nation's capital to pursue my studies in Journalism. Upon graduating, I realized the industry had taken a giant turn towards digital media, leaving newspapers and publications across the country to downsize and shift. That meant I, too, needed to shift. Instead of getting discouraged, I leaned into my love for the online space and started working in digital marketing and social media. It was the best decision I have ever made, thanks to trusting my intuition and following my passion.

While maintaining my marketing career, I found time to tap into my creative side and began making nature-inspired jewellery. Perhaps it was to pass the time during school or as a nod to my hometown, but what started as a late-night hobby flourished and became a successful brand adored by nature-lovers across Canada and beyond. Birch Jewellery, my entrepreneurial venture, continues to be my favourite vehicle for creativity.

Throughout my journey to womanhood, the thing that has endured is the heart of that little girl, who used her big imagination to create beautiful things. Whether creating a social media campaign or a new accessory, my inner child will always be included in my pursuit of happiness. From my backyard to the big city, to who knows where next, I believe that the universe will lead me to where I am supposed to be.

Sherrice Kirby is an artist. The canvas and the page are her tools for the translation of how life and nature speak to her. She hopes you are met with beauty and calm in the presence of her work.

Sherrice Kirby

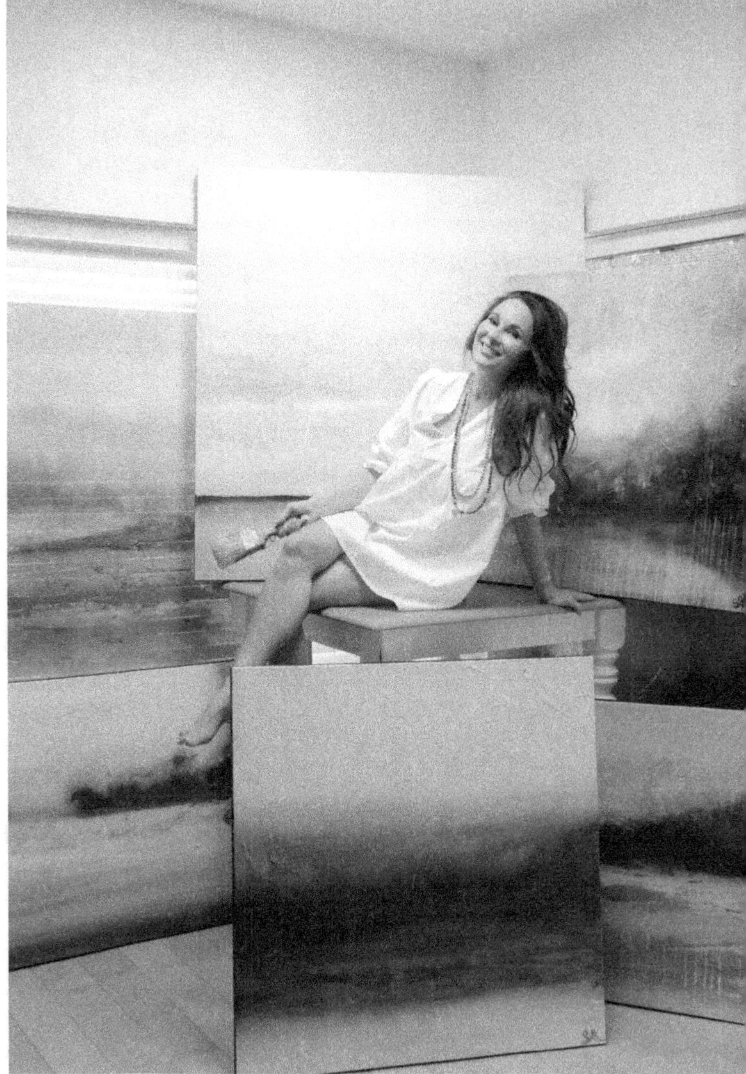
Photo Credit: Julia Loglisci

Wisdom, Creativity & Contentment

I'm meeting the beautiful precipice of fifty this year. Attuning deeply to the idea that, depending on perspective, and the unknown, this journey is approximately half over. Experiencing the end of what represents youth, fertility, and endless pursuits. I reach for gratitude that is not easily attained for the wrinkles on my face and the pain in my joints.

Although, my attention is taken by what has been created in the wake of the chase to arrive somewhere. I reflect on this life, seeing a family, a home, a million memories, and a deep understanding of how to cultivate creativity into every corner of my life. This is where I find my peace, and beauty nestles up to meet my ego's lust for something more. I've come to have profound respect for every emotion that flows through my system, and the awareness not to attach to any as a permanent residence in my body. Life has shown me that to stay sane, I must stay creative. In the hours that require resiliency, having a space to etch the pain may be the only relief that can be found when there is no soft place to land. What I know is that there is no festering in the wounds of perceived failures and what was not achieved.

There is a hard-won freedom in no longer yearning after outcomes for visions that are not my own or seeking a happiness that was not designed for me. Contentment is the friend that has been waiting for me to know and understand her. It is a relief to be courting the wisdom of my years and honing my discernment muscles for truths that are my own. I know my seeking nature will never stop wondering what is possible. So, when the muse stirs, I go to the canvas, listen to what she has to say, and commit to the next movement. A masterpiece or a mess, it's all mine.

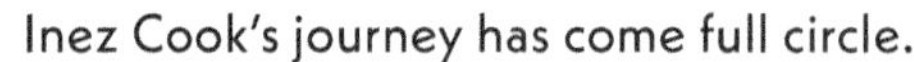

Inez Cook's journey has come full circle.

Inez Cook

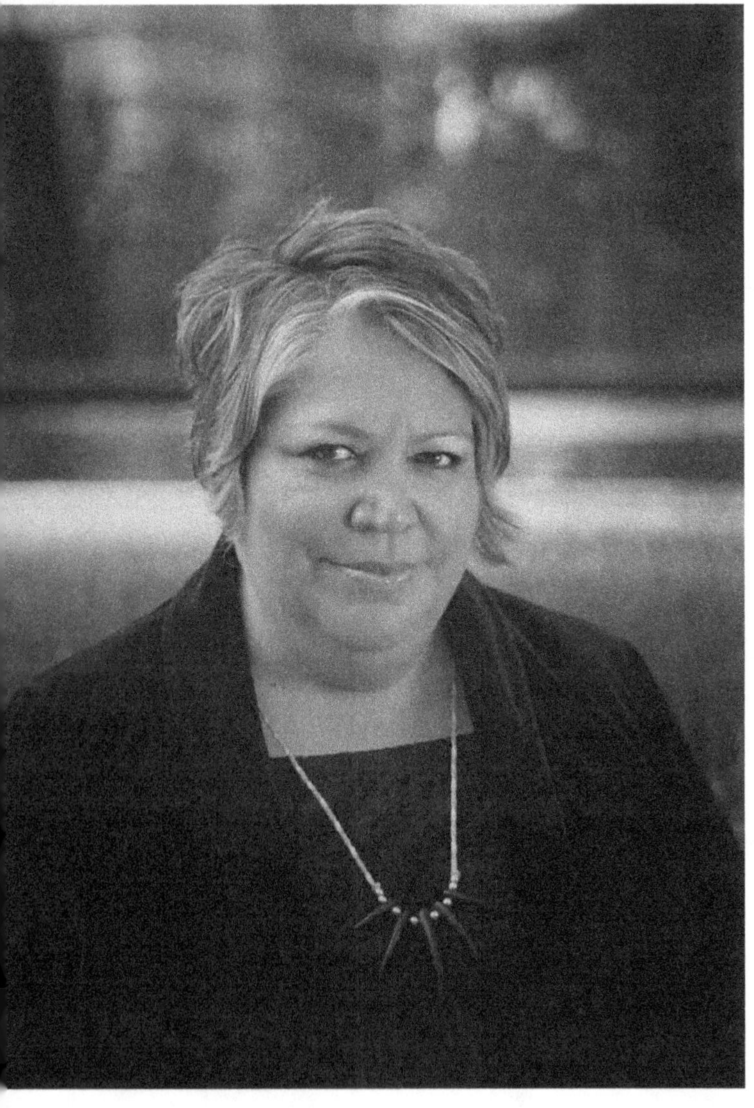

I started my Flight Attendant career thirty years ago. It has given me the opportunity to meet the world and celebrate the culture I yearned for. My dream was to open a restaurant and take people on a journey to experience what I had been able to in my worldwide travels. I wanted guests to feel like they 'got away' through a dining lens.

After five and a half years abroad, I was ready for a change. I got hired with Air Canada and moved home to their Vancouver base.

It was just before the Vancouver 2010 Olympics; the whole world was coming. I had just returned from Kelowna, where had seen an Indigenous restaurant, and was surprised there was no longer one in Vancouver. I shared this information with a close friend and thought it was time to celebrate my heritage. We worked day and night and opened Salmon n'Bannock Bistro on Feb 15th, 2010.

There was a lot of media attention with the new Indigenous bistro and it was printed everywhere that I was Nuxalk (New-halk). Being part of the Sixties Scoop, I had been adopted out and no one in the Nuxalk community knew me. The Nuxalk community thought possibly it wasn't true, maybe I was choosing a culture just far away enough that no one would ask questions.

A lady came in, snapped questions at me.

I knew my biological mother's name.

I told this lady, she got on the phone, and when I returned with her tea she was standing with her arms extended and said, let me be the first to welcome you home.

We are family.

11/11/11 I went back to Bella Coola for the first time as an adult. I was reconnected to my community at a three-day Potlatch. I received regalia and my traditional name Snitsmana. This is the first time in my life I truly felt like I belonged.

My dream restaurant was to take people on a journey, I had no idea the journey I was taking them on was my journey within. Full circle

Melanie Phillips makes the choice to be free and runs toward possibility.

Melanie Phillips

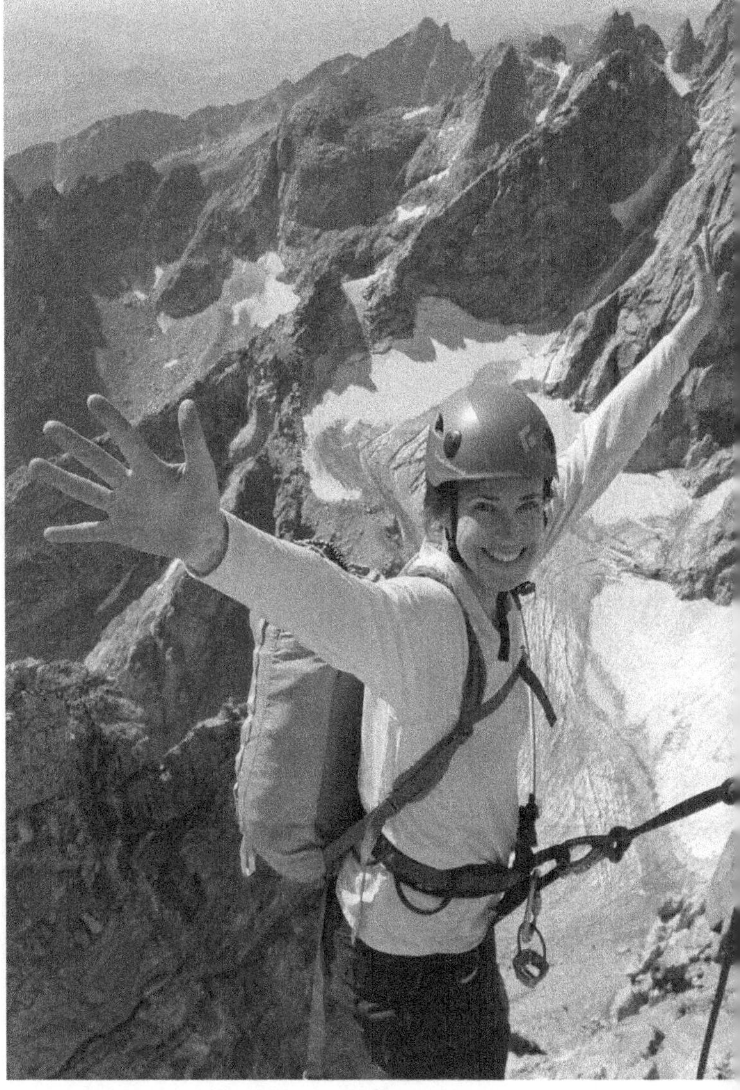

"I'm going to have a great fucking life."
These are the words I spoke to my doctor through heaving sobs as I sat in her office, tormented by the sudden and unexpected suicide of my beloved. I didn't fully believe it, that I would ever live again. The pain of loss was excruciating. All I wanted was him back – our life back – our home and family together again.
I thought I'd passed through the toughest storms of my life. I'd already navigated a decade long autoimmune condition and gruelling divorce. Clearly, I was doing something wrong. Clearly, I was being punished by the Universe. Otherwise, why would my life be filled with so much suffering?

What I've discovered is that life will bring us experiences that expedite our growth and awakening. Big challenges mean you can handle them. Big challenges mean you're on the fast track of internal success and expansion.
I began to reclaim my life and create a world that I love. After my partner's death, I began rock climbing and mountaineering in my forties. I was confronted by the remnants of post-viral fatigue syndrome and was scared that I wouldn't have the energy. But mostly, I came up against my internal fears.
One rock face at a time. The determination of my fingers pinched on a hold. The articulation of my toe placement. In situations beyond my capabilities. Not seeing how I could finish the climb. Terrified looking down. Yet an inner voice whispered, "Keep on going, keep on going. There's always a way."
Life wants us to be an example of what's possible and transcend the known.
When we live from possibility instead of limitation, we allow ourselves to be who we truly came here to be in this life.
There's no time to waste living in outdated versions of ourselves. I've dedicated my life to liberating myself from my past and assisting my clients and students to do the same through spiritual mentorship and energy healing.
Your past doesn't define you. No matter what challenges you've faced, they're not who you are.
Are you being the most optimal version of yourself? The time is now. Rise up to meet your essence and your magnificence.
Life wants you to be free. Freedom is a choice, and it's an inside job.

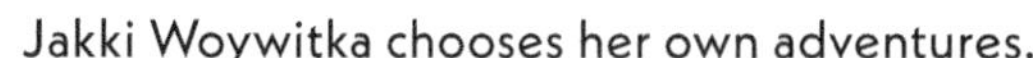

Jakki Woywitka chooses her own adventures.

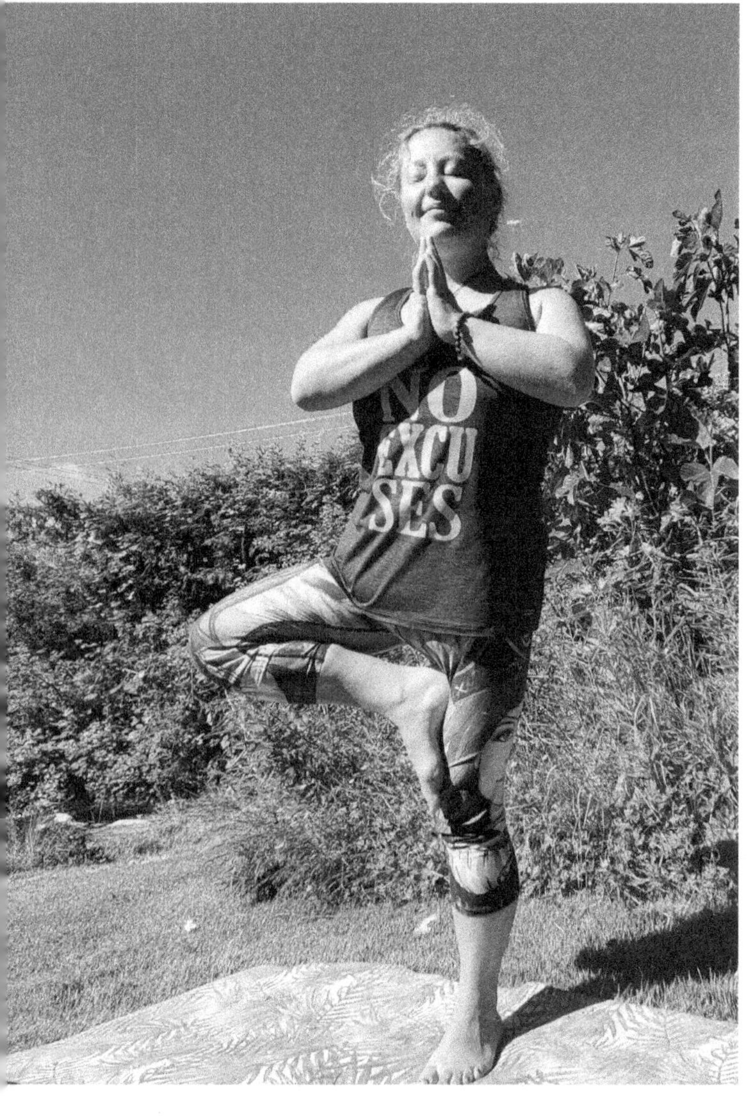

Jakki Woywitka

Fitness fanatic and adventure-loving, thirty-six-year-old, Jakki, was devastated by the diagnosis that she was in Congestive Heart Failure. She felt her dreams ripped away. What would her life feel like without sports, travelling, and working overseas? Would she still be able to complete her goal of visiting every country on the planet?

During her first appointment with a Cardiologist, she was told that she would be on medicine for the rest of her life. She was told that all the side effects she was having were not from medications and that she was being psychosomatic, and to just deal with it.

Driving back home, she had to stop more than once to control the sobbing. Stopping at a trail, she ran as fast and as hard as she could. How could this be happening to me? Why was my heart failing me? This can't be my life from now on. Why am I taking medicine that is only making me sicker? I hate my life! I just want to die! She tripped and tumbled onto the ground. As she lay there in a sobbing, muddy mess, a light bulb went on. This didn't have to be her life. She had a voice. She had a choice. Life isn't about what happens to you, it's about the choices you make. In that moment, she made the decision to change her story. She joined natural healing groups, researched, and talked to others. She came to one conclusion; there are many different treatments, there is no wrong or right way to deal with a chronic illness.

The only thing she could do is listen to and trust herself.

Now, two years later, she is medicine and medical device free, back to being an athlete, and is on a mission to help others with Heart Disease live their best life.

Her advice to those with Heart Disease and other Chronic Illnesses is: Learn to listen to yourself. Nobody else is in your body. Get expert opinion, talk to those who have been through it, do your own research, and check in with your body. You matter and deserve the best that life has to offer.

If you had told Mellisa Mills a decade ago she'd be at the helm of a growing plant-based cheese empire, she'd have laughed in your face. After all, she'd been fired from just about every job she ever held for insubordination. But it turns out, she just needed to do things her own way.

Mellisa Mills

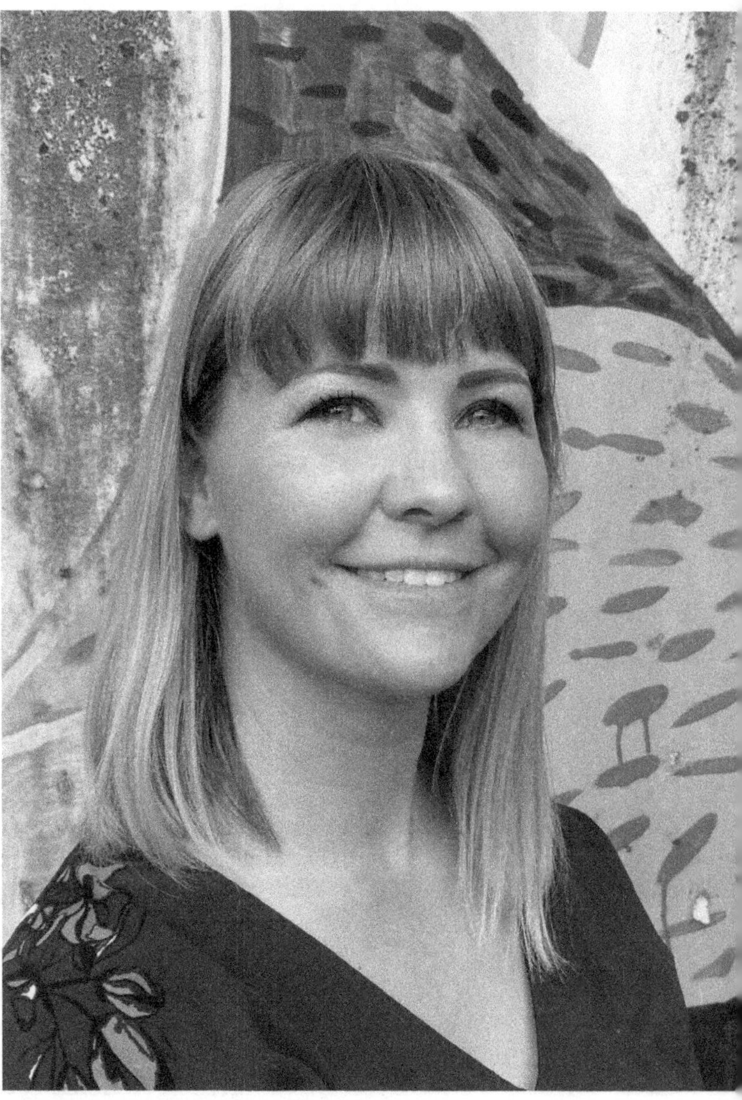

What a story it has been so far. With a lifetime of plant-based eating under her belt and a strong entrepreneurial spirit, Mellisa has some serious veg cred and she put it to good use. In the lively hub of her family's kitchen, she got into the culinary game at an early age. Later, in between the many jobs that never seemed to stick, her DIY spirit and curiosity about nutrition and plant medicine combined with her love of quality ingredients to create Spread'Em Kitchen.

Mellisa first turned a blender, a bicycle, and $500 into a thriving farmers market stand in Vancouver. And several years later, this little passion project turned into much more than that. It moved into its own industrial facility, where it gradually grew into a celebrated manufacturer of plant-based dips, spreads, cheeses, and other dairy alternatives.

Before long, retailers started calling. First, it was small independent shops, then specialty natural food chains, and finally, conventional grocers lined up for a chance to stock what has since become a household name and staple in many kitchens across Canada.

As the CEO, Mellisa remains in command of the company's innovation initiatives. Drawing from international flavours inspired by her extensive travels, she develops and perfects recipes held up by the twin pillars of nutrition and taste, She also passionately spearheads the company's community and sustainability initiatives and remains the face and voice of Spread'Em Kitchen, sharing its mission of creating delicious food that's good for your body and the planet.

She lives in Vancouver with her partner Luke and their hilarious little cannonball of a toddler Benjamin. You can still spot her at local farmers' markets on the weekends unless she's busy experimenting in her home kitchen.

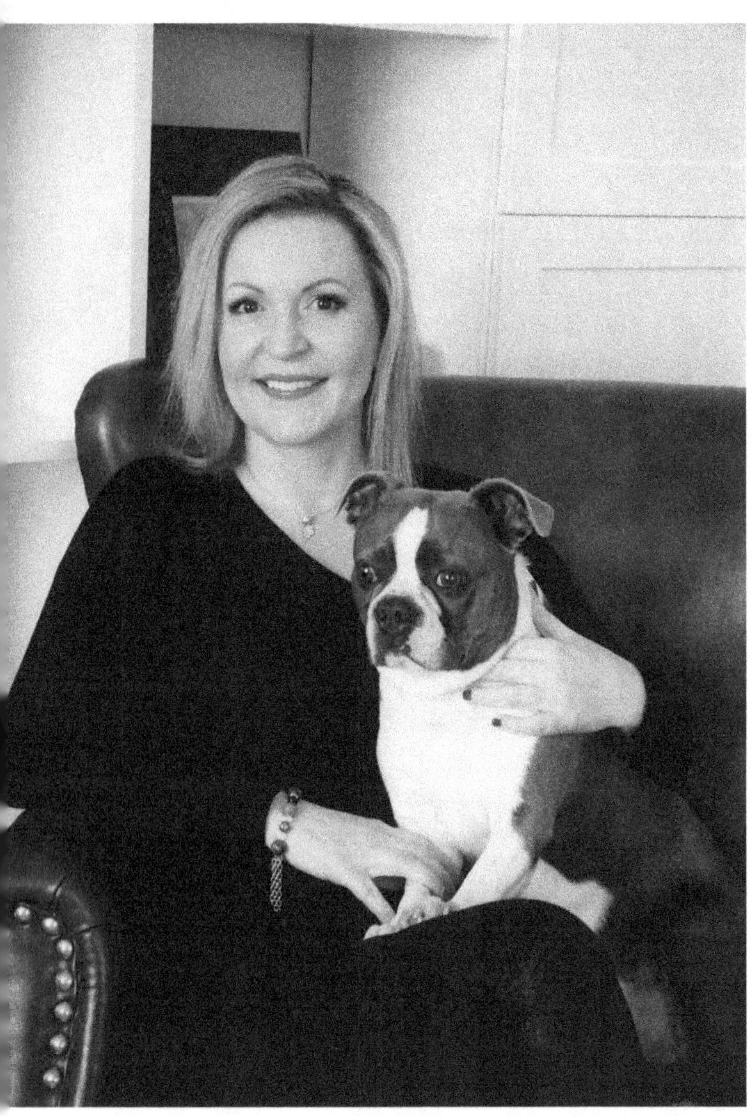

Olivia is a passionate, intuitive, self-renewed intriguing woman, who in her long journey of self-discovery, found a unique talent that can help others in their own path of self-discovery and purpose.

Olivia Repnicki

At a very young age, I have always believed in the mystical powers of stones and crystals, but it took me nearly forty years to understand the healing gift I have in me to help others find their path of happiness and success. I have always been highly intuitive but shield away from it. I could feel people's energy deep into their souls. The feelings were too strong for me to face them, partly because of my own struggles through adult life. I often felt misunderstood.

At the toughest point in my life, I opened my soul to this journey. Discovering my inner self through crystals helped me to overcome my fears and learn to feel joy and embrace my life. I believe in the mystical powers of stones and crystals and I know that there is a special crystal for everyone and for every stage of one's life journey. I think of crystals and stones as powerful talismans that can help us through any obstacles or challenges and can shine light on what we are seeking in life.

Today, I see myself as a creative, caring soul and a certified Reiki Master, who has a unique gift in helping others find answers in their own life's struggles. The ability to heal others from the inside out is my passion. With my psychic and mediumship abilities, helping individuals find answers to their own inner peace, health, and happiness, has become my purpose.

My journey of discovering my inner need to help others, lead me to Crystal Obsessions. Combining my gift of intuition with my love for crystals, I create healing jewelry, blessed with reiki energy, that I want to share with the world.

Reiki is a Japanese ancient healing technique for stress reduction and relaxation. I call it a "massage for your soul."
I combine my healing energy with love and dedication into all of my jewelry designs, to offer you peace, health, happiness, and guidance on your path to self-discovery and purpose.

Dawn Williams is a successful engineer and loving mother.

Dawn Williams

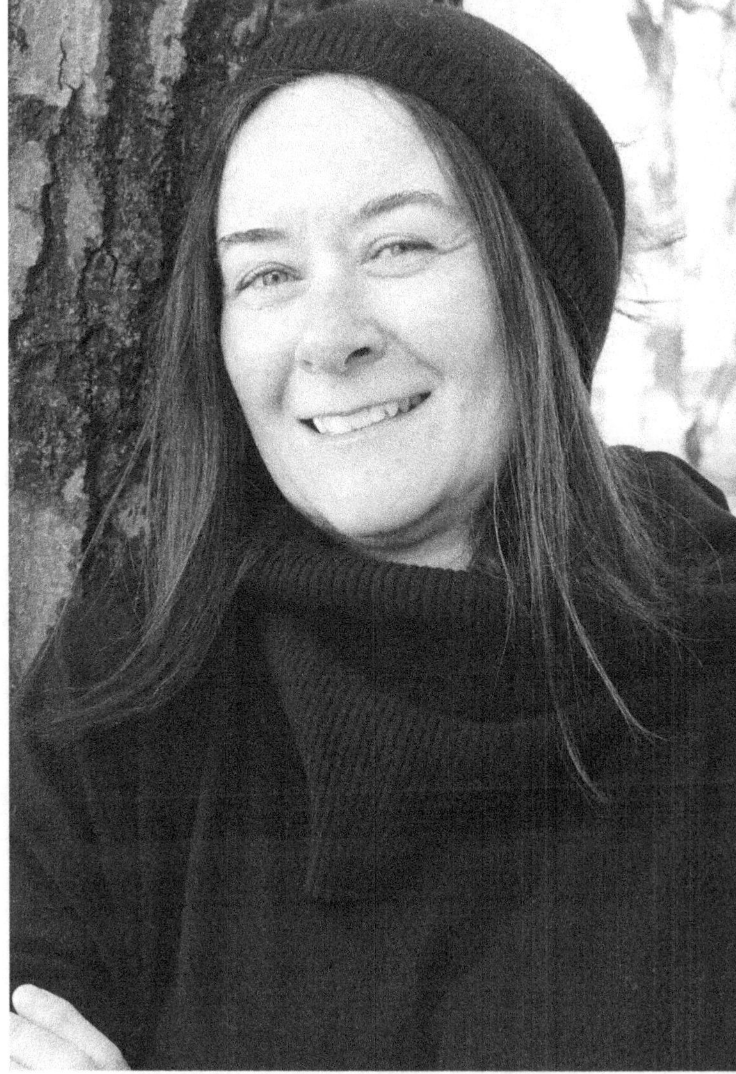

Finding balance is the key to living a happy life. We can't sacrifice our own meaningful pursuits to the responsibilities of work and family. We must endeavor to retain our sense of self so we can fully participate in all aspects of our lives.

While not being a goody two shoes my whole life, I have always had a healthy respect for the rules, and my mum. Due to my rule following tendencies, I struggled to leave a marriage that functioned for a relationship that truly made me feel alive and happy. Following my heart, I found the courage to leave and ultimately married a wonderful man and had two awesome children. Soon after I began to flounder and lose myself. I became a mum first and forgot to be me. Holding firmly onto my small group of high school and university friends, I didn't develop new friendships. Living at a distance, I didn't see my besties often. Life became all about my work and my kids - both wonderful, but over time a sense that something was missing became apparent. To combat the feeling, I immersed myself in work and my kids. My husband and I drifted apart.

Recently, the struggle to manage this has grown, and I find myself thinking about what I want and who I am. I take more time for myself, putting myself ahead of work and the kids. Entrenched in old habits, this doesn't come easily but the results are worth it. My kids mean the world to me but making time for myself is making me a more present mother. My kids are my joy, but they don't define me and will benefit from my self- care. While I thoroughly enjoy, my career, it can't come at the expense of my personal happiness.

Finding the right balance ensures I am true to me and happily available to others. My journey is new and not complete and realizing that I matter is a gift that I have given to myself and my children. I knew it once and am finding it again. Finding balance is how I am pursuing happiness.

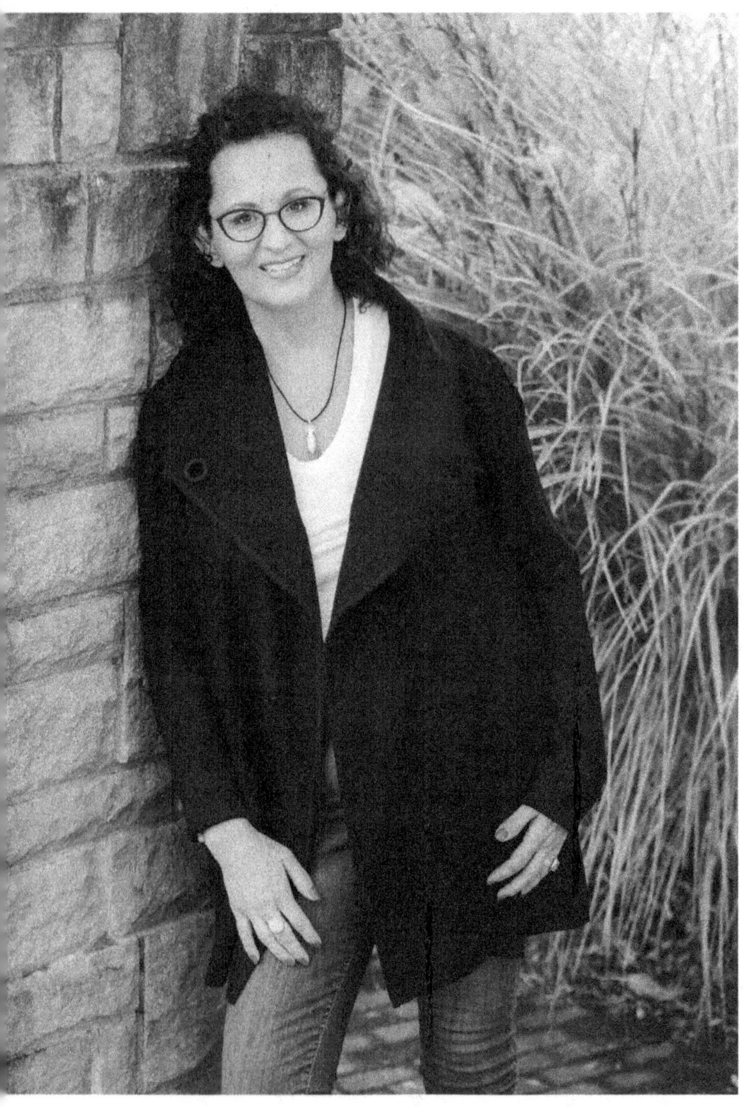

Sharon Storoschuk is an intuitive coach, energy healer, medium, craniosacral therapist, and Reiki master.

Sharon Storoschuk

Growing up, I used to say that I wanted to help people. Never in my wildest dreams did I think it would be as an intuitive coach, energy healer, or medium. I didn't even know what those things were!

Looking back, on my incredible life, my accomplishments are many; three degrees, global travel, and a successful career in public health. Yet, I've lived a large portion of my life in darkness fearing my own power. Deemed too sensitive during youth, I shut down, not crying for twenty-five years. Being caught up in the doing of life had me forget how to just be. After several relationships, I finally married at forty-two but my marriage ended after only four years.

Many of my adult years were lonely, paving the way for emotional and physical health problems. There had to be more. It wasn't until I tapped into lost emotions that I took responsibility for my life and found my true power, allowing me to fully enjoy life!

Moving to Vancouver was pivotal. The discovery of Reiki coupled with weekly visits to women's groups reconnected me with my emotions. I tuned in to my own intuition and trusted it. Learning that everything is energy and that I create my own reality, changed my life. No more sitting in the shadows, now my Divine Feminine could shine!

Discovering that I am not my degrees, my job, or any of the roles I assume, but that I am a Divine Being having a human experience was enlightening. The last twenty years spent trusting my intuition and leading with my heart have led to joy. The unlearning of societal norms and eliminating destructive self-thoughts have allowed me to accept myself and find happiness in service. Discovering that real power comes from within, is what released me from my role as a societal minion and allowed my evolution to Powerhouse of the Divine Universe. I can't make you happy, but I can help you get there. My passion is helping women find their voice and create the life of their dreams. I am powerful beyond measure and so are you!!

Sue Clement is a Business Strategist who helps entrepreneurs expand their visibility, increase their impact and profitably scale from six to seven figures.

Sue Clement

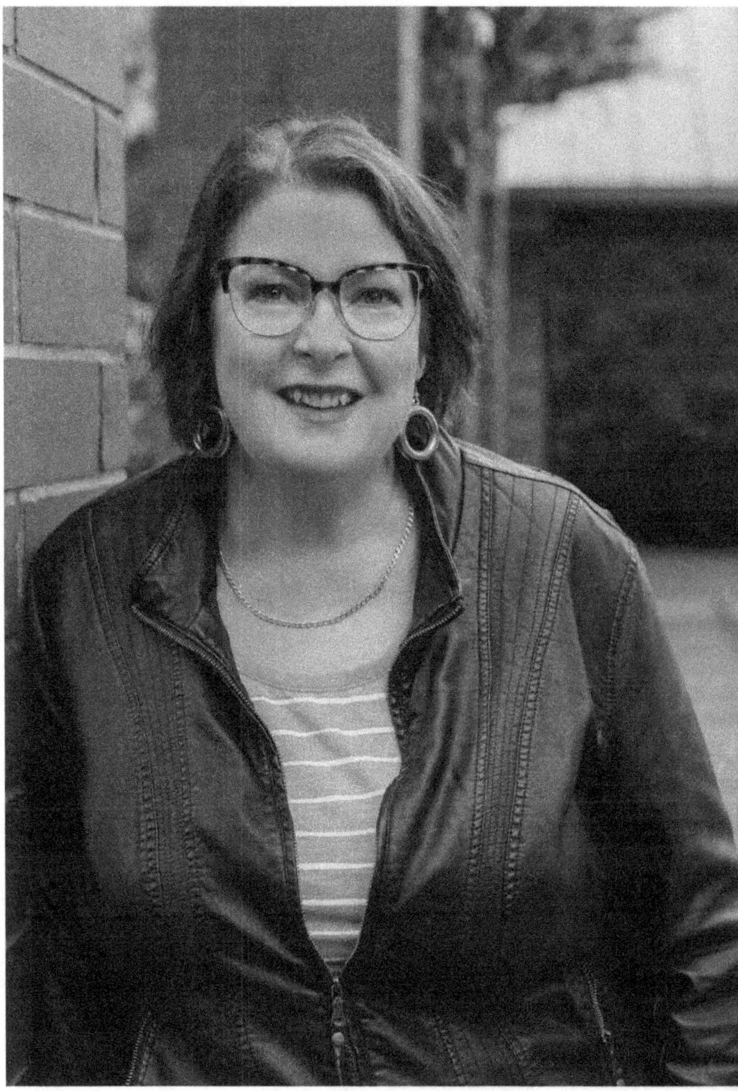

When I started my first business, an employment agency, I struggled greatly. I was hanging on by my fingernails when the dreaded phone call came.
"Sue, your rent is ninety days late. If you miss your payment on Monday, the Sheriff will padlock your business doors."
I was instantly thrown into "deer in the headlights" panic mode. Fear stuck deep, and then shame rolled in. What would I tell my employees and clients?
That was nearly thirty years ago. I'm relieved to say that after numerous sleepless nights, I got better at running my business and turned it around. In nine years, I grew the revenues to 5.2 million dollars and then sold the company.
I'm often asked how I went from the brink of bankruptcy to creating a profitable, thriving business. The biggest shift came quite unexpectedly. Driving to my office, swaddled in fear of failure and shame, like a lightning bolt of inspiration, the thought "I am not my business" boomed loud in my head. In that moment, I untangled my identity from the business, releasing myself from the potential failure. Yes, my business may fail, but I wasn't going down with it. This simple thought broke me free from the confines of fear. I became bolder, took more risks, and gained the confidence to sell to bigger companies and projects. Almost overnight, I was transformed into a self-confident businesswoman on a mission. And it worked.
After selling my company, I started Business Coaching. For the past twenty years, I've helped struggling entrepreneurs transform into successful CEOs with profitable businesses. I've found at the heart of success, or failure, is fear. Fear is a sneaky devil, often cloaking itself as doubt, procrastination, perfectionism, confusion, or shiny penny syndrome. And I've experienced them all! Success comes from the ability to call fear out, to stop playing small, and to be brave enough to go all in. Ultimately the best antidote is action, no matter how tiny. Having the tenacity, commitment, and mental toughness to fall in love with the process and do the work is key.

Remember, no matter what life throws your way, you are stronger than you think and more resilient than you believe.

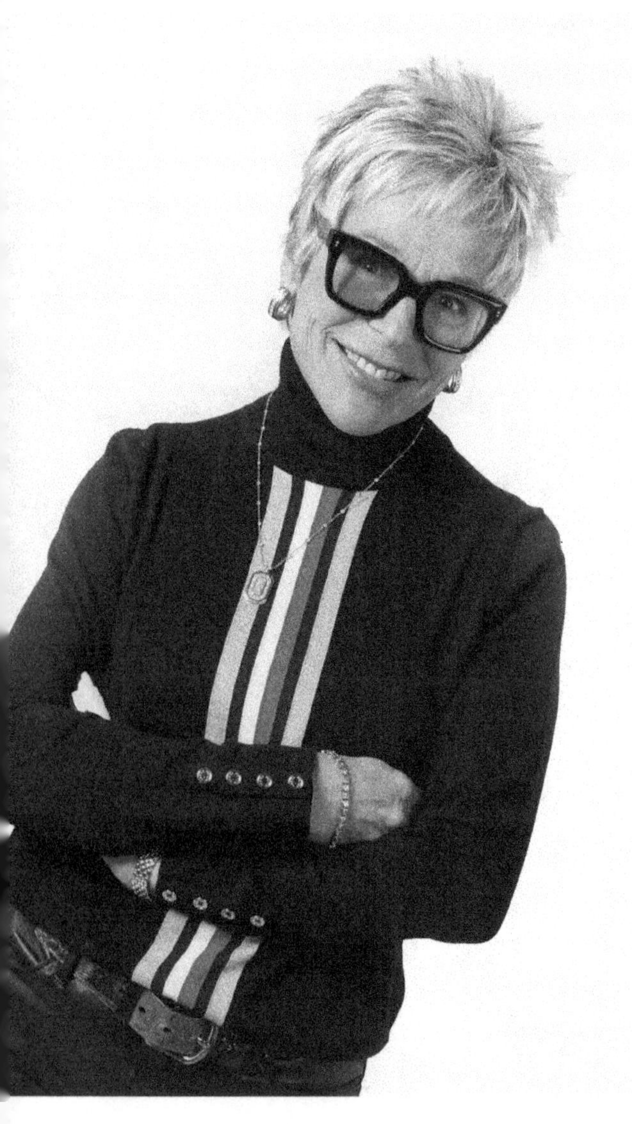

Suzanne Sendel is the founder of the Suzanne Sendel Agency, a distributor for multiple high-end eyewear brands, and creator of The Original FTG.

Suzanne Sendel

Inspired by strong women in my life, I was raised by two resilient and driven women who were Holocaust survivors, my mother and grandmother inspired me to be ambitious and never give up on my dreams.

For the greater good of my business career, I have reinvented myself several times over the years without ever looking back. I have worked in the fashion and design industry and have always been driven by creativity. On vacation, my sunglasses broke, and as they were being repaired, I discovered my future right in front of me! The purchase of an original hand-painted frame changed my life. For the next year, I was approached by hundreds inquiring, "where are your glasses from?" I took this as a cue to contact the manufacturer. Three months later, I resigned from my job and reinvented myself as an optical distributor. Always moving forward and believing in my entrepreneurial skills, I began my most passionate journey.

Today, I carry the most provocative, luxurious, story-telling collections of eyewear. Priding myself on my work ethic, I have built a strong following and have customers across the globe who appreciates my tenacity, honesty, and commitment.

On a summer day, I awoke from a dream with a novel idea. The next morning, I sketched it out and began developing. I soon launched my own addition to the optical accessory market with a must-have solution to an old problem. My optical pouch, The Original FTG, stores multiple pairs of glasses while preventing loss and damage. Many people wonder why nothing like it exists. Building my brand by reaching many through social media platforms, my quirky videos have caught the eye of the optical industry's top influencers. I have won various awards including one from the LinkedIn Town Hall ceremony, here in Montreal. I even made the top ten list of the most prominent podcast series in the optical industry. Surmounting the challenges along the way, I am elated to see my dreams come to fruition. I am confident that this product will open the door to many more creative opportunities.

I have always associated myself with phenomenally successful, confident women, as I am honored to be tconsidered among them.

Kelly Trerise spent two decades as a professional makeup artist in the TV and film, fashion and magazine industries, before founding Gloss Boudoir.

Kelly Trerise

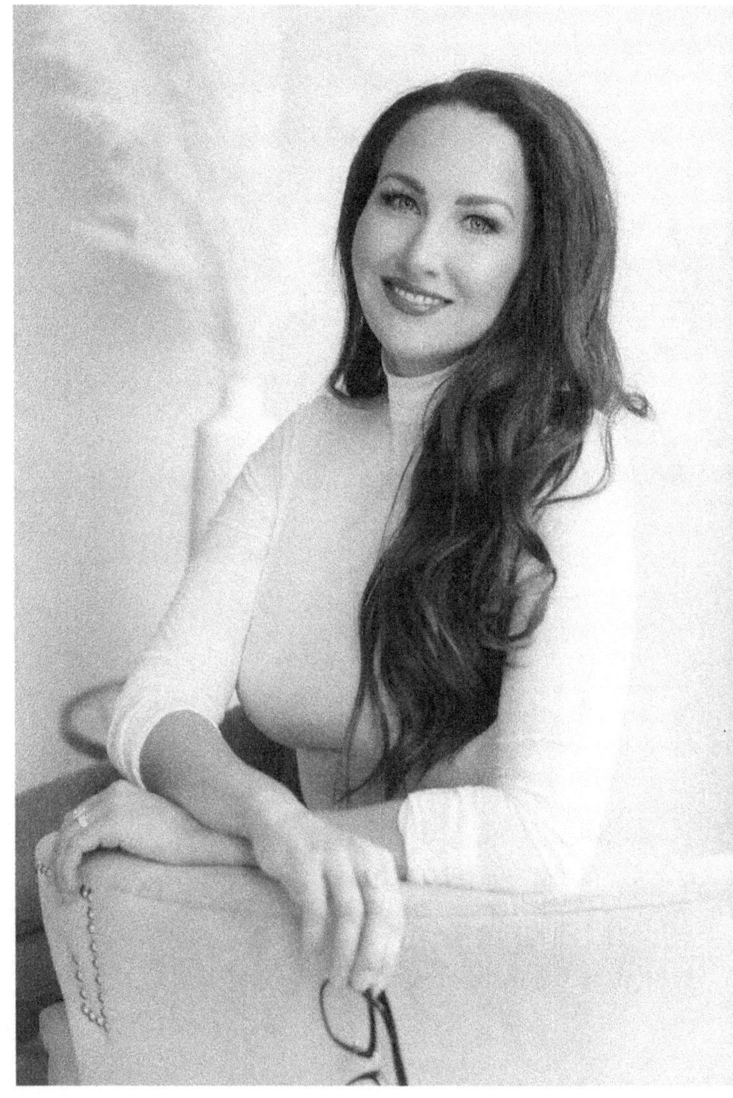

I felt a lot of pressure to be successful when I was growing up. My Dad was an Olympian and a senior partner in a major law firm, and I watched my Mom build her thriving music agency from the ground up. I admired them both but also was never sure I'd be able to live up to their greatness. When I was in high school, we had a 'take your kid to work day'. My parents' careers didn't interest me, so my Mom enquired with a makeup artist friend of hers, and I got to spend two thrilling days on the set of a popular TV show!

Those two days changed my life.

I started to practice makeup artistry on anyone who would lend me their face, and I developed a deep passion for transforming women with my brushes and seeing genuine happiness in their eyes when they looked in the mirror.

Several years into my career, I found there was something still missing. I was in a ten-year relationship that was debilitating yet addictive. I looked for attention in unhealthy ways and was dying inside from sadness. At twenty-five, I found the courage to leave and decided to spend the next few years exploring myself and indulging in what made me happy. I sold everything I owned and traveled the world for a year, visiting sixty-eight countries! I unraveled who I was; what I stood for and learned more about humanity than I could ever imagine. That time abroad was exciting, terrifying, and complex.

I arrived home to Canada a new woman: powerful, open & fearless. I wanted to create a space to provide that same energy for other women. Seven years ago, my business partner and I opened Gloss Boudoir Studio. The studio focuses on helping women build self-confidence in a safe and judgement-free space. I label myself a feminist. I built my life around empowering women, employing women, and creating a niche market in which women can thrive. With the unwavering support of my husband, I'm living my own greatness and realizing, years later, that success has everything to do with who I have become and not what I do.

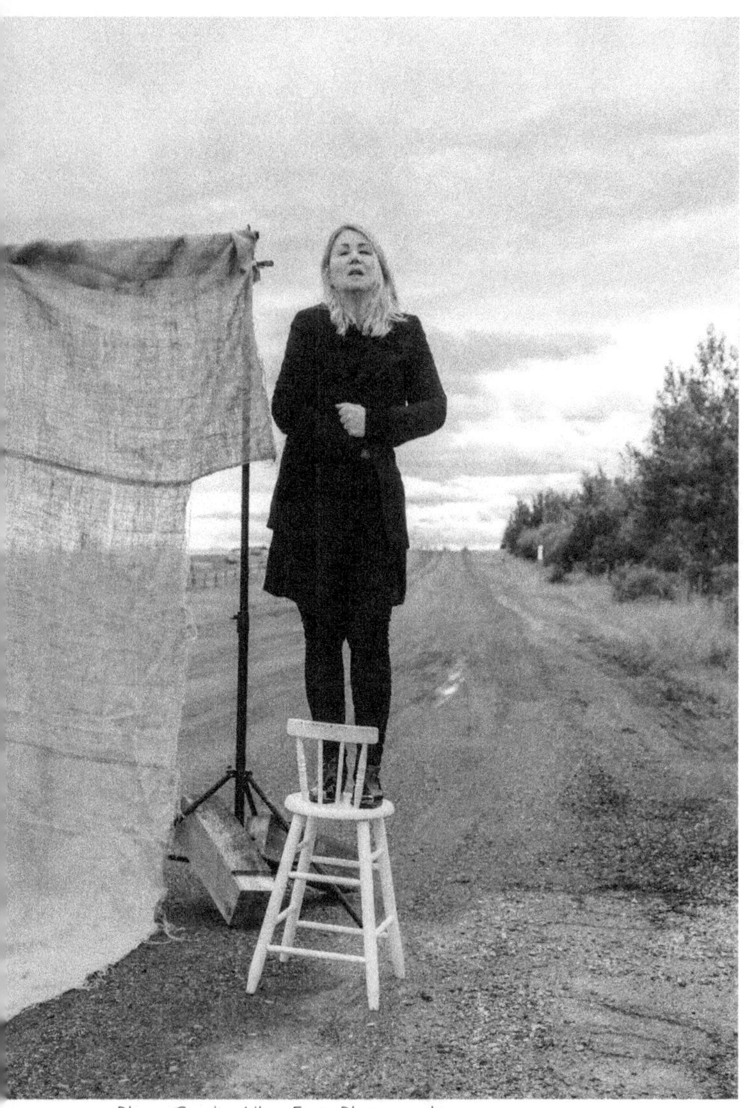
Photo Credit: Alkan Emin Photography

Jann Arden is an award-winning multi-platinum singer, songwriter, actress, broadcaster, author, and an inductee to the Canadian Music Hall of Fame.

Jann Arden

It's not easy being a person. It takes decades to figure out what you're doing. In fact, I would venture to say, we never REALLY know what we're doing until it's too late. We learn more from despair and disaster and disappointment and failure than we do anything else, so yes, it is indeed hard to become a person.

You have to be willing to fall over and over again. After a decade or two of tripping yourself up at every turn, you realize that the missteps are quite worthwhile and that the obstacles provide a kind of giddy satisfaction. It makes me happy to overcome- to figure out-to solve- to achieve to ACCOMPLISH. Triumph isn't a triumph at all unless it's earned. People often take the time to tell me, 'How lucky I am.' I answer back without missing a second. "I'm not lucky at all. I work hard. If you want to be lucky, you have to work hard." The conversation is short. Anyone that thinks that luck is what makes things 'happen' in their lives would be mistaken.

That's not to say that I've planned anything in my life. Working hard and having a plan don't always belong together. They can exist without each other. I've never planned anything, and anytime that I did, life had its own idea of what was going to happen. Good things come out of bad things. I've told this story many times, the one about how I ended up becoming a singer and a songwriter. It was because of a very bad thing, and I'm pretty sure that makes people tip their heads wondering how a bad thing could make itself useful.

My dad was a terrible drunk.

In order to stay out of his way, I was either outside until the sun fell behind the trees, or in our very dingy concrete basement. There was a record player down there. A guitar. Hundreds of LP's. It didn't take me long to copy everything I heard, learn a few chords and start making up my own songs. Without dad's alcoholism, NONE OF IT WOULD HAVE HAPPENED. Good things come out of bad things. Believe it.

Hillary Samson owns Transforming Ventures, where she supports entrepreneurs to connect with the soul of their business. She believes sacred guidance is available at all times.

Hillary Samson

Every one of us is constantly receiving guidance on what actions to take for our highest good, but so often we are resistant to hearing this divine voice. About three years ago, I became committed to listening to, and acting on, that powerful guidance. There are many names for this still quiet voice guiding us – intuition, higher self, divine feminine, and voice of God are but a few. It has transformed every aspect of my life, including my relationships, happiness, and success at work.

For many years my work has been rooted in the left-brain, masculine world of wrangling spreadsheets and crafting business plans. So, for me, it is still very much a step-by-step journey to listen to this sacred inner voice, especially when it speaks to a different path than my logical brain thinks is best. I continue to practice with these steps:

ASK: Every morning I ask for help to reduce resistance to hearing this sacred guidance. If I have a specific challenge, I ask to be shown the next best step to take to resolve it.

LISTEN: We hear this guidance not with our ears or in our minds, but in our bodies. Once I learned to recognize what a "yes" and "no" was in my body, it has become a powerful tool to help me live in the beautiful flow of life.

ACT: We all have perfect free will, and each moment we can choose to act on the guidance or follow another path. Start with small acts of listening (i.e., What should I have for dinner?) and build awareness over time.

Through this practice, I have observed hundreds of times how things have unfolded perfectly when I listened to this guidance, and perhaps more poignantly, how they went poorly when I ignored it. This powerful practice is available to every person; we are one, and we all benefit, individually and collectively, when we say yes to acting on this loving guidance to bring more flow and joy into our lives.

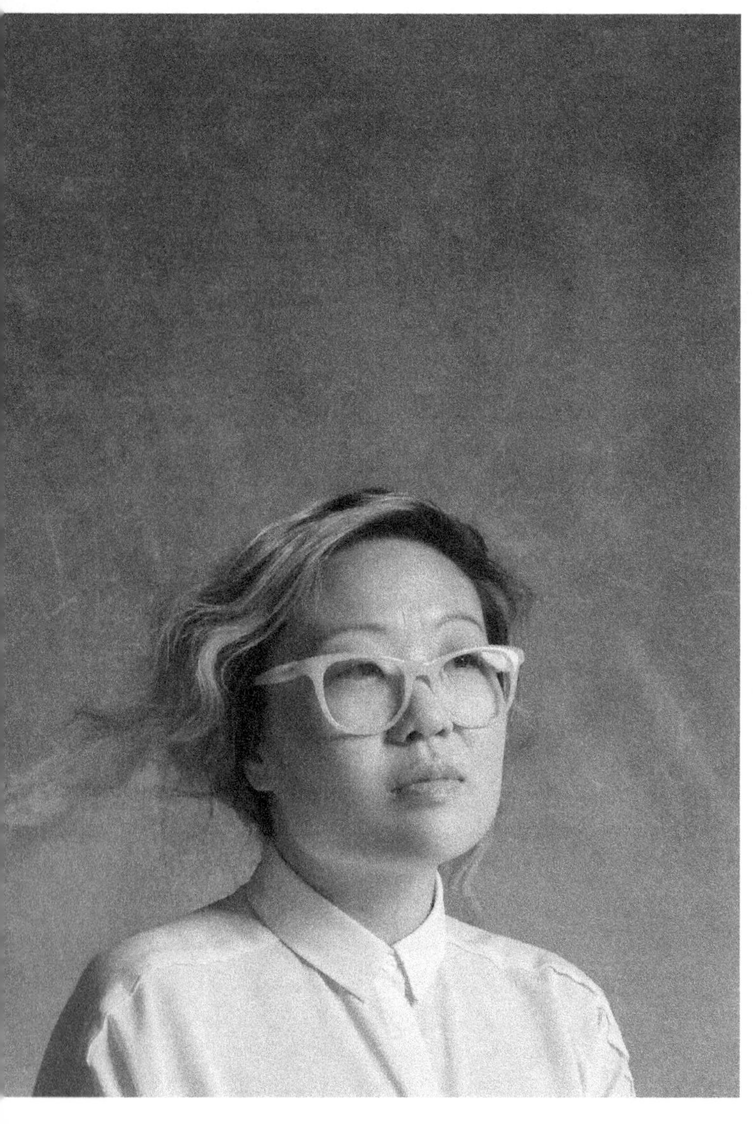

Julie Kim is a Film Director and Cinematographer based in Vancouver, British Columbia. She worked her way up the industry ladder through a predominantly male camera department.

Julie Kim

2020, a year of elevating women, has ironically been the demise of a couple of key men in my life. My relationship of eight years ended with my partner's infidelity, and I lost my father suddenly to an un-COVID related death. I was precariously moving through two different heartaches at the same time. Pain was absolutely testing my faith in happiness.

I've been working with men in a male-dominated industry my entire adult career. There just weren't many women in my department at the time, so I became part of an exclusive boys' club. One that taught me how to fix my taillight, how to pack $10,000 cash, and the importance of talcum powder on a sweaty summer day! Beyond that, I learned the tricks I carry with me today; lighting with less, how to be a graceful leader, the art of "fake it till you make it," basically, it pays to believe in yourself. My mentors were invaluable in guiding me to this point in my career, and I pass on the same integrities to my assistants.

New choices led to new relationships, including a renewed and deeper sense of self. I generated the courage and strength to love bigger, to embrace vulnerability in vital ways, and to focus on things I have let lay dormant for too long. Deepening my relationship with others and myself, fully and unconditionally, breathes new life into me. These challenging times have highlighted one thing that would never let me down, and I found always waiting for me, my creativity.

In the "pursuit of happiness," you accept the pain, the joy, and keep doing what you love. Simple or profound, humans are social creatures. We are here to connect regardless of the outcome. Directing gives me that opportunity to reflect on this.

As a filmmaker, I am honoured to seed my vision within the stories and passions of others, specifically for the broader good of our youth who need that critical voice and encouragement. I would say to be a woman in film isn't about standing exclusively with women, but more about standing as a woman with your beautiful creative tribe.

Christina Rose is a Mindset and Manifestation Coach and Subconscious Mind Expert who uses unique subconscious mind modalities and a "whole"-istic approach to transformation, to help women release their limiting beliefs and embrace the totality of themselves.

Christina Rose

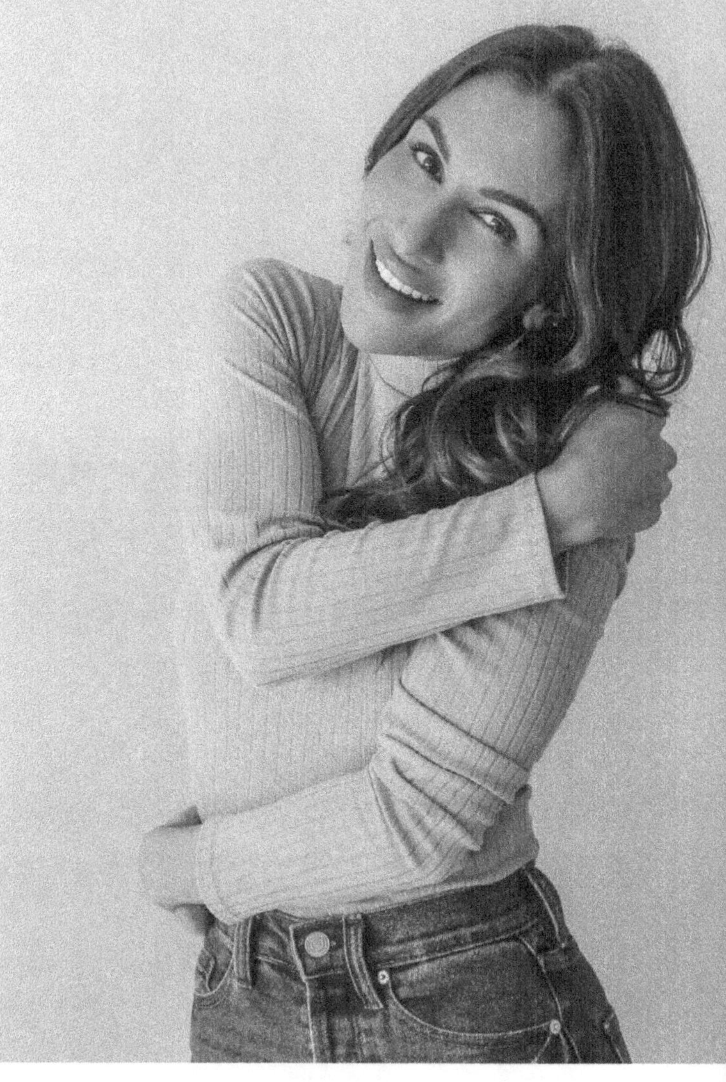

To know me is to know that my pursuit of happiness exists within the paradigm of my conscious expansion and my journey toward reclaiming my most authentic self. I consider my life to be a remarkable story of personal triumph. From childhood issues of deep insecurity and a teenage illness that almost took my life; to enduring emotionally toxic relationships, struggling with disordered eating habits, and having paralyzing anxiety in my twenties that left me defeated and hopeless: There was a time, as I approached thirty, when I sincerely questioned whether my dark days would ever end.

But I never gave up on myself. Somewhere inside I knew, buried within me, beneath the layers of insecurity, deep-rooted shame, and feelings of unworthiness, was a truer and more authentic version of myself. A version that so desperately wanted to be revealed and expressed in the world. A version that loved and accepted all parts of myself, in all the ways I am, and in all the ways I am not. A version that was empowered by the notion that, despite my past, by choosing to be at cause for my life, and taking back my power from all my life's circumstances and the people in it who impacted me negatively, I could tap into a divine and powerful force within me and create the life I had always wanted.

I embarked on a journey of personal growth and transformative inner-work to dismantle my learned conditioning, subconscious limiting beliefs, and the adopted "protective patterns" of my psyche that ultimately, were not serving me as an adult. Unearthed was the essence of the woman, leader, coach, teacher, wife, daughter, and true force to be reckoned with that I show up as in the world today.

Through my personal pursuit of happiness, I have discovered my own resilience, cultivated a deep sense of self-acceptance, and have come to understand the great wisdom of embracing my humanity in its totality. It is an honour to serve the world by helping other women do the same.

Here's to a pursuit of happiness that endures all!

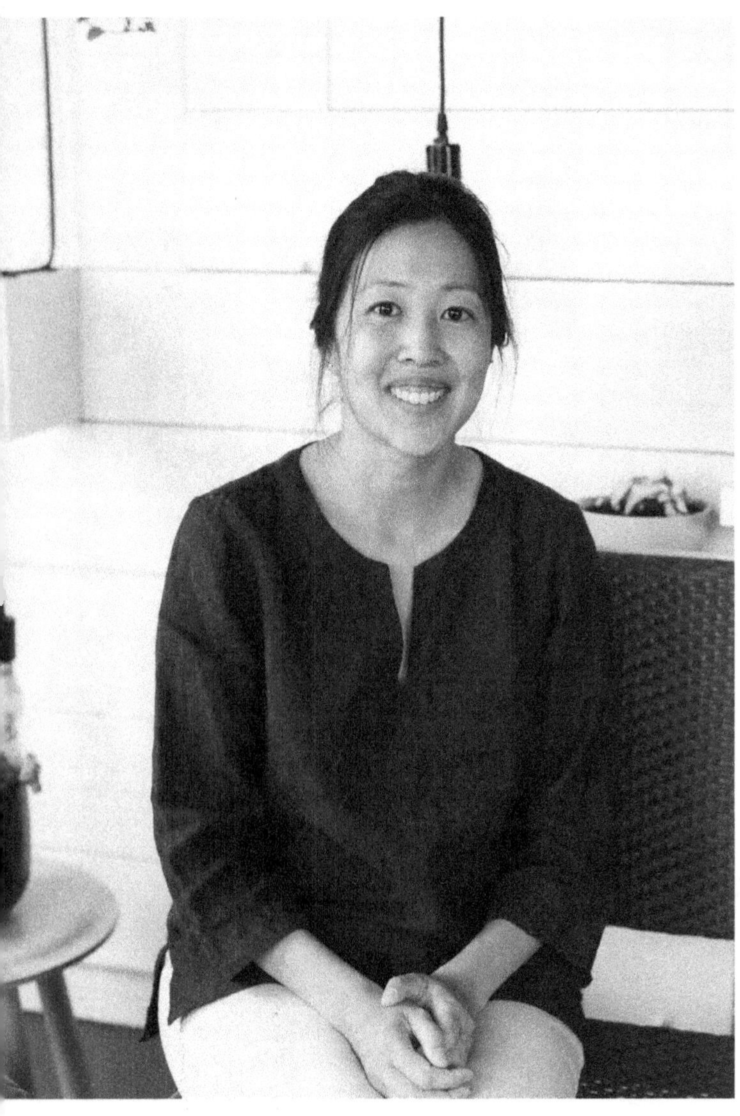

Sara is the owner and entrepreneur behind Illo Leather. She designs and makes beautiful and timeless hand-stitched leather bags and accessories in her studio in Calgary, AB.

Sara Nishi

My partner describes me as "strong-willed," but he definitely means stubborn! After a bit of reflection, I realized there isn't anything I've really wanted to do that I haven't done or somehow made happen. I truly never say 'can't' to myself. In my younger years, I was flying overseas, working random, fun (and not so fun) jobs, and living in new and exciting places. In my thirties, things changed after having our two boys. Becoming a mom was a bit of an adjustment, to say the least. What saved me from me was accidentally falling into leatherwork. I loved it and thought, "yes, I can." So I started a business.

What I love about leatherwork is working with my hands using centuries-old techniques to create modern and enduring pieces. I refuse to use machines and, although my work is more labour intensive and time-consuming, I believe the quality and artisanship are worth it.

I write this in my fortieth year, and Illo Leather is now almost six years old. I run my business like I run my life, saying yes to things I want and no to things I don't. I couldn't pass up the opportunity to collaborate on this book. To be connected to all these incredible women in print form is so comforting. Also very daunting as I'm a woman of few words.

Due to my "strong-willed-ness," it's probably taken me a lot longer to get to where I am. I like spending my time creating and do the bare minimum when it comes to anything online. (Apologies to everyone still waiting for an email and my total inconsistency of posts. Thank you to my wonderful clients who spread the word for me.) Overall, I feel good about the progress I've made and proud I won't have to compromise myself.

Patricia Wilson is a writer, poet, a musician and was born on the same day Elvis recorded "That's All Right Mama," so, she is always looking for the roll in rock and roll.

Patricia Wilson

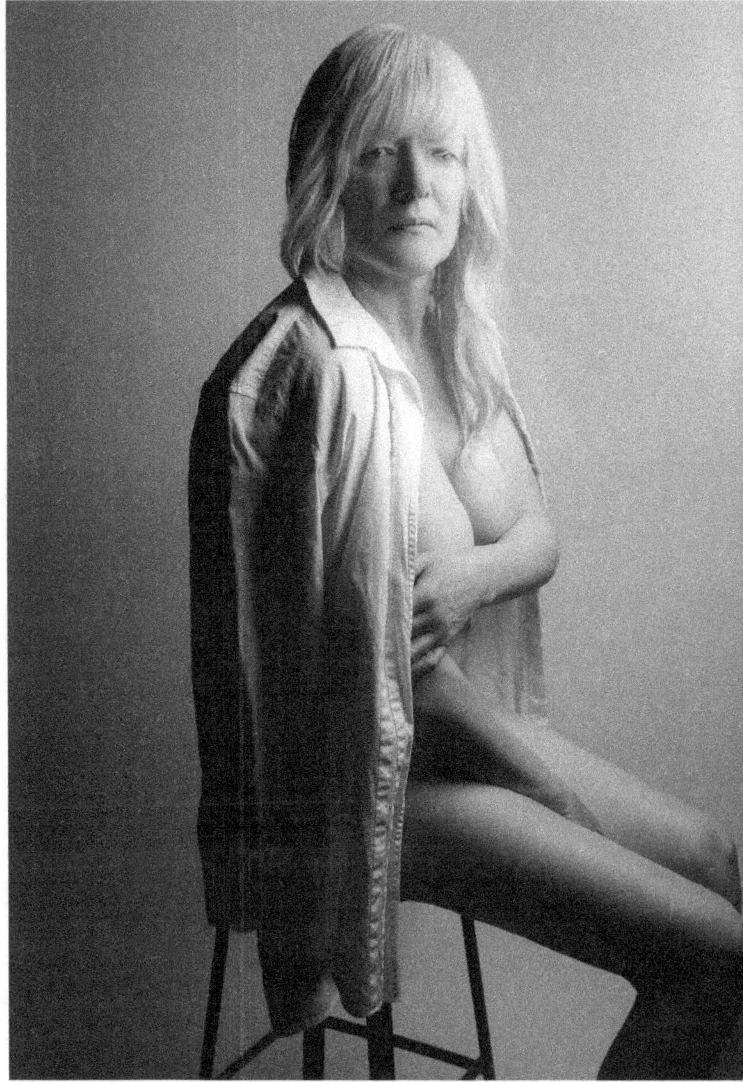

Photo Credit: Alkan Emin Photography

Life's a continuing journey, and it takes from us, gives to us, creates who we are at any given moment. Anyone who has walked this human mile can tell stories of deep pain, struggle, joy, and love. A life's bouquet that sits in front of our soul's morning mirror as we reflect on all it took to get where we are now. Sometimes I can live my whole life in a bite of food. Dinner cooks in stages, and I scribble the beginnings of poems and stories. Can't wait to see Hélène when she gets home, and we can share food together.

The woman I am today is on a different journey to womanhood than most women I know, not any better or worse, just a different road for the woman I see in the morning mirror at sixty-six years old. I was never a thirteen-year-old girl, or young woman dealing with the gasping hardships of being female against a male-dominated world. That path is not part of my female psyche.

Experiences that most biological women have dealt with, and have risen above, become who they are right at this moment, and the importance of that in their journey, I do not share. I struggled in my own way, and that is a story to be told somewhere else. I am fortunate to call myself a woman physically for over thirty years. I have been with the same partner since 1992. She is a babe and a constant source of learning and love for me.

My meandering point here is - every day is a day filled with the past, propelling us forward to the future to give us direction. Yet, the present is a steady hand that focuses us and fills us with the knowledge that, right now, we are all we should be in this moment, filtered through whatever different emotions we as humans have been gifted. We are who we are right now. What a great way to start a new day, a new year with a new journey of self as we exist right now. We must share our gifts in acts of kindness, it's what makes us truly human.

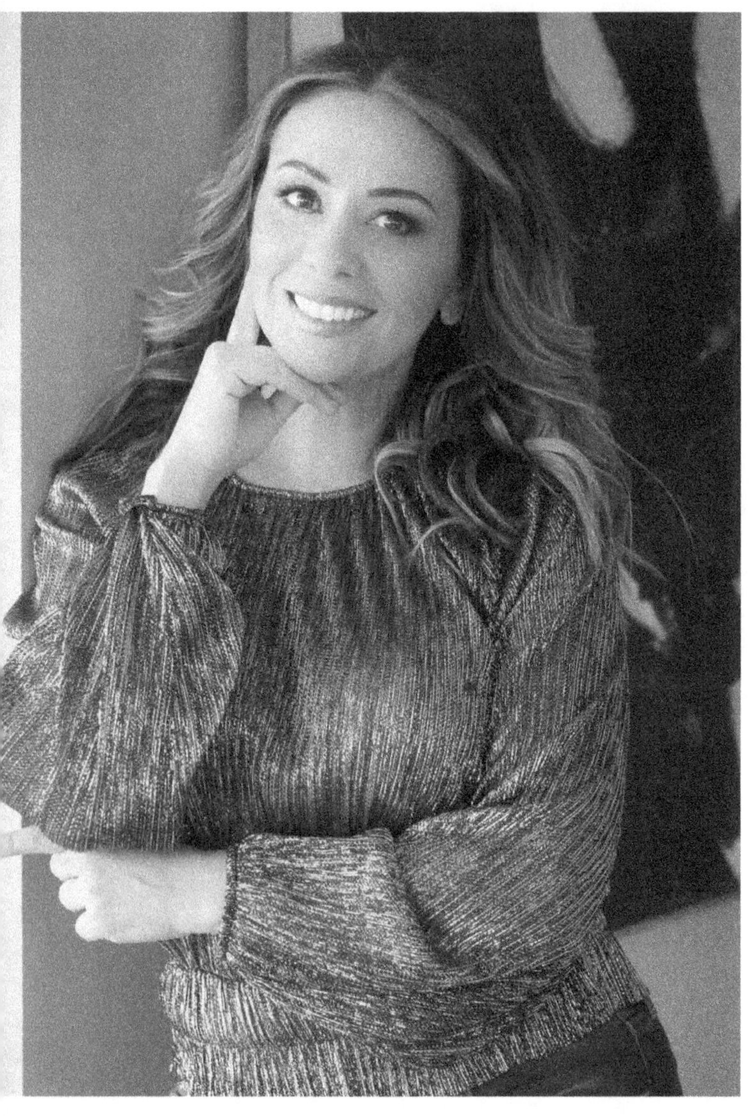

Maria Kritikos is the founder of the Ladies WHO Lunch® Network, one-half of The Real Estate Sisters, and author of Girl With A Plan.

Maria Kritikos

I went from being a reserved girl in high school who experienced a very sheltered upbringing to marrying into a very prominent, influential family. I lived a very comfortable, some would say fairy-tale-like, experience until I unexpectedly found myself a single mom of a two-year-old, homeless, and sleeping on my mom's couch. That was a very dark and challenging period of my life until I realized there was only one person who could save me and put me on the road to happiness.

My greatest power came from realizing that I had a choice about how I was going to respond to what was happening around me. I could give up and blame others for putting me in this situation, but the truth was, there was only one person who could save me, and that was the person I looked at in the mirror every day. It was really nice to finally meet her, to get to know her, and to know that I would be living with her for the rest of my life.

I want to encourage you to take responsibility for your life. Take action each and every day towards creating the life you desire. Persist until you succeed. Always take another step, even when you're tired, even when you don't feel like it or when you're not in the mood. Then take another, and yet another.

You know what happens when you take responsibility for creating your own happiness instead of relying on others to create this for you? No one will ever be able to take it away from you.

Keep moving forward, even if all you can see is five feet ahead of you. Action in the direction of your dreams is imperative. Consistent action must be taken daily. Most of us stall because we are not sure how our big dream is going to unfold or how it's all going to work out.

You can accomplish anything you want if you just give up the belief that you can't and stop relying on others to give you what you have the capability of creating yourself. Keep putting one foot in front of the other and dream with your eyes wide open. I'm Maria Kritikos, and I believe in you.

Amanda Doucette is a self-proclaimed foodie, spin class, and Pilates enthusiast - and a tax lawyer.

Amanda Doucette

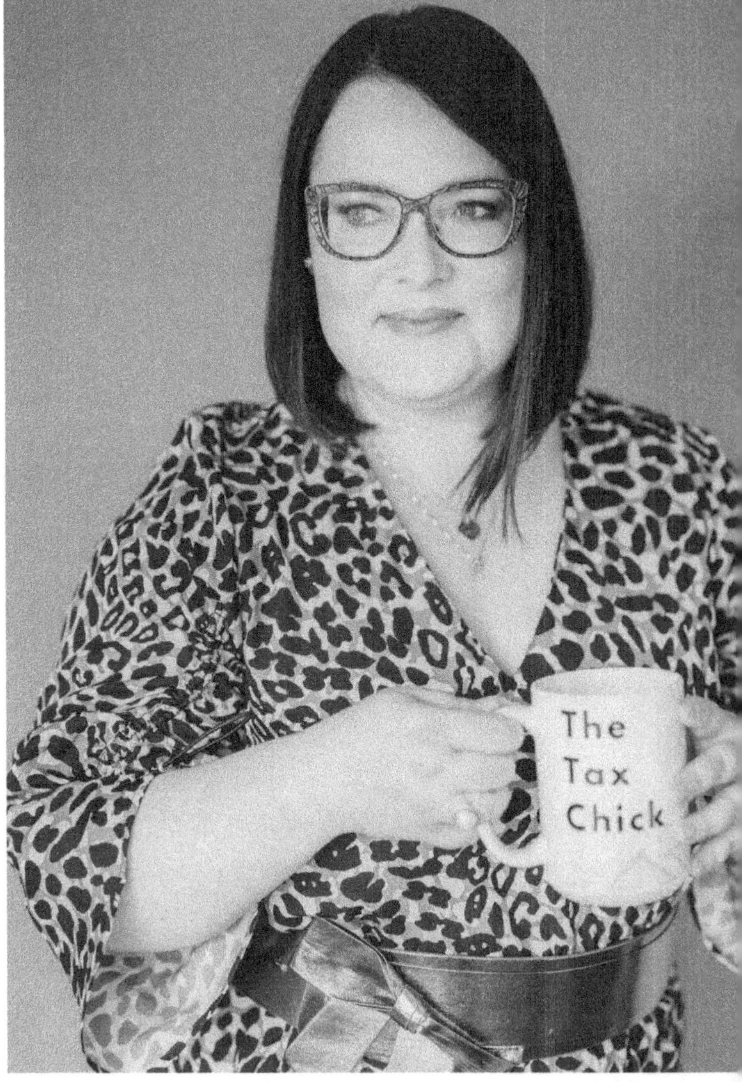

Math, spreadsheets, and numbers in general, are not my favorite things. If you gave me the choice between reading through five boxes of documents or analyzing one spreadsheet, I would be diving into the first box before you finished your question. Turns out many of my clients feel the same way.

So, what are my favorite things? I love to learn. I love to be challenged. I love to laugh. I love conquering something that seems insurmountable. I love teaching. I love empowering others. I love to bake. I get an endorphin rush from organizing a closet or a drawer. And as it turns out, I also love learning and talking about taxes.

I did not seek out a career in tax law. Instead, tax law found me. Saying "yes" to practicing tax law was scary. And yet, it was the best decision I ever made.

The truth is that I do not always fit the mold of what people expect when they hear "tax lawyer". That used to bother me. But in 2020, I took the leap and decided to share my unique take on my profession - through the creation of "The Tax Chick Blog" and "The Tax Chick Podcast."

The blog and the podcast have become an outlet of creative expression for me. Writing and speaking about taxes in this way has allowed me to indulge in some of my favorite things – curious conversations with new people, learning new things, teaching, and a lot of laughter. While I have not yet incorporated a baking element or spin class into the podcast or blog, I am not ruling this out for the future!

I challenge you to embrace your uniqueness. Laugh when it feels good. Be curious. Welcome the opportunity to try something new even if you are scared you might fail. Instead, focus on how great you will feel to have stepped out of your comfort zone!

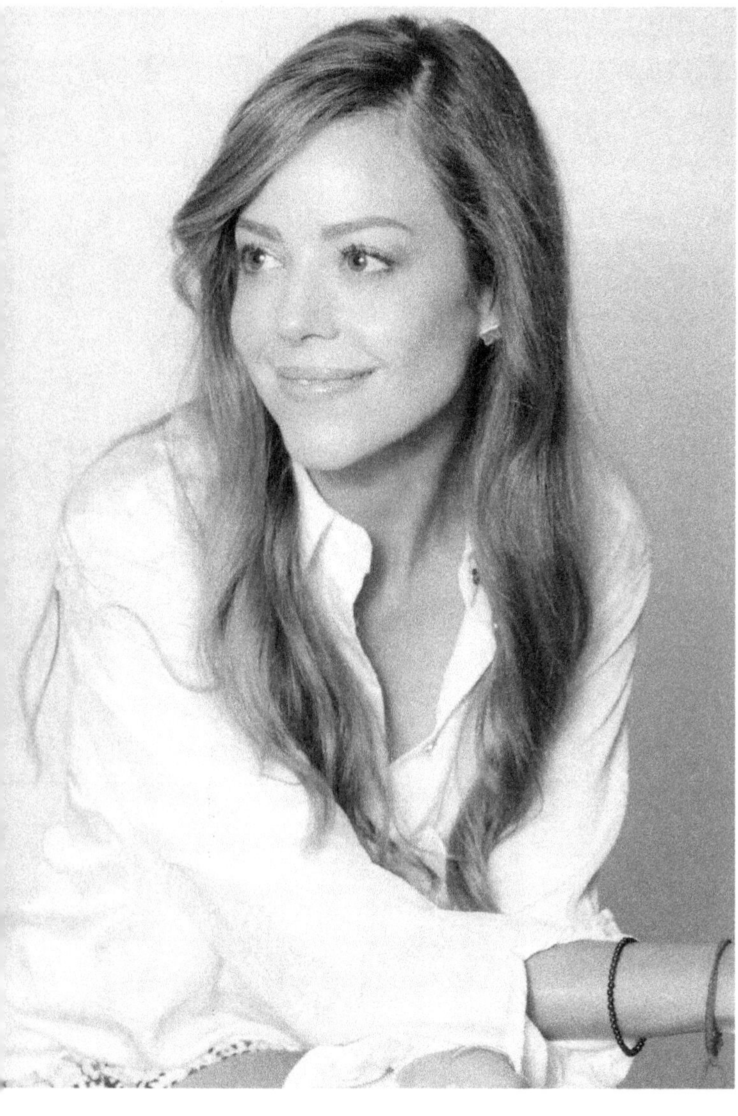

Stephanie Gust is the founder of Benesse Health. There is one word for her, and that is PASSION.

Stephanie Gust

I am profoundly moved and amazed by almost everything. The unique geometric pattern behind a leaf on the ground fascinates me just as much as the latest building by Alberto Kalach. And I can literally talk about each of them for hours, what can I say!? Some of my earliest memories have to do with this profound sense of inquisitiveness that drives a desire in me to know, understand and feel!

I think the word feel is so important! I will never forget, in university, I remember my professor stopped me in the middle of my enthusiastic presentation and corrected me; "don't say I feel, say instead, I think." I obeyed and shifted my wording, however, it didn't feel right. It stuck with me forever. So much value is focused on dense intellect alone. What's the point of a choice without a feeling? After all, and at the core of our ambition, it's a feeling we are after, isn't it? I have come to realize, especially in the last four years, after shedding quite a bit of egocentricity, that feeling your way through decisions, people, observations, and transitions is a high form of intelligence. One that is connected to our most inner authentic self and has never proven me wrong. I always ask myself; how does this make me feel? It's a great compass.

The most comfortable thing for me has always been being me. I'm black or white, bold, convicted, creative, adaptable, outspoken, and I've been called "aggressive" by timid personalities and "passionate" by strong ones. At the very core, my essence is not vastly different from when I was four. Above all, however, I believe my passion for life has honestly saved me at times and has given me the courage to take risks; like making leaps from one profession to the other and eventually owning my own business, all while being a full-time mom!

It's the passion in the seen, but most importantly, in the unseen that propel me forward. When I don't know when to start, I start anywhere, as I know that one thing leads to the next and that motion is necessary for progress. We are continuously expanding and never get it done, really... I love it!

Karen Reid Sidhu is a mother, a wife, and a mentor who focuses on helping others find the strength to overcome adversity and is the Executive Director of Surrey Crime Prevention Society.

Karen Reid Sidhu

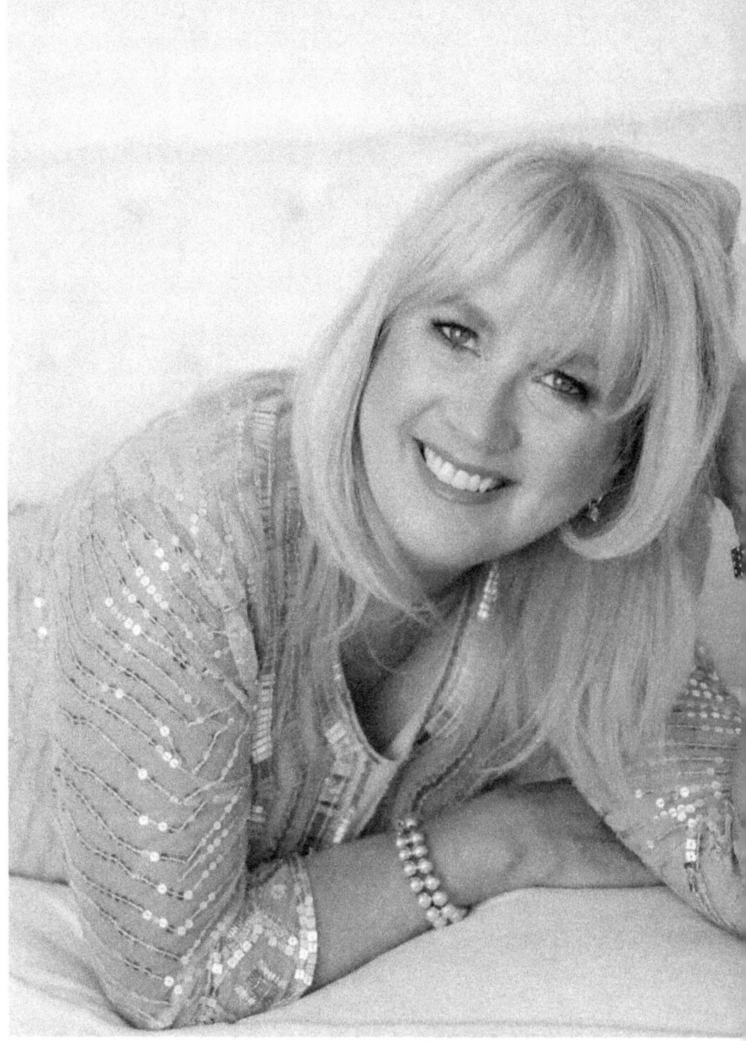

Healing. Life experiences made me who I am today, some good and some bad.

As a survivor of sexual abuse as a child by a family member, then a family friend, when something this traumatic happens to a child, their world becomes distorted. Certain life choices I made definitely added to my pain, and surviving domestic violence was the final moment I realized changes needed to happen.

I finally found the help I needed to overcome the deep wounds that were infecting my life.

Being a survivor takes work but more importantly, strength to face the demons and shame that live deep inside.

It's not easy to move past the memories, but I did it, and today I have the courage to share my story. What happened doesn't define me as a person, but empowers me to be strong, the strength that others at one point tried to steal from me.

There are so many women with these wounds and are either too embarrassed or ashamed to talk about their experiences. I understand, but know, there is help. Part of the healing process is being allowed to grieve the loss of innocence. Healing takes place when you realize it was not your fault.

Over the years, I have met so many strong women who helped me find the courage to face these demons. Now, my focus is on helping others find the strength to overcome adversity. One of my passions is a mentorship program for vulnerable youth that I oversee, and I have witnessed so many youth overcome adversity – very proud moments.

It will be thirty-four years this year that I am married to my amazing husband, and the day of the year my story resides on is our anniversary. I have a daughter and two sons, who I am very proud of. Life is a journey that no one ever said was going to be smooth. I have seen some serious sinkholes but managed to climb out with a full and complete life. I have only one regret to this day about what happened to me as a child – to face the two people who sexually abused me – they are both deceased.

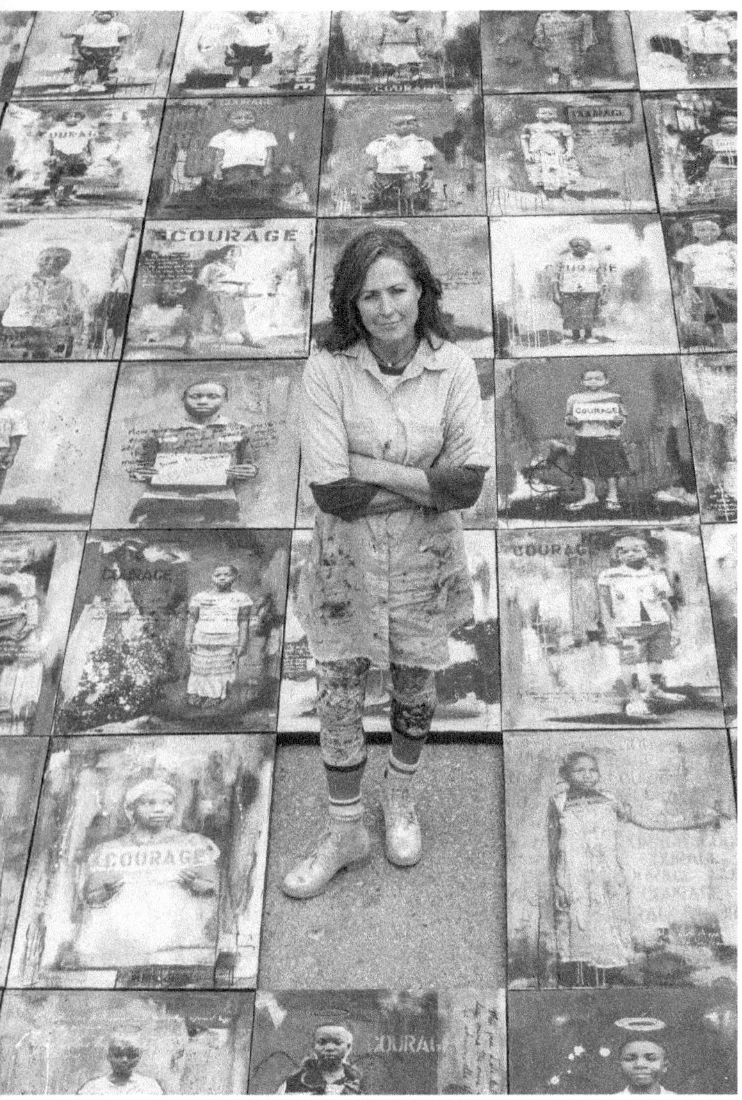

Heather Haynes is an artist, partner, mother, sister, daughter, and friend.

Heather Haynes

My life has been a steadfast pursuit to find the balance of these roles. I list artist first because that is how I define myself above all else. It has taken me a long time to be able to admit this, although I have recognized it forever. The drive to create will burn inside me forever. But for me, art is much more than creating something pleasant to hang on your wall. My artistic career has led me to some of the darkest places on Earth, with a drive to tell stories you've likely never heard before.

From 2013 to 2015, I created a monolithic art installation entitled Wall of Courage, dedicated to orphans in the Democratic Republic of Congo. I had put myself in front of stories of extreme violence, torture, rape, and sometimes the more merciful - death. These children I was meeting had lost everything. As an artist, I did not instantly know what I could do to help them. I soon became convinced that if I could somehow show the world they existed, perhaps their fates could be altered. All of their stories are that of courage and resilience, and I am honoured and humbled to know them. I want others to know them too; for their faces to be seen and for their stories to be heard. The Universe presents us with many options every day. We can choose to grab them or let them slip on by. This one I grabbed ahold of and I held so tightly that it became a part of me.

Wall of Courage has since inspired many initiatives that are changing the lives of these children and their communities. The project is much bigger than "me," and it is not limited to these eighty-one children depicted on the Wall. It is a planet Earth project.

I have made a lifetime commitment to support these children with my Congolese brother, Kizungu Luanda Hubert. Through touring Wall of Courage, we have garnered support and funding to provide for over 140 orphans and educate over 700 of the most vulnerable children living in the Democratic Republic of the Congo.

Laura-Lee is a daughter, a sister and a mother who believes that each choice you make is an important building block. Laura-Lee concedes that even if your goals take longer than expected – simply focus on your next best step.

Laura-Lee Lofgren

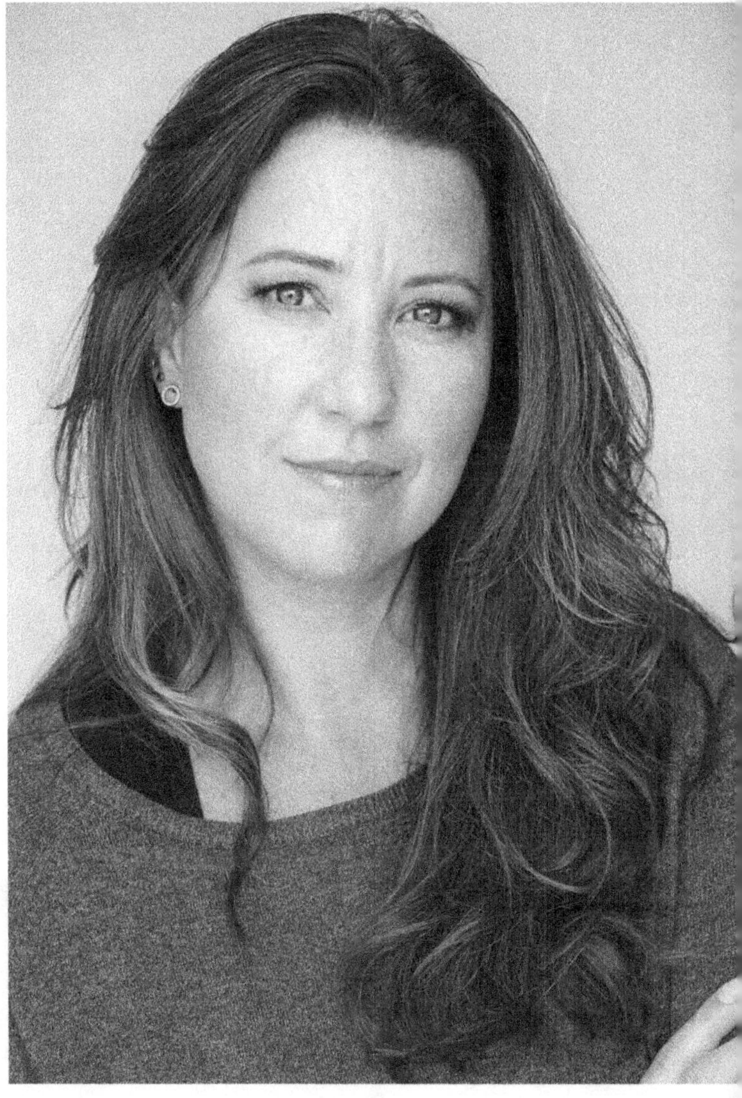

He was "our Dad."

My dad married my mom, who was a widow when they met. She had two boys who were six and three when they married; then I came along. Biologically, my brothers are my half-brothers, but you wouldn't know it – we are just brothers and sister. I had a great childhood that I recall right up until alcoholism took over the days and conversations.

When I was thirteen, my dad's job changed dramatically. He had become the Chief Engineer on the Vancouver fireboat when I was born. He had always worked away on boats, but he wanted to be closer to his family, so this job was perfect. After Vancouver sold the fireboat to San Francisco, my dad had to complete basic training to re-earn a position with the Vancouver Fire Department, just to be offered a desk job that he didn't care for. I remember how hard it was on him and how hard he worked for it. My dad always impressed a good work ethic upon me. He also always had a drinking problem, which became magnified under the stress of losing the job he loved. Alcoholism is a family disease, but people didn't see what we went through, or didn't believe it.

Lying. Hiding. Enabling. Hallucinations. Hospitalizations. Car Accidents. **Shame.**

Ironically, I never saw him drink – he was a closet drinker, and the disease was unpredictable. However, he did go for help because we asked him to. It was clear he didn't want to disappoint his family, but deep down he didn't truly acknowledge that he had a problem. One night, ten years later, he died of alcohol intoxication. After all the family turmoil, that night I felt at peace. I felt guilty for feeling that, but I knew he was also at peace. Only days before his death, I had decided to forgive him and let go of the anger I felt towards him. Instead, I was intending to love him for all of who he was.

I didn't get the chance to tell him. I was his only daughter, his only child, but he was "our Dad."

Acceptance. Forgiveness. Love. Empowerment. Choice. Healing. **Empathy.**

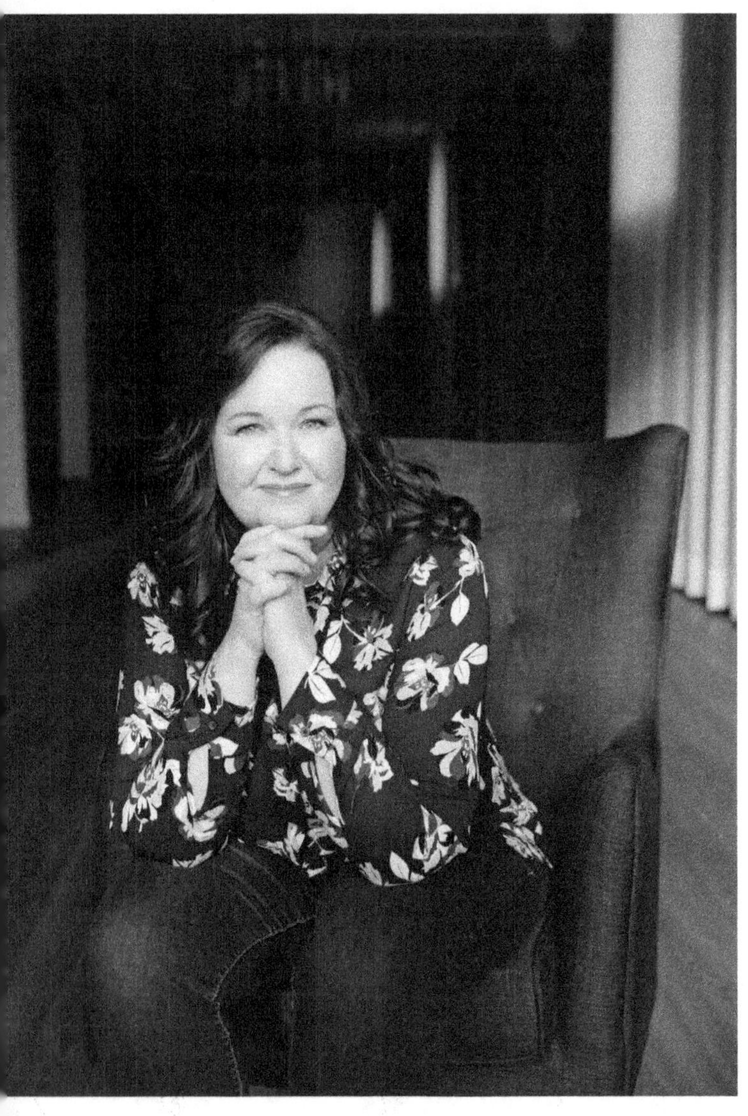

Kim Page Gluckie is a tenacious midlife, no crisis Gen Xer living her legacy. Recognizing that life is unpredictable, she is on a mission to champion women to prioritize themselves, in spite of the grind of real life.

Kim Page Gluckie

I am approaching fifty years old with excitement! I am an established business owner, mother to three daughters, and trailblazer for other Gen Xers with the GenXO community. I am also a career communications professional, passionate connector, and growth expert with wisdom, learned and earned from a gamut of experiences – raising toddlers to teens, navigating an exciting career, and being blindsided by setbacks at exactly the wrong time!

My life was dramatically interrupted by a car accident over five years ago with lingering physical and emotional impacts. It upended my business, which broke my heart. And recently, surprisingly, suffered another interruption with an unexpected stroke! But this process of falling apart and putting myself back together again simply reinforces my clarity we have to try to live a life of joy and purpose, even during the rocky bits.

Now I know, without doubt, that self-care is more than the cure after falling apart. Being highly self-interested is the very thing that holds us together. The notion of prioritizing ourselves, however, is very difficult. This is the premise of GenXO – a community to encourage Gen X women to establish their stories and build their legacies, before, frankly, it's too late. Many women have been so busy working hard on life, not raising a fuss, that a genuine dedication to self-interests has landed way on the bottom of the priority list. Shockingly, we're often considered the underwhelming, forgotten generation, between Boomers and Millennials... which is unfair since we're the glue, silently straddling overwhelming pressure to hold everything and everyone together. Except ourselves!

It is well past time to break these societal views and normalized challenges.

This means being more purposeful in creating opportunities, braver in telling our stories, more responsible for our well-being! I want other Gen Xers to be midlife, no crisis too!

The Gen X journey should be louder, braver, and more fun! And it should not be alone. My mission with the GenXO community is to provide knowledge, support, and space for Gen X legacies to grow.

Katherine Dines is a broadcaster, public speaker, actress, and voice artist in radio, film, television, and video games. Katherine shares with thousands daily on one of the top radio stations in Canada's capital. She amplifies the voices of those who are vulnerable. She knows what it's like to be silenced. A strong voice for mental health and survivors of abuse and assault.

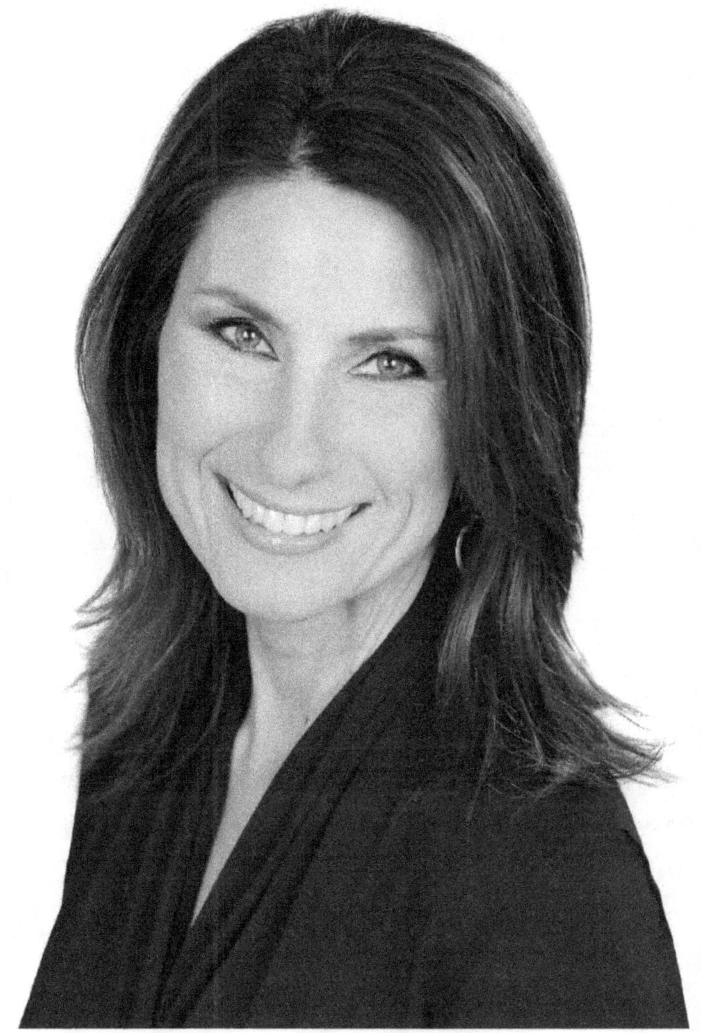

Katherine Dines

I've had a colourfully challenging life. Often called a black sheep, a rebellious teen. I developed an eating disorder, and vices to numb the pain of trauma that remained undiagnosed and untreated until I was well into adulthood. I tried to erase myself.

My dearest gifts and greatest teachers are my daughters. Being their mother helped me realize I needed to be healthy for myself and for them. But the curve balls became faster and more frequent. A diagnosis of a genetic heart condition while I was expecting my second baby girl sent me to the rock bottom I thought had already smashed me to bits. My marriage crumbled and suddenly I was alone with a newborn, toddler, and no job. Adjusting to a heart disorder we all shared. I was spiralling.

I finally reached out for help and received several diagnoses of mental illness including complex PTSD. Knowledge is power and I finally started learning how to take mine back. I also learned the value of being alone, loving my own company. I started sharing my story publicly because women who had heard me in private therapy groups thanked me for sharing in a way they were not yet able to. They said knowing they were not alone helped them feel validated. They told me, it gave them courage and hope. I never imagined I'd have an impact like that on someone. They'd given me a gift in sharing how it made them feel. Another reason to keep going. A way to turn the pain of the past into a healing tool.

There are infinite possibilities, opportunities to learn and move forward in every aspect of life. Every day is a new adventure, sometimes filled with disappointments. Learning to find the blessings and always with love, gratitude, and forgiveness. That's true success for me.

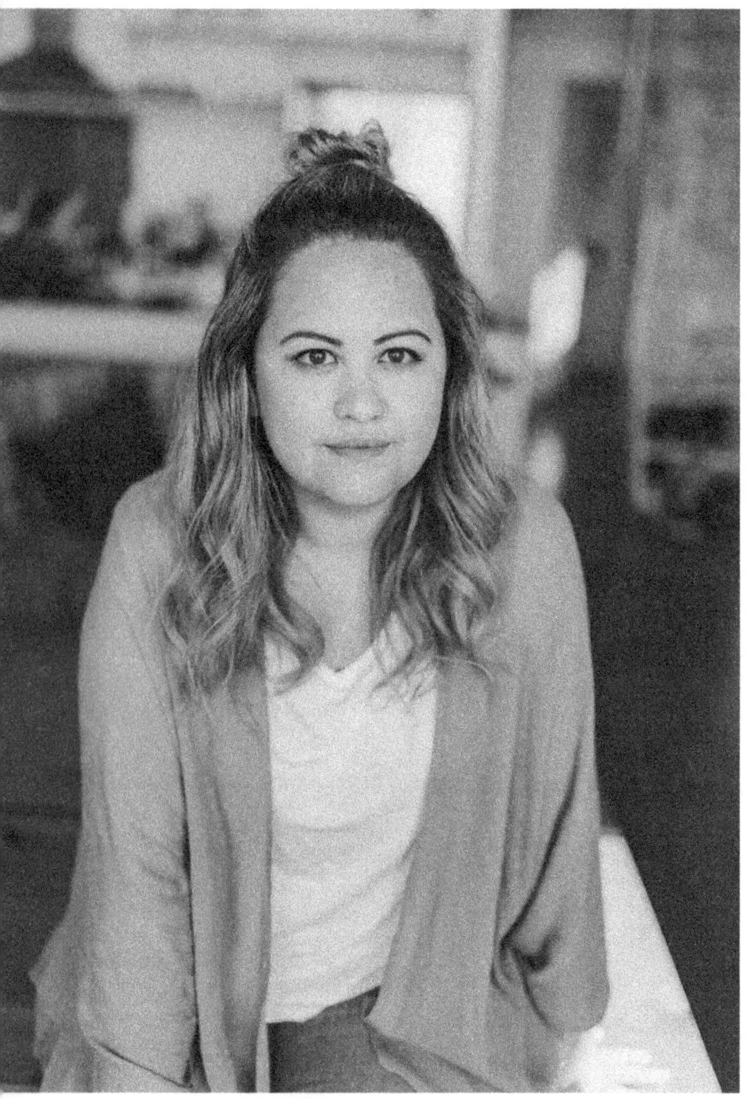
Photo Credit: Diana Battung

Kristy Powers is a multi-passionate entrepreneur who is best known for her work as a photographer and is incredibly proud to have some of her work featured in this book. Her journey has led to her becoming a certified ADHD Life Coach with a focus on female entrepreneurs who have ADHD.

Kristy Powers

So how did I get here? If I told you all of the businesses and jobs I've done or the groups and events I've been a part of, I might take up most of this book. I used to hold a lot of shame around that, and now I embrace it. I realized that not only was I in the pursuit of happiness, I was living it all along.

Whether I was showing up to a home party selling jewellery, opening a co-working and event space, or creating images for someone's new website with a personal branding shoot - the core has always been the same. I thrive in connecting with people, holding space, and creating an experience.

But behind all the successes and failures in both personal and professional life, there was still a struggle that I didn't understand. Why hello, undiagnosed ADHD! This discovery was my missing link. Something that was holding me back from my full potential. I've learned to work my strengths and manage my weaknesses. Now as a coach, I have the training, tools, and knowledge to help others do the same.

Looking back, I haven't been "all over the place," I have been creating a powerful body of work. Give yourself permission to embrace change.

Kym Klopp is an entrepreneur and environmental activist.

Kym Klopp

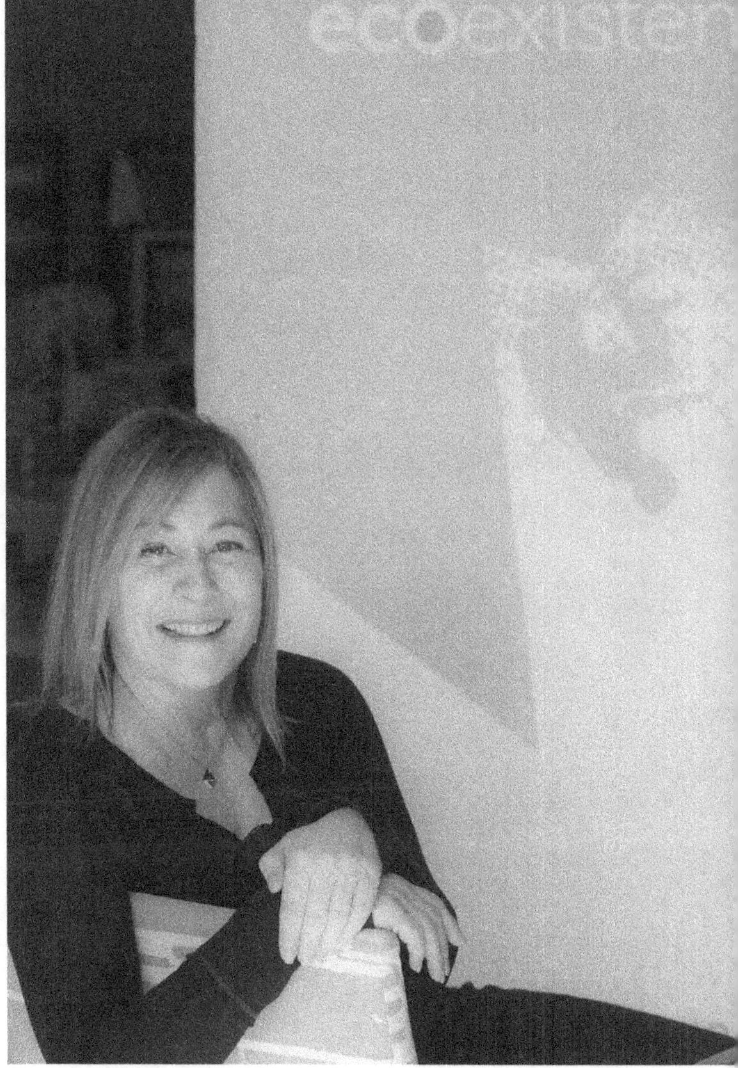

Photo Credit: Michele Crockett Photography

From a very early age, I had a passion and curiosity for all living things. Animals, people, the planet, whatever it may be! These passions and curiosities acted as the headlights on my journey through life as I ventured through many careers looking for the one that made the most sense for me. After years of working in the downtown district, I recognized that my passion lay within my neighbourhood. I wanted to live, work and contribute to my community in a positive and meaningful way.

When my dog died, I took a month off of work. This life-changing experience heightened my curiosity and passion for supporting those who surrounded me. It allowed me to open my eyes to recognize that my purpose in life is helping others so that we as a community first, then society can work toward creating a place that is supportive of all things living!

At this point, I realized my next step in life was to open my own shop in the Toronto neighbourhood I live, with the environment in mind. I wanted to offer alternatives to conventional products that we use in our homes and on our bodies. I aimed to educate my community on the harmful, yet conventional products that were out there, and illustrate the benefits of making the change to living a more sustainable lifestyle. My goal was to expose my neighbourhood to what is out there and provide them with a platform to make the change, hoping it would create a chain effect throughout the city.

At my shop, I strive to create a warm and knowledgeable place where I hope to inspire people to ask questions and vote with their dollars. This is my lucky number thirteenth year. Throughout the years, I have been witness to the rise in awareness to the point where many sustainable options are now considered conventional and many individuals are conscious of their purchases. While I don't pretend to have solved the world's problems... what feeds my passion to continue creating betterment is the pride I hold in my community. They now embrace many of the issues and concerns I value and collectively, we can continue to strive for change on a global scale.

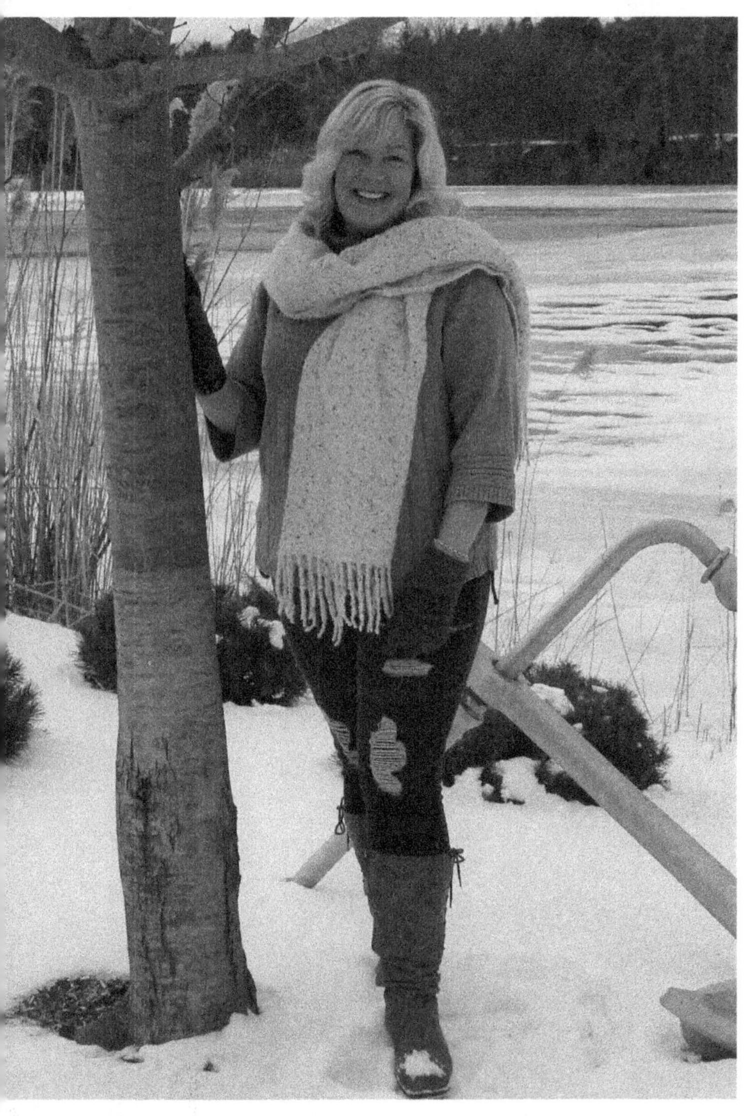

Shantel Taylor is a hairstylist and mother, who dedicates her life to family and those searching for INNER PEACE through their "journey of the heart."

Shantel Taylor

Could the passion inside of us be the catalyst to finding the courage to follow our dreams? Maybe it's not the outcome nor completion of a task to acquire accolades and recognition, but the journey that we travelled instead? Living with an open heart and true devotion to ourselves, the path we follow will become a more natural and instinctual journey. I believe this is the best route to creating and realizing our purpose, and in turn, finding personal success.

At an early age, I learned to believe in my dreams. My mother's unconditional love for us was the one constant in a childhood that was often tumultuous due to domestic violence. Moving a dozen times in a dozen years didn't stop my belief that someday we'd live in a beautiful place and have a big, happy family. My prayers were answered when my mom found peace, love, and security with my stepfather. This experience taught me to be forgiving, take chances, and keep believing that I can manifest my dreams. The turbulent years taught me resiliency, resourcefulness, and to have an open heart. I have eternal gratitude for these lessons. As a profession, I chose hairstyling which, although exciting and financially secure, terrified me! Experiences from instructing to owning a salon taught me my strengths and weaknesses. I love helping others and sharing in our personal growth.

Through this growth, my biggest dream of being a mom came true! I felt blessed and followed in my mother's footsteps. With a home salon, I was able to dedicate my life to my children and family. The balance this created also allowed me time for volunteering in my community. I have immense gratitude for these years with my children and recognize that it is responsible for my healing and purpose. My own childhood had taught me the value of a mother's love and the gift of having three of the most amazing sons is my most cherished blessing. They have taught me pride, humility, leadership, sacrifice, and love. It is true that believing in our dreams may help make them become reality. But, believing in ourselves and helping others find their dreams is what gives ME inner peace.

Amy Spadafora learned at age five, when her parents divorced, the importance of resilience, to help her navigate the upheaval. Having a strong-willed mother also taught Amy the coping skills to face any challenge that she'd face in life.

Amy Spadafora

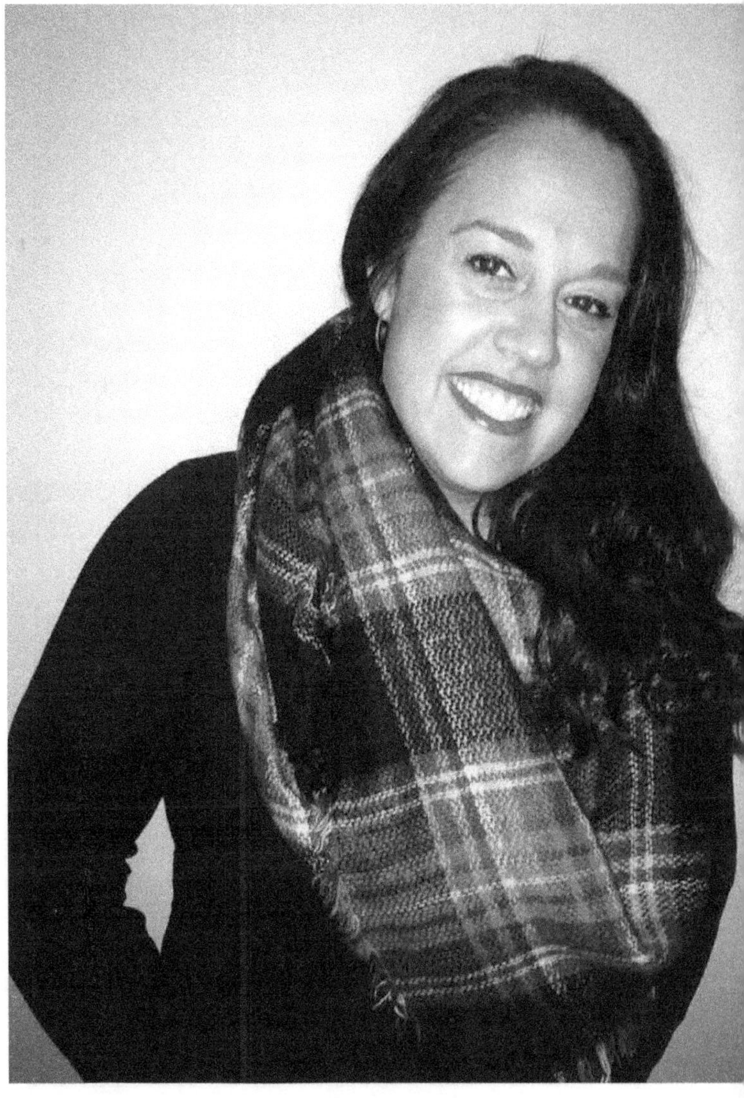

I believe in planning for everything. When pursuing a goal, it's vital to have a plan A, B, and even C because rarely do things go the way we anticipate. Without a backup plan, unexpected roadblocks can threaten our chance for success, but being adaptable to trying different paths can lead to rewards we've never considered. Game plans help me to survive; they're how I've overcome anxiety from the fear of failure. Staying the course and accepting that there will be setbacks is important, just as knowing that you're not alone can give you strength.

As a player and captain in various sports, I've met many people and gained friendships throughout life who later became a support network to lean on in times of self-doubt. I try to empower others by being inclusive, since each one of us has a gift to contribute. Success has come through all the people who have shared in my life.

Having someone in your corner helps move you forward which is why I became a Recreational Therapist for children with special needs - to provide the support to achieve their best, using abilities they possess, not what others believe they should have. Never letting others dictate my direction is huge for me! I'm proud of the fact that when others made me feel I didn't belong, I never gave up; never let anyone talk me out of being "me!" Not everyone plays fair, but the good-guy can win and I take that with me always!

No one else knows my passions, my strengths, my worth, but I really scored big when I married a partner who supports me and takes every risk along with me; shares my interests and believes in me and my plans. My family inspires and motivates me to be my best and I'm genuinely grateful that they've helped me realize that I am important, because I have value, purpose, and vision - as a woman!

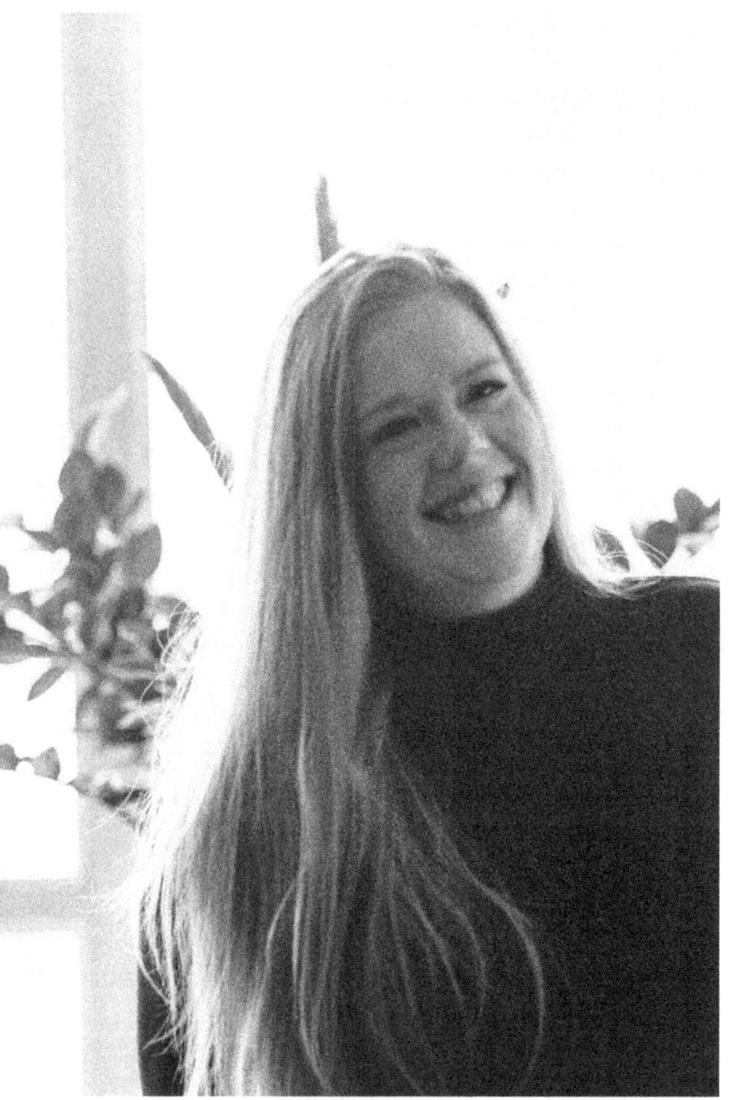

Charlotte Elspeth Hill has suffered great losses earlier in life than some. Her strength is in her DNA though, and she claims surviving her biggest fears as a child has liberated her as a woman.

Charlotte Elspeth Hill

I am the third generation of Elspeth on my mom's side. The name to me is synonymous with strength. My grandmother, Elspeth Hughes, was a trailblazer. She defied gender norms and was one of the first women in Canada to get her pilot's license. My mother, Elspeth Hill, raised two children while caring for a husband who battled cancer three times. While my dad was sick, Mom worked three jobs at times to make sure we had what we needed, all with the brightest smile on her face.

Mom and Grandma set the tone for my life. I grew up a tomboy and Mom and Grandma celebrated that I was nonconforming. When I didn't want to wear dresses to school dances, they made sure I had the new pair of basketball shorts or the runners I wanted. I lost Grandma in my early teens, yet her legacy has never faded. When I was twenty-seven, I lost my dad. It was sudden and I wasn't ready. My grief was untameable and wild. Mom and I got through it together. It was only five years later when she was diagnosed with cancer. I dropped everything to take care of her, but she was gone in less than three months of diagnosis.

I couldn't understand why I didn't grieve the way I had with Dad. Why I was calm and seemingly ok. The greatest love on this planet is between mother and child. She set me up to make sure I'd be ok. I was holding her hand when she took her last breath and all the strength and beauty, she has, she had transferred to me. I carried on, the way she did so many times throughout her life. I am in mourning, of course; I will be for the rest of my life. But the gift of strength she got from her mom, and that they both passed down to me, is the most critical piece of my being that has allowed me to overcome the greatest hurdles in life.

Is that in the name? Of course not, but having Elspeth as my middle name is a reminder of that strength I still hold.

Donelle Clarke creates hand-fabricated fine jewelry using both traditional silversmithing and metal clay techniques and ethically sourced materials.

Donelle Clarke

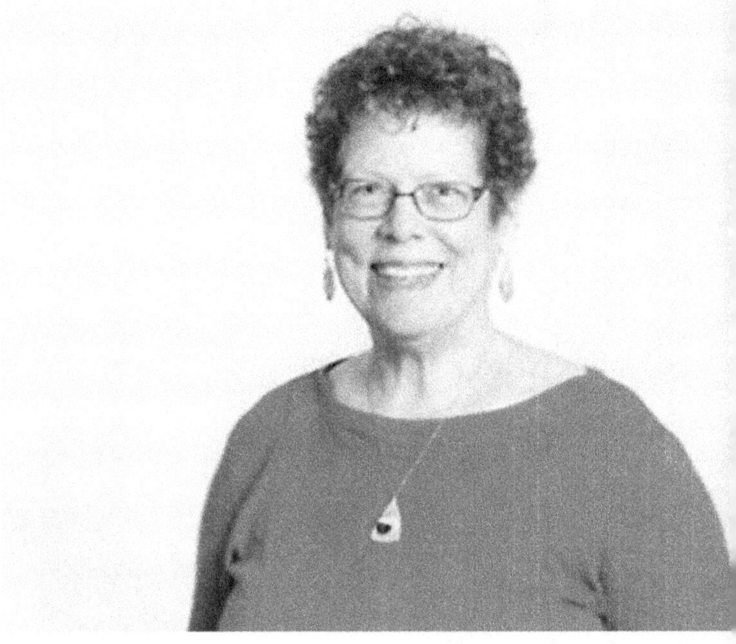

Have you ever noticed that life shifts from everything going well, to falling apart on you? That's how my life feels. This strange year started out great! I've been making jewelry for seven years now. I enter jewelry contests to push myself to keep improving. This year, one contest had a Roaring Twenties theme. I researched period fabric designs, found one, redrew it, and then carved it in Metal Clay. And thrill of thrills! I won an award from Metal Clay Europe for this pendant!

I started my adult life as a neonatal nurse in San Francisco, advancing to a specialist. While still a student nurse though, I was in a terrible car accident. Nobody was killed, but years later effects showed up from that accident that prevented me from working. I was losing feeling in my legs. I flew up to Canada every three weeks for treatments from a brilliant chiropractor. Eventually, I moved here for a job. The culture shock surprised me, but I adapted and expanded my areas of nursing expertise, doing research, palliative care, and teaching master's students at UBC. But government cutbacks in the '90s meant hospitals were laying off nurses with master's degrees. My whole life revolved around my work, so I really didn't know where to turn next.I ended up at the other end of the nursing spectrum as Director of Care for home care and geriatrics, and a certified Dementia Consultant.

As retirement approached, I wanted to give my creative side room to flourish. I took a jewelry-making course in silversmithing and found myself totally enraptured. That led me to work with Metal Clay. I was totally enamored and began the journey to find my own voice in this medium. Silversmithing involves constant learning, definitely an important thread in my life. I love how happy people are when they find a piece of my jewelry that is a true fit for them!

The pandemic has interfered with so many lives. Community markets, my main source of income, were shut down. But I've just designed and built my own website! I'm getting ready for the next upswing!

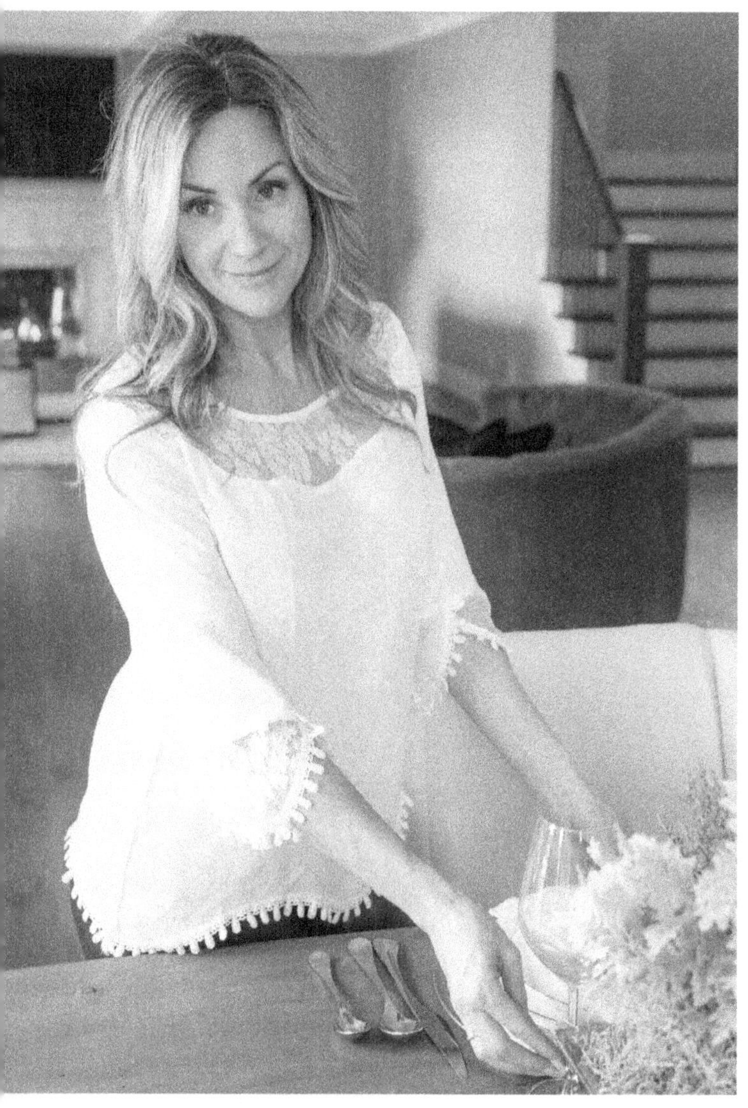

Tara Lavoie is a Manifestation and Success Consultant whose passion and purpose is to help burnt-out professional women who have lost all meaning in their work and life discover their long-lost dream job and rekindle the love in their personal relationships. She is also the Owner of a boutique Interior Design and Lifestyle company. What matters most to Tara is her family, her life partner, and their five beautiful children. She is happiest when in the kitchen making dinner with her family.

Tara Lavoie

What brought me to where I am today – coaching entrepreneurial women exactly what to do to clear up their mindset, invite in abundance and build the life of their dreams. That defining moment in my life happened in 2015.

In 2015, I had found myself as a forty-year-old stay-at-home mom of three with a passion for interior design. Over the course of a few months, I realized I was not living a life of truth and integrity. Although the decision was the toughest I have ever had to make, with all the courage I could muster, I packed up just a few of my things, and with my children close by we made a space of freedom and opportunity for ourselves. I poured over hours of mindset work and started the process of defining my "new" life's vision.

I was passionately motivated to build a legacy for my children. I grew to realize that my life, up until this point, was not littered with mistakes; rather, every experience was a necessary step in my journey. That I had made the best decisions I could have for where I was at that time in my life. I felt grateful for my marriage instead of sadness for it ending, and I let go of blame and my limiting beliefs about it being a failure.

My passion and purpose in life now are helping other women to locate the most beautiful peace, love, and connection within themselves, their careers, and their relationships. I help clear up their mindset, invite in a higher level of abundance, while simultaneously building their dream life full of purpose and fulfillment.

Tammy-Lynn McNabb's success is measured in teardrops and milestones.

Tammy-Lynn McNabb

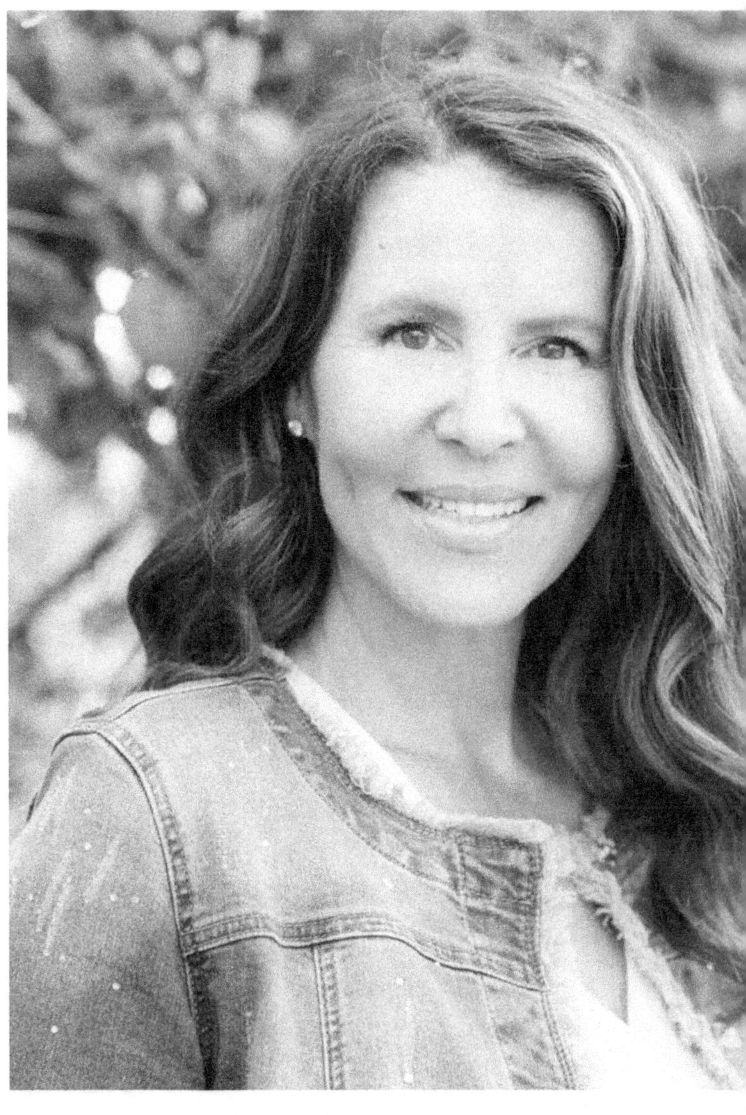

Fifty-three years ago, I was born to a teenage mom who was seventeen, and a wild child father who was twenty-one. Though both were excited about being parents, there would be years of adversity and challenges to follow. We grew up poor, though I never really entirely knew it. When we left Manitoba in 1971 for British Columbia, my parents looked at the move as an opportunity for something bigger and better for their small family. Only being able to afford a one-bedroom apartment in the West End of downtown Vancouver, my dad built a bunk bed for my brother and I in the apartment's broom closet. We thought this was the best fort that a dad could ever make a kid and was typical of my parents forever turning lemons into lemonade.

Years of living in social housing, I learned the value of a dime and what hard work meant. There wasn't a day that my parents didn't work hard. We could have fallen into the trap of poverty. My parents chose another path. Seeing them complete their GEDs and then go on to college, set the stage for me to always challenge myself, at any age, to be better than I was the day before. This feeling sparked the entrepreneur in me.

All these years later, I understand the heartache, stress, anxiety, and fear these two young parents went through. I admire them for taking less and giving more. In moments that are meant to break us, we come together and push through.

I look at my life and the desire to always do more, make more, see more, travel more, experience more. I do it so that my mom and dad know that everything that almost broke them wasn't in vain. I include them in everything, so they know what FANTASTIC feels like. I know my love of life and my determination in my business pursuits are foreign to my mom and dad, but deep down, they know that everything I do, I do because of them.

So... Mom and Dad, today I dedicate July 22 to the two of you. Thank you for every moment in making me the woman that I am today. For all of the lessons taught and learned. For every tear, every smile, and every achievement. As life begins to get shorter, we now know that it has all been time well spent. I love you both.

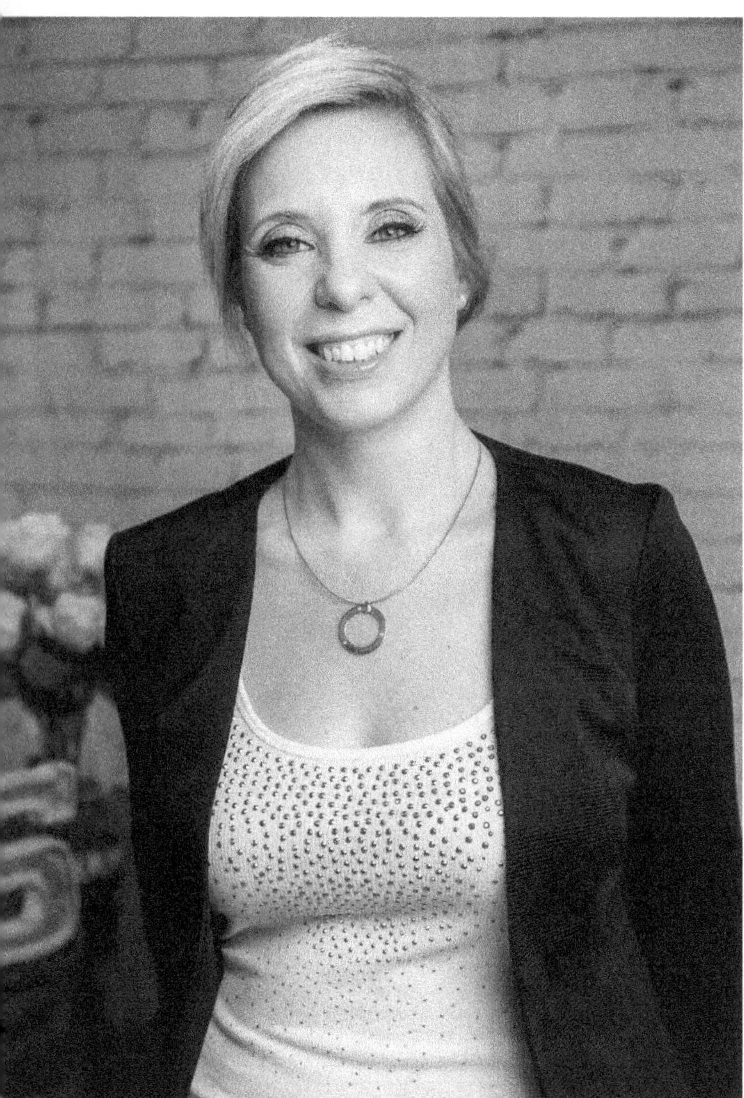

Photo Credit: Linda Mackie Creative

Shelley Essery is an Author, Entrepreneur, Certified Professional Life Coach, and Certified Law of Attraction Facilitator.

Shelley Essery

"Just keep going!"

These words became my mantra during the difficult years following an unexpected job loss, only seven short years from full retirement. I even had them engraved on a pendant I wore daily to provide much-needed encouragement. As a result of suffering the devasting effects of financial loss, my husband and I made the terrifying decision to follow our dream and launch our own business. Against all odds, we forged ahead despite the fact that neither of us had any experience owning a business. Our journey to success was a long and bumpy road that ultimately taught us the secret to surviving financial loss, the art of self-reinvention, and how to shift from survive to thrive!

Sharing my knowledge to help other entrepreneurs and dream builders shift from an ordinary life to an extraordinary one is not just a passion; it is a privilege. My philosophy that success comes through personal growth is at the centre of my own achievements in business and life and is the motivation, purpose, and love behind my book "Life Revived – The Business of Living Life" and ShelleyEssery.com.

When I began my journey, finding the information I needed and getting answers to my never-ending questions was half the battle. Having a trusted resource or place of inspiration and encouragement would have saved me a tremendous amount of time and energy. My goal is to support people, who like me, are starting over with a committed desire to live an inspired life and pursue their dreams. I believe success is available to us all. The secret is in finding the courage to embrace what makes us exceptional and becoming vulnerable enough to share it.

"Life is like the very water that sustains a physical body. You can try to cup your hands and hold on to it, but in the end, it will slip through your fingers leaving you with nothing but an experience, a moment in one person's life and if you don't share that moment then it dies with you, and then what did any of those experiences really mean?" ...Shelley Essery

Christina's greatest lesson has been that it's your HEART, not your mind, that will lead you to your authentic self and a greater purpose in life.

Christina Weizmann

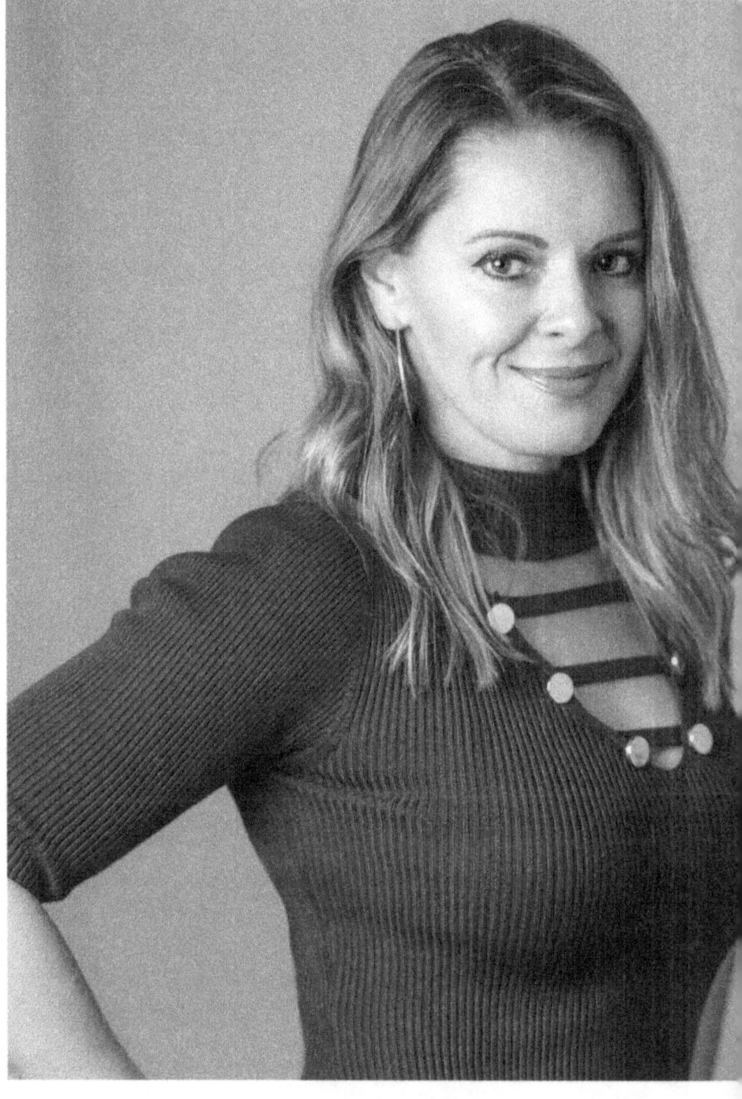

Looking back on my "fabulous forties," the highlights were getting married and becoming a mother to our sweet Doodle and wonderful daughter. I switched careers from creative director to diamond dealer and became a bestselling author, as well as a vegan. The greatest shift came when my marriage was hanging by a thread, I had a miscarriage, and I took my first ever ambulance ride with an inflamed (broken) heart at forty-five. I ended my marriage because, without my health, I knew I would end up with nothing. I moved with my girls on the 8th day of the 8th month into suite 808.

I knew it was the right move when I saw a car sticker parked outside our new building that said, "Olivia's Loft." My daughter is Olivia. The Universe had my back.

I spent the next eighteen months starting from scratch, finding my voice and shifting my mindset amidst a pandemic. I embraced every thought leader on every life topic and took more courses than I can remember. I was exhilarated but lost – not yet heeding my intuition. We are told to calibrate our mindset, but without aligning with our "heartset," we continue to sabotage ourselves. I realized that the guidance of my much wiser, more powerful heart is smarter than the noise and clutter in my brain. Our heart is what will truly transform us. Only then can we change the world and be a titan for humanity – living for a cause that's bigger than ourselves.

All people are born pure and creative, and as we age, we often lose that deep connection to ourselves because of the outside noise. When an evolutionary woman has the heartset of saying YES to the impulse urging her to create and follow her passion, it expands and becomes her main source of guidance. An evolutionary woman fixes the problem by empowering others to look within their own impulse to create and soar. The major crisis we are facing globally today is giving the human species the possibility of evolving to a higher culture.
I invite all of us to become a new kind of leader in the world as an Evolutionary Woman.

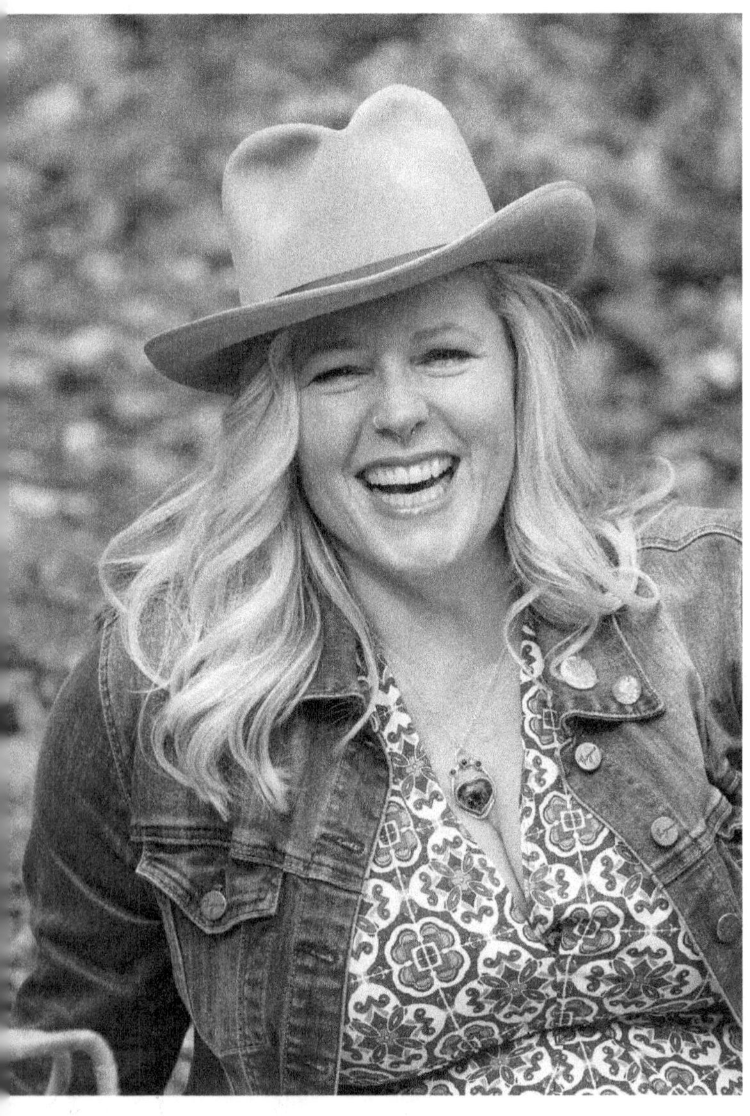

Jessica Séguin is a mother, coach, and businesswoman, who helps women gain clarity in their personal & professional lives to maximize self-empowerment & own their experience rather than fall victim to it.

Jessica Séguin

As kids, we fail repeatedly; it's through failure that we learn. Something happens as we grow older, as though we expect ourselves to automatically know how to perform, be or do whatever it is, that we begin without allowing ourselves room to grow into mastery of any subject.

Despite having no formal business training, I began my first venture into entrepreneurship in my early twenties, and that project never quite got off the ground, neither did my second one. When a third opportunity showed up, I was firmly refusing to even entertain the possibility when it was offered. When asked why, I answered, "I've failed at entrepreneurship before," and the reply was, "Why does that mean you'll fail again?"

Past failure does not equate to future failure. Overnight success is never truly overnight.

Guess what? I didn't quite succeed in THAT venture either! But the lessons began to take root within my being, and I started to see the common thread that connected my training over two decades and those previous ventures. Each one of those failed businesses had, at their core, supporting and helping vulnerable individuals from an emotional, physical and spiritual standpoint. This is when I tuned in more clearly to my talent and began to learn where my entrepreneurial gaps were. I honed these skills while simultaneously working a 9-5 job, and when my position was eliminated, I knew this was the time to fully commit to what had been calling for nearly thirty years.

I was terrified of failing again, even with the lessons that past failure had taught me, but I harnessed that fear and propelled myself into a place of faith in myself. It took six months of consistent action, zero clients, zero income, wondering how rent would get paid, and how I would put food on the table for my kids. My faith wavered, and I almost took a government job, something I had vowed to never do, but that fear was triggering my survival instinct again! On the same day that government job was offered, I landed my first true client, and I tossed the need for security aside and embraced my true calling.

Connie Peters is an entrepreneur, mother, wife, and pet-lover in suburban Vancouver who wants to encourage you to start where you are, right now.

Connie Peters

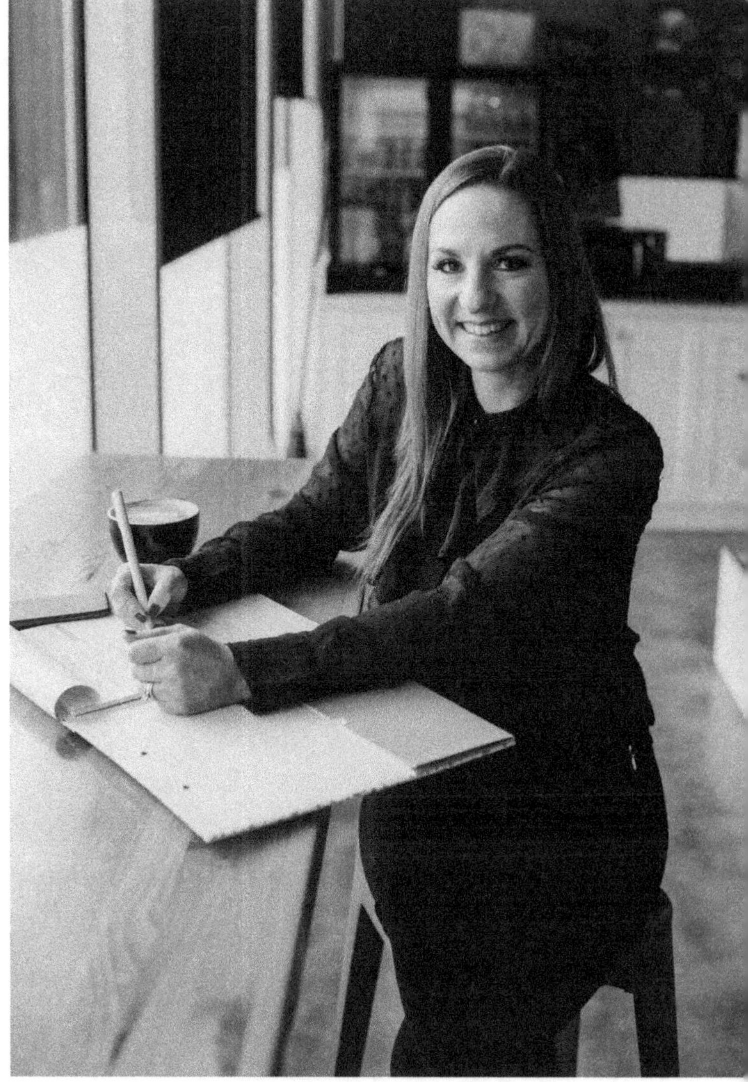

My favourite quote is, "Start before you're ready." I can't remember where I heard it, but I love it. I tell women who want to be business owners or start something new these words all the time.

I started my entrepreneurial journey by creating a mom-focused events business in 2008 to get myself out of the house and meet other new moms. That business grew to twelve cities, a print magazine, and a mom blog over twelve years before I sold it. It was my first entrepreneurial pursuit and won't be my last. Since I sold Modern Mama, I've been focused on helping other women entrepreneurs learn social media, grow their businesses, and help them work on their business behind the scenes. I also am an automotive journalist and content creator, which keeps me learning, driving, and creating.

When I discovered Boss Ladies Association, a large and growing Facebook Group, last year, I just knew I wanted to be part of it, grow it, take it on. So, I did! I bought the business from the savvy gal who started and had grown it to that point. I am now working to provide valuable networking and learning resources for women-owned businesses through the group and website. We now have a locally focused digital magazine in four locations: Edmonton, Okanagan Valley, Greater Vancouver, and Fraser Valley, BC. The purpose of the magazine is to help local women learn about locally-owned, and women-owned businesses in their communities, and to support them. I want to grow this magazine and Boss Ladies Association to many new locations in 2021 and beyond!

If you're thinking about starting a business, if you've been dreaming about an idea for years, and you're waiting for just the right moment in time to start, this is it. Start before you're ready, just start where you are.

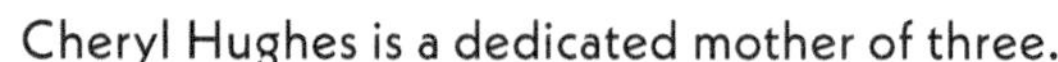

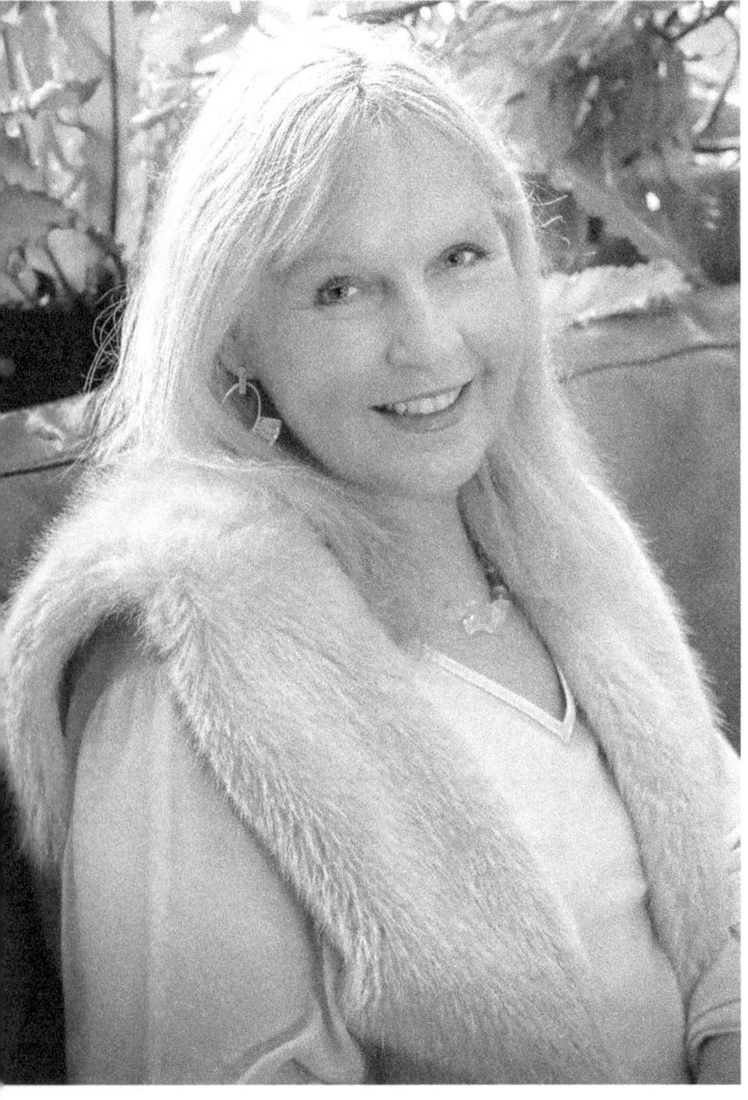

Cheryl Hughes is a dedicated mother of three.

Cheryl Hughes

Addicts Mom

This is not my pity party; I already had that party. This is my reality. I started out raising three boys, soccer mom, boy scouts, basketball, and class trips. Life was what I thought it should be; routine, curfew, and bedtime stories.

But that all changed. A rebellious middle child, ADHD diagnosed. That was ok, medication for that. When he was sixteen, he was at a concert and broke his jaw crowd surfing, off to the hospital for surgery and a prescription for oxycodone.

That was the beginning. That was sixteen years ago, and oxycodone was just becoming the drug of choice, it made him feel normal. Over time oxycodone was not enough. He stole and became homeless. It felt like his only thought was how to get high, and he did not care who he destroyed to get drugs.

As a mom, I tried to walk the thin line of helping and enabling. I was not particularly good at it; I did not know where the line was. Every phone call distressed me. If he called, it was some outlandish story of pending death if he did not pay a drug dealer. Then, if he did not call, I thought the worst. I gave him money. I did not know what else to do. What if he robbed someone to get money? I felt responsible. I became addicted to my addicted child; I would blame his friends, and I would blame myself! I was between terrified and depressed. I just wanted him better.

Then he got arrested. Six and a half years in federal prison. I felt guilty to say that I was relieved. I felt that at least if something happened, I would be informed in a few hours as opposed to him being on the streets, and I may never have known what happened to him. It has been a year and a half since he went to jail. We talk daily.

This has opened my eyes to a different world, a world of situational awareness. I felt helpless and became the victim.

But not anymore.

Voted "Most Original" in high school, author, speaker, and award-winning TV producer Andréa Fehsenfeld has forged a creative life living up to that distinction.

Andréa Fehsenfeld

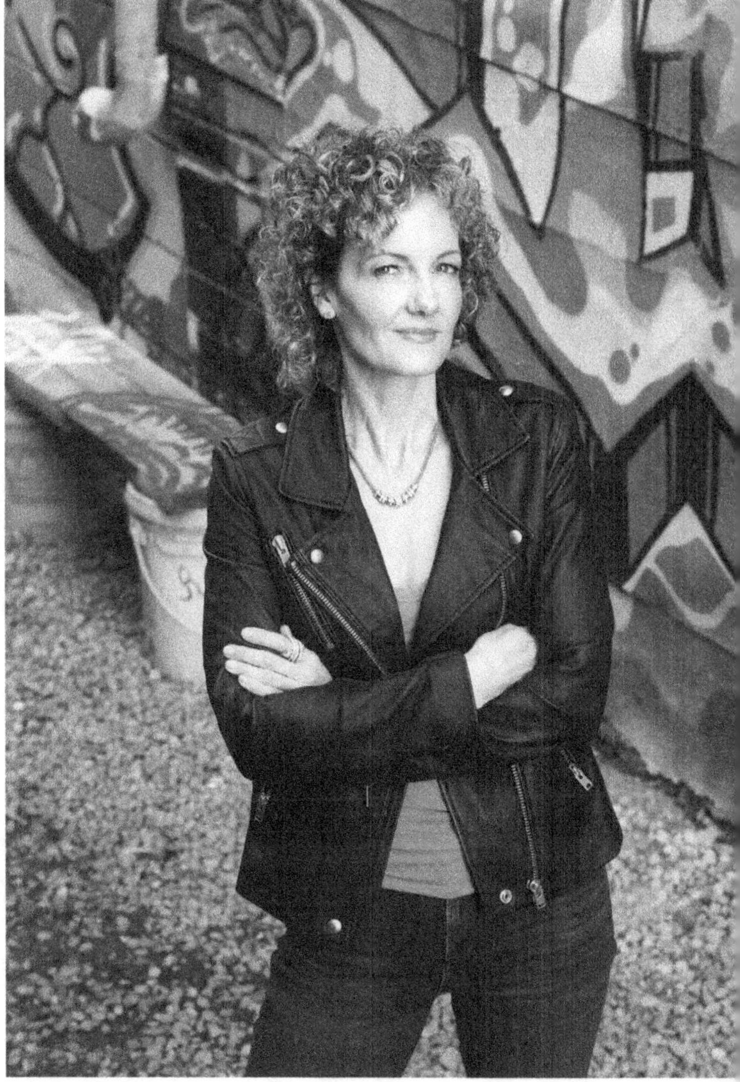

Being original, however, isn't always smooth sailing. Society creates boxes for us to fit into at work, play, and home. But what if I don't want to fit into any one box? I've struggled with this conundrum my entire life.

Fifth grade is when the realization truly hit home: I wasn't like the other kids. More importantly, I didn't want to be like them. The pack mentality turned me off. Being popular, or toeing the line, felt safe and limiting. At that age, I could already identify, but not yet fully understand, the invisible force of convention. How it shapes and influences. How it compartmentalizes. How it can make us fearful.

As I developed as a woman, I decided not to live my life as a popularity contest. I like pushing boundaries. I like expressing myself in ways that buck convention. It's a bold decision not to conform and marching to the beat of my own drummer has created challenges, personally and professionally. Falling on the wrong side of conformity usually does. But I embrace those hurdles because if I'm not living who I am inside, what's the point?

From the screen to the podium to the page, my goal is to tell stories that make people feel. If they get uncomfortable or unsettled with what I conjure, that's okay. It's also okay if, a week later, they're still thinking about what I said or wrote. And it's more than okay if they email or write a review telling me how my work has impacted them.

It's why I do what I do.

No surprise then, one of my favorite quotes comes from the famous advertising executive Bill Bernbach, "Rules are what the artist breaks; the memorable never emerged from a formula."

I encourage future generations of entrepreneurial women to remember that quote. In the end, there's only one life. Embrace yourself!

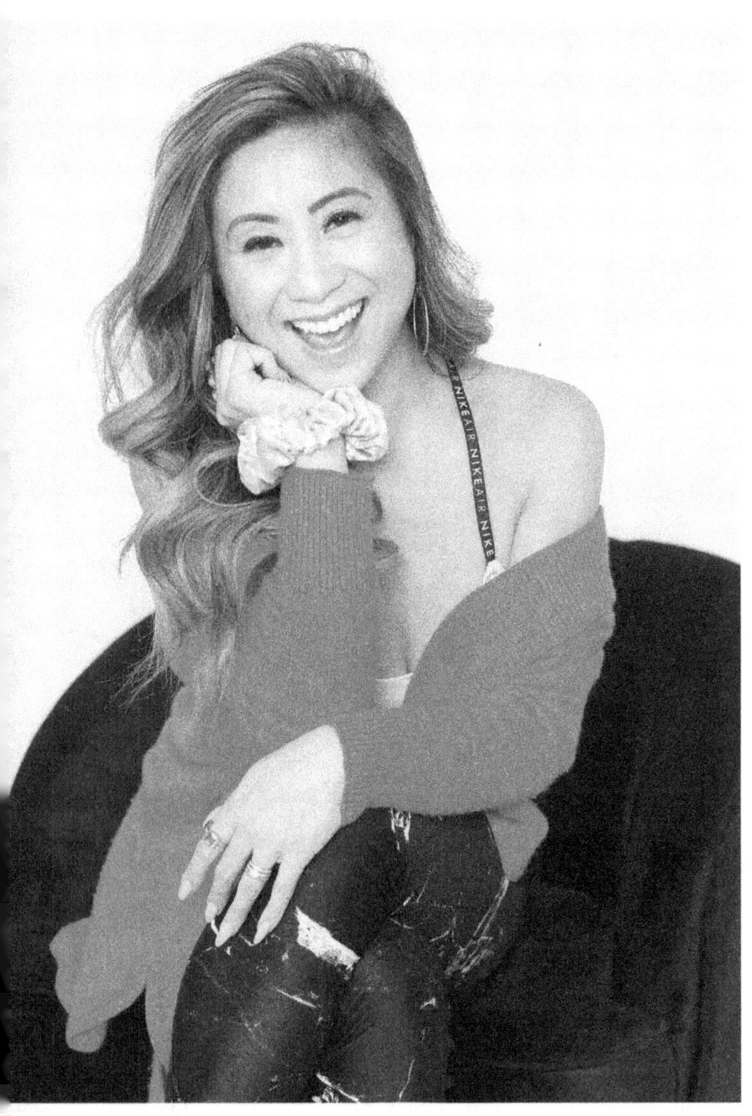

Genicca Whitney is a soul-shaking entrepreneur, body love activator, and manifestation master. She's on a mission to raise the vibration of the Universe with her Trifecta Transformation Method. She believes - you can have it all.

Genicca Whitney

There have been times in my life where I fell victim to my circumstances, where I allowed my external world to dictate who I was - and the kind of life I would live. The pain I endured in this mentality became a detriment to my evolution, and I fell to my knees with despair. It was in this moment of darkness that I experienced an undeniable light. I was ready for a new way of being, thinking, feeling, creating, choosing... and living.

I surrendered my fears and rediscovered my power, cultivating a deep faith in the Universe. It was the birth of my two girls that ignited a fire within me. Because of their presence in my life, I decided to turn my pain into purpose. I invested thousands of dollars to reinvent my mindset, to heal the wounds of my spirit, and to come back home to my body. It was the inner work I chose to commit to that changed the trajectory of my life. For once, I realized what it meant to have it all, regardless of what was happening outside of me. I stopped looking for evidence that my dreams were possible and became the only evidence I needed. For me, having it all means becoming the kind of person who knows who she is at the core, who is brave enough to walk with fear, dances unapologetically with self-worth, and plays in the present with purpose. It's not an end goal or a physical manifestation; it's a daily decision to fall in love with the life we are living and having an unshakable faith in the life we're creating. I profoundly believe that when we fuel our mind, our spirit, and our temple with the crème de la crème - we can heal the world. This is the Trifecta Transformation Method, and it is wildly potent and powerful. Decide today to become the catalyst for radical change. You are safe. You are called. It is time.

Daniela is originally from Buenos Aires, Argentina. She is an Emotional and Energy Healer, Wellbeing Coach, Entrepreneur, Worldwide Competitive Ballroom and Latin Champion, Black Belt in Kickboxing Martial Arts, and a blessed mom and wife to a beautiful family.

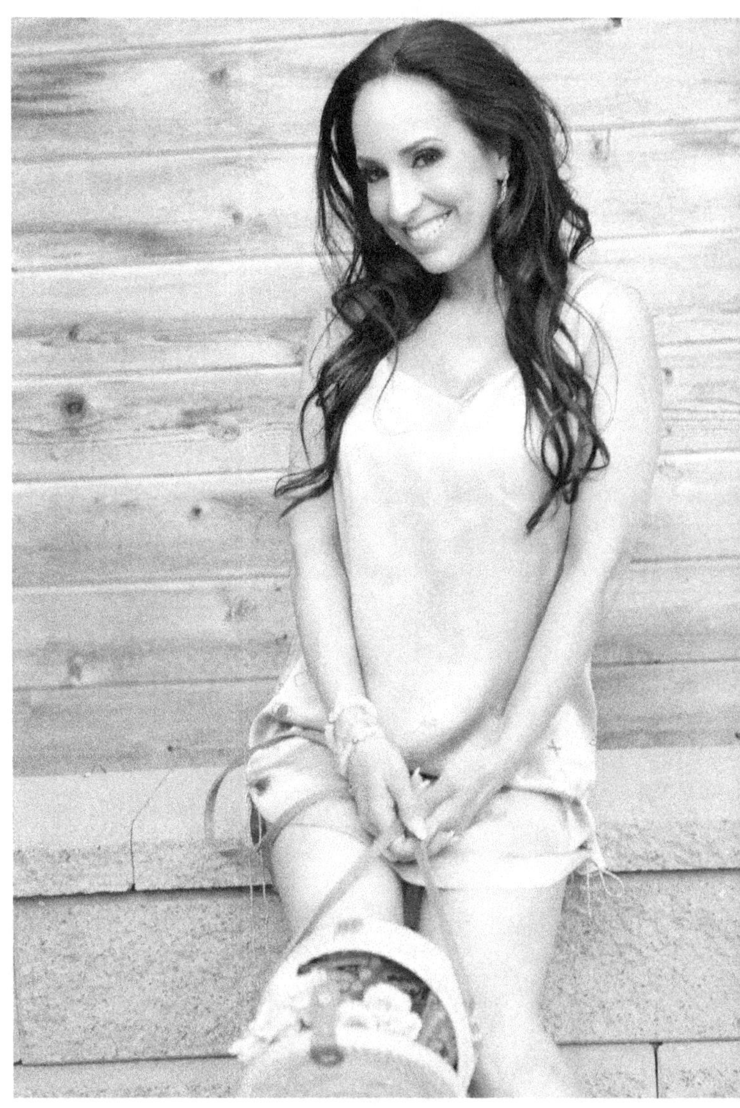

Daniela Fisher

From a very young age, Daniela expressed curiosity and was fascinated by the wisdom of the Universe. She has been studying and practicing spirituality and wellness for thirty years. She says: **"listening to my heart has always been at the top of my list!"** And this is how, Naturally Given, was born four years ago.

Daniela creates unique products that heal the emotional body, and her services are a fusion of Angelic Reiki Healing, Aromatherapy, Chakra, Crystal, Colour, and Flower therapy, which are ancient forms of healing methods to bring awareness, raise vibration, and create transformation in humanity.

Why "Naturally Given"? Because she believes our souls were given two gifts: **1) Free-will** and **2) A unique talent that no one can do it better than you.** YES, we are all a **"limited edition"**, she says, and our souls occupy a very special place on Earth! We are all spiritual beings in a physical body, therefore, we are all made out of energy, love, and light which make us one with Source. If Source is unlimited, then it makes sense that we are also unlimited! The only thing that limits us, is our belief systems. **"If a thought can make you sick, then it makes sense that a thought can make you well" – Dr. Joe Dispenza.**

The Universe believes in you and wants to help you release wounded beliefs that don't serve you and that are not the truth of who you really are. It's time to trust LOVE more than your fears because **"Everything you need to know is within you!"**

Daniela's "key" elements to her transformation were daily gratitude, grounding, meditation, physical movement, doing more of what she loves, living in the now, and creating a strong positive mind.

LOVE is the most powerful force that there exists and is the key to open our hearts to unleash our highest potential and therefore create a planet of love - what she calls - **Heaven on Earth!**

Your Divinity is your birthright! Just Be You because You were born to shine!

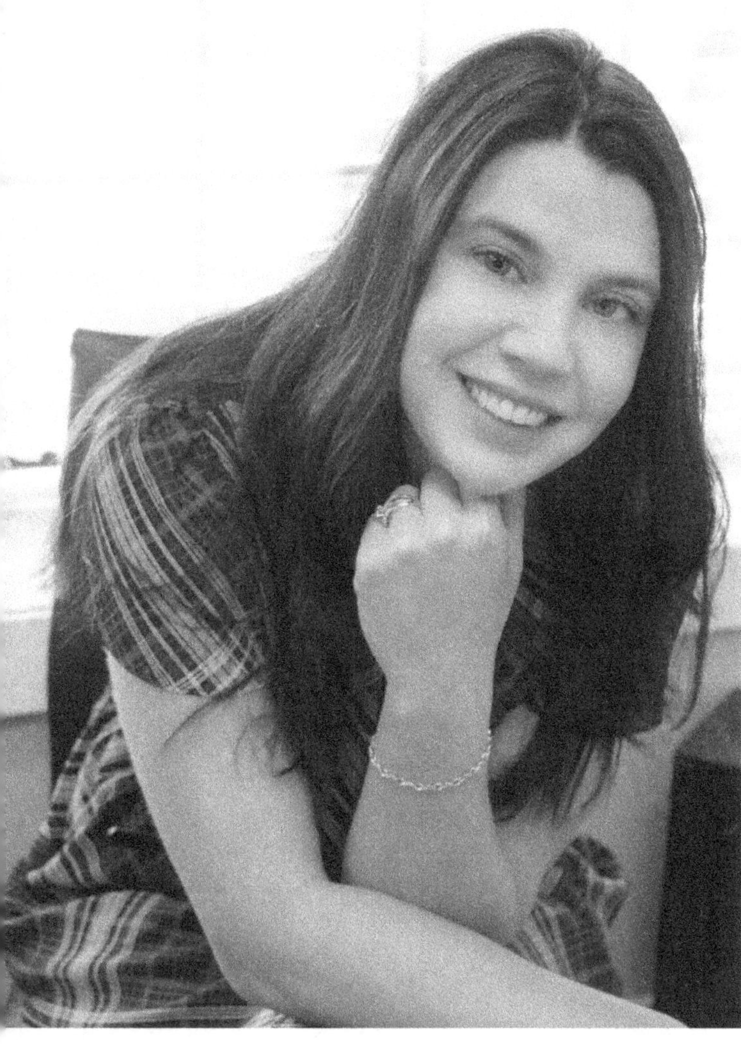

Dale-Lynn Desabrais helps empower people to find joy through financial freedom.

Dale-Lynn Desabrais

Growing up in Alberta, family was everything. I had little concept of money, or the value of things. My father, a brilliant mechanic, often worked for free or discounted rates. He wanted to help people while raising his family and worked hard for every penny he earned. When he wasn't working, he was spending time with family, making memories. He was full of JOY. Because of my humble beginning, happiness and stability were paramount to me when I started my own family. Losing parents at a young age taught me the value of the transfer of knowledge. My children experiencing joy and having financial security were integral to me. In my pursuit of this, I found my life's calling.

In the first few months of my career, fresh out of business studies, I found this new world where there was an abundance of money. Not coming from money, I was both surprised and excited at the prospect that with knowledge and education, not only could I help others find financial freedom, I could also do so for myself and my little family. So began my journey for financial stability and the pursuit of JOY, intertwined!

I learned quickly that financial freedom doesn't mean having a lot of money or making the correct investments, it means having a plan and making the right decisions. I learned that financial freedom doesn't have to come at the cost of happiness and joy.

Armed with this knowledge, I began my career goal – helping others in their own financial pursuits. I teach my clients that to achieve financial gain, they need not sacrifice their joy! We can achieve both!

With this came Desabrais Wealth Management, the firm I created. I utilized both my education and experiences and incorporated my own bit of passion. In this, I have an outlet for human connection where clients become like family; where I spend my time pursuing JOY while my clients chase theirs. I'm most powerful when I'm helping clients, family and friends plan for their futures and live their dreams. I aim to EMPOWER, EDUCATE and create FINANCIAL FREEDOM for clients so they can pursue their dreams, as I am mine!

Jessie Lyon is an entrepreneur.

Jessie Lyon

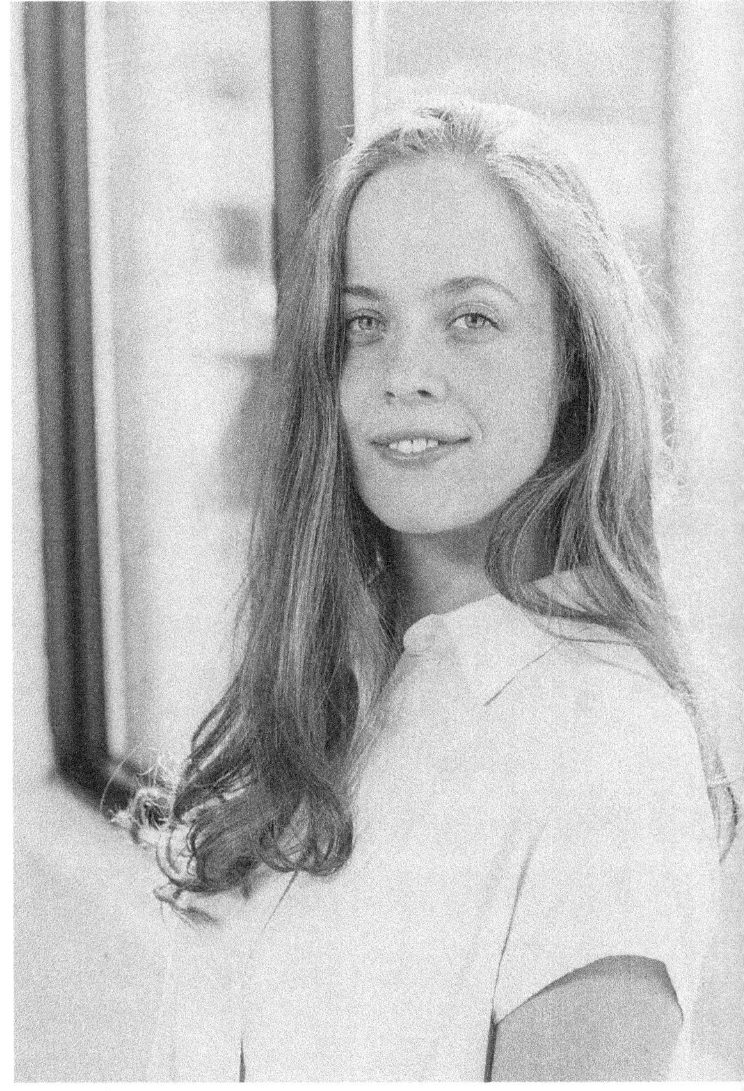

I started being a business owner because I was looking for a way to marry profit with ethics, something I believed in. I met my business partner, we had an idea to start a give-back artisanal lifestyle brand, and then, we did.

According to the 2017 American Express OPEN Small Business Monitor, 81% of business owners say their happiness is due somewhat or entirely to being an entrepreneur, and 94% of entrepreneurs say they are happy with their lives. Why?

I asked myself this many times throughout my ongoing journey. When I was operating out of my boyfriend's old, stick shift, gold Volkswagen Jetta and pitching boxes of blankets to shop owners across the Ottawa Valley, I often asked myself, what am I doing? When my first warehouse was a storage unit without electricity, I asked myself, am I missing something? When my partner and I were the only two people doing all the jobs at our company, there were many dark days that brought this question forward.

So why?

I'm an entrepreneur because it is my natural state. I trend toward grey zone, the thing that we're aiming for but cannot see, that gap makes me excited. I'm an entrepreneur because I know the power that business has to change. I'm an entrepreneur because I never give up. What began as me selling to my neighbourhood boutique, has, step by step, grown into a brand represented by shops across Canada and the US, a network that supports over 100 artisan partners. Not overnight, but every day, driven by something hard to describe, that feels most like an unwavering commitment to my task, and its greater impact. I'm an entrepreneur because my community supports me in doing so, I would be nowhere without them.

So why are entrepreneurs so happy? We're happy because our thoughts, feelings, and actions are aligned, and every step we take is governed by our gut. The humility and grit that the entrepreneurial journey forces us to take makes us constantly reassess who we are and what we're standing for. That definition and drive feeds you, and it feels really good.

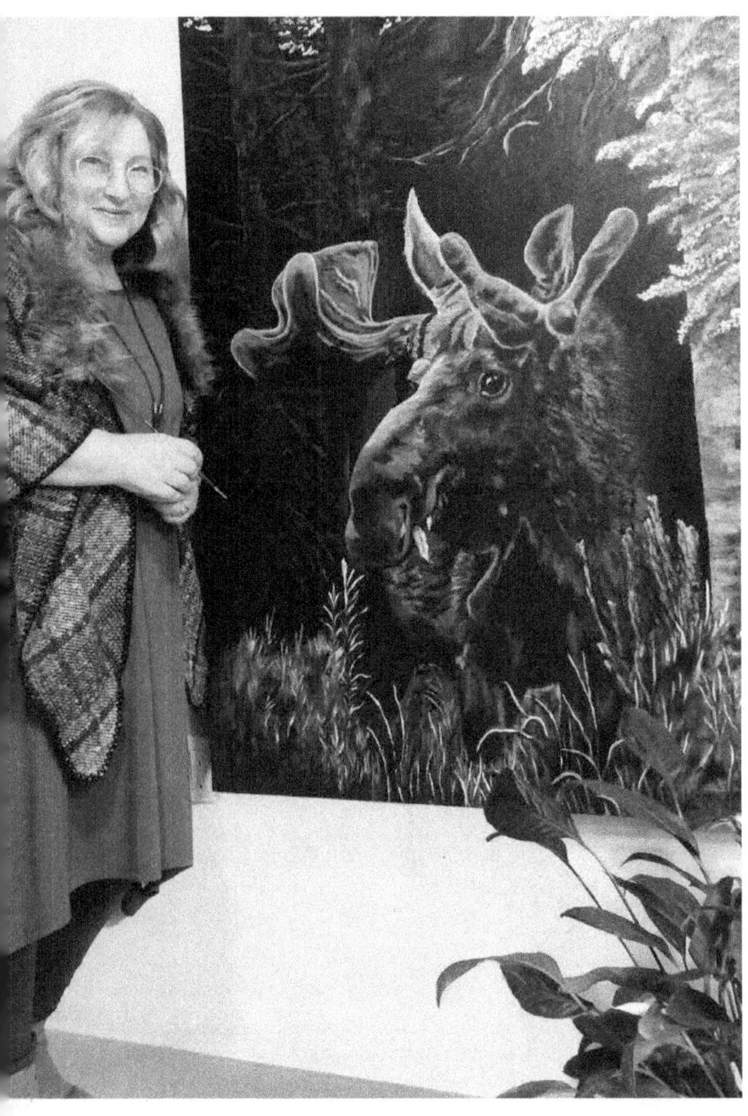

Achieving abundant awards throughout her lifetime, artist, Lynda Moffatt, has honoured the legacies of her father and grandmother, who taught her how to express gratitude for the world around her.

Lynda Moffatt

Having a father who loved to sketch and being my artist grandmother's namesake, I felt that becoming an artist was my birthright. Still, it's taken a lifetime to develop the skills that shape my personal style yet still respect techniques of the old masters of realism. Whenever challenged, I've always felt guided toward furthering my education and knowledge.

Travelling extensively, I realized the benefit of networking, so I joined artist associations in different communities, which led to jobs that taught me curating, the history of art, designing and framing, and the business side of the arts. Studying oils under New Albany Arts Council founder — Harold Cooper — proved a pivotal phase for me.

Being commissioned to create a public mural — the first acknowledging the history of black peoples in a parliamentary building — set my career on the path of self-employment.

Most every day, I wake up wanting to create; I paint even when not feeling my best, a testament to the value of art therapy! By incorporating my other passions — boating, diving, and history —my art reflects inspiring places I've explored, both in and around the Great Lakes.

I've never let fear stop me from starting a project, and diversifying my skillset across several disciplines primed me for teaching others to explore who they might become as artists. Believe in yourself and trust that any roadblocks you encounter may be necessary for you to learn and grow!

My greatest success comes from taking chances and trusting my intuitions but also God, family, and especially my partner, Kevin, helped me get to where I feel I'm meant to be today — living my purpose!

"God gave artists art so they would never be lonely." This quote inspires me and reminds me I'm not alone, even in a solitary studio. When given a gift, I believe we cannot take it lightly, especially if we asked for it! We're meant to work on it every day and never take it for granted. Ask yourself - what is your gift to share?

Amanda Lavery is an entrepreneur and the CEO of CoCaBee, Canadian skin care brand famous for the Antibacterial Lip Balm.

Amanda Lavery

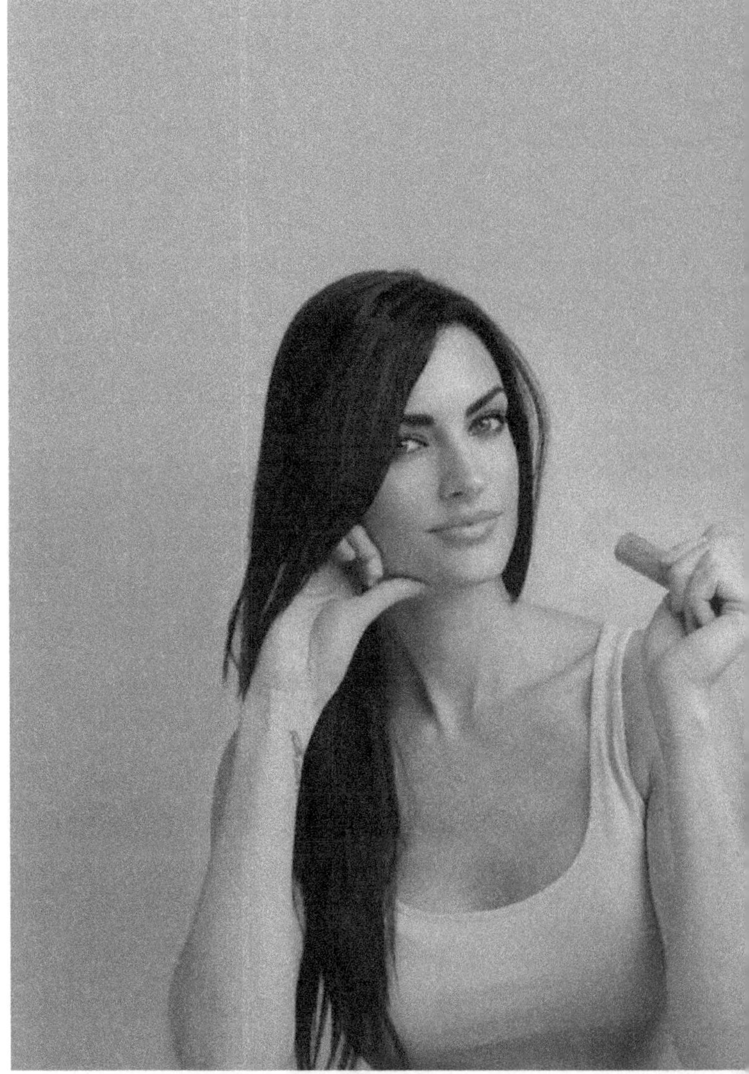

Not too long ago, I found myself becoming more and more cautious about my health and what I was putting in and on my body. I started reading more labels, checking the ingredients, and researching the methods of how products we consume are created.
To put it mildly, it's a little scary sometimes to find out what we are really taking in from everyday products.

As a result, I changed many of my consumer habits, but I found that I did not have a truly organic option for lip balm. I decided that if I had no organic option for my beloved lip balm, that I would make my own!

With a lot of passion and tenacity, I started researching various recipes, and their organic ingredients, and through trial and testing I eventually came up with something great! It wasn't only organic, it was smoother, more flavourful, and longer-lasting than any lip balm I had tried before.
Eventually my friends, family, and even coworkers noticed I was using something different and asked about it. Turns out there are lots of lip balm lovers out there- and when they tried it for themselves, they loved it so much that they asked me to make them some too. From there, the idea of CoCaBee was born

At CoCaBee, we believe that amazing beauty and skincare products don't need to come at the expense of animal testing.

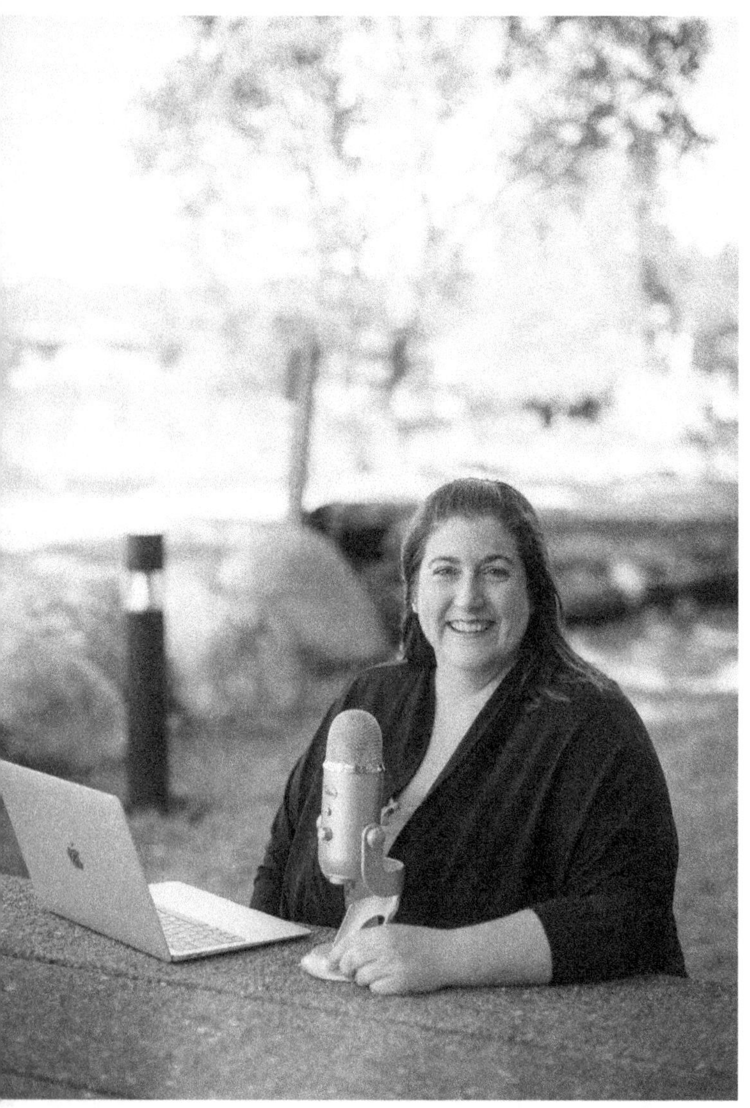

Michelle Elise Abraham is an international speaker and a celebrated podcast producer.

Michelle Elise Abraham

"Go Confidently in the direction of your dreams, live the life you have imagined" Henry Thoreau. That quote my parents chose for me for our yearbook, my graduation year. Little did I know the impact that quote would have on my life.

From Au Pairing in Switzerland to sky diving in Mexico, scuba diving in Fiji, 4x4ing in Australia, and bungee jumping in NZ. I lived in ski resorts in Europe and worked on Cruise ships from Alaska to the Caribbean. I was living my dreams. forty-seven countries, a collection of friends and memories, I was reminded that the world was indeed my oyster!

After a tragic loss at nineteen, while backpacking Europe, I travelled for years. I went all over the world in pursuit of happiness only to find it was always there inside of me. The moment I stopped, slowed down, and turned inwards for validation, love, and acceptance was the moment I realized, I do have everything I need, want, desire available to me, right here, right now. It was then that I met the love of my life and started to see what business success was really like.

I realized I have gone confidently in the direction of my dreams, found the confidence to leap, taken risks, and never looked back or gave up on myself. I became comfortable being stretched out of my comfort zone. I said YES to me and Yes to adventure.

It hasn't always been easy. I have struggled, had failed businesses, big debts, ended relationships, and gained a lot of weight, but I kept going. I vowed to only do work I love and to use my voice to make a difference.

We all have a story to tell, a story to inspire action, and one to make an impact on those who hear it. As a Podcast Producer, I have the privilege and honor to help thousands of stories be told and to celebrate our High Vibe Leaders who are making a huge impact in this world with their stories. Now is the time to celebrate YOU and you too have a message to share with this world, time to speak up, let us hear you!

Fiona Forbes is an award-winning TV host and producer.

Fiona Forbes

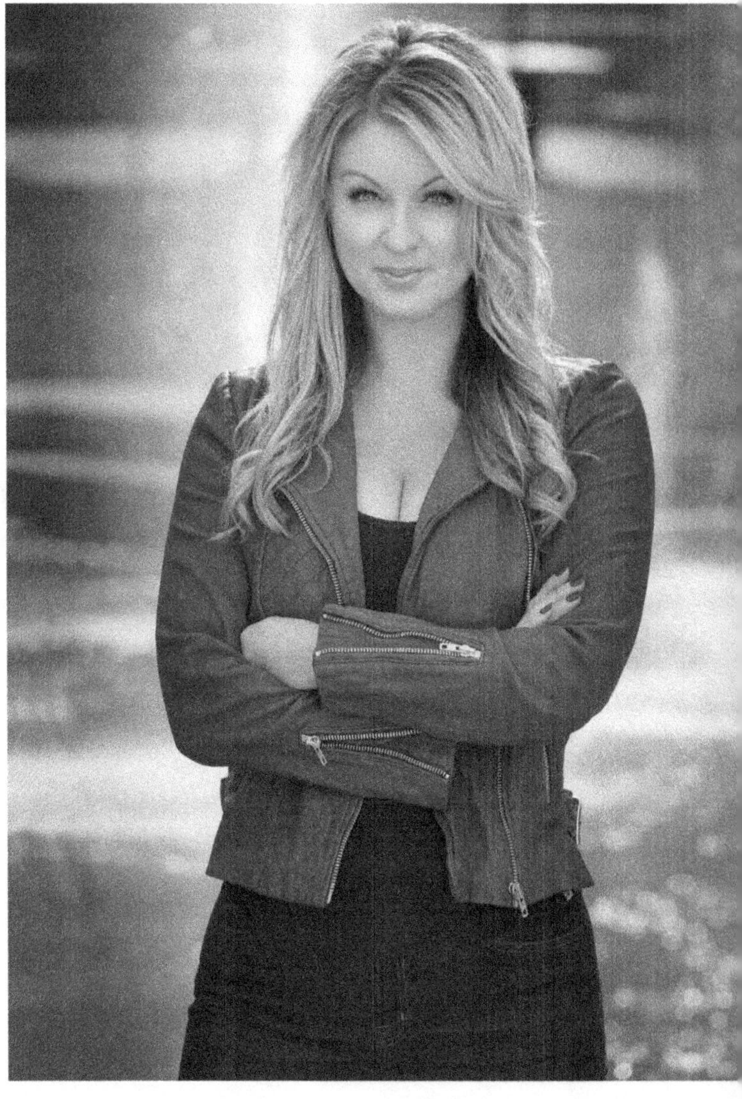

Panic. Anxiety. Stress. They plagued me during my youth. I really didn't know what a panic attack was when I first had one. Couldn't breathe. Dizzy. Claustrophobic. Drowning. The world was closing in around me. It's like you're completely losing control.
I was in class at UBC, and the panic overtook me... I ran from school and raced home. It happened again on the bus... I yelled at the driver to stop. I didn't care if everyone thought I was crazy - I had to get out.
My panic attacks continued for months before I decided to see a therapist to uncover the cause.
The stress of school and life was a little too much for me, and it was manifesting itself in anxiety. With my therapist's guidance, I learned what was happening to me and whyThe school stress was a given...that age old question of "what are you going to do with your life" was a huge part of it. A toxic and abusive relationship that I needed to get out of, but didn't know how. Once I knew these were the triggers, I dealt with them head-on. It wasn't easy but I'm happy to say I came out the other side and learned to cope with what was bothering me deep down. Back then, I was a shy nerd who was planning on going to law school, and the thought of speaking in front of a courtroom was something unfathomable to me. My dad suggested I face my fears and take a broadcasting class as a tool to get over my shyness. On the first night of the course, there was a posting for an audition to host a TV show. On a dare, I auditioned to tackle my fear of public speaking. I went to the audition with no intention of being on TV, got the job, and a week later I was hosting a live television show and discovered I loved it. I felt at home. I'm still in the TV biz today and haven't looked back since.
Do I still get nervous? Hell yes! But armed with knowledge and the confidence I never had in my youth, I've learned that fear is really the same adrenaline that we get when we're excited and it's all about channeling it in the right direction. When it comes to toxic relationships, it may be hard, but extracting those people from your life is the best thing you can do for your soul.
Today, panic attacks are more widely understood and discussed, but back then, they were something you simply didn't tell people about, so I suffered in silence for far too long.
To all the shy nerds who get nervous, panicky, and anxious – I'm here for you – let's talk about it!

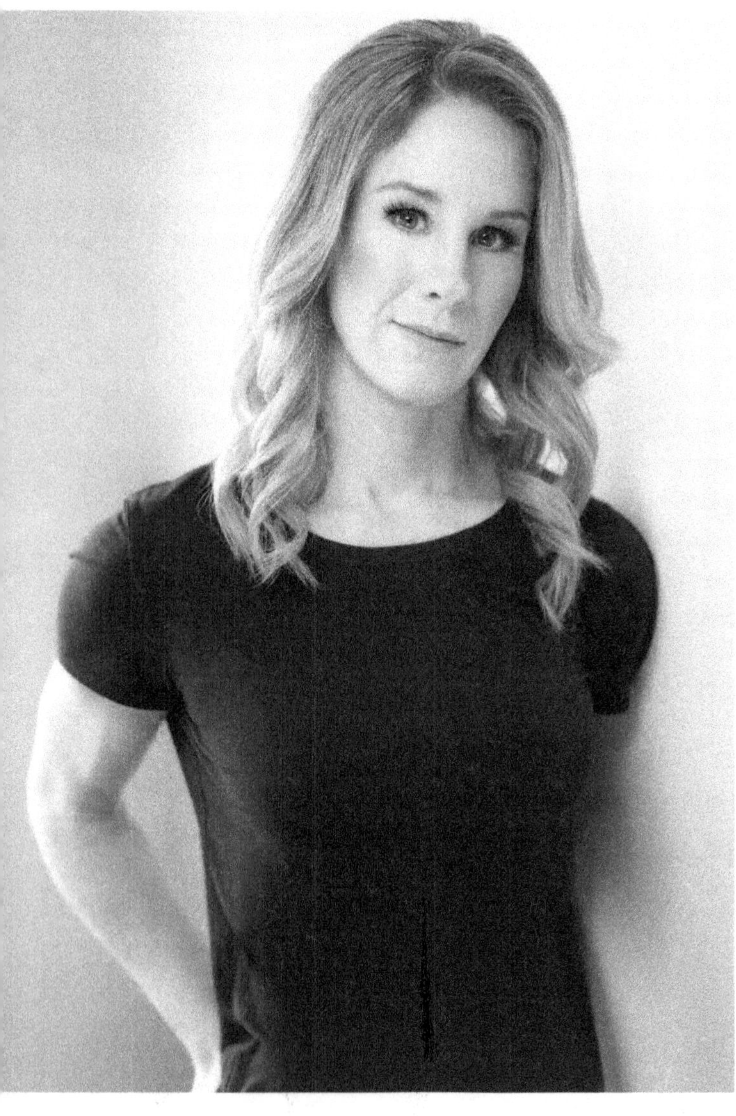

Andrea Ross is a Canadian stunt performer in film and television.

Andrea Ross

I am a Canadian stunt performer in film and television. On camera, I get the awesome privilege of fighting, flipping, and falling for some of today's top actresses. Off-camera, my free time is filled with kiteboarding, mountain biking, skiing, and hiking in my own backyard of Squamish, Canada. I have been an athlete my whole life, and I like to consider myself a skill collector. Always wanting to learn something new from others with expertise to share.

The thing that motivates me to get up and going most days is knowing that if I am not putting in the work, someone out there is. I believe my hunger for success comes from my father. He was an entrepreneur who built his company into what it is today, while simultaneously attending almost every athletic or academic event for his four children. From him, I learned the value of building something for yourself, and giving back to the community that helped you get there.

The biggest lesson I have learned from my own failures is to find ways not to fear them. To trust that it holds a place in my journey. To learn what I can strengthen to succeed the next time. To enlist help from one of my many resources to overcome the obstacle, or to deviate and honour a different path. Not easy to learn, but it has been most useful.

Over the past year, I have co-created the Live Your Fierce Project with my former boss and long-time friend, Amber Read. The LYF Project is a community and leadership platform where women find their fierce, share their journeys with other women, and find ways to live their fierce in their daily lives.

I am lucky to have built my coaching and stunting career off of the mutual energy, guidance, and enthusiasm of other women who are killing it in their respective pursuits. I think it is so important to share one's journey. The impact has a rippling effect, and I believe more and more women are finding ways to pursue their own success, their own fierce. I believe the LYF Project and this book are wonderful examples of just that.

Tamara Spence is a mother, wife, coach of many, former nurse, athlete and artist searching for an authentic life.

Tamara Spence

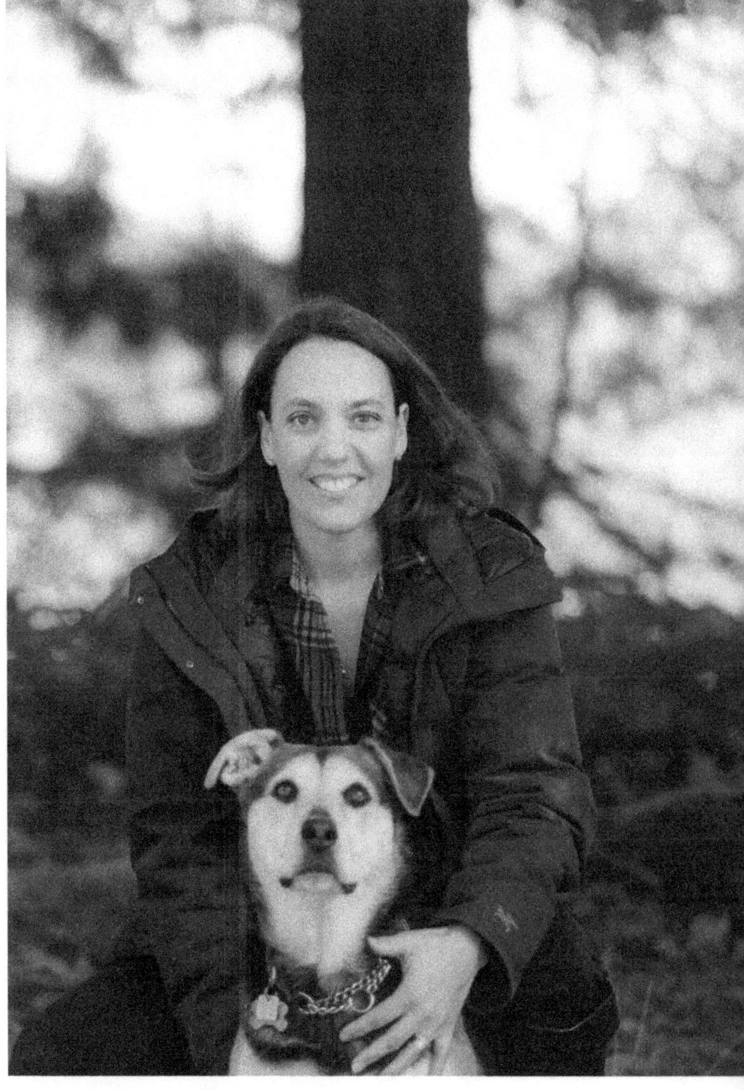

Artistic process, like life, is a journey of discovery. Layers of life build over the years, each with its own emotional trials, creations & celebrations.

Mine began in Vancouver, born to my father, a sculptor and my mother, a nurse. People and career paths that both influenced me greatly. Growing up as first a city and then a Salt Spring Island girl, my childhood holds memories of spending precious time creating alongside my father in his workshop. As an artist myself I sought, yet did not find, positive reinforcement from him. When I lost him at 27, I found myself left with a deep sense of self-doubt, criticism & struggle to create meaningful work in my life.

Driven to play hard by both my father and older brother, I found enjoyment in sports, specifically volleyball. Injuries plagued me, coaching youth fulfilled me, training educators taught me what was not for me. Layers of life, lessons galore, that led me to my greatest joy, my husband Chris, with whom I share our 2 sons, Ethan & Cody.

Still my search for meaning continued. At a crossroads, Nursing fulfilled my mind's love of science, but not my artistic soul. Years of battling depression, layers of anger, frustration, more self-criticism built up, all compounded by trauma both personally and professionally. There were moments where I would sink my hands back into different mediums, still seeking that outlet of joyful expression. Turning to a hypnotherapist to process my grief and self-doubt, I was finally able to start creating without my inner voice telling me it wasn't good enough, that I wasn't good enough.

Beginning with black and white abstract drawings to circumvent the negative talk, I created madly until I needed more meaning. Painting with acrylics, I discovered my desire for things to be colourful and bold. Choosing to combine my abstract line drawings with watercolours led to my creations of abstract realism. I enjoy manipulating the components in a design, to create the composition and impact I want, without the critical voice rising up to distract me from my process of discovery.

I am happiest when creating with meaning. I am a meaning maker.

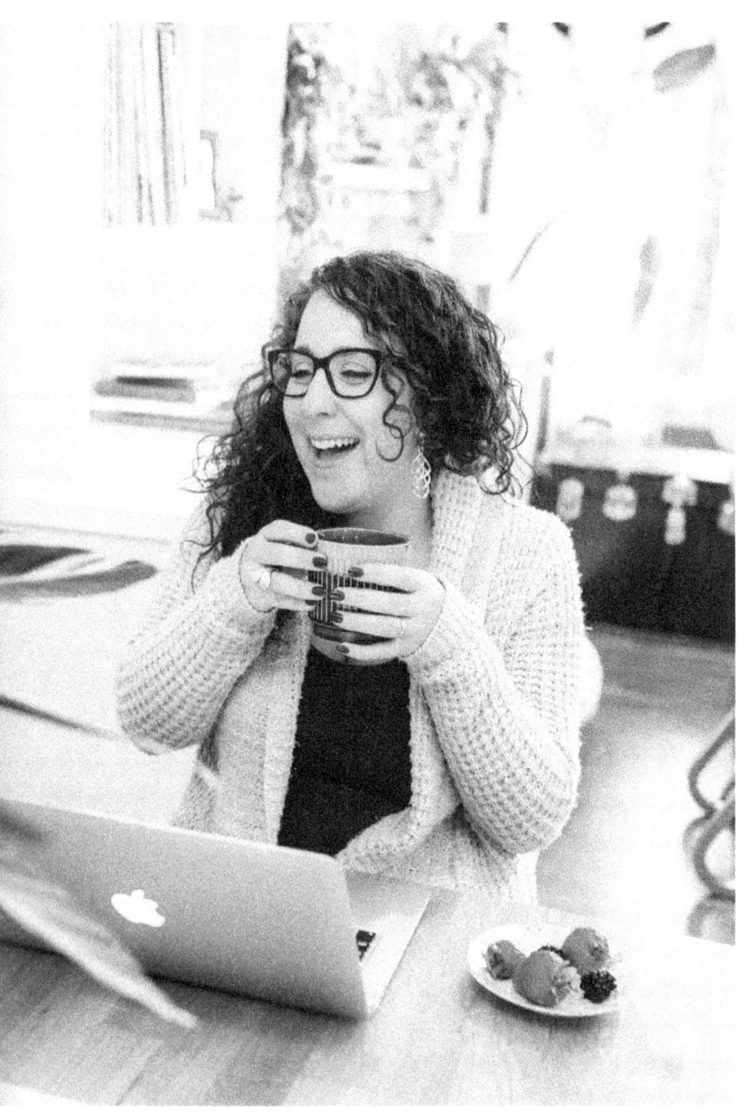

Blair Kaplan Venables is a social media marketing expert and mentor. She is an international speaker, Founder of the "I Am Resilient Project" (iamresilient.info), #1 best-selling author of Pulsing Through My Veins: Raw and Real Stories from an Entrepreneur, and one of the most resilient people you will ever come across.

Blair Kaplan Venables

When I was a young girl, my Aunty Heather gifted me a $10 shopping spree for my birthday. She took me to a fascinating wholesale dollar store in my hometown of Winnipeg. She told me that I could buy anything that I wanted. I can't remember what items I spent my money on, but my mother often reminds me that I ended up buying only gifts for others and nothing for myself. This event was one of the first signs that I was born a giver and destined to make a difference in the world.

The I Am Resilient Project emerged from a need to heal deep wounds from my past traumas. Every time I would tell my story about my relationship with my father, forgiveness, and acceptance, I could feel my wounds healing, and my resilience muscle growing stronger. I knew I had to gift this powerful and therapeutic experience to others. Our community is where people can read, listen and share stories of resilience to overcome their challenges. This community is a project created to help others and has been a guiding light on my journey through darkness.

Something else that you should know about me is that I literally came into the world blaring. I was given the gift of the gab and am known to embody an extremely wild imagination. I'm from a long line of passionate entrepreneurs. I am surrounded by motivated and ambitious friends and family members, so it was inevitable that I would find creative ways to help and inspire people. I can do just that as a social media expert and through the I Am Resilient Project.

Through writing, speaking, and creating, I fill the cracks of my heart with gold, and my words may do the same for you.
I am resilient, and so are you.

Madeleine Marentette is CEO of Canada's multi-award-winning Grail Springs Retreat Centre for Wellbeing which she founded in 1994. Bestselling author, speaker, and metaphysician, Madeleine is a passionate visionary dedicated to the transformation and wellbeing of people, animals, and the planet.

Madeleine Marentette

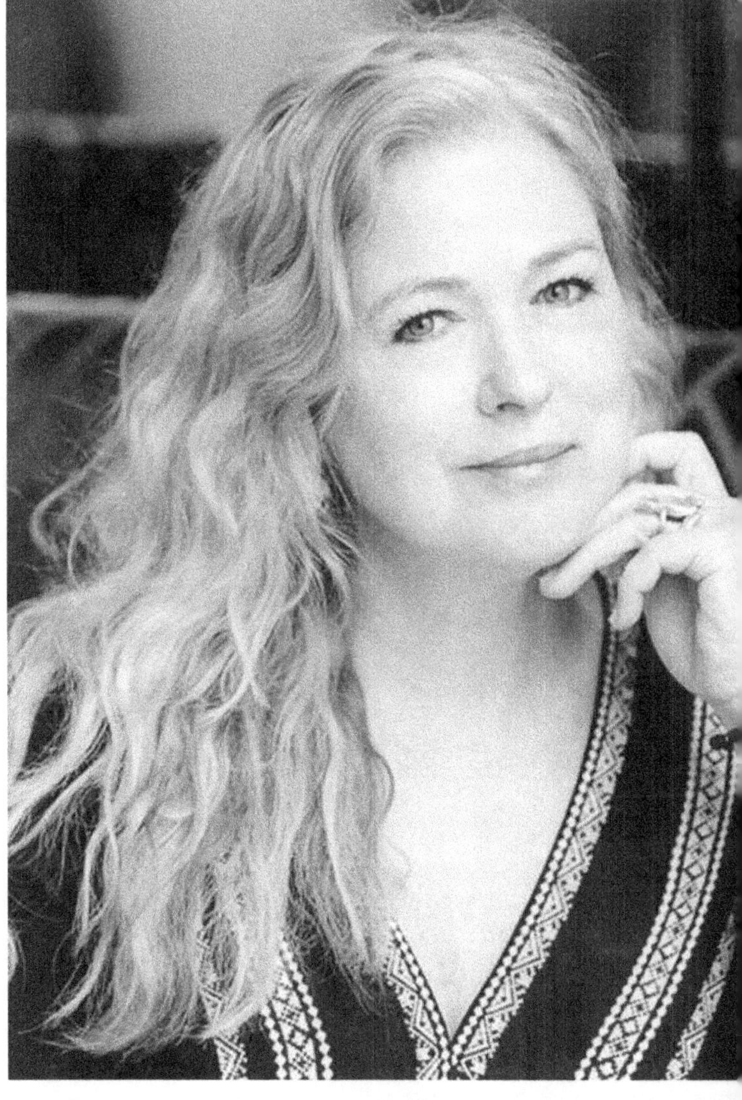

I began my career in the hospitality industry in Toronto while supporting myself through college, studying art history, interior, and architectural design. All would serve me well in the future in ways I could not yet imagine. I grew up with an excitable appreciation and love for beautiful spaces, excellence in design, our connection with nature and the animal kingdom, all influenced by summers in Germany living with my grandparents. Hikes under the canopies of the Black Forest, adventures to mountaintop fortresses, castles, and medieval monasteries fueled my continued thirst to uncover life's mysteries. Stories of rescues, secret passageways, hidden treasures, magicians, and noble knights, had me awaken to a commonality we share; the quest for peace, beauty, and wholeness.

It was in the final months of college when I was catapulted into a health crisis that became my own life-challenge to overcome, heal, and become whole again. The changing moment in that crisis was delivered in 1988 when I attended a discourse given by His Holiness the Dalai Lama at Convocation Hall at the University of Toronto. An inner revelation and realization about the mind's profound connection as the mediator and the medicine, between cell and Spirit, led me to a full healing while immersing myself in the life-study of Raja Yoga, the science of mind, meditation, the soul realities, and metaphysics.

That healing journey from illness to wellness became the very catalyst, philosophy, and foundation for the manifestation of Grail Springs Retreat, today a thriving and beauty-filled sacred space to support the human-soul potential. I believe we are each the embodiment of the Holy Grail, a symbol of complete wholeness. We have moments in our life when our cup is empty, when our cup is full and even overflowing, and everything in between. It is our will to seek and find that which will bring us happiness, meaning, purpose, and wholeness to our life.

The Holy Grail is a promise: Seek, and you will find.

Cathy Kuzel is a dynamic speaker; best-selling author; Business Development expert and Founder of The Connected Woman Association.

Cathy Kuzel

"Beauty begins the moment you decide to be yourself."
~ Coco Chanel.

Do we really know who we are? Taking the time to learn more about ourselves can be life-changing. In the pursuit of creating the life I am currently living and the joy that comes with it, I'd like to share some of the things I've learned along the way.

When you are being yourself, what is really important to you becomes clearer. Being yourself does not mean you are narcissistic or selfish. Being yourself means you like and respect who you are, and choose to live your life your way. You're not afraid to let your freak flag fly!

Be confident with who you are and what you do. Doubting yourself happens when you are always comparing yourself to others or listening too intently to outside opinions. It becomes quite easy to second guess yourself. Confidence in yourself and your decisions will inspire confidence in others.

What people think of you is a reflection of their own shortcomings. When people speak negatively about you, they are saying more about themselves than they are about you. The reverse is also true. My mom used to say that when you point a finger at someone, there are at least three fingers pointing back at you.

Walk Your Talk. Build your credibility, integrity, and confidence by taking action and do what you say you'll do. If we've committed to doing something, we need to "Stand Up. Stand Out. Step Forward." No excuses. None.

Know and protect your boundaries. Learn to say 'no.' It's not like we can place a "No Trespassing" sign on our foreheads. Setting our boundaries protects our health, well-being, and builds our identity. Pleasing others can be a nice thing to do, but don't make it a habit.

You are who you surround yourself with. Knowing how certain people impact your life allows you to create a cycle of self-improvement and bring more joy into your life. Choose to spend time with people who are genuine, possess empathy, and are not quick to point a finger.

Oscar Wilde said it quite brilliantly. . . "Be yourself, everyone else is already taken."

Crystal Bonnet is an International Raw Food Chef and Instructor teaching others to create healthy dishes that not only taste great but look beautiful.

Crystal Bonnet

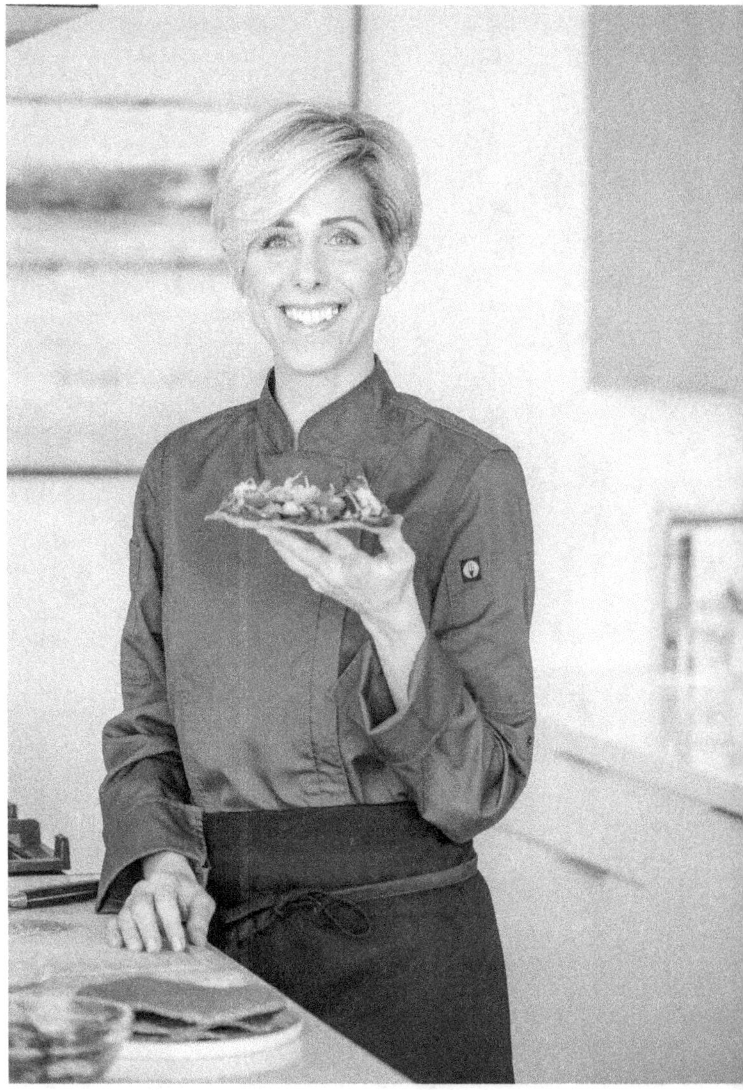

"With knowledge, anything is possible!" With these words, I empower those around me to strive, achieve, and realize their dreams. As a woman in an industry dominated by men, I will not stand in the way of anyone's success, and will continue to grow alongside those who share my passion.

Through the strength of character and single-minded pursuit of perfecting my craft, I am now an internationally recognized raw food chef, highly sought-after professional instructor, and the author of multiple cookbooks - but it was not always this way. Believe me when I say that it was a challenging, incredible, and beautiful journey that brought me to a place where I am now in the laudable position of teaching others through the digital **Crystal Dawn Culinary** custom courses. As a graduate of the highly respected plant-based and raw food nutrition programs at Matthew Kenney Culinary Academy and the Pure Joy Academy, I learned the importance of culinary aspects and nutritional elements of creating with living foods.

When I was younger and embarking on the journey to discover my true spirit, a career path in raw food nutrition was not in the cards. Ultimately, it was the deterioration of my physical self that forced my mind to make some hard decisions. Even today, when I look back, I am saddened that our society places a low priority on health and mental welfare, and pledge to myself to never fall back on old habits.

Pursuing this path of clarity brought many great adventures to my life. The abundance is real! Opportunities materialized. Soon, I found myself in demand to develop unique plant-based menus for exciting new restaurants, design and cater multiple international health retreats, and collect my recipes into well-received eBooks.

Although it took a strong push from those I love, my raw chocolate and dessert business's launch brought such satisfaction and sense of accomplishment; **I felt liberated knowing I would always be my own boss.**

If you only have one take-away from my story, I would love it to be a piece of advice for all who are doubting their potential—**believe in yourself**. You have more strength than you have been led to believe!

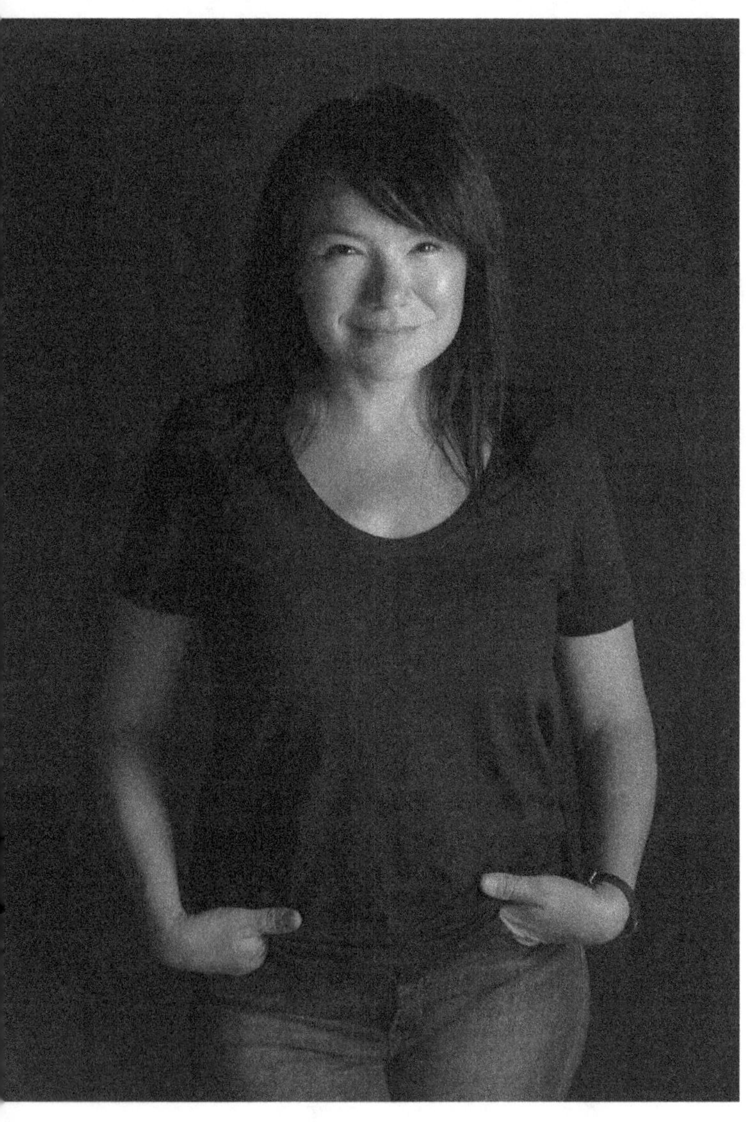

My name is Jennifer Podemski. I've never really felt comfortable identifying myself by what I do and more recently I've realized that what I do is actually inextricably connected to why I'm here. So, let me begin with that.

Jennifer Podemski

My name is Jennifer Podemski, and I am here to amplify and celebrate the voices of the underdog. As a mixed Anishinaabe woman, growing up in Toronto, I witnessed my mother, a beautiful, brown Anishinaabe woman from Muscowpetung First Nation, be ostracized because of her race. I harboured shame and resentment and struggled with my own sense of identity. As a mixed girl myself, I always felt alone, on the outside, never quite fitting in no matter where I went. I was still quite young when I began using my own sense of "otherness," identifying it in others as a way of connecting.

As I built my identity as an actor and performer and entered the professional realm, I quickly realized that there was an absence of Indigenous people. Even when we were there, those stories were being told through a white, colonial lens. It didn't take very long to realize that the same skills I acquired through my childhood would be required in my professional life.

By twenty, with enough professional experience under my belt, I began to mobilize. I travelled across Turtle Island (US/Canada) teaching workshops to Indigenous youth, encouraging them to get into the film and TV business. I began plotting my infiltration into an industry as a content creator who spoke up for the voiceless and the invisible, working exclusively in the Indigenous space. It's important to note that there were other Indigenous people who came before me who worked tirelessly in front of and behind the camera to lay the foundation and groundwork from which I was able to work. By twenty-five, I opened my first production company with my colleague, Laura Milliken, and together we created space to amplify the voices, perspectives, and experiences of Indigenous People while training and mentoring those who would later forge their own distinct paths.

For many years I identified myself as a writer, producer, actor, and director, but I'm also the manifestation of my ancestors' dreams, and I've been given the tools and the platform to speak up and speak out for the underdog by reclaiming space and harnessing my gift as a storyteller.

Janine Jones is a free-spirited creative, mother and creator of beauty and a Resident Artist at ROAM Gallery

Janine Jones

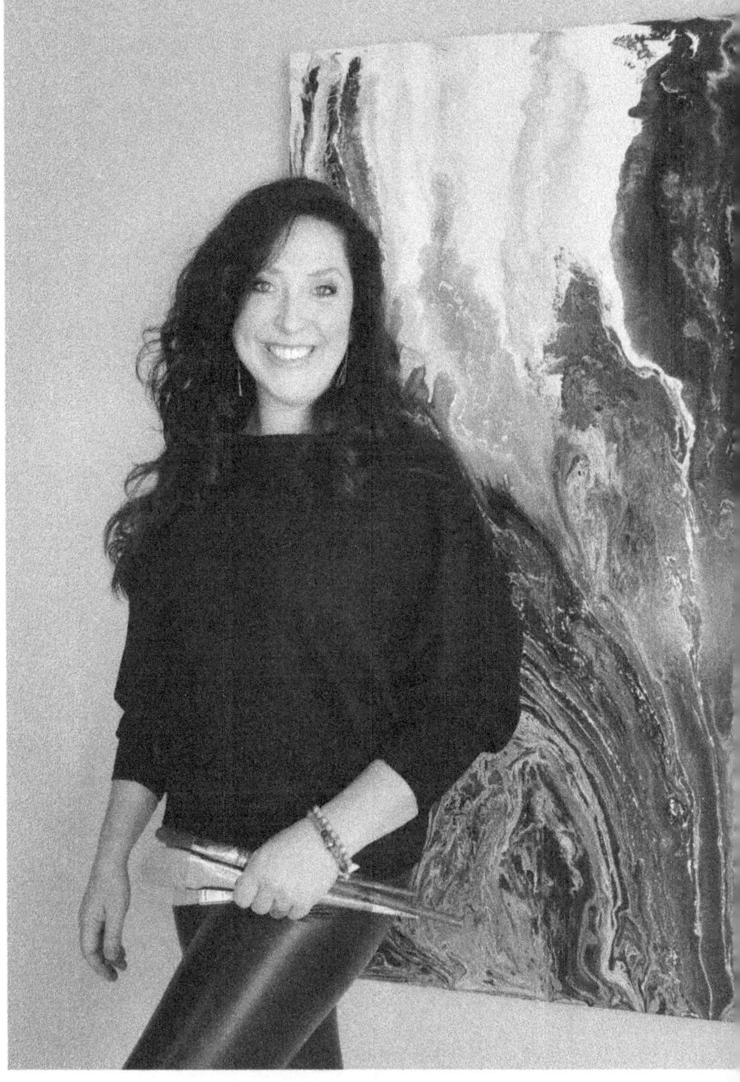

Dreams mean a lot to me. I have dreams for myself and my son. I have a rich sleeping dream life. I am also guided by vivid or sometimes unwanted dreams that fuel my artwork. I use these moments to envision what I paint, transcribing self-aware recaps of my life and the people around me to a canvas for all to see. A creative soul with a foundation of childhood memories sprinkled with elements of myself, love, and pains that blossom into life on a canvas.

Growing up in a diverse and complex family, rich in history with an unconventional upbringing, has led me to live a free-spirited life. I sometimes lose myself in relationships, yet I always survive — but I want more than just survival for my son. I choose to raise my son on my own, so I can provide a stable environment, rich with multiple chosen influences for him to grow. My pursuit of happiness is linked to my son's wholeness and wellbeing. Like me, he is free to share and be creative, to express his emotions through multiple mediums without shame, and to know that acceptance of his self-awareness is what drives me to be a better woman each day.

Nature, along with my dreams, provides the fire for my soul. Like my nomadic life, my inspiration sometimes wanders. The ocean on the west coast inspires the most in me, but Lake Huron holds my heart. I format thoughts from feelings and visions and bring them to fruition through art. My current works are inspired by the emotions and words of others, capturing moments in time from their lives, bringing forth new strength in visual imagery, which then takes the viewer on a journey through the minds and hearts of both creators. Through capturing these precious moments of love and time, I aim to inspire others to shatter their fears, live their dreams, be free of social norms and, dare to express what's deep inside. If I live by any words, it is live free and live your dreams!

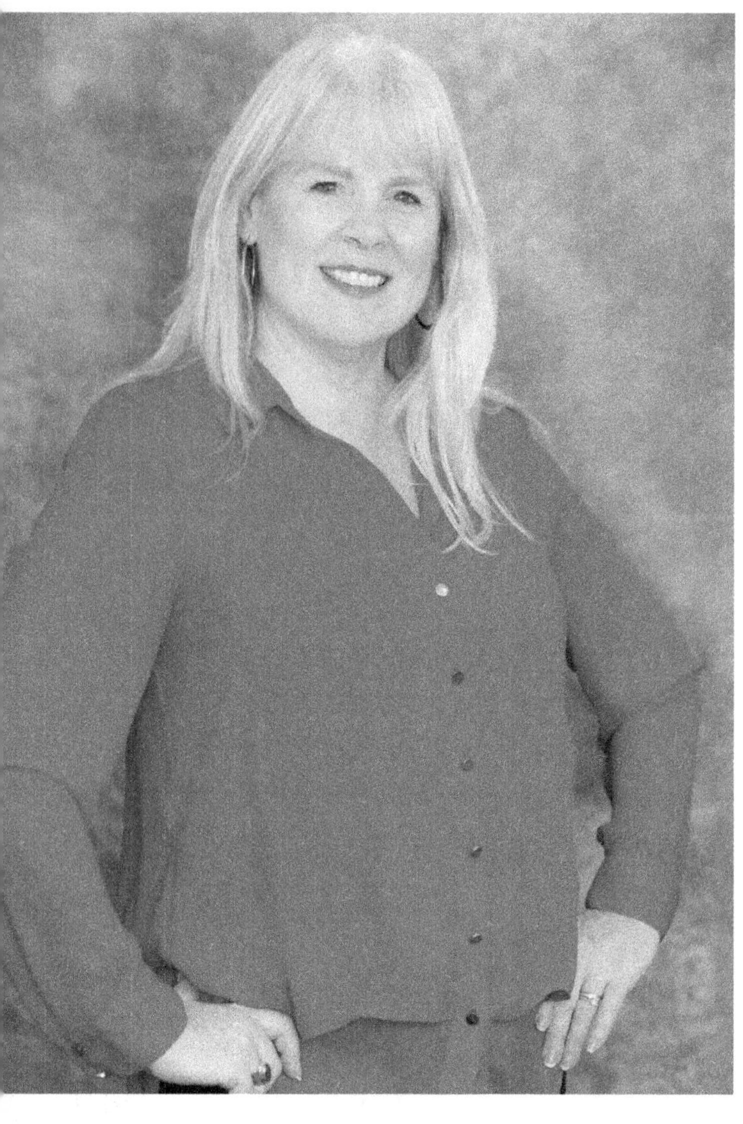

Patricia Lapeña is a business owner and leader who creates success through commitment and resilience.

Patricia Lapeña

I grew up in a very conventional family environment in Vancouver. What was instilled in me growing up was a far cry from a mindset of abundance, but a girl could daydream. At a young age, I knew that money was important. I was the kid with the lemonade stand and the table with the beach seashells to sell. I once took a bag of toys from my closet and went door to door to sell them. I was a born entrepreneur but never knew what that meant. I spent hours dreaming up business ideas, planning for the day I had fame and fortune. I could see it. At some point in my early adult life, my desire for a big life and success was jaded with indecision and procrastination to the point of stagnation. I was full of ideas but no results. I lacked the ability to follow through and see my ideas go to fruition.

In my pursuit of happiness and success, I realized I was heading for a lifestyle of complacency, when something finally clicked. The biggest turning point in my life happened in Africa at age forty-five. Climbing Mount Kilimanjaro was an immense challenge, both physically and emotionally that changed me forever. On the final push to reach the summit, where all I could do was take one small, exhausted step at a time, I had a revelation. It was life-transforming – for the first time in my life, I clearly understood what commitment and resilience were. I could do anything.

Soon after, I dove headfirst into my personal development journey with the goal to dismantle my limiting beliefs that held me hostage. It was time to call that little tenacious girl selling seashells on the sidewalk, back. I would be the person who could obtain success! In fact, I had to fast track my progress, to make up for lost time.

In difficult situations, I pull from my experience on Mt. Kilimanjaro. I have become a leader in my community and a business owner with the financial freedom that I had envisioned. Today, I continue to seek new opportunities as I did not come this far, to only come this far.

Dianne Watts is a corporate board executive and former politician who has found her role in supporting and empowering women.

Dianne Watts

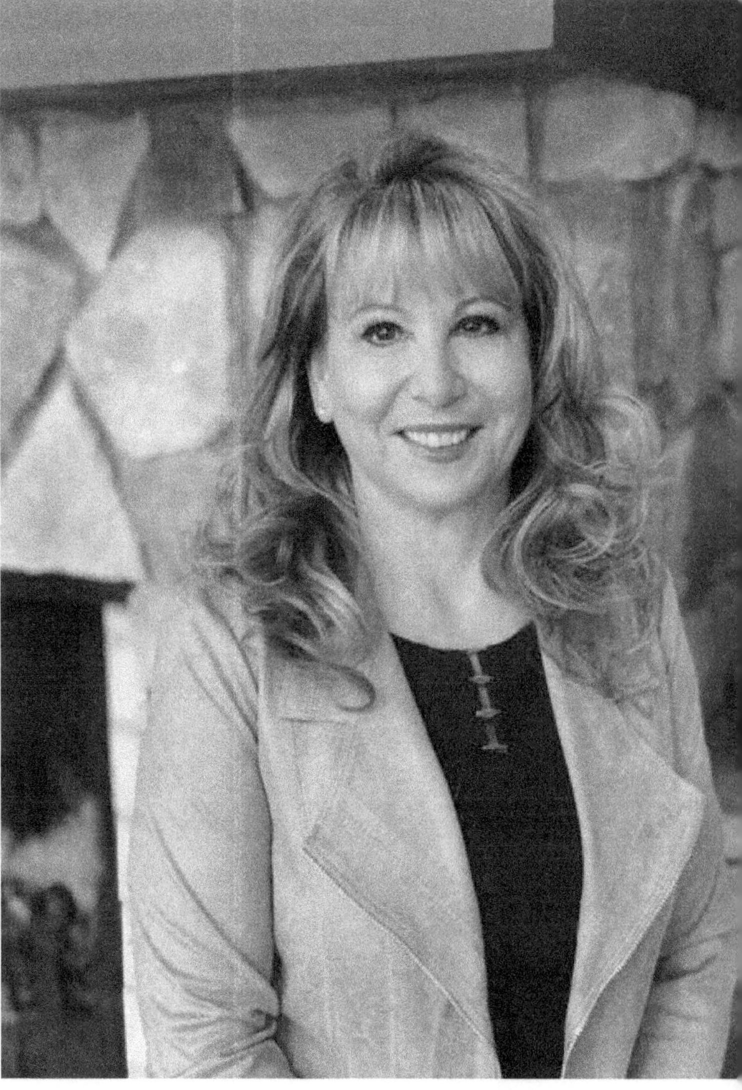

I have held many titles along the way, from a businesswoman, CEO, Board Director, City Councillor, Mayor, Member of Parliament, Political Contributor to name a few. However, these are just titles; they are what I do, not who I am, and certainly not what defines me. A strong sense of self, a strong sense of purpose, and being true to my core values are what defines me. I have been a Buddhist for over thirty years, and each day I strive to be my most authentic self. Say what you mean – and mean what you say!

There is no doubt in my mind that the most difficult times in my life have taught me the greatest life lessons and have been a catalyst for immense personal growth. I also know that you do not walk down the road in life on your own. Many people have been alongside me, some I did not care for, some who were very aggravating, and others whose kindness and love have kept me going.

No matter what role people play, there is always an opportunity to learn life lessons, and sometimes the people who make us the craziest are our greatest teachers! And, I certainly have had a few of those!!

It has been very important for me to understand and reflect on what I create and manifest in my life because I am creating my life story. However, we all have things that happen in life that we do not have control over. This is why we cannot lose sight of the fact that everyone has a life story; some more difficult than others, and this is where compassion and empathy come into play.

I believe so strongly that we need to support each other, empower each other, and work collectively to ensure the next generation of young women feel loved and supported. Especially the young girls and young women who are at risk and who are struggling. As women, I believe we have a very important role to play using the lessons and the tools we have developed to affect change within ourselves and the world.

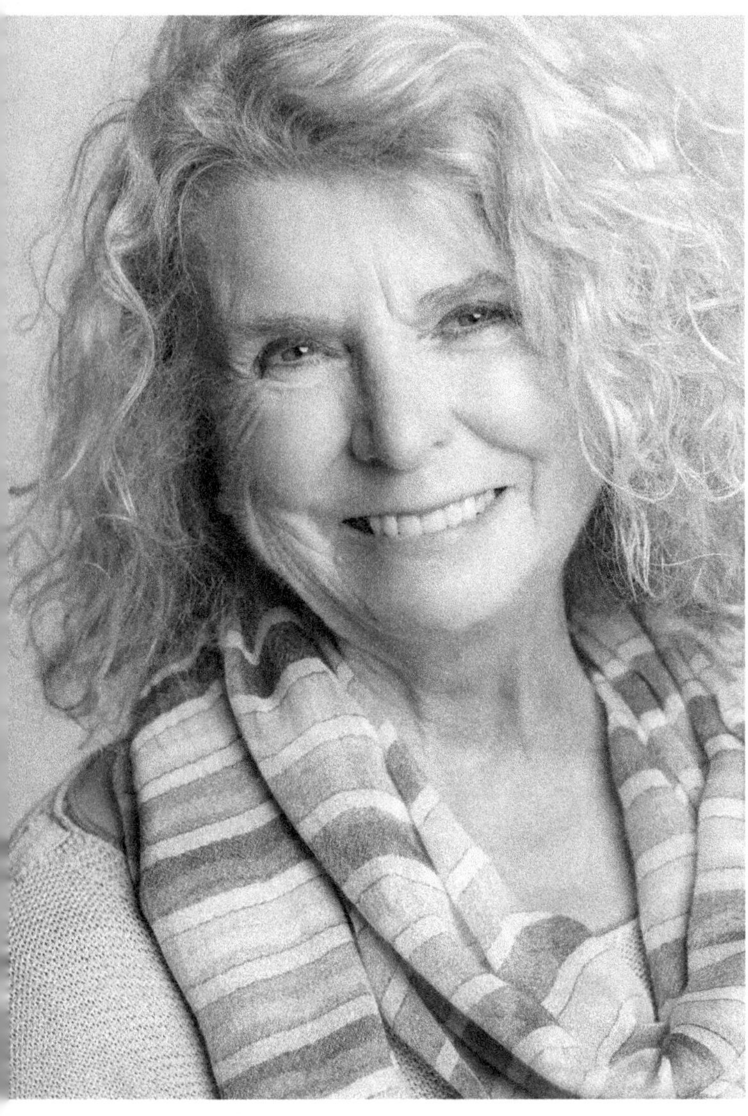

Mary Daniel is living her life as an educator, artist and traveller.

Mary Daniel

I say "yes" when opportunities interest me. Learning to say "no" was more difficult, and it took time to be skillful at this!

I was beginning my eighth year as Principal of a diverse large high school- my favourite position of many I had had. I was fulfilled here, part of the vibrant hustle and bustle of the school. At the end of each day, "I felt truly alive!". Was now the time to forge a new path?
I believed it was time to shift, but to where? To what?
I had an artist's studio that was sadly being used as a recycling area, and as I headed off to work each day,
I would see this beautiful space I thought of as my sanctuary and ask, when?

"Beginning is the most important part of the work" - Plato

Where to start? I said to myself, "take some time - there is no rush." I wanted to re-imagine myself as a full-time working artist. I would become a learner again and knew this would take focus, dedication, and just plain hard work. I was renewed by challenges, but it was not easy for me to begin. Plato's advice can also intimidate – what if I failed?

I just had to begin.

I knew, as in many ventures, suspending judgement while exploring the beginning of work was critical. I needed to develop my practice of opening my mind. I said "yes" to the opportunities to apply for international residencies to work alongside artists from around the world, explore cultures and their inspirations, failing and learning, discovering and renewing myself and my practice. At times, I have found this to be close to a state of grace and in a meditative flow and, at times just pure frustrating. I give myself time, let my art rest, contemplate, and know things will shift – I just give it space.

After ten years, I am finding my voice as an artist and know there will be more missteps as well as many joyful occasions in my studio sanctuary.

I like it here.

There are three words that best describe Lisa. She is an uninhibited OPTIMIST, unfettered FUTURIST, and unapologetic PLEASURE SEEKER.

Lisa Chan

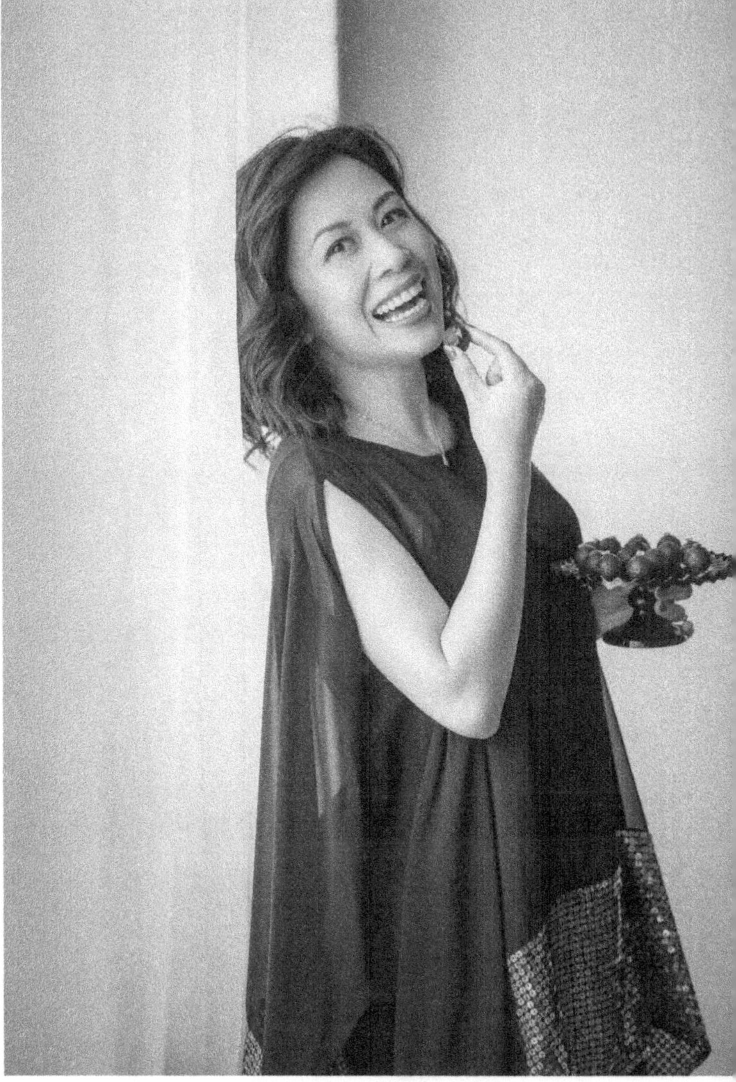

My life has gone from conventional to adventurous in a few short years. I met my husband when I was sixteen, and now I'm on my fourth marriage to the same man. Many of us have at least three to four significant relationships in our lifetime. Some of us, including myself, recreate those relationships with the same person.

I didn't know how much I had been missing out on living life until I was forty years old. Some would call it a mid-life crisis, but to me, it was more like mid-life boredom. The thought of being with the same man, having the same till death do us part sex made me question, "Is that all there is to life?" I realized to transform my life. I needed to take responsibility and own my sexual pleasure. So, I decided to experiment with Cannabis as an aphrodisiac. After many trials, I concocted my own pleasure-inducing, THC chocolates called TrufElle. These incredible truffles took me out of my head and into my body-transforming mediocre maintenance sex to mind-blowing vacation sex at home!

TrufElle has helped me let go of some of my ego, and this helped build intimacy in all my relationships. I had a relentless commitment to radical transparency and authenticity, which allowed me to be seen at my core. As soon as I was able to be vulnerable with others, it brought down the walls and enabled others to be authentic with me.

Thanks to my discovery of Cannabis, I'm now living my most authentic life. I have the most passionate, intimate relationship with my husband where I can feel safe to say what I mean and mean what I say without fear of rejection. In addition, we have magical moments with friends and the closest bond with our family. My vision is to create a movement to help women ignite their sensuality. The key to attaining erotic freedom is by owning your sexual pleasure. I believe that all women have the right to discover mind-blowing orgasms!

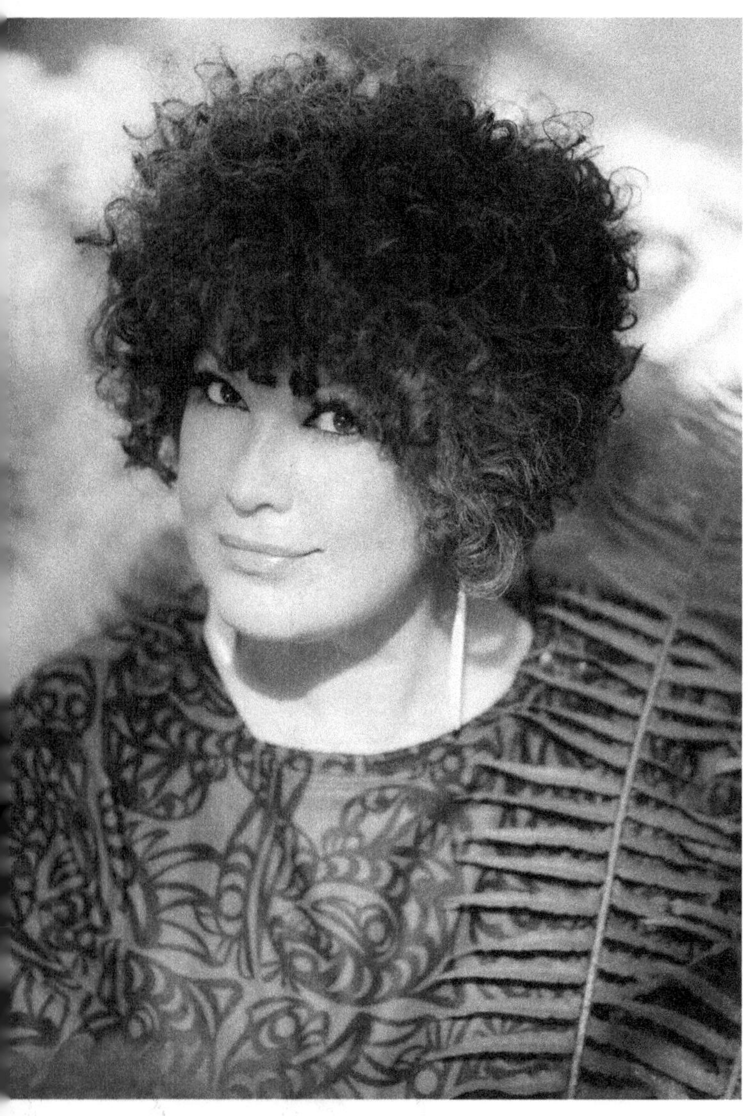

Heather Nightingale is an internationally acclaimed makeup artist of over twenty years. She creatively finds love and happiness everywhere!

Heather Nightingale

Gifts given to me include the desire to seek the truth, the ability to embrace change, and the courage to follow my heart.

Change is the one thing that existence guarantees; life is change, and change is life. As children of the Caribbean, my three brothers and I lived an idyllic life, with a stay-at-home mom and a father who worked as a Chartered Accountant. Days were spent climbing fruit trees, riding bikes, and visiting loved ones. Appearances were deceiving, and at nine years old, my life changed forever. My mother, me in tow, departed for the airport. I watched, heartbroken, as my brothers receded into the distance. We boarded a plane with a one-way ticket to Montreal. Coming to Canada changed my life in unimaginable ways and I am forever grateful that my mother had the courage to board that aircraft. Each experience, both traumatic and beneficial, allowed me the opportunity to reflect and grow. I have discovered that the greatest moments in time have occurred because someone, somewhere, changed something.

Joy, change, and trauma have always been processed through the lens of my artwork. I use drawing and painting to work through emotions and reflect on lessons learned. It is how I express my innermost thoughts. Leading with my heart, I search for the truth! I am relentless in my pursuit of resilience, strength, happiness, and love. On my journey, I have been blessed with a loving husband, mentors, and all-around amazing human beings, who have shared their stories with me, and guided me to the path of self-discovery and truth. From them, I have learned to love myself and build trust. I now maintain solid relationships with my most wonderful and extended family. Art, my greatest gift, has given me the freedom to express myself and transform my life with love, happiness, and joy! Now, I give back by empowering others to find their light. My restorative journey acts as a blueprint to help others heal. While following my heart, I acknowledge, accept, and even embrace change which is a practice for life!

Tina-Marie Springham plants seeds and shifts perspectives. She'll tell you "Yes You Can," offer a perspective you had not yet considered, then with a nudge, encourage you to step boldly into your truth, live it truthfully and say, "now...watch what happens."

Tina-Marie Springham

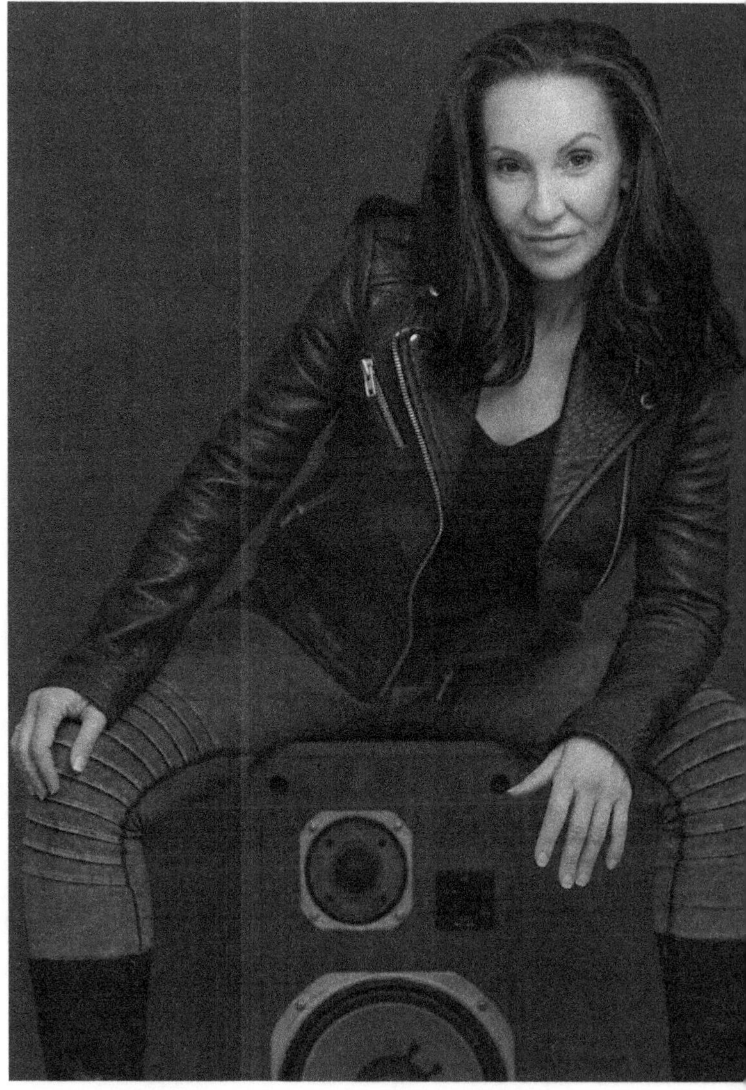

I believe your words are mighty, your perspective, your superpower. That is what I live. That is what I teach. #seebeyondwhatyousee.

I don't motivate, nor do I wish to be motivated. Motivating is making someone do something that they don't want to do. Rather, I want to inspire and be inspired. That happens by doing what you love. When you do, you tap into your gifts, this ignites your mind, heart, soul, and spirit. That radiates your light out for the world to see, causing a ripple effect of inspiration for others to be inspired.

The greatest lesson I've learned from failure is that there is no failure. There are attempts at things in life. Some work, some don't. With either, comes knowledge. Your perspective, along with "choice," and this newfound knowledge, are what equip you for what's next. Things not working out are a gift for another attempt, pivot, or change in direction. How can any of that be called failure?

I've had to pivot, shift, transform from then to new, old to now, many times. Each time serves to teach, grow, and reward me, to lay the next steps in my journey, painfully or passionately, but all with purpose.

What makes me feel most powerful in life is my relationship with God. From that comes my faith and inner peace, which I'd wrestled with in life. But I've been able to get out of my own way, and with His help, really put my money and calling where my mouth is, figuratively and literally. In 2019, I boldly shut my business down and simultaneously committed 110% to my dreams, and as Peter Dinklage said, "I will, from now on, for **better** or **worse**, be a **working actor.**" This pivotal decision set me up for 2020. My faith has helped me withstand the storms. It's all led to here. I am now a working voice artist, actor, and teacher of kids, about to embark on even bolder steps in writing and directing in 2021.

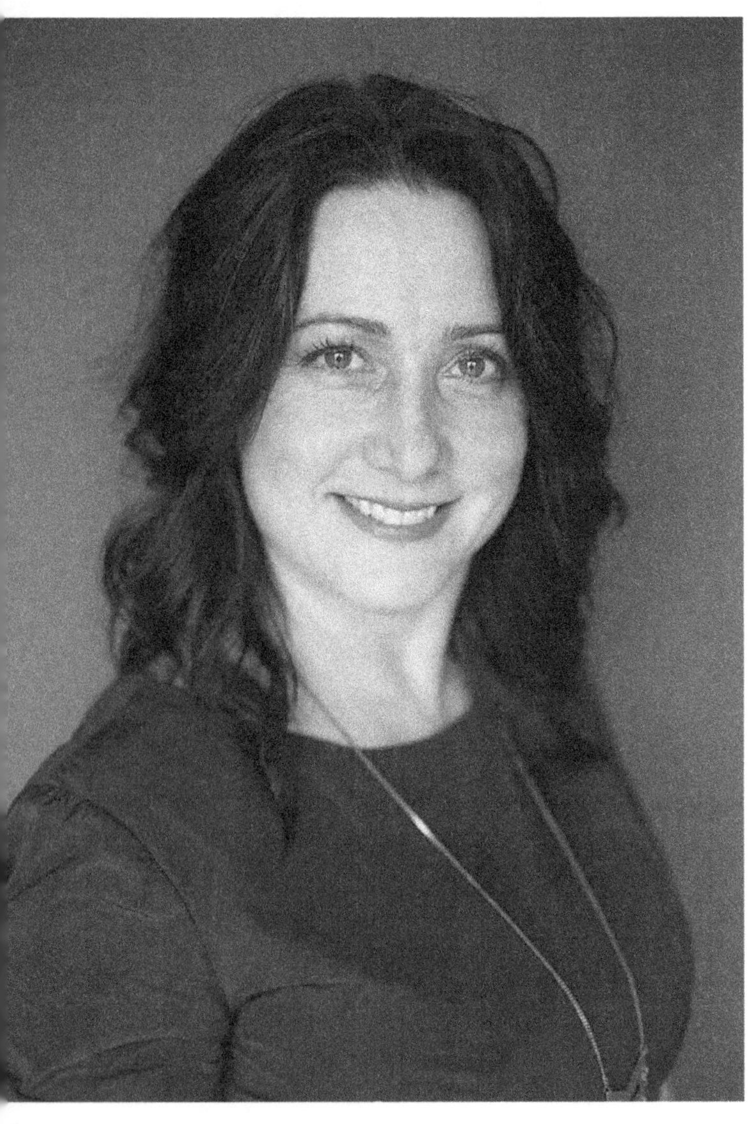

Lisa Holly is a driven serial entrepreneur, focused on natural health, human rights and passionate about helping Canadian families achieve their dreams via mortgage lending.

Lisa Holly

My mother told me when I was very young that I could do anything I could dream of in life; what she forgot to tell me was I couldn't do EVERYTHING!

For that reason, I've led a fantastic and full life. I was first a classically trained ballet dancer, then a teacher, and finally a performer. In my late teens, dabbled in old-school landscape architecture before auto CAD was a thing, having worked on the SkyDome! I started at an early age in lending, which has led me from Toronto, across the country to BC, and back to London ON, where I run a successful mortgage business with Dominion Lending Centres Forest City Funding, the top mortgage origination franchise in the Country!

I am a very proud mother of identical twin eighteen-year-old daughters, Marlo and Lauren, who both recently began studies in Kinesiology at Western University.

Whole food and fitness have been a passion of mine for twenty years. Given the opportunity, I may pursue functional medicine in my later years for the sheer joy and understanding of how the human body works.

I once read a quote by Sir Richard Branson, "If somebody offers you an amazing opportunity but you are not sure you can do it, say yes – then learn how to do it later!" Inspired by this, three years ago, my girlfriend approached me to open a yoga studio with her, and in an attempt to balance out my stressful work life, I jumped at the chance! I'm now also a proud owner of Evolation Yoga London. I've learned so much more than about yoga, to be an employer, a mentor, a health coach, and I found my tribe in the process. My greatest achievement is when I ask how other people know each other, oftentimes, it was through the studio!

My favourite sayings are; just breathe, have faith, everything is as it should be.
My mother also said if you're feeling down, put some lipstick on.

I dig deep, live passionately, and hopefully along the way, inspire other humans to live from a place of love, with grace, humility, and the same fire that drives me to be the best I can be.

Daria is a designer living in beautiful Victoria, BC, who loves helping clients create a home they truly love, and that brings them joy and comfort.

Daria Bunting

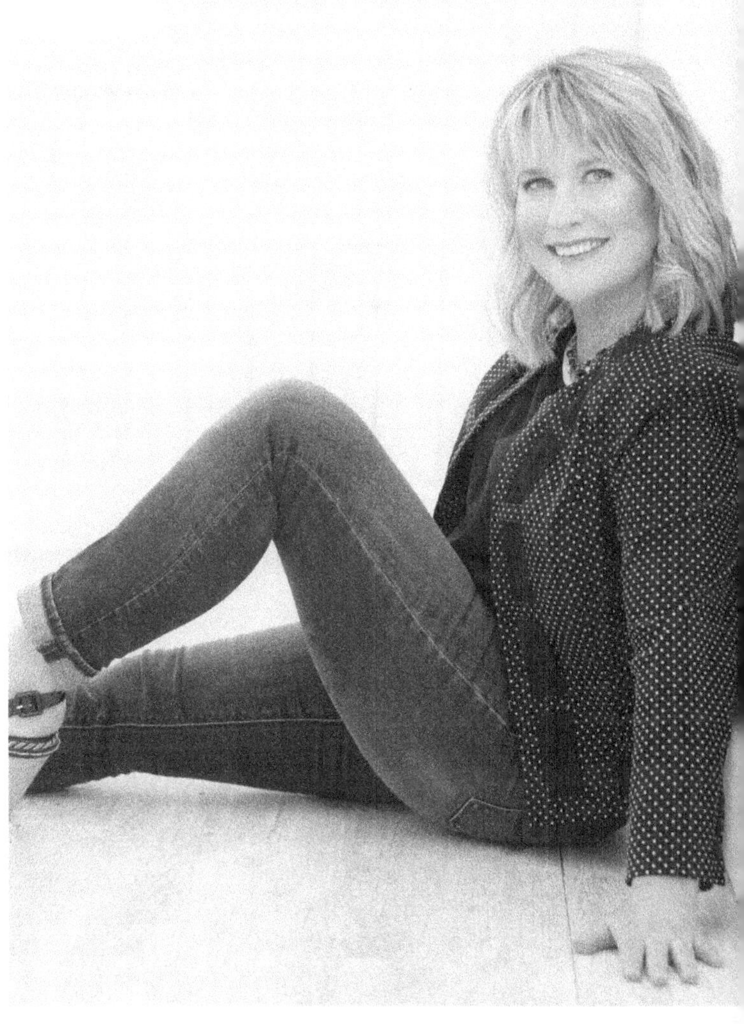

My journey thus far has taught me some lessons that I want to share and hopefully enlighten you to live a fulfilled life, full of passion, doing what comes naturally to you. I struggled for years, wondering what I would be when I grew up. At thirty, I was still figuring it out, and at thirty-four, I went back to school studying Interior Design. In my first class, I realized; this is my place. All my life, I loved being creative and making things look beautiful. It dawned on me that it felt good to do what I loved and was naturally good at instead of the thing I should do to pay bills. As one of my favorite poems says, The Road Not Taken by Robert Frost, "I took the road less traveled by, and it has made all the difference." So, I decided to take a leap of faith and left a good city position to try and find my way by following my heart. I wanted a career where I could use my talents, and that brought others joy. I loved helping to create beautiful homes that people loved to be in.

We all have different talents, interests, and desires which make us all unique. I say follow your heart; it will always lead the way to your ultimate happiness and success. Remember, every moment can be a new beginning. So, if you try something new and it turns out not as planned, try again, do not give up. My path has taken work, and there have been ups and downs. It is all about the journey; if you are doing what you love, then it is worth the ride.

This day is my birthday. I always make time on my special day to celebrate me. I share this to remind you to celebrate you on your special day and every day! We are all here to make a difference, let's show our gifts to the world to make this a better, more beautiful place.

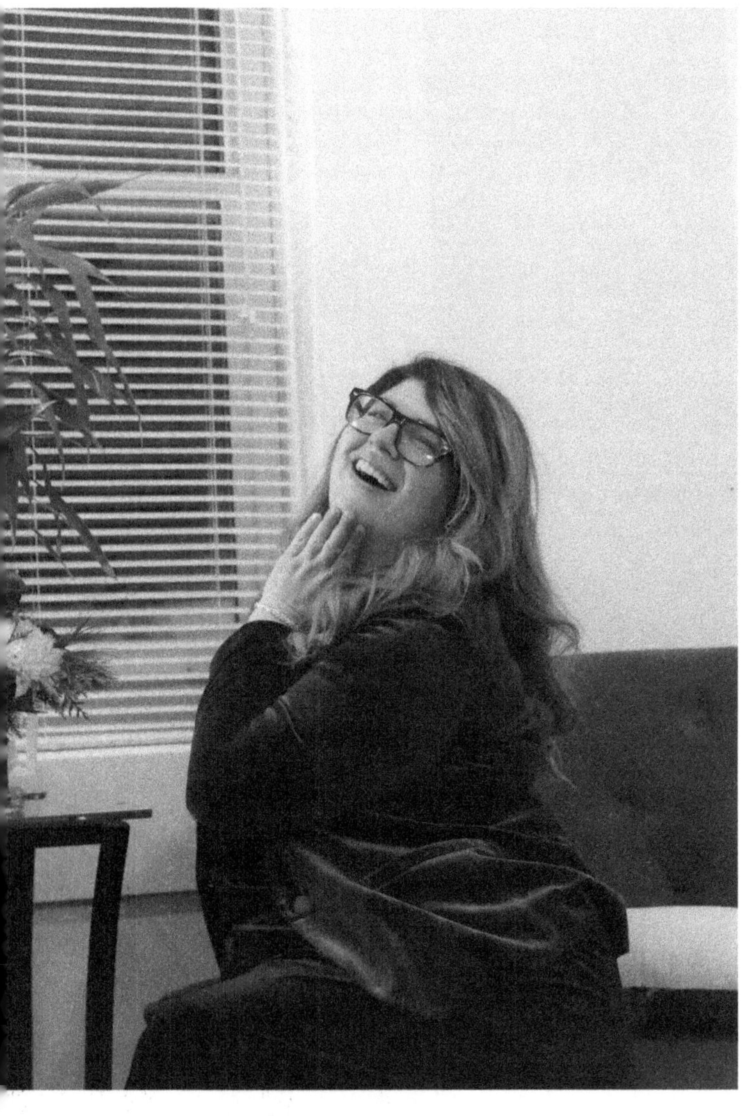

Debra Schubert has walked through the storm with patience to move forward in healing

Debra Schubert

"Sabr el Muftah, el jenna" is my favorite Arabic adage. It means, "patience is the key to paradise." My name is Debra, and unless we've spoken about it, you would likely never know that I am Muslim. In 2002 I started a twenty-year journey toward paradise - peace within myself.

This journey stems from having experienced my fair share of oppression, many acts of which I inflicted on myself. I am not here to compete in the oppression Olympics, except to say that for a very long time, I believed that I was not worthy of tasting the sweetness of life. When I converted, I felt that I could never be completely celebrated as a Muslim, and I was torn about my relationship with the hijab (scarf). Verbal and non-verbal body language let me know that I was seen by the wider society as deviant and a traitor. Even now that I removed hijab, I am somewhat perfidious, because I'm not easily categorized. I am acculturated as an Arab Muslim but socialized in Canadian society, and my family encompasses all Abrahamic faiths. I have been told that I am a renegade appropriating a culture that is not mine; and to my fellow Muslims, I am a Jewish Zionist and can never truly be trusted.

I have worked diligently correcting the tropes that I had come to believe about myself as a Muslim convert, and in May of 2015, I packed up my socially constructed box and threw it out the window. It has taken me decades, but in 2020 I officially stepped into my power. In doing so, the biggest lesson I learned was that in order to heal, you have to walk through the storm with patience. This doesn't mean passively await change because patience is a verb. It's a muscle that I had to train to taste the sweetness in life that I had been looking for. And it's okay to slip or regress - in fact, it's a necessary part of the journey. Just make sure you don't stay there. Take stock of where you were, acknowledge your achievements and give yourself the grace to move forward, peacefully and with beautiful patience.

Stacey Wells is blurring the lines between fantasy and reality. WELLS.

Stacey WELLS

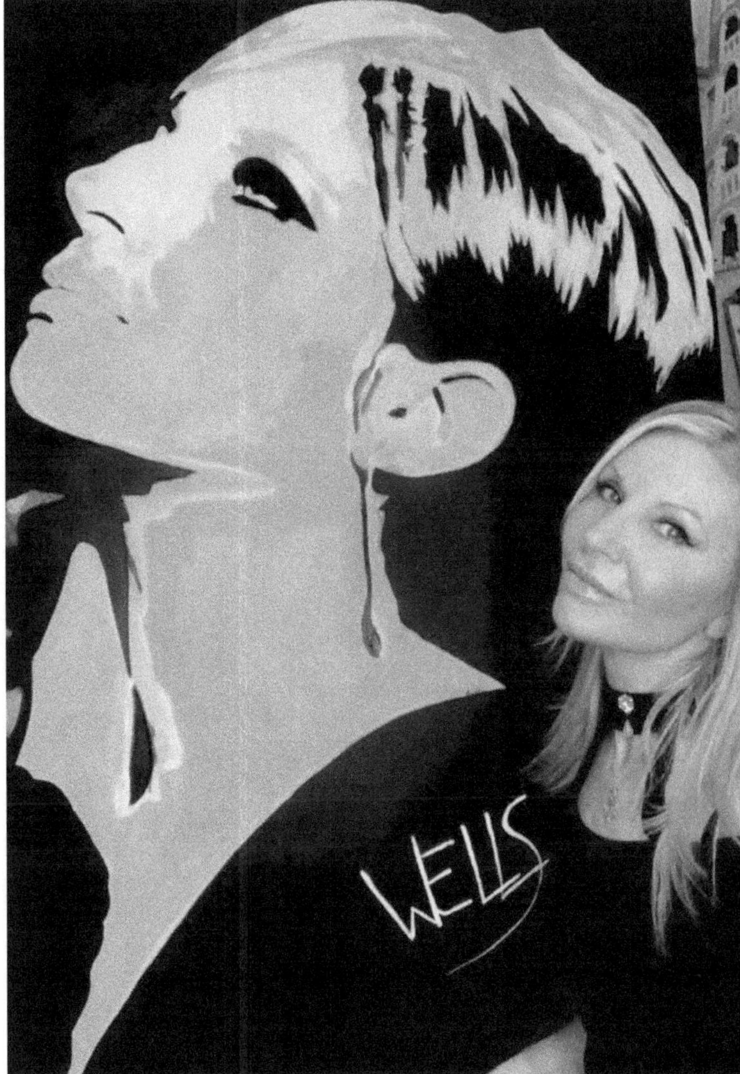

My dad was killed in a plane crash when someone put a bomb on the commercial airplane, he was piloting. As a child, I knew that life can be short. I wanted to live each day to the fullest, having as much fun as possible. My mom gave me the gift of rose-colored glasses and the freedom to be myself. I ran with it.

I love being me. I'm not referring to my physical being, but my mind. I can get lost in my imagination, I feel happy alone in my thoughts, like a secret garden that is filled with adventure, incredible beauty, vibrant colors, great music, and the feeling of happiness.
I feel like the luckiest person in the universe.

I am a mixologist of music, wine, humor, and pop culture, blending them to create art that starts conversation, and brings people back to a moment in time that makes them smile. My art is a mind trip for the viewer, a moment that they can escape to enjoy a memory, a special moment that makes them smile.

People say I have an innate talent for capturing the essence of my subjects. I believe that I am connected with people; I see and feel things that others don't. It's a gift that gives me an insight into people's souls, which helps me tell their story with my art. My art can be found at galleries across the US and on art collectors' walls worldwide, including a few celebrities. I've worked hard, I've created my every opportunity, and now opportunity finds me. It was such a thrill to get a call from the Hard Rock Hotel International saying, "We love your art," and they commissioned me to create artworks for their hotel!

I followed my dreams fiercely and never gave up. When I was diagnosed with a rare and aggressive cancer, I never told a soul. Instead, I spent all my time in my studio, and during chemo, I created art to help others which raised over $50,000 to help kids. I am a survivor as an artist, an entrepreneur, and in life. I am a survivor.

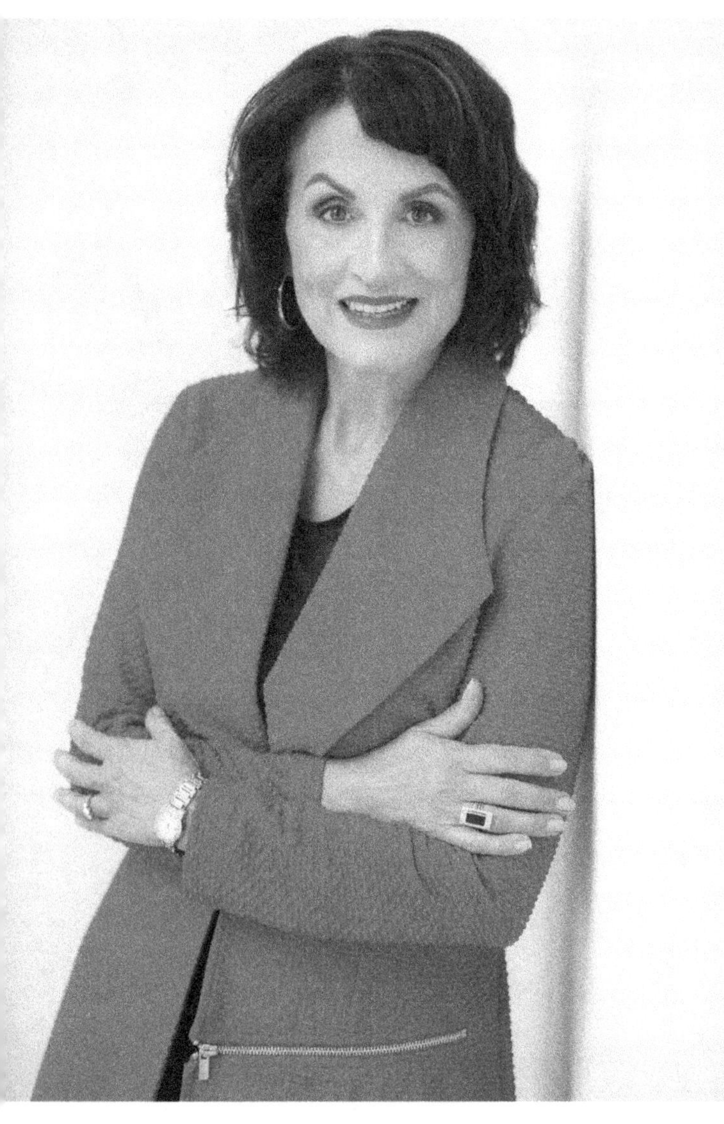

DeeAnn Lensen is a five-time best-selling author, award-winning advanced esthetic educator, master coach, and spa consultant.

DeeAnn Lensen

My life changed when I realized that I was essentially living in my own little castle surrounded by a moat. The next level of success and fulfillment glowed just beyond the other side, and I kept working on building a bridge to get there. But I repeatedly gave up and allowed the bridge to rot after convincing myself that I was "too busy" for it and that I was okay where I was. Subconsciously, I was holding myself back so I wouldn't have to face my insecurities or risk failing.

I am an international spa consultant and skin care expert, as well as a certified coach and NLP practitioner. I added coaching to my business because I realized that people go to the spa to feel better, and that spa staff needed to have an understanding of their own self-esteem if they were really going to be effective in providing that. Once I received my certifications, I understood that I also got into coaching because I needed it! It was only through coaching that I fully realized how my upbringing had created a set point for success and happiness. When I rose above it, I was accosted with unconscious excuses not to continue—there is safety inside the moat!

Almost every woman I know or have worked with has struggled with the same thing. They find themselves stagnating in their career or their goals, unable to find the motivation to move forward, or constantly running up against self-imposed roadblocks. They don't realize that their ego is trying to protect them from failure because this reasoning feels powerfully authentic.

Want to explore your potential? Start with noticing the way you talk to yourself and work on replacing self-criticism with self-compassion especially when you apply your skin care! The messages you download are a deal maker/breaker, so upgrade your internal perception of yourself and watch your life improve!

Changing these messages on your own can be challenging, so if you find yourself faltering, consider reaching out for support. Something I offer that can be very beneficial is group coaching. In these groups, we support members to shine a light on their current reality & build their own bridge to the other side of the moat.

Diane Webster is the Owner of Cuervo Boutique, supplier of confident, curated clothing.

Diane Webster

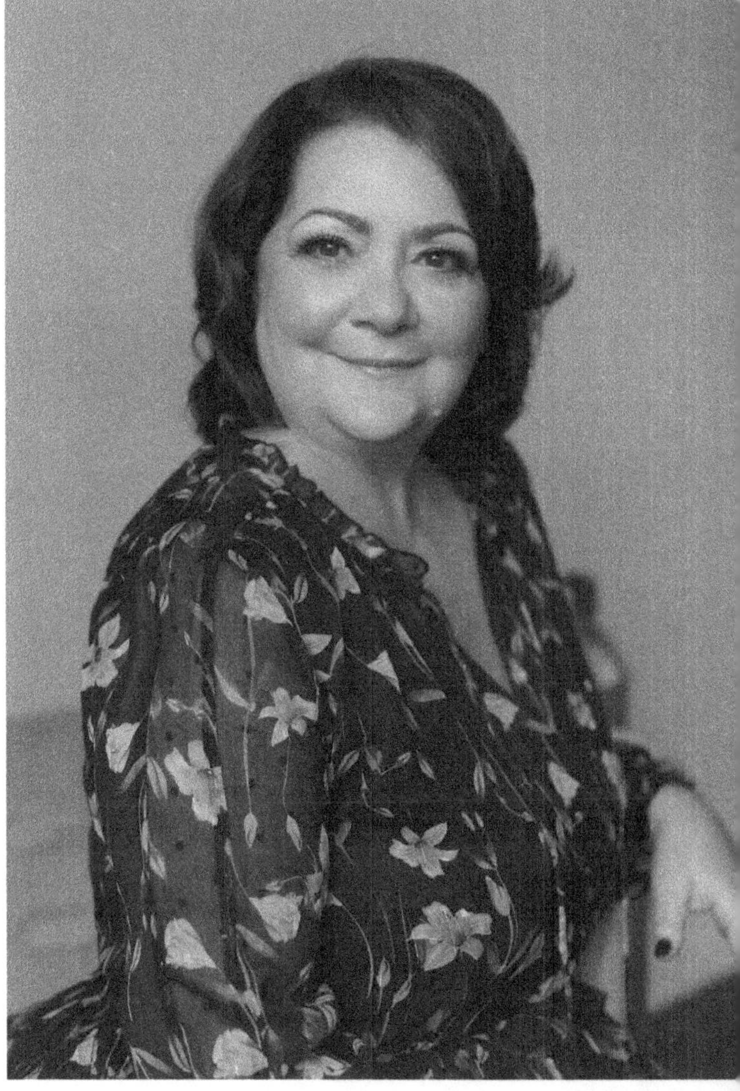

When did I start to feel invisible?
Every day I was feeling myself becoming more and more invisible, I felt myself shrink inside, and it was soul-destroying.

Shopping in department stores and boutiques, I was ignored by staff or worse, told that there is nothing there for me, while the sales associates approached the younger clientele. Finding clothes was another story; fashion and my age did not seem to match.
To make matters worse, I was without my career, one I had worked in for close to thirty years. A career based on beauty and anti-aging skincare. I was forced back into the traditional workplace and unable to find a job, despite a lifetime of experience, which did not seem to matter as much as my age did. I was no longer seen as relevant or of any value. Aging is not easy on anyone.

Having your existence devalued is one of the most painful things that you can experience. However, it also fueled a fire within me and put me in the driver's seat. I asked myself, am I looking for a job in the same industry because it is the only thing that I think I can do? I made it here to my sixties ... it was not an easy road, but I had continued to demonstrate my resourcefulness and resilience throughout my life, so why would I stop now?

Luckily, a door opened that I choose to walk through. I was presented the opportunity to study Small Business and Entrepreneurship. What business model could I create that would differentiate my business from others that are similar? My experiences over the years had shown me that the inconsistency of fashion and age made it difficult for women to find suitable clothing that matched how they wanted to feel.

I decided to open a clothing boutique in a neighborhood setting where I could reach women, provide an atmosphere of inclusiveness, create connection, and make my store a comfortable environment where age was not the issue. A place where when they leave, they will feel inspired and confident. You are only invisible to people who do not deserve to see you.

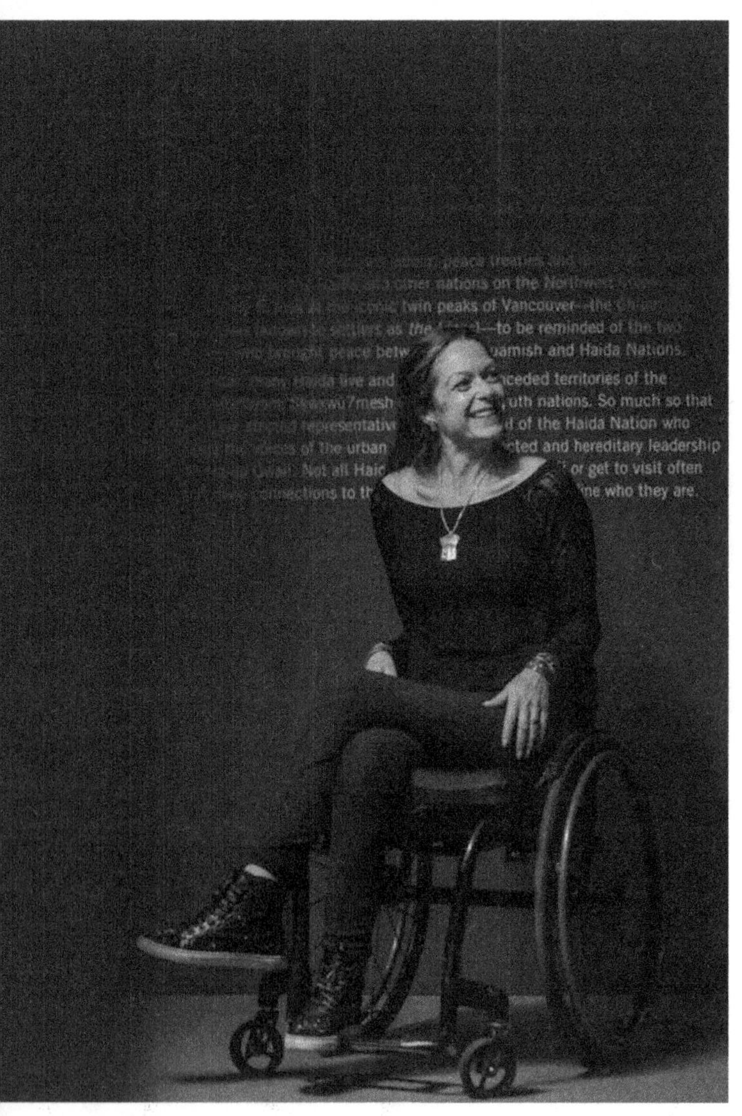

In Chloe Angus's pursuit of happiness and success, her greatest lessons have been defined by "doing it right because it's the right thing to do."

Chloe Angus

My fashion label, Chloë Angus Design, is a Vancouver-based, independently owned, collaborative Canadian brand that has dressed movie stars, media personalities, politicians, and princesses. My designs have graced runways and red carpets around the world, and in 2018, (after recovering from a spinal cord injury that left me paralyzed from the waist down, that is a story for another day) I had the honour of being awarded The Industry Innovation Award recognizing my contribution to growing the fashion industry. My career is everything a successful fashion designer could dream of. But there's always more work to do in the sometimes-dirty world of fashion. And doing it right, just because it's the right thing to do, remains a turbulent, but worthy journey. In fashion, body image, ageism, even racism impacts the industry. For some, fashion and style equate to being young, thin, tall and white. In doing it right, my brand leads with diversity and inclusion. I show models of all ages, shapes, sizes, identities, ethnicities and mobilities. I say it takes little talent to design for young, tall, beautiful people; true talent lies in designing for all shape and sizes, for everybody who wants to feel strong, powerful, and included in fashion.

I also care about our Earth and do it right by choosing natural and innovative fabrics that are better for the environment. Growing up on the pristine BC coast, on an organic seafood farm, consideration for our environment is second nature to me. I support sustainable change in all areas of my business, from packaging to promotion. We stand proudly Made in Canada, in step with Canadian labour standards and their associated costs.

But my most profound honour is doing it right in my collaborations with Indigenous artists. I have committed my career to changing cultural appropriation in fashion; my collaborations strive to set industry standards for working with Indigenous artists around the world. Through honest, fair, transparent collaboration (licensing, compensation, representation), we ensure that collaboration equals inclusion and celebration; that it eliminates appropriation and elevates reconciliation. When done right, fashion can uplift and empower the wearer, giving them the confidence to go out and to do what they're born to do. I was born to do fashion, born to help uplift and empower others through my confidence in doing fashion the right way; not the easy way, but the only way that makes me happy and successful.

Tonia LaRiviere turned her difference into positive change as she advises on issues of accessibility.

Tonia LaRiviere

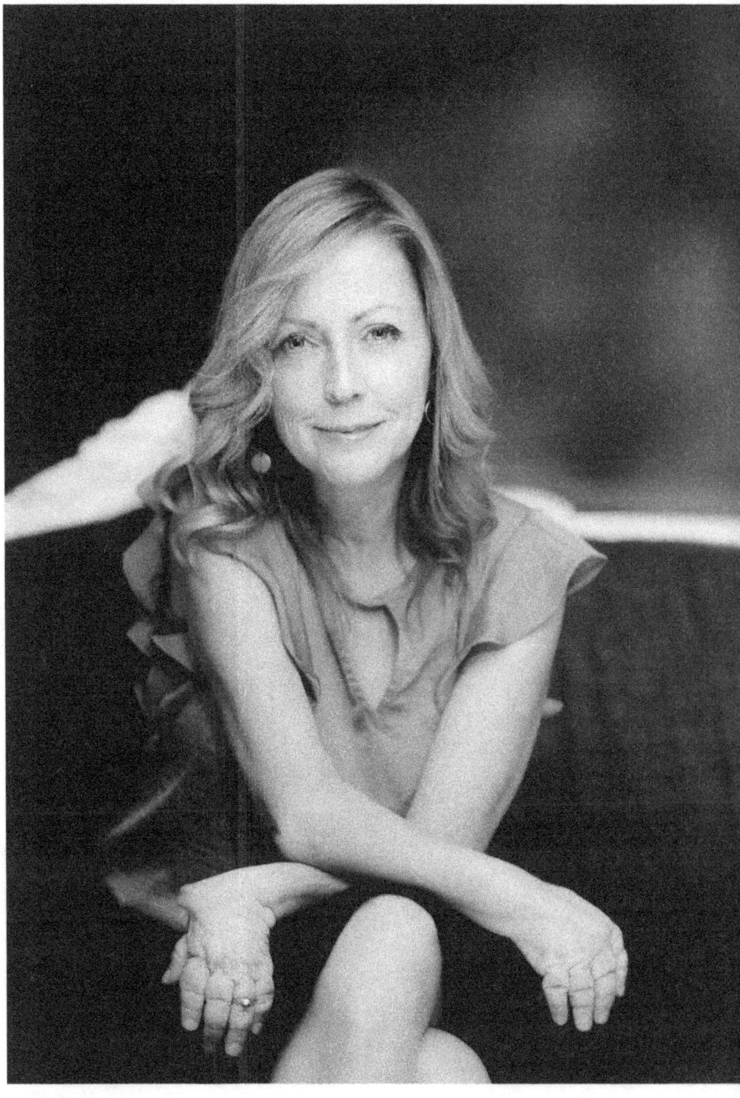

I was diagnosed with Juvenile Rheumatoid Arthritis when I was twelve years old - my life was turned upside down. It affected every joint in my body, including my jaw and neck. I was a normal, active kid, living a normal life, and within a couple of weeks, I was bedridden from pain, unable to move a finger by myself - my life would never be the same. At the time, I was angry, resentful, defiant, and stubborn. I didn't want to be treated differently. Three weeks prior, I wasn't different, I was able to go to school, be physically active, and play with my friends. Three weeks prior, I was able to get out of bed, get in a bathtub, and dress myself.

When I was eighteen, I was diagnosed with clinical depression; my biggest challenge yet. I was physically, emotionally, and now mentally depleted, but I managed to fight every excruciating minute of my days. I survived.

In those earlier years of my diagnosis, I experienced bullying, social exclusion, and lack of understanding with few supports, with the exception of medical supports. To date, I have had twenty surgeries, all a result of arthritis, and there will be more in my future.

I got involved with the Steadward Bears para-swim team. It was the scariest thing I have ever done. All of my intentions and achievements were in defiance of my disability, which served me well. I had worked in film, television, event planning, communications, and makeup artistry. This was different; I was changing my narrative. This experience was profound in my personal growth and self-awareness.

I now embrace my difference in a way I never have, I value my perspective, I am in a position to use it for positive change. I was a board member for the Arthritis Society and continue to share my story in an effort to educate others on the realities of arthritis. Currently, I am in my most meaningful role to date as the Chair of the Accessibility Advisory Committee with the City of Edmonton, advising City Council on issues of accessibility, and contributing to policy advancements and education... just don't ask me to put on my socks.

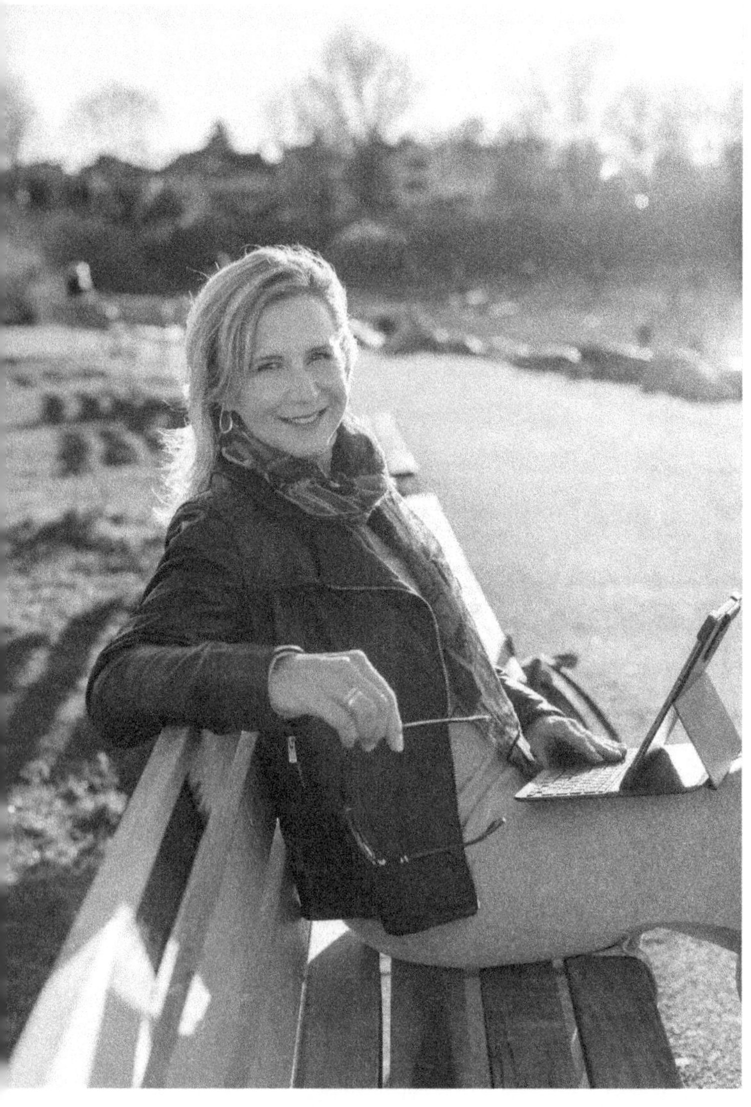

Deciding her life story was not going to read like a victim impact statement, Susie uses joy as her GPS.

Susie Doré

Like a predator, he would come hunting for me, tiptoeing as only a drunken, foul-smelling monster can. I'd curl up in closets and hold my breath, flatten myself under beds, bury under piles of coats at adults' parties—anything to hide—but he would find me. From five to eight years old, I endured sexual abuse by a family friend. Living in silent terror and believing his threats to stay quiet, I was a shattered little soul with a shameful secret.

At fourteen, I was blindsided, learning my abuser played in my mother's curling league, but felt strong enough to finally tell her. Queue the movie called "Let's Pretend It Never Happened," where my alcoholic parents chose to do absolutely nothing. In the betrayal of the family cover-up, my voice was silenced again, and my already damaged soul, destroyed.

How do you come back from that? As survivors of sexual abuse and inevitable PTSD can attest, you have to push through the pain until it hurts less. I buried my aching emotions and got busy building a healthy life and career, until my mid-thirties, when repressed memories surfaced and brought me to my knees. Almost thirty years after the fact, I went to the police and pressed charges—letting justice take its course. My now-sober father had my back, and witnesses that were interviewed recounted key details that validated mine, but the case was dropped because my mother refused to corroborate my testimony.

By this point, the ripple effect of trauma had impacted every area of my life—from bad business and financial decisions to toxic relationships I tolerated because I didn't think I deserved better. I was broken, and it was time for a reckoning.

I drew a line called dignity and decided my life story was not going to read like a victim impact statement. I chose to lean in to the healing energy of self-love and forgiveness, to celebrate courage and resilience, to surrender to vulnerability, to surround myself with loving friends and family, and most of all, to choose joy.

My story is still unfolding, and with joy as my GPS, it's now a purpose-filled brand platform for growth, transformation, and big dreams.

Roseanne Parke is a wow-man!

Roseanne Parke

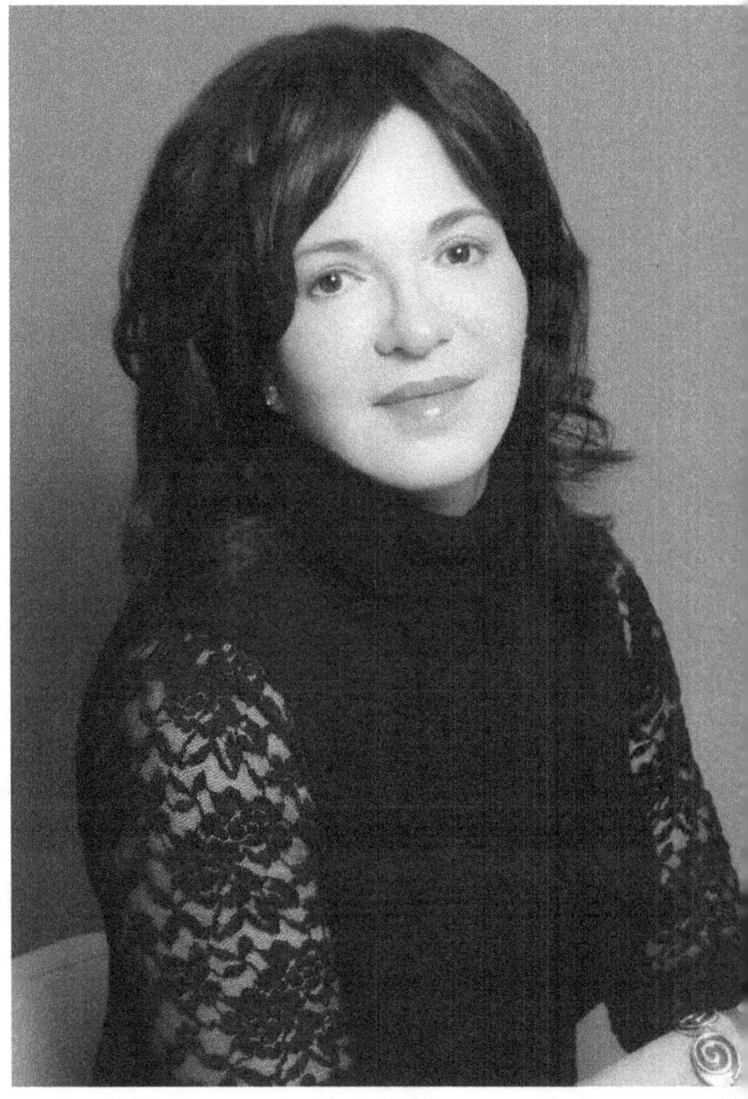

I am a wow-man! My daughter coined that term in a birthday card a few years ago. In that instant, I knew all the sacrifice had been worth it. Until that point, I was simply a nurse who left the bedside to pursue a corporate sales career. When that market became unreliable, I opened an esthetic clinic - my third career in my fifties.

Money and job security were my initial drivers, but in the process of 'selling my services,' I had to ask questions to uncover my customer's goals and needs. Listening to them, I began to see a common thread of underlying health signals that needed answers, e.g., why do some women not lose weight even with dieting; how can you look like you're on the top of your game physically with diet and exercise yet rely on caffeine to keep you going during the day, and wine to unwind at night.

All too often, women miss these subtle signals and attribute them to 'just life' or getting older. I started my new journey researching articles, attending conferences, and talking with experts to understand what might be lurking deeper.

You know the motto, "build it and they will come"? That's what I did. I pitched my vision of 'healthy inside and beautiful outside,' and I found doctors with the genius, shared passion, and willingness to move from traditional family health practice to join an integrated clinic. Here, they would help our clients achieve their goals of optimal health and natural beauty.

There were challenges. Although I was passionate about developing this model of care I had very little business intellect to guide us. There were the inevitable bumps in the road, but as tough as the lessons were, I persevered. I am inspired by a quote from Martin Luther King, "The ultimate measure of a person is not where they stand in moments of comfort and convenience, but where they stand in times of challenge and controversy."

I am a woman who questions run of the mill thinking when it comes to disease and aging. I don't sell services; I provide information to empower my clients to make the right decisions for their journey.

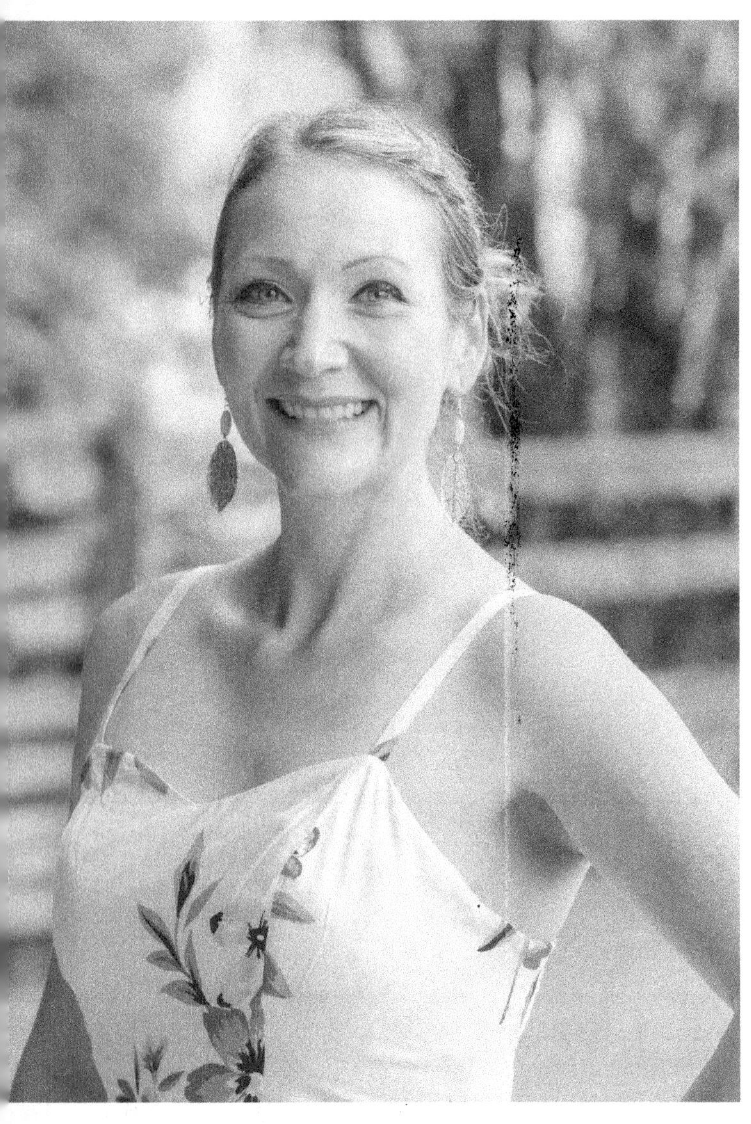

Kristal Barrett-Stuart was the founder of The Sparkle Project BC (a non-profit initiative to empower young girls to share their unique sparkle with the world) and co-author of the book "Sparkle: An Inspirational Handbook for Young Girls" Unfortunately, what Kristal thought to be her path turned into a whole different journey, a journey of deep healing.

Kristal Barrett-Stuart

In 2015, at the height of launching The Sparkle Project BC, releasing the inspirational book, music video, and empowerment events for young girls, I noticed an unusual round circle bite. I quickly made an appointment with my MD in fear of Lyme Disease (antibiotics are required as soon as possible). I used to believe that doctors had all the answers and knew everything health-related, boy was I wrong.

My Doctor quickly dismissed the bite and said, "We don't have Lyme Disease in Canada," which was the start of my long and painful journey to remission. I walked out of that office that day with full trust in my doctor and missed the critical window in receiving the antibiotics that could have stopped it from becoming chronic. Two years later and with over 100 insane symptoms, I was diagnosed by a Lyme literate Naturopath Doctor with "chronic, neurological Lyme Disease."

What I want to share more than anything is HOPE and to empower women to be their own health advocates. I realized we give so much of our power away by listening to Medical Doctors and not listening to our own innate intuition. We have become so programmed to believe there is only one way, the Western Medical way when in fact there is a whole world of incredible healing modalities out there that we aren't told about that truly define the world of health and healing.

Please know, you are not alone, and that healing is a puzzle that requires a balance of mind, body, and spirit. In the last five years, I have been to two different countries, had a stem cell transplant, spent weeks at a hospital in Mexico and underwent Hyperthermia, and have tried over eighty different modalities, many of which have blown my mind.

True healing is in your hands; you are your own healer.

Verna is an accounting professional but her passion with fashion and personal styling overflows that she needed to share it to the women who has the same heart as she has.

Verna Bohn

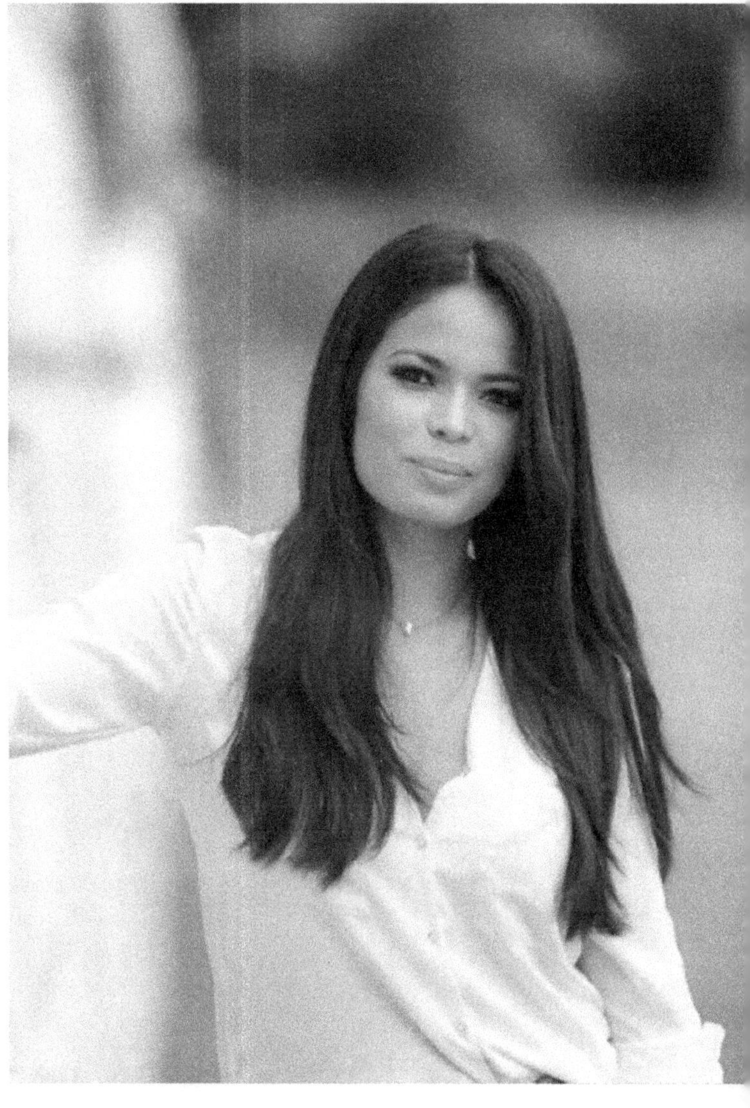

A few years after immigrating to Canada, Verna founded an advocacy company called Curves Is Fashion.org. It was first launched in February 2012, and Fresh Magazine was one of the media sponsors! Initially, the organization put together a revolutionary fashion show; a personal style fashion show where women of different sizes, shapes, walks of life, professions, and personalities were showcased on the runway displaying their very own personality with style. All the clothes from the runway were from Verna's own wardrobe and each look was styled by her.

Verna is an accounting professional by trade, but her passion is style. This passion overflows, and she channels it into empowering women and instilling a positive personal outlook in individuals with style. For Verna, beauty comes from the inside, and style is the expression of that beauty. It comes in different shapes and sizes, and all women are beautiful. "My group of friends always thank me. When they are with me, they feel beautiful. I will make sure you feel beautiful whether you're around me or not."
Verna co-created and co-managed several fashion events over the past few years within the Filipino community in Vancouver, Canada, and abroad. The core purpose of each endeavour is the empower women with a positive perspective of themselves through style.

Project: The Amazing Her is Verna's latest project with Curves Is Fashion.Org. This initiative helps empower a group of young girls between the ages of twelve and twenty-five from a specific tribe in the Southern Philippines. She is working hard to make this new project happen – like a new baby. Verna is looking forward to bringing people together to support these women through her website www.curvesisfashion.org where she shares her passion with you.

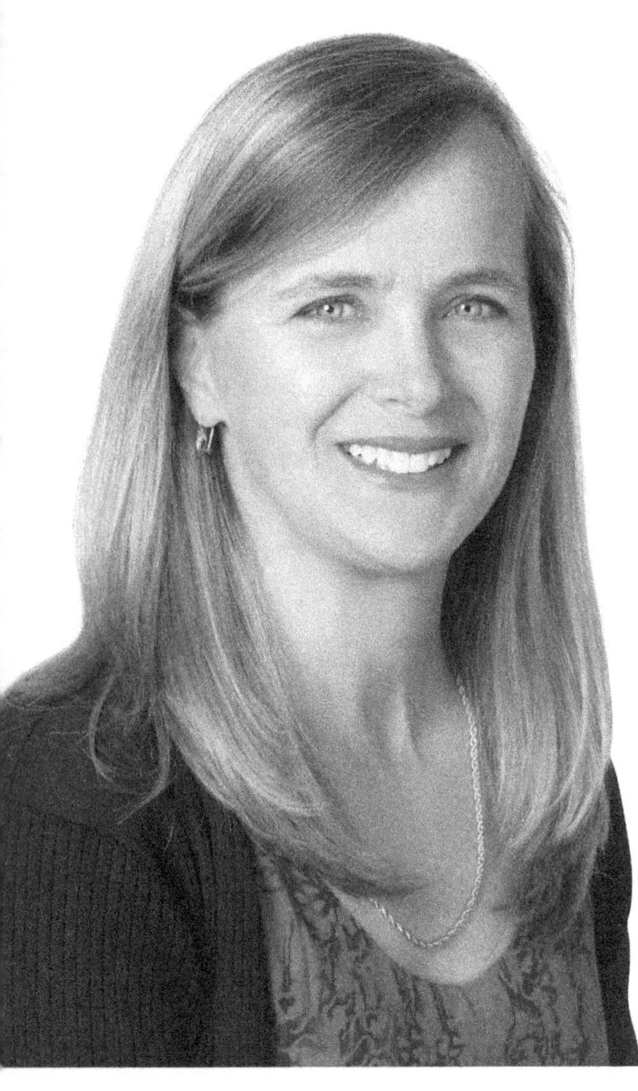

Dr. Diane Lacaille is a rheumatologist and the Scientific Director of Arthritis Research Canada/ Arthrite-recherche Canada.

Dr Diane Lacaille

I've spent my life at the intersection of medical practice and research. It's a unique space that I feel privileged to call home. As a rheumatologist, I see arthritis patients and their daily challenges. As a researcher, I find answers to questions that arise from my clinical practice. It's the perfect marriage and one that allows me to see an immediate impact on patients' lives. Arthritis is a misunderstood disease. Many assume it's no more than aches and pains and only affects older people. It's actually the leading cause of work disability in Canada and doesn't discriminate based on age.

Pain is one aspect. But how pain reaches its tentacles into all facets of a patient's life is most concerning. How do you work with arthritis? How do you care for young children? How do you stay active and lead a fulfilling life? It's not easy.

At Arthritis Research Canada, we work with patients to find solutions to these problems. Their needs are at the centre of everything we do as the largest clinical arthritis research centre in North America. We may not be able to cure this disease but we can reduce pain, prevent joint deformities and disability that comes with them. We can give people the tools and treatments to live full lives despite arthritis. Our mantra is practical research for everyday living. Helping patients today, not decades from now.

I started my research career 21 years ago as a trainee with this organization. I saw a gaping hole in the treatment of arthritis patients, which focused mainly on controlling the disease with medications. I wondered, what about the social and emotional upheaval it causes? I dedicated the next decade to addressing challenges arthritis patients face at work and developing tools to help them thrive.

Research is the producer working quietly behind the scenes of medicine. It doesn't always get the recognition it deserves, but without it, patients' quality of life would be drastically reduced. I now lead the organization that gave me my start and a team of outstanding medical doctors, research scientists, and trainees who are the future of research. I honestly believe the future is bright for arthritis patients.

Kim Appelt is a celebrity fashion stylist, YouTuber, and content producer for brands. She is also a champion for everyday women.

Kim Appelt

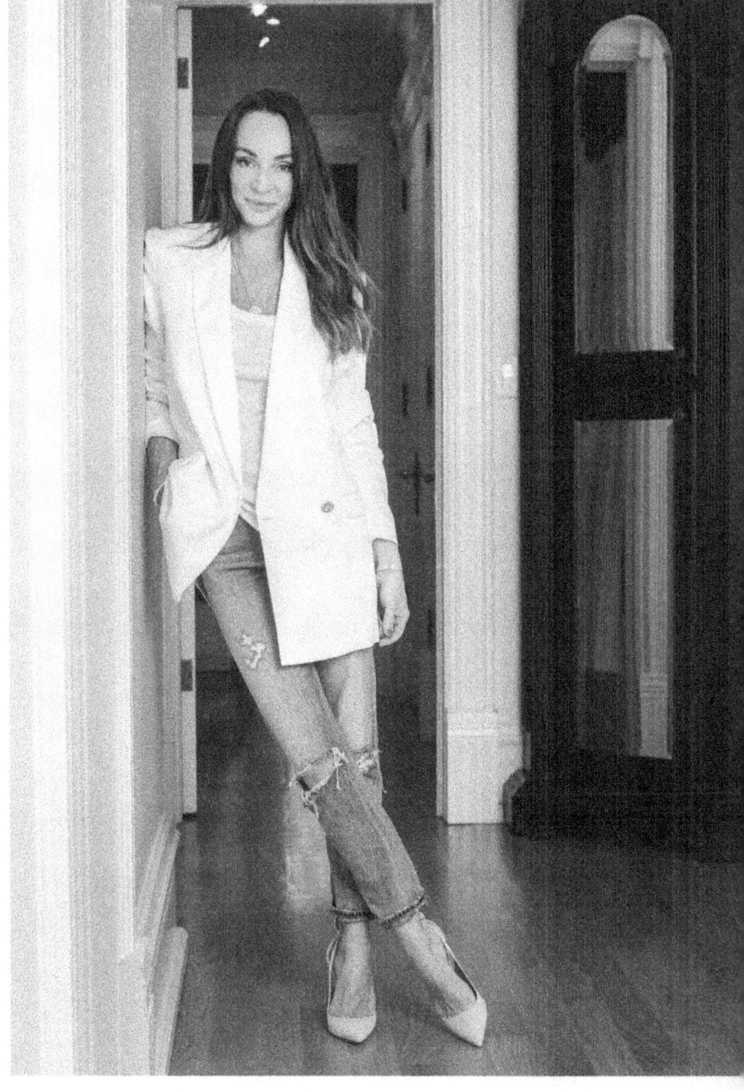

For as long as I can remember, I have been dressing people. My first and very willing participant was my little sister, Kristen. I would place my mother's nylons tightly on her small head to create an imaginary long Elsa-like braid. The smile on her cherub face as she got in her "wheelbarrow-chariot" with her beautiful braid and outfit made my heart beat faster, and it was then a desire to dress and create was born.

Fast forward many years, I did what everyone told me to do. I received two sensible degrees in university, got married, had three beautiful children, and stayed home to raise them. I dreamed of going back into fashion, dressing people for the red carpet, and helping the everyday woman. The woman that was also at home raising kids, working on her career, the one I wanted to show that you could do anything and feel good every day in your clothing. That everyday woman that was me; I needed to help her.

Everyone told me I couldn't, but I started dressing myself and taking pictures for a blog with hopes to inspire. I withstood the criticism of the women around me that didn't understand my larger goal. I took a course in styling, and one client at a time, doors started opening, and I just kept saying yes. I said yes for my kids so they could see the importance of following your dreams, for the other moms that also wanted to turn their dreams into goals, and for the everyday woman so I could eventually reach her and encourage her. Over time, more doors opened, I styled celebrities for magazines and red carpets. I turned my blog into a YouTube channel that has millions of views, I have a pending book deal, and a TV show in the development phase.

I now have the ability to reach every woman, to encourage her, help her dress, and help her feel confident in her clothing. The moral of the story is; if you have a dream, pursue it, live it. Write it down and become it. Everyone is built with a purpose; pursue yours. Mine was the everyday woman that lives in all of us that wants to look and feel her best, that wants to contribute to a higher purpose. I am here for her, cheering her on.

Tracy Valko is an award-winning Canadian mortgage professional and the Principal Mortgage Broker and Founder of Valko Financial Ltd.

Tracy Valko

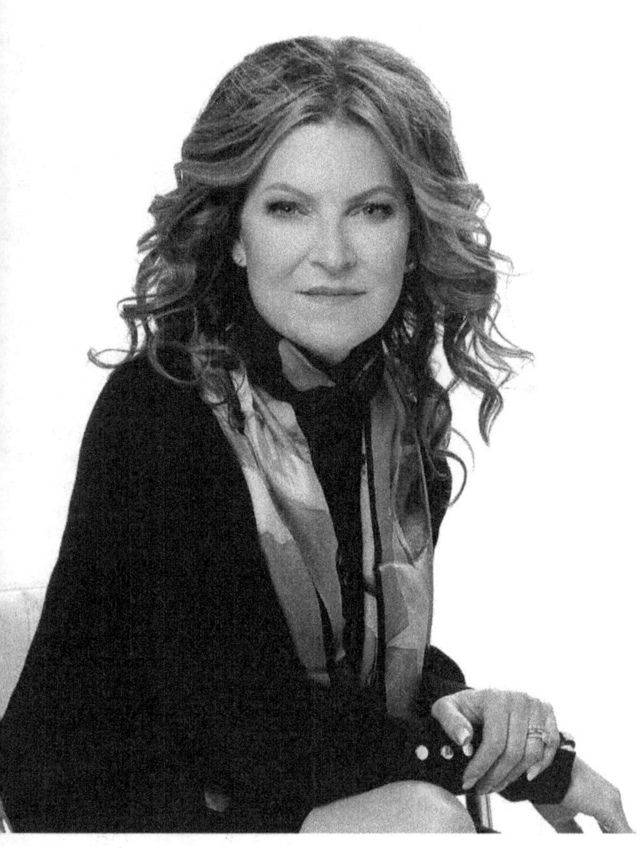

From the outside looking in, Tracy's office walls are stacked with awards and certificates acknowledging her success and growth in the mortgage industry. From the inside looking out, you'd be a woman who was told early on in her career that she'd have to choose between being a successful professional or mother. You'd be a brave young woman starting out in a very male-dominated industry. You'd also be a woman who (to this day) doesn't listen to anything but her own intuition.

Growing up in a time (as most of us did) when people didn't talk about how they "feel," and mental health wasn't a hashtag yet, Tracy had an intense desire and an incredible ability to connect with others.

As she slowly built her business, one connection at a time, she left lasting impressions on people with her honesty, integrity, commitment, and professionalism. Serving and guiding people through some of life's toughest and most difficult financial situations, it's impossible to not become genuinely invested in their lives and their positive outcomes.
Broker/Owner of Valko Financial, The Valko Team, and enormously proud mother of two, Tracy literally jumps out of bed in the morning with more purpose now than ever before. The pandemic caused great difficulties locally and globally, that cannot be ignored. Amplifying and expanding her efforts on social media to connect with local people, businesses, charities, and organizations, Tracy has become a community pillar of kindness and give-back, always putting the people first.

In 2020 Tracy began speaking publicly on her personal journey of mental illness and the impact it has had on her own family. As a panelist at GTACC's 2020 Women in Leadership, Tracy had the opportunity to speak honestly and openly about the things that have challenged her. She was featured on Roger's Blue Monday broadcast, encouraging more dialogue and accepted conversations around feelings and wellness. She has hosted financial wellness, mental wellness, and family wellness webinars on her social media completely free of charge to her following.
Mortgage Professionals of Canada named Tracy Valko Broker of the Year (2017) and Canadian Mortgage Professionals inducted her in late 2020 to the Hall of Fame.

Vicki Saunders is the founder of SheEO, a serial entrepreneur, award-winning mentor, advisor to the next generation of change makers and leading advocate for entrepreneurship as a way of creating positive transformation in the world.

Vicki Saunders

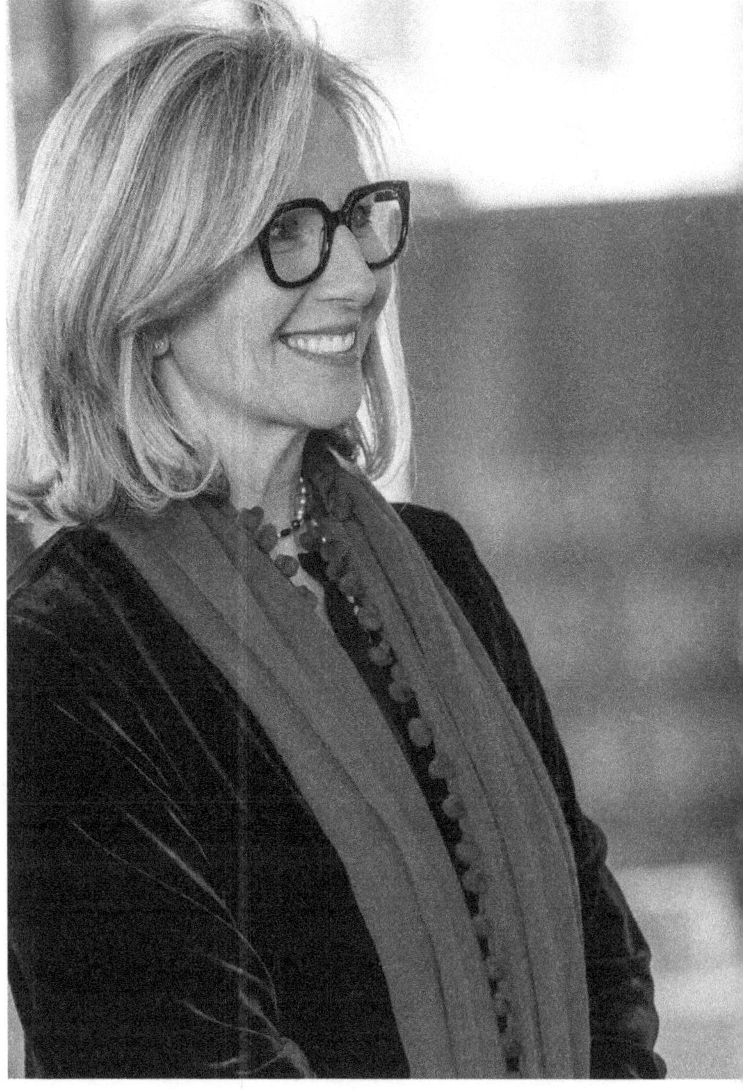

I am always obsessed with the equation of energy for impact. What can I do for the least amount of energy that will have the maximum impact? After decades of experience, learning and reflection here's the most impactful lesson I've learned.

In the past six years with SheEO, we have all been practicing Ask/Gives: asking for what we need help with and giving what we can offer. The giving part is easy for most of us in the community. As women, we are conditioned to tend to others and to give openly.

The hard part of Ask/Give, we all thought, is asking for help. Whenever I ask in crowds of people, "who would be willing to help someone in the room if they asked you right now?", nearly everyone's hands go up. When I ask, "who loves asking for help?", the hands are few and far between. Turns out, the hard part underneath the ask, at least for me, is the willingness to receive.

In 2018 I was out to lunch with an Activator, Colleen Abdoulah.
After lunch, we went to her favourite store and she said, "Pick something." "No thanks," I said, "I'm good. I don't need anything." "PICK SOMETHING," she said again. I dug in. "No, really," I said, "I don't need anything."
This went on, back and forth, several times.

Finally, she walked over to me, grabbed my shoulders, and shook me, vigorously. "RECEIVE!!!!" I felt this through my whole body. I realized... I was blocking her gift. **By not receiving, I was denying her the ability to give to me.** WOW.

I was so brainwashed in the culture of "I should be able to do this myself!", "I know she offered to help, but she's so busy!"

And on and on with the excuses, conditioned in me, not to receive support. **Receiving is at the heart of our connection with one another.** It is the action and the practice that opens us up to realize that, together we can do anything. When you practice receiving from others, you'll see everything change around you and realize that you have all that you need to achieve your dreams.

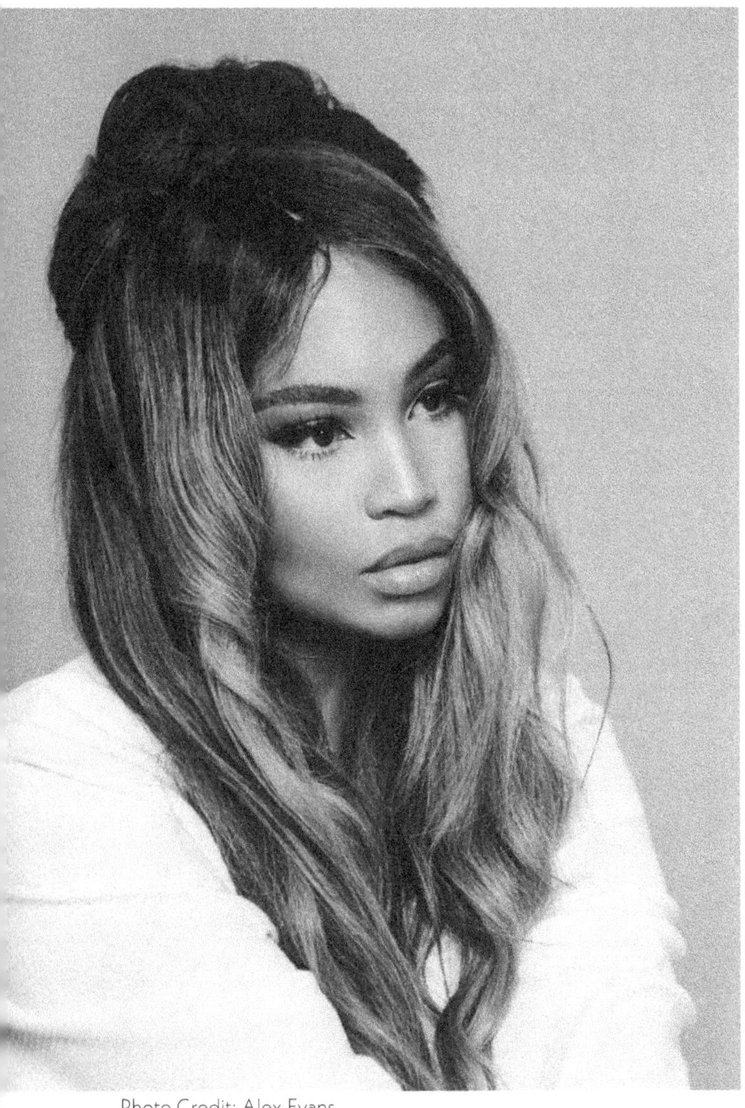

Photo Credit: Alex Evans

Krys Lunardo is a product of the creative forum – host of ET Canada's "Beauty Beat with Krys," co-founder of clean beauty skincare brand, Sistine, founder of luxury lifestyle print magazine Dauphine, and mother of two vibrant little ones.

Krys Lunardo

A native of the Bahamas — I was raised on a landscape that nurtured my creative prowess. Intrigued by the nuances of design as an adolescent, it was organic for me to immerse myself in the studies of architecture and fine art history at the University of Toronto.

Although my studies offered a diverse background in the premium business landscape, I was constantly compelled to search for other innovative platforms that afforded creative freedom. While my European travels and exposure to fashion led to celebrating five years of my print publication, Dauphine — it was my curiosity of clean beauty and environmental impact that prompted a paradigm shift in skincare. Recently recognized by Coveteur, Refinery29, Fashion, Hypebae, Women's Health Mag, The KIT, and Seventeen magazine, Sistine has already made its mark on the beauty space in just fourteen months.

Of course, unwavering dedication to all of my endeavors built the verifiable success of my enterprise, but it's the synergy of those combined aspects that is fulfilling. They all share this appreciation of provoking human beings, fine arts, and inclusivity while embracing culture. It's the exploration of the beauty in all things — including flaws, failures, rawness, and ambiguities that add to the structure of happiness for me.

Uncovering vulnerabilities through trial and error can often distort our outlook on life. The silver lining is that we become more resilient without even knowing it. It's a theory I hinge on — a constant reminder that success is abstract and cannot be applied to all of us with the same stroke. As women, the odds are evidently stacked against us, incredibly so for my fellow WOC, and as time progresses, our active willingness to work together to impact change certainly adds to social success.

Through it all, nurturing the root of the future generations – my little ones – to understand the multi-dimensional concept of life and all of its offerings, while applying good stewardship, brings me happiness. Life is on borrowed time, so let's make the most of it while our feet can still touch the ground.

Margarita Romano is a certified equine-facilitated coach that partners with horses to create a safe space to help heart-centered entrepreneurs, leaders, and teams overcome the stories of their life - past and present.

Margarita Romano

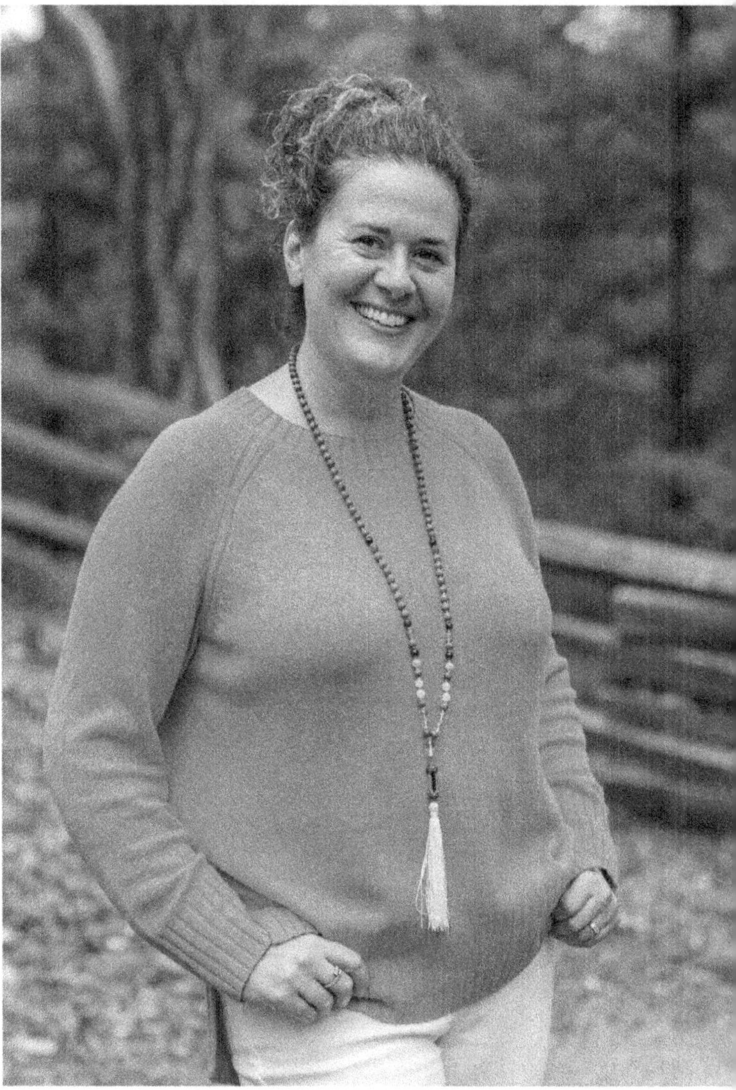

I have always had a connection with bringing love to tense situations. I was voted "peacemaker" in my high school senior year, and just a few years ago completed a personality test that divulged my strongest personality type as, you guessed it, peacemaker. It is safe to say that I have peacemaking in my DNA as it has stood the test of time. I have always successfully played the role - diffusing arguments between loved ones, between coworkers, hell even between strangers!
I do not enjoy conflict and always encourage people to communicate from the heart.

So, why do I partner with horses? The finely tuned instinct of a horse allows them to be mirrors for us and reflect what we are holding inside energetically every second. This highly effective form of feedback helps people move forward with a loving connection to themselves, and to others, allowing people to live the life they truly want. In pursuit of success and happiness, I have learned that both will effortlessly flow if I follow where my heart is leading me to be AND take the time to connect from the heart. To really see, hear, and understand people.

When you focus on showing up where you are called to be, you are filled with a level of happiness that is so profound, true success in all areas of life then finds you. The importance I place on holding a loving space for people helps me dilute conflict for myself and for others, hopefully increasing joy in this world - one connected moment at a time.

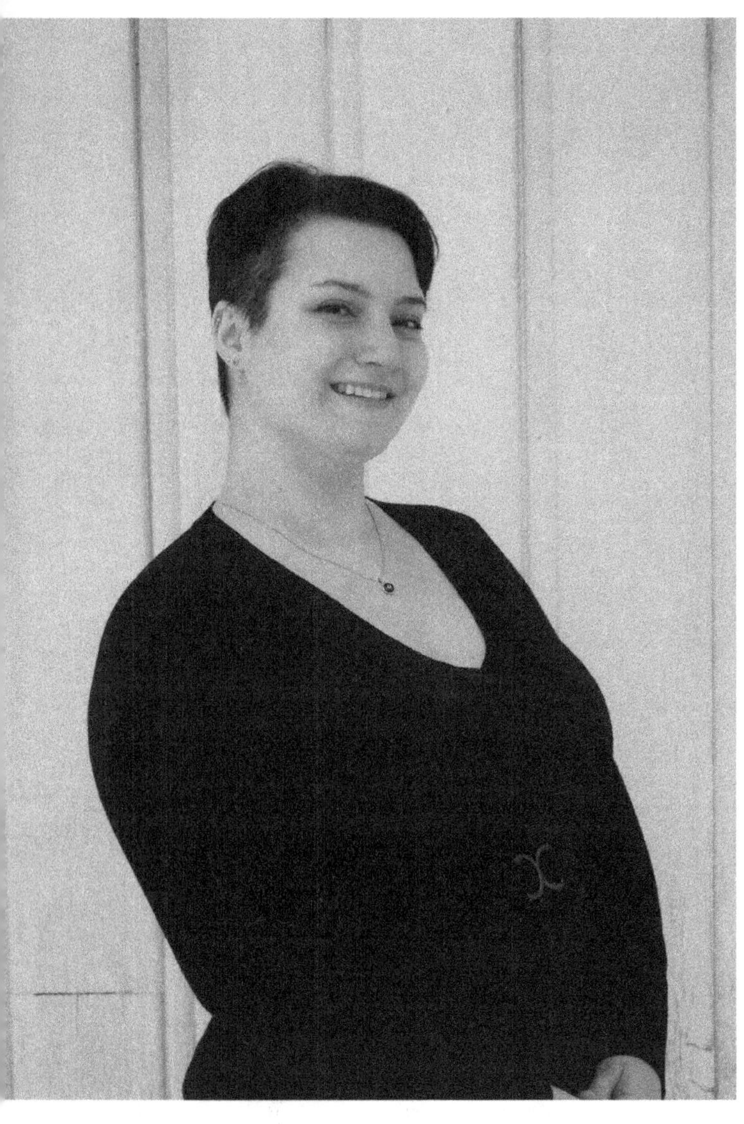

Jacinta Sarpkaya is well known for many things, but above all else, she's known for having too many hobbies.

Jacinta Sarpkaya

At any given time, I have a half-dozen projects on the go, and none of them is the same medium. Of all the hobbies that have ever consumed me, however, my love of stories has always prevailed. Whether fiction or fact, myth or modern, stories have taken me through the hardest times of my life, and I have learned that stories can bring people together. I have made good friends with stories: rolling dice at a table, sharing fandoms, even sharing trauma. And although I've always struggled to tell my own stories, I've discovered in them my voice and my power.

For every trauma, every mistake, and every injury, my stories have taught me about myself and allowed me to connect with others. The hardest times of my life have given me the insight and perspective I need to help others, and to help myself. Bullying and the challenge of making friends gave me insight into the value of kindness, and the importance of inclusivity. Disordered eating and a BPD diagnosis inspired my passion for mental health support and the end of stigma. Two debilitating injuries taught me how to get back up again and again, and in the aftermath of rape at the hands of men I trusted taught me that even in the darkest moments, I have champions, I have the right to be heard, and "No." is a complete sentence. In heartbreak, I discovered gratitude for having loved intensely. Every cloud maintains a silver lining, and for me, that always included a lesson.

From every story filled with pain, I have pulled a lesson of hope and a drive to keep going. As I continue my journey as an artist and a writer, more than anything I want to share that with others. Though I've not yet crafted the story I'll share with the world, I can feel them being woven together. Whether that story comes in a book, in a painting, or in a conversation with a stranger, I know my story is powerful. We learn the most from the stories that are the hardest to endure. If I can help just one person by sharing mine, the pain will all be worth it.

Karen Kristjanson is an author, a co-parent, and a life coach who nourishes and inspires courage in parents through her words.

Karen Kristjanson

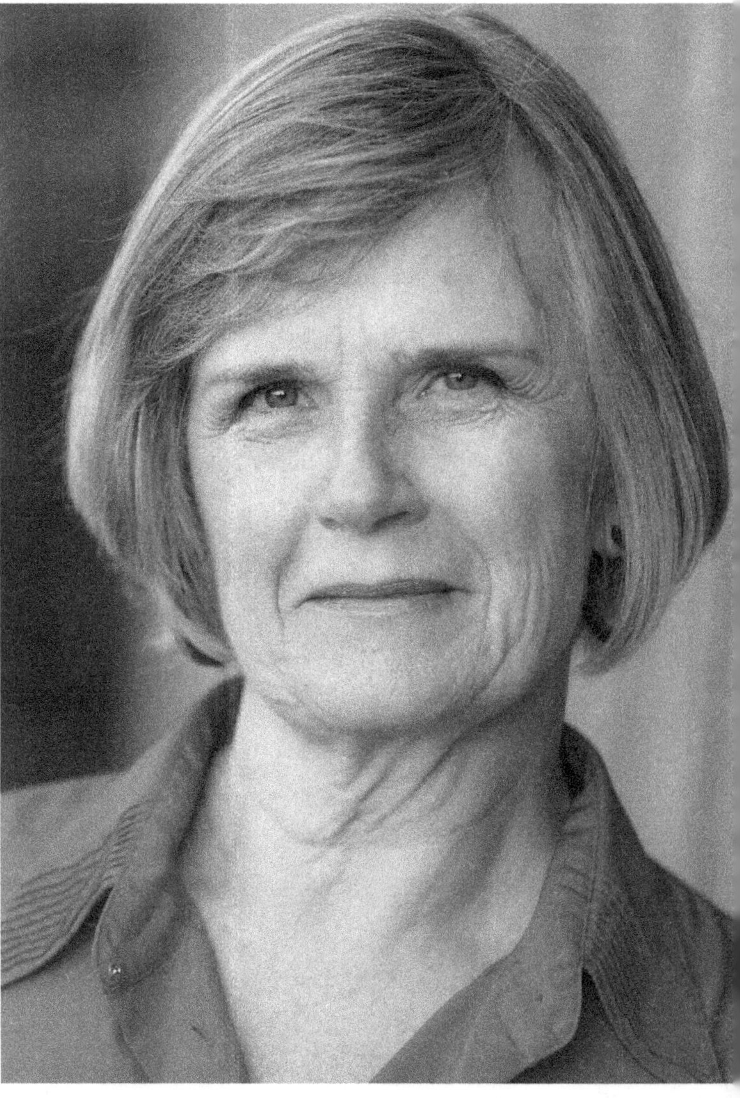

"Everyone's normal until you get to know them." That's one of my favourite sayings. When we feel weird or less than we want to be—remember we have lots of company! Yet it's our unique combination of strengths, passions, wounds, and life circumstances that propel us forward. Our uniqueness lets us shine and contribute. For me, shared parenting after divorce became a focus because I co-parented my now-grown sons.
It was the best choice for them and for me.
While it's not easy, my experience showed me it's an important option, because children want to love and know both parents. My first two years post-divorce were the loneliest of my life.

When I discovered the story of another mother's experience co-parenting, my relief was immense. I was not alone! However, one story was not enough—I wanted more. I determined to discover other stories myself and offer them to the world. Could I do it? My drive to offer co-parenting stories to divorcing parents, combined with my skills as a master life coach coalesced to "Yes." I needed every smidgen of courage and determination I could muster in the nine years of researching, writing, and finding a publisher for my manuscript. I found parents to interview by word of mouth. Their stories challenged and inspired me. Some held such sadness they were difficult to hear. Others taught me about lives different than mine: parents of children with special needs, lesbian moms, high-conflict parents.
The thread of hope weaving through them was growth, as parents described how much they had learned about themselves and about being a parent. This was my first venture into serious writing, so getting the support of other writers was critical. The manuscript completed, I sent my book proposal out, week after week, to potential publishers. Now it's thrilling to know these stories are out in the world to support others co-parenting.
Aside from raising my sons, my greatest sense of satisfaction comes from my book, Co-Parenting from the Inside Out: Voices of Moms and Dads. It's where my deep personal goals, life experience, and skills meet what the world needs. Where do your goals, skills, and life experience come together?

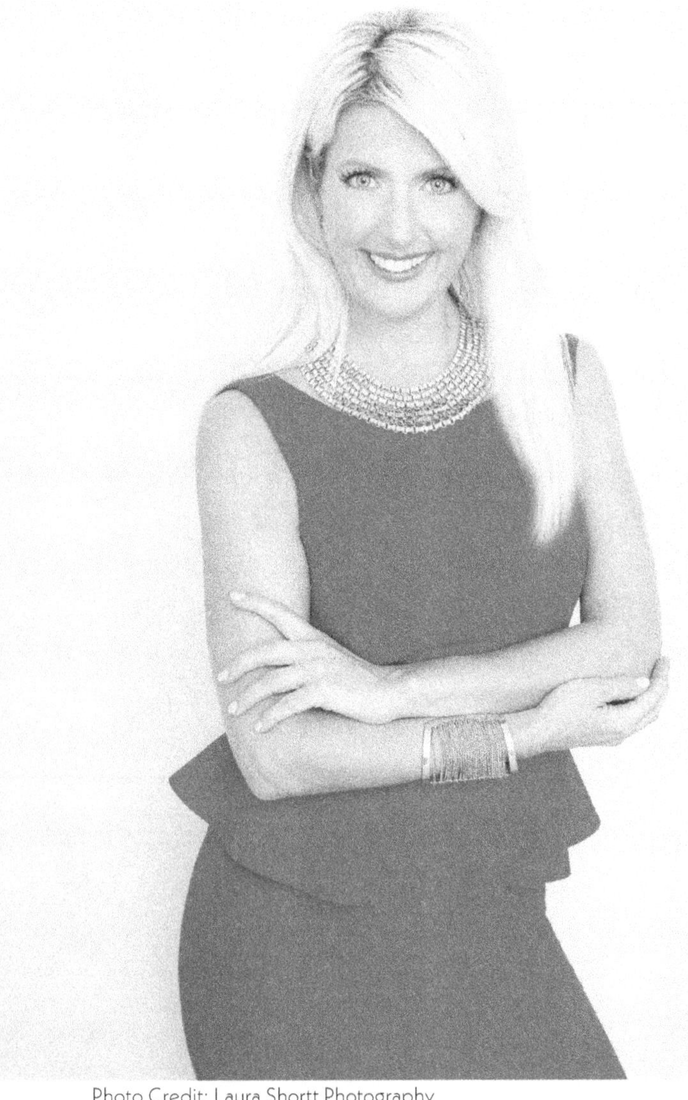
Photo Credit: Laura Shortt Photography

Janice is a multi-passionate entrepreneur with fortes in business strategy, integrative healthcare, and women's leadership coaching. She has unshakable Joie de Vivre – fueling multiple life transitions, and journeys to seven countries, to save her own life! Often referred to as "the exception," she is here to connect you to why you are an "exceptionn-elle" woman, too.

Janice Skoreyko

Remember who you wanted to be when you grew up? Take a moment. Open your heart and think back... smile. This was, and still is, your personal invitation; your first "Elegant Move."
Over the past three decades, I've discovered no matter how far away you feel from this invite, there's a series of "8 Elegant Moves" you can use to create the exceptional life you were meant to live now.

The second move is to "Check Out the Show." As a young person, I was literally a suffocating, fragile, flower, struggling with COPD and low bone density. I carried this identity into adulthood; showing up fearful, dimly lit, and weak; which had to change. Alone in China, following my near-death experience, it became abundantly clear that self-care was not selfish; it was essential – enter move number three: flipping my to-do list on its head, I found my "Indulgent Transformation" tasks on top; dancing, laughing, loving, and chocolate-making – move number four.

Still feeling constricted, I discovered that I had been framed! My own mind had me living inside a painting titled "Tiny Existence." Stepping outside of the frame – move number five – I awakened to the world of possibility, the ability to "coeurageously" create my masterpiece, living outrageously from my heart – move number six. The most rewarding relationship in my life is with the Universe. We celebrate and converse daily – move number seven. Giving from a glass that's half full is so passé. I invite you to be the glass at the top of the champagne tower, give from your overflowing flute – move number eight.

What I know for sure: if you don't give your heart a reason to keep beating it won't. There's an abundant difference between a fear-based script and coeurageous, exceptionnelle living; champagne towers are essential and flight school was amazing.

You too are an exceptionnelle woman; I am here for you. xo

Bif Naked is a Canadian actress, motivational speaker, poet, pop and rock singer, and songwriter.

Bif Naked

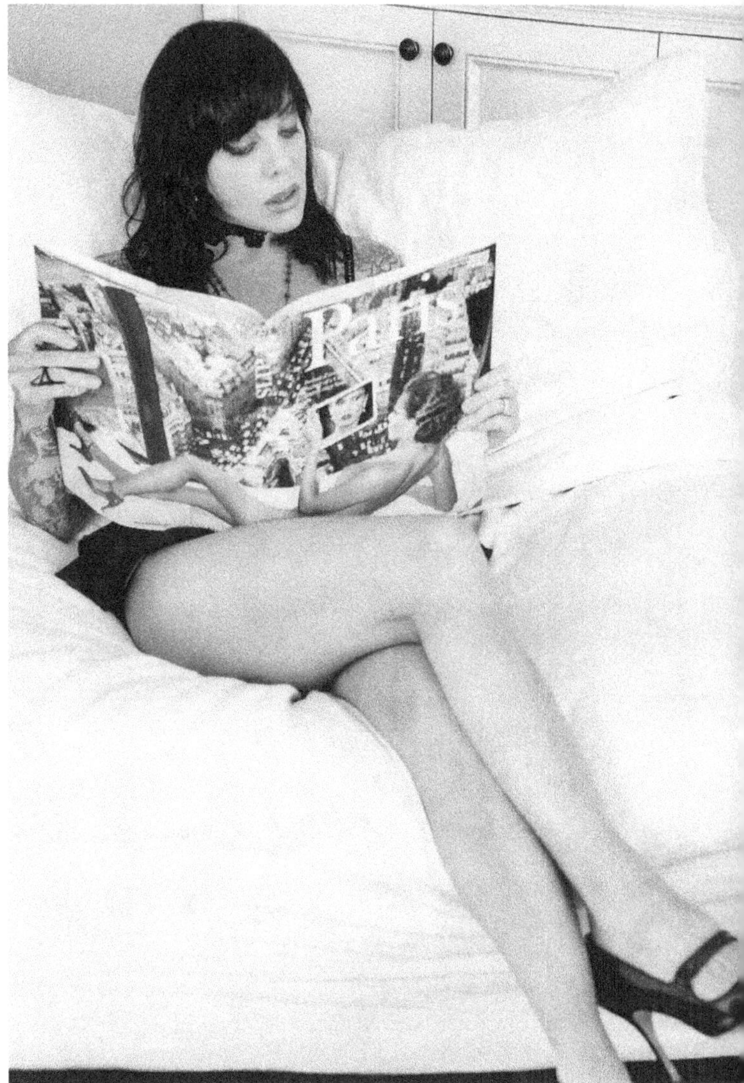

Photo Credit: @CocoandKensington

As I go through life, I live in enormous gratitude and awareness. I have always felt incredibly blessed, not just as an adopted kid, but as an eternal optimist. And, with a true awareness that I am forever learning and aiming to be a better person. Like many of us, I guess I have always tried to evolve, or grow, whether or not I knew how, or even had the grace to do it. But whether or not the journey was a hard or happy one, the truth is that "grace" never really helped me. Only self-discipline did. It's a lesson I learned and carried with me my whole life.

When I was in the sixth grade, I was the class clown, and I got into trouble frequently. My teacher felt that the best punishment for me was to write lines. Like, a thousand lines per offense. At the time, I felt incredibly persecuted and quite sorry for my twelve-year-old self. But the truth is- it was the best training I ever had.

The repetition of these lines not only perfected my famous, curvy handwriting, but drove the message of these lines home. Decades later, I still remember the line:

"Self-discipline requires doing what is necessary when it should be done, whether it is a pleasant task or not"

It is the best advice, and I STILL live by this! Nothing ever comes easily. Growth, either personally or in our businesses or art, takes work. Sometimes, it is very hard, and for most - it would probably be easier to just give up. But having the self-discipline to keep at it, stay consistent, and remain on our path is what makes the biggest difference in anything we do. Because evolution and change are hard, and take all of our commitment, no matter what!

Self-discipline is our truth! And it takes authentic, steady self-discipline to achieve anything we do in life. As the line says, "Whether it is a pleasant task or not." The reward is finding joy in the journey and finding our grace along the way.

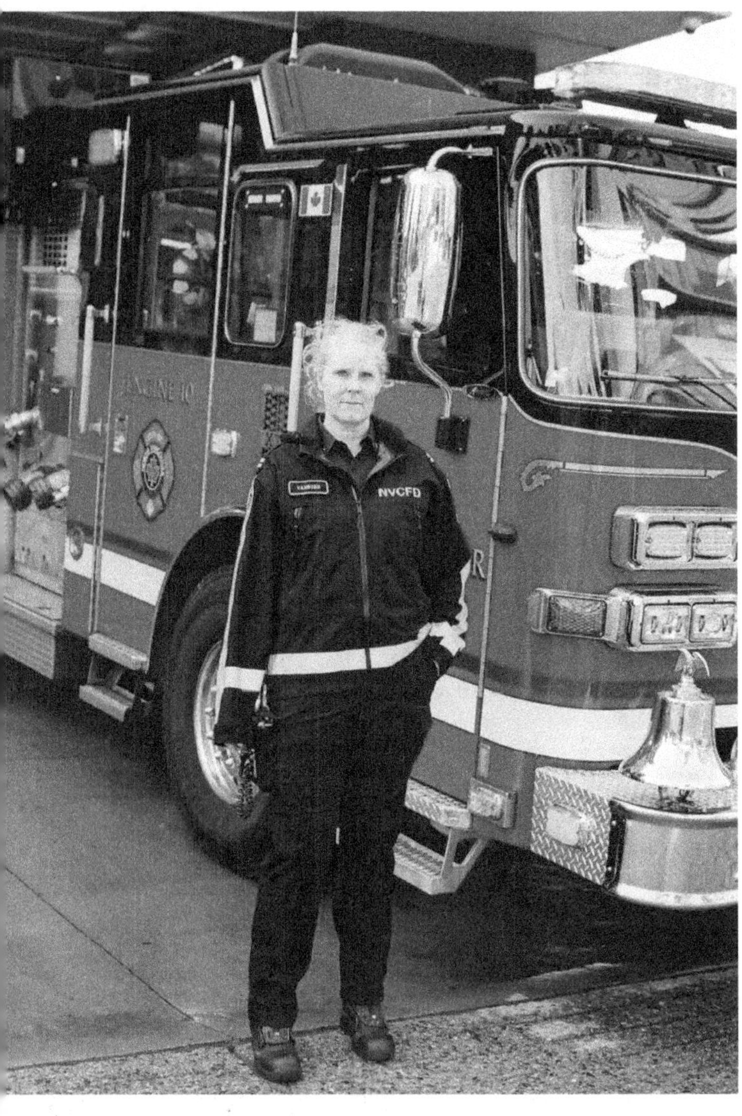

Sam van Born is a Captain in the fire service, a health & wellness entrepreneur specializing in immune support, CBD, and a kick-ass single mum.

Sam van Born

My daughter, family, and friends tell me some of my greatest strengths are that I am caring, helpful, hardworking, strong, and resilient. There usually isn't a time where I am not busy doing something, and that something usually involves helping others. That is my fuel; that's what drives me to do what I do. If I can help someone in any way, it fuels my soul. Being in the fire service usually doesn't give me the closure I crave. We help people during their worst moments and usually don't know the outcome, and because of that, I sought to venture into the health and wellness realm. Now, I help people deal with their root causes and try to help prevent disease on a cellular level.

I have been through a lot; an abusive marriage, bankruptcy due to my ex gambling – a debt I am still paying – and moving six times in the last ten years. If it weren't for my daughter and some amazing people in my life, I'm not sure where we would be. I feel now we are on an amazing path.

It's hard to stay positive in trying times. What I have learned from my biggest failure, and what I try to focus on, is putting positive thoughts into the universe. I truly believe what you put out is what you get back. I ask a lot of questions and try to manifest what I want in my life – and helping people is just that.

I wanted to be part of this amazing collaborative book because I want people to know; you are not alone. There is help, and things will get better. Helping people realize that if you don't feel well, it doesn't have to be forever. I dealt with my gut health and when that was healed, everything started to change. This is what I am great at, and especially dealing with a pandemic, your immune system is key. Let's meet for a coffee. I'd love to chat and see if I can help you too.

Marisa Pothier is a dedicated entrepreneur passionate about helping animals and educating people on how to live a vegan lifestyle.

Marisa Pothier

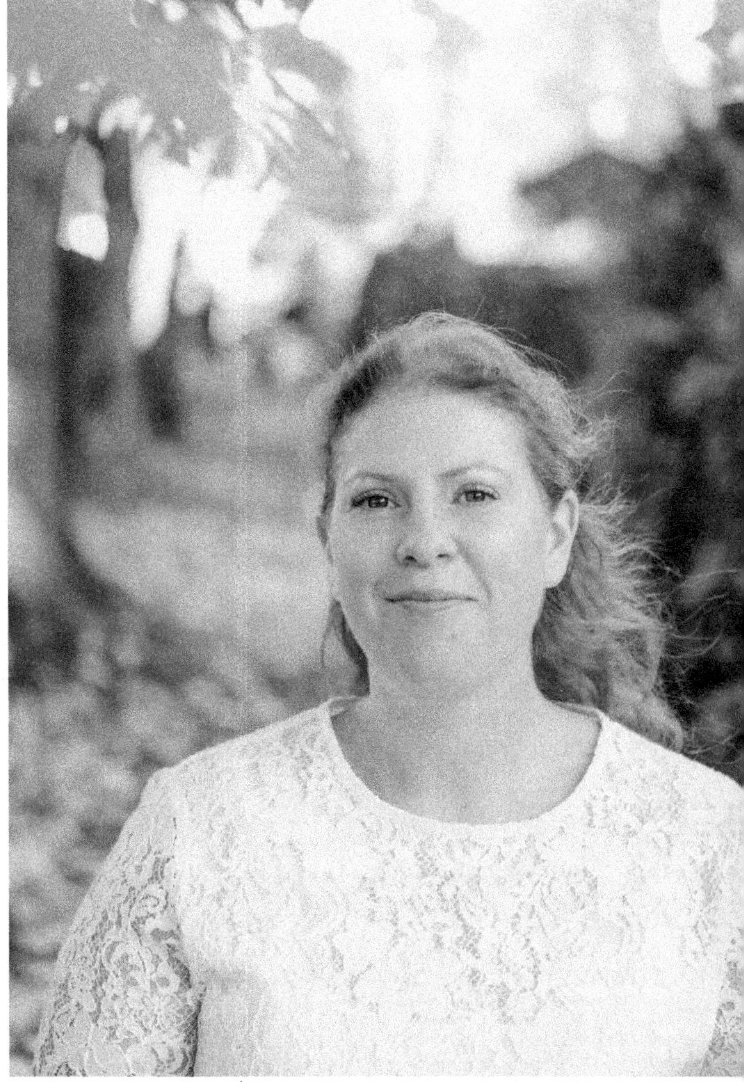
Photo Credit: ToshaLobsingerismyphotographer

She is the business owner of Honest Cleaning and Services, based in beautiful British Columbia, Canada. Her focus is to educate others about green and animal-free alternatives to harmful store-bought cleaning chemicals, which are often tested on animals and not good for our own well-being.

After working a career in education with young adults, she saw a huge demand for change for the future, and wanted to share her veganism as a tool to help show others that using and eating animals will be a thing of the past.

While making the switch to eating a plant-based diet, Marisa learned about the conditions that animals face when they undergo testing in labs for cleaning products. Many household cleaning chemicals are very toxic and harmful to our health, so she saw this as an opportunity to bring veganism and safer options for use in her business model.

She started working for Saje Wellness and learned about the benefits of essential oils. Soon after, Marisa took her knowledge and experience and started making eco-friendly green cleaners to use in her side gig as a housecleaner.

In her role as a house cleaner, she quickly learned that she enjoyed the independence and responsibility of making her own life for herself. She struggled with high stress and long demands while working with children in the education system. It was clear that she needed to follow her passion, and she decided to start Honest Cleaning to better live a life with more freedom and flexibility.

In her spare time, she is often found enjoying animals and nature. She likes to go hiking and road trip in BC and will often be sharing on social media about yummy vegan eats along the way. She is a proud vegan of four years that enjoys helping others make the transition and show people that living a cruelty-free life can be simple and rewarding. Her goal is to leave this planet a little kinder for all of us.

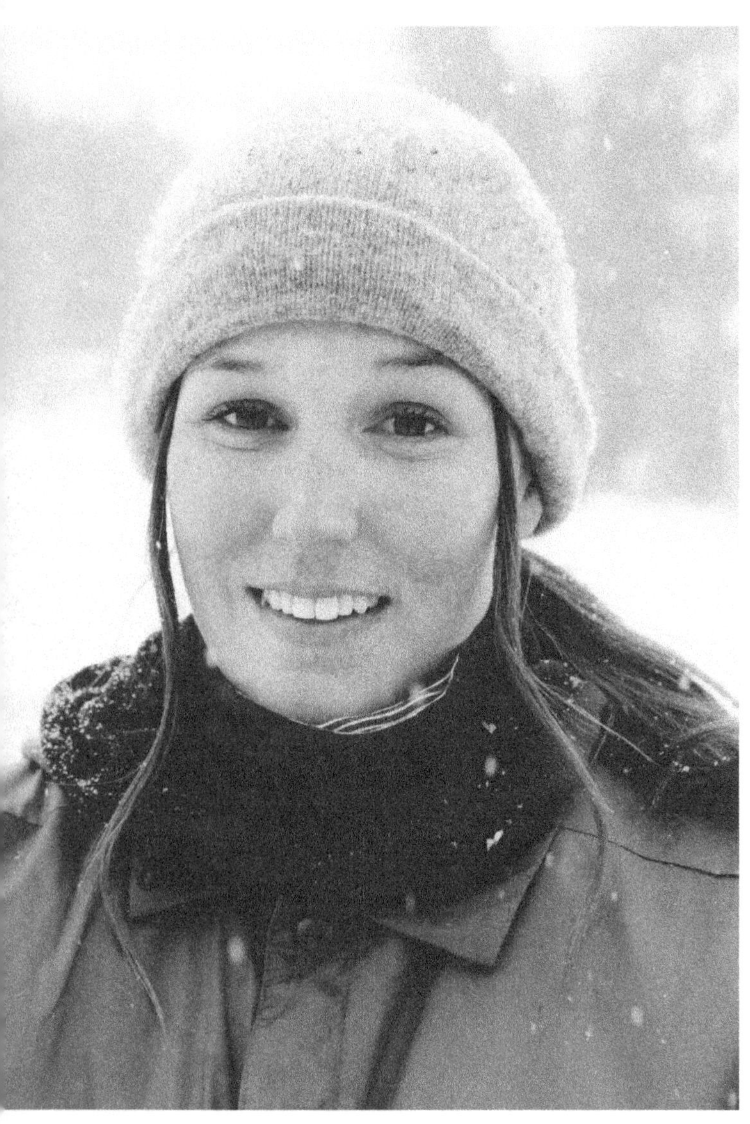

Spencer O'Brien is an Olympic snowboarder and spokesperson for Arthritis Research Canada who lives with rheumatoid arthritis.

Spencer O'Brien

I was twenty-four when the aches and pains began. It started small; stiffness in my knees when warming up for a workout, little pinches in my shoulders while riding. I ignored the pain and chalked it up to getting older.

In 2013, I became World Champion in my sport for the second time and qualified for my first Olympic Games. I was plagued by joint injuries and pain that year, but I pushed through, eager to earn my ticket to the 2014 Sochi Olympics.

I qualified and breathed a sigh of relief. But I was still in pain every day. All I could think about was snowboarding and getting to the Olympics. As my condition worsened, so did my mental health.

I fell into a deep depression, angry at my body for betraying me. I could hardly train, and despite spending every day in physio and at the gym, I was the weakest I had ever been. By November 2013, just two months before the Olympics, I had not snowboarded in seven months. I struggled to get out of bed in the morning. I could barely walk down a set of stairs. I felt like a ghost of myself, and the Olympics seemed like an impossible feat.

Then I was diagnosed with rheumatoid arthritis. My first thought was, "how? I'm so young, that can't be right?" My second thought was, "how will I snowboard?" I broke down into tears in the doctor's office, fearing I'd never snowboard again.

I was wrong. I did snowboard again, and since that day, I have attended two Olympic Games, won an X Games Gold Medal and have continued to do the sport I love so much.

For a long time, I was afraid to speak out about my illness. I didn't think it could happen to someone like me. I'm now the spokesperson for Arthritis Research Canada because I want people to know that dreams are still possible when you have arthritis. Thanks to arthritis research, I have regained a quality of life I wasn't sure I'd ever be able to get back. I want the same for millions of others living with this debilitating disease.

Debra Bromley is a unique soul - an entrepreneur, a landscaper, a sports enthusiast, a friend, and a dreamer.

Debra Bromley

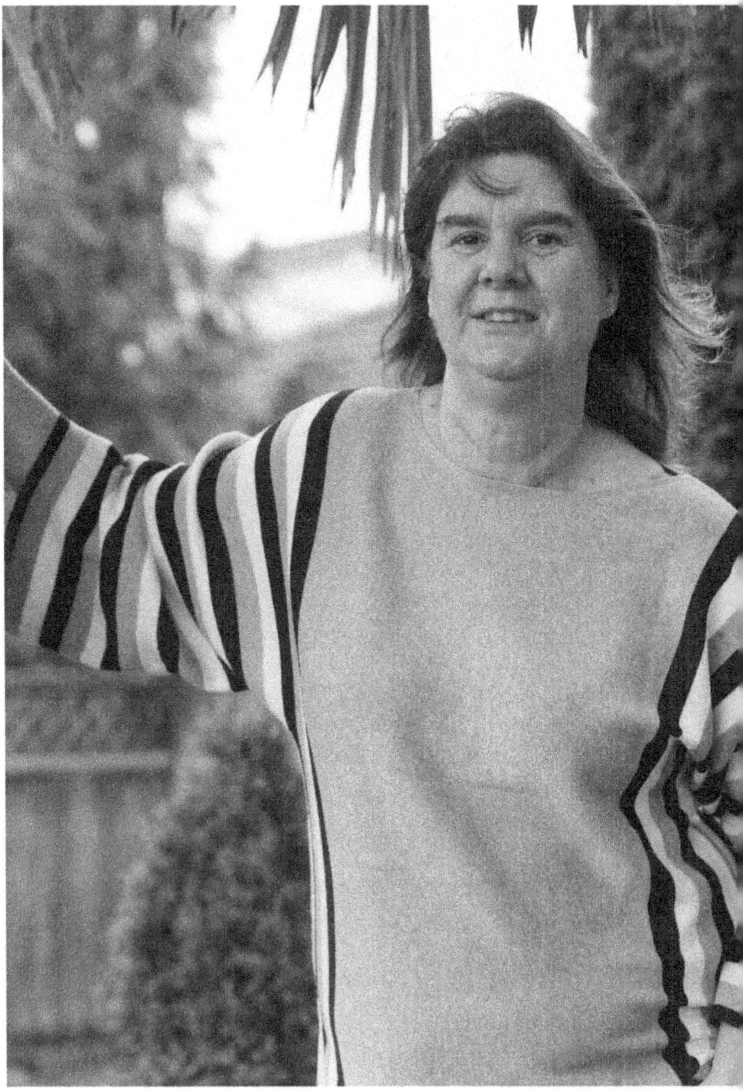

My life has been filled with strong passions - some easy, some challenging. While I have not made lifelong careers out of all of them, I can say that I followed my heart and tried them all, even the ones that may not have been conventional for a woman.

Growing up, I had compelling desires to play ice hockey, football, surf, and ride motorcycles - not necessarily the average female activities. I was determined and ventured into all of them. I also had a love for acting and found myself in at least one stage production.

Graduating from university was a dream of mine that came to life with a Bachelor of Arts degree from UBC. That led to running my own landscaping business, which has gone on now for thirty-five-plus years. I find myself more passionate about landscaping every day. I love being an entrepreneur. A few years ago, I was able to expand my business into the U.S., - a lifelong ambition of mine coming true.

In amongst it all, I was blessed to have had three daughters, all born at home with midwives. My visions growing up never left me. I told my cousin in California not long ago that even today at the age of fifty-five, I still have the same fantasy of moving to California. So many wonderful memories were made there over the years. Throughout everything, my greatest joys have been spirituality and friendship. I have been very fortunate to have had such close friends to laugh with. I believe my best friend was truly a gift from God.

I have heard that I have been a mentor to people. I hope this is true in the sense that I have helped them, but most of all, I hope that I have been a friend to them. There is nothing like the feeling when you see people look inside their hearts and follow their passions - tremendous inspiration.

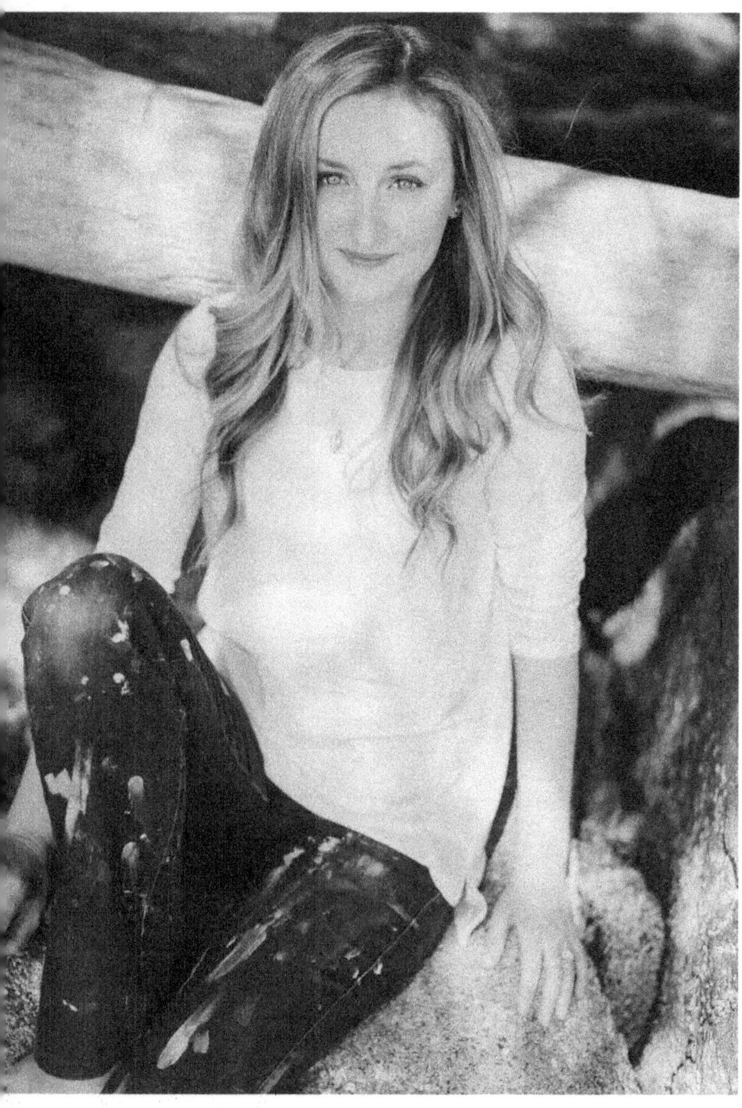

In pursuit of a forgotten dream, Tiffany Reid found love...

Tiffany Reid

With tears in my eyes, I slipped off the ring and disappeared into the night. What I thought was the worst moment of my life turned out to the best decision I ever made. My father once told me this story: Once upon a time there was a man who proposed to a woman. She said no and lived happily ever after.

I took a year for myself and pursued my love of art. Painting, taking classes, and allowing myself to find myself emotionally and artistically. I didn't necessarily know where the journey was leading me, but my inner self kept telling me it was right.

It was during this time that I fell in love with two special people who encouraged me to follow a forgotten path.

Corey lost his wife to a tragic battle of cancer, leaving him alone to raise a toddler. Despite everything, Corey had made a conscious choice to pursue happiness. After many cocktails and a terrible Elvis show on our first date, we were smitten. That was the easy part. There were many mixed feelings of grief and guilt. One of the biggest hurdles I had to overcome was being an insta-mom. Tantrums, sleepless nights, picky eating... it all hit me like a ton of bricks. I went from the indulgent single life (eating Doritos out of my belly button and sleeping in) into full steam motherhood! But Lyla had the ability to melt your heart with her sweet "I love you's" and morning snuggles. Our love was bigger than grief, and with patience, we became a family.
Lyla and I grew especially close through art. She was wildly creative, and while I was teaching her to grow up, she was teaching me to be a child. My art is often inspired by connecting to the inner child and enjoying the simpler more abstract parts of life. Corey gave me the courage to dream big. He thought I was truly talented and encouraged me to take my art to the next level. Art has made me truly happy, and by pursuing something I love, it has led me to love itself.

Mandi Sellers is an accomplished business owner, an inspirational leader to those around her, and a loving mother of two talented daughters, Mandi Sellers has been able to harness her strengths to achieve her ambitions.

Mandi Sellers

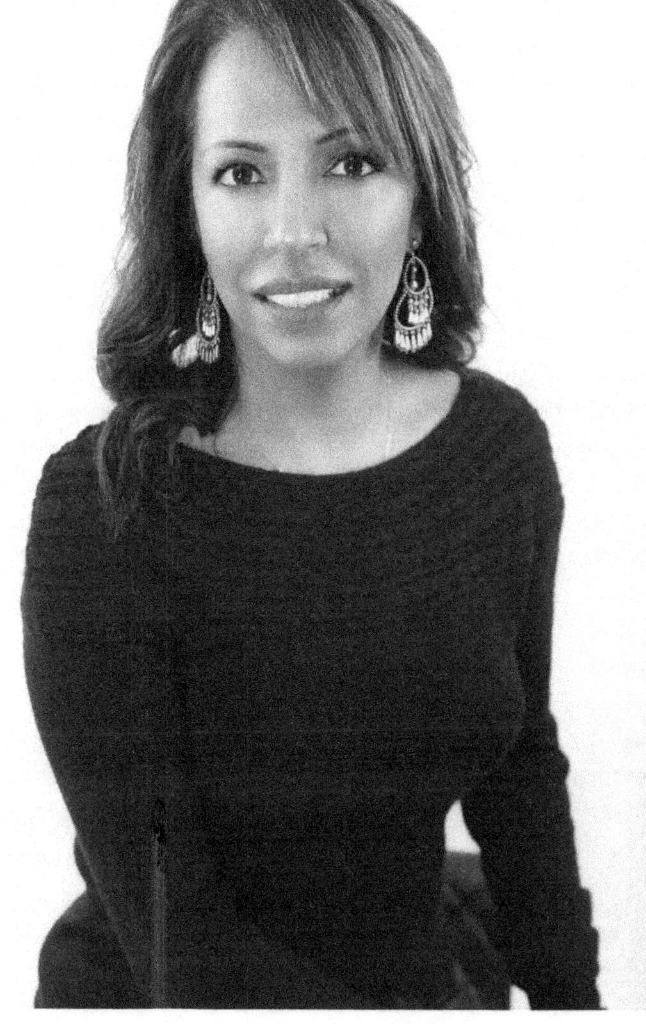

Arriving as an immigrant from India with her parents at the age of three, she had to maneuver between her Canadian life and Indian roots to find her authentic voice in an intricate and delicate cross-cultural dance.

Growing up without a voice, she was determined to give others one. As a girl, she was exposed early on to an unjust system that favored men and diminished women. Embracing imperfection in her journey, she had to make difficult sacrifices that, for years, impacted her relationship with community and culture.

Transforming her grief that resulted from loss, shame, and guilt for being a woman with defined choices and a bold outlook, into deepened compassion and awareness for self and others, she was able to create ground-breaking programs that empower women and Indigenous people. Advocating for other people serves her life-long learning goals and facilitates her own self-empowerment. She has learned to heal with people and grow together. Continuous personal growth and development remain the prime inspiration and strength behind her ongoing efforts to serve others.

Her programs are currently offered to over eighty Nations, communities, and friendship centres province-wide, and her company is recognized in both public and private settings for its exceptional services. Mandi's finely tuned compassion, empathy, and intuitive insight combined with exceptional business acumen, yields long-term successful results for her clients and those she serves.

Driven by this authentic passion to help others and a desire to give back to her community, Mandi is constantly developing innovative ideas to foster her devotion to society's personal and spiritual advancement. Her team members describe her as someone who empowers those around her, a woman of action, and one that can quickly turn a 'no' into a 'why not?'.

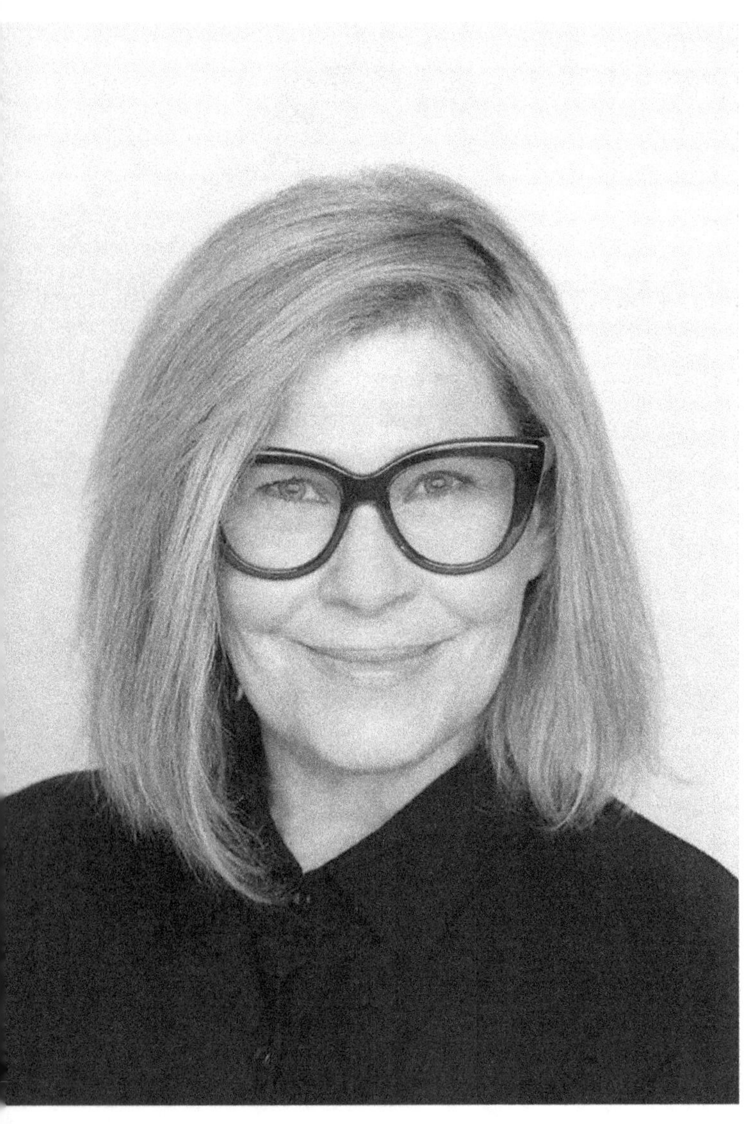

JoAnn Fowler is an entrepreneur, an Emmy nominated makeup artist, and the founder of Sappho New Paradigm Cosmetics - challenging the patriarchy every step of the way.

JoAnn Fowler

The more I live this life the less I know I know.
There are times in my life that I have had the seemingly right answers to the right questions. There are times in my life that I have not even known that I need to ask a question in the first place. There are times I am proud of myself, my actions and my reactions.
There are times I fall woefully short and I feel shame
And the path is never linear
Rather it ebbs and flows, and the goal becomes to stay vigilant to stress and to strive for kindness, to myself and others. I once went to a talk that the Dali Lama gave, he answered a question of how he deals with his anger towards the Chinese in Tibet and he said,

"I meditate at 3 a.m. every day for 4 hours - I take all the anger in and I turn it to love and put it out."
You could hear a pin drop – everyone was in awe
And then he said
"And some days it works
And others it doesn't"
We do the best we can with the skills and knowledge we have
And we know that change is necessary
I strive to be a better student.
Happiness comes to me when I feel purposeful, when I am being of service, when I am creating.
My company is my apology to the next generation.
It is my intention to leave a legacy of transparency, authenticity, fallibility, vulnerability, creativity, equality, sustainability and ultimately hope.
For the good of all.

"Walk confidently in the direction of your dreams and live the life you imagine, and you will meet with success unexpected in common hours" – my version of Thoreau's longer statement.

Gladys Loewen is a retired manager and educator on disability resources and inclusion.

Gladys Loewen

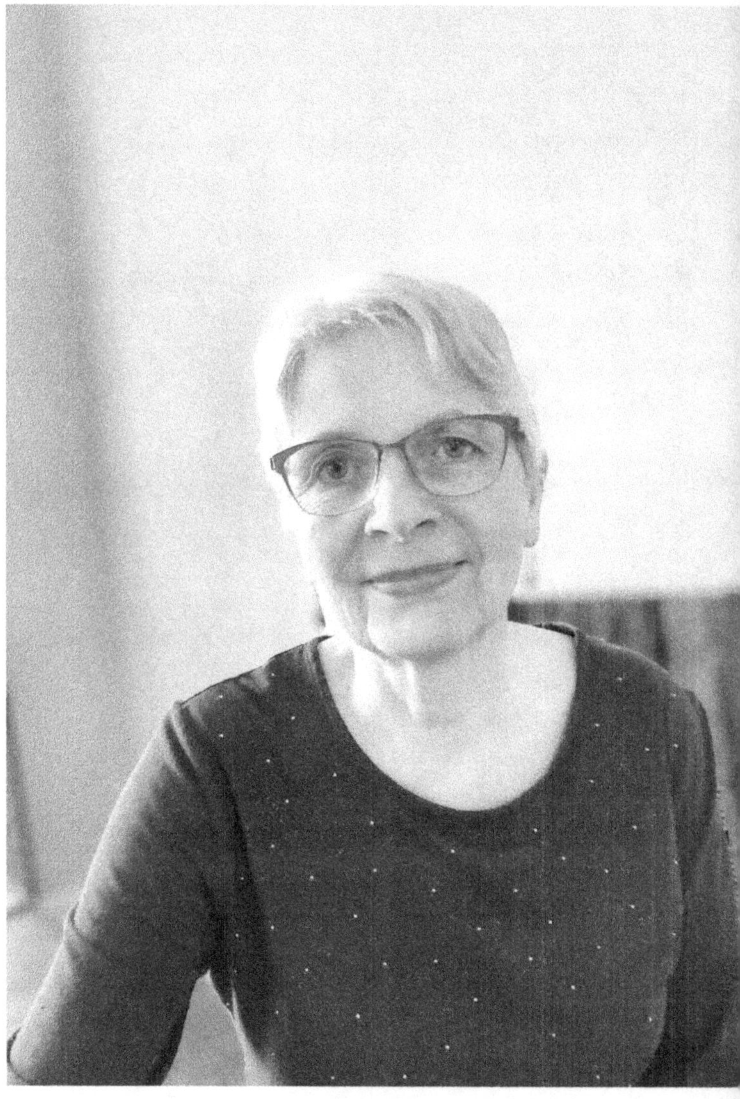

It is so common to be asked, "What do you do?" as an identifier in social conversations that I wondered how I would transition to retirement without my professional identity in hand. Surprisingly, retirement offered me a path of "rewirement" where multiple learning opportunities and challenges abound.

This path has concentrated on health, taking classes, and volunteer opportunities. Physiotherapy and Pilates facilitated my transition from using a cane to walking independently; from lifting two pounds to lifting my grandchildren as infants. With greater mobility, I can indulge my love of travel and culture which has included trips to Siberia where my mother was born, Colombia where we lived as children, and the Marquesas Islands for an adventure. I sing in a community choir, revisiting my lifelong love of music, treasuring the connection of that shared, musical experience.

Through volunteer work in Guatemala for a charitable organization, I am a "madrina" (godmother) to three Mayan students whose educational fees my husband and I underwrite. I offer reading glasses to women who can no longer thread a needle, a real problem as Mayan women typically clothe themselves and their daughters by sewing their huipiles (blouses) from their hand-woven textiles. When they successfully thread a needle, their faces glow with excitement, knowing they can still sew and embroider.

Returning to my Mennonite sewing roots, I take quilting classes, making quilts for my grandchildren, teaching them sewing skills. Quilting has led me to an international quilting project where, using two red XXs, people commemorate each of the 70,273 disabled people gassed by the Nazis in 1940-1941. I made quilts for the project, introduced others to it, and currently coordinate six volunteers doing data entry to document 2260 quilters and crafters from around the world who participated in making 860 quilts. As a consultant, I offer training on reframing disability to create inclusive environments in higher education, guided by principles of social justice and diversity. My former career provided the springboard for this avenue of training.

Hence, today when you ask me, "what do you do?" I have the pleasure of deciding which of my rewirement identities I want to share with you. Being open to opportunities allows me to define who I am.

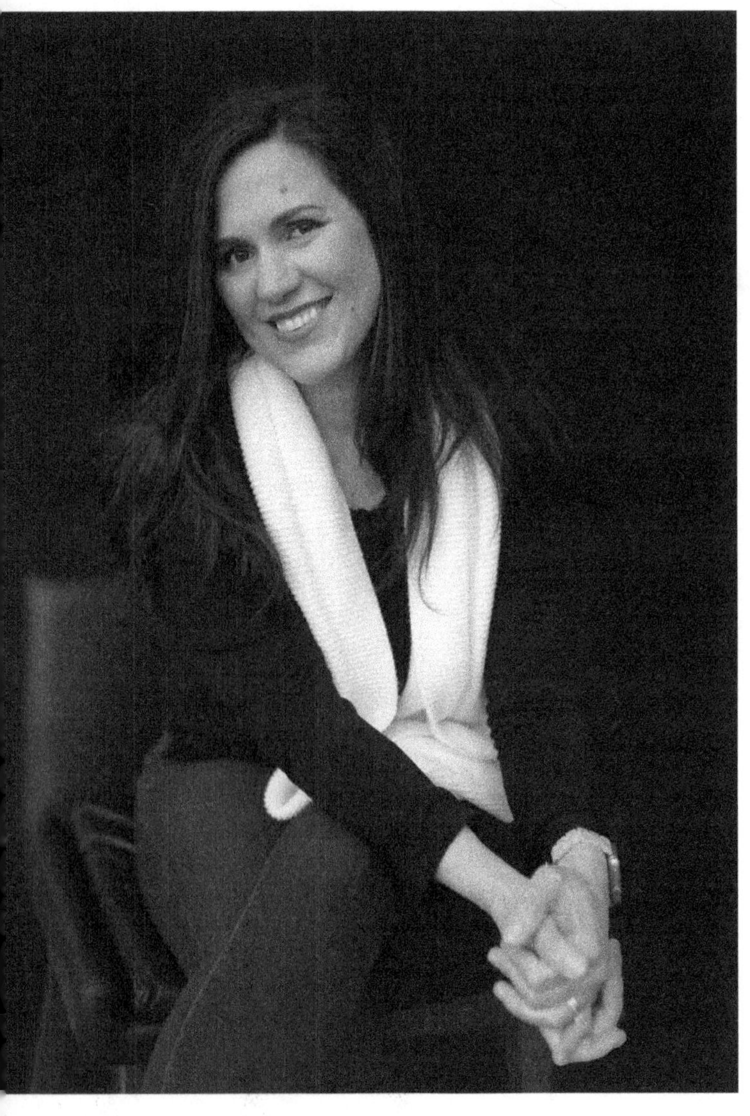

Danielle is the top-performing Realtor® in her market, mother of a hilarious and witty 4-year-old, one half of a dynamic duo, and living her best life, with gratitude, in the glorious Coastal Mountains of BC.

Danielle Menzel

From a young age, I had big plans, big dreams. I was going to leave my mark on the world! I wanted to be a lot of things; a veterinarian, an environmental lawyer, a sociologist, an activist, maybe a politician... but "real estate agent" was never on my list.

I did not identify with the stereotypical agents you saw on TV. You know the ones; the sleazy salesman, the high-rolling agents on reality shows, or the made for tv movie variety, shallow, part-time agent/bored housewife. So, when I fell into the profession by chance, it took me a long time to come to terms with the difference between how pop culture portrayed people in my profession and reality. Let's be honest, I still cringe a little when someone introduces me as a real estate agent - knowing that the stereotypes exist, and some people still believe them.

I have always been a people person. I wear my heart on my sleeve, I am not particularly thick-skinned, and I care a little too deeply what others think. I am not financially driven. I hate small talk, and I love learning what truly makes a person tick. Reflecting on this makes me realize why this career is such a natural fit. I become invested in my clients' outcomes early on. I love to help people. My clients' goals are practically as important to me as they are to them, and this requires no effort on my part - it is simply how I am wired.

So, here I am leaving my mark; not in the big ways I anticipated, but in important ways, nonetheless. Sometimes all it takes is a shift of perspective to realize that the little things have a large and cascading effect on other individuals and their future. You can have a meaningful impact on others' lives and the world in ways you could not have predicted, and it does not always have to be grand gestures. Often the seemingly insignificant and mundane has the most influence. A huge step out of my comfort zone landed me in a career that has been more rewarding than I could have imagined.

Mélanie Bernard is an entrepreneur, teacher, mother, total hype woman, and co-owner of MINI TIPI.

Mélanie Bernard

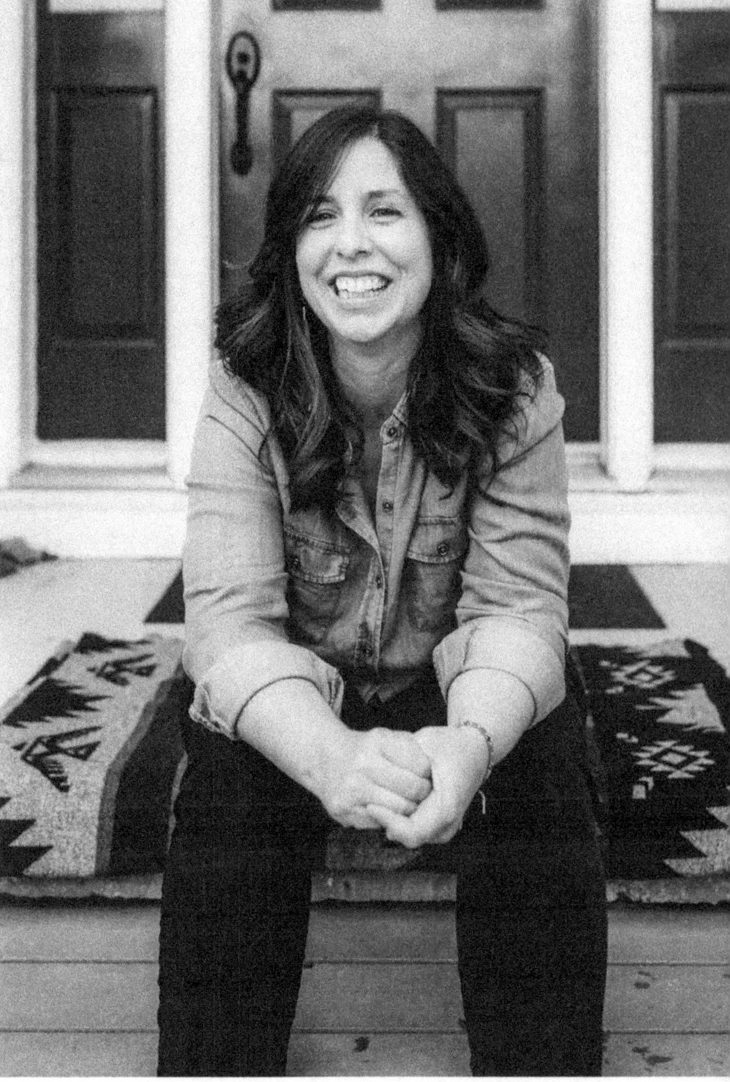
Photo Credit: Wild Dawn Photography Crystal Dawn Cook

My dream started while I was a stay-at-home mom. I worked on my passions at night while my kids were sleeping. Now I work full-time doing what I love. I've seen our business grow, and I get to hire other incredible women who have a similar vision as mine. Being able to show my children and community that they can follow their dreams like I followed mine is so important to me.

On tough days, I wake up remembering that I have created my dream job. Every day I get to work with incredible people I admire, and my work makes a difference in my community. There's nothing more motivating than that!

Things do get overwhelming as a business owner. One thing I say when failure happens is: "no one is going to die." It helps the perfectionist in me stay resilient. It puts things in perspective and motivates me to look forward and face challenges with an open heart and courage.

I believe curiosity is the spice of life. There is always something new to learn. What I love about being an entrepreneur is getting involved on multiple levels. You get to learn new skills, sometimes in a painful way! Knowing I am a lifelong learner keeps me hungry for success and pushes me forward. The phrase the more you know, the less you fear, reminds me to stay curious and motivates me in my pursuit of knowledge.

I have learned that everyone looks like they are pros at what they do. But they all started somewhere, trying to figure it all out, having both successes and failures. We are all messy and complicated and just trying to figure it all out. Don't let the fear of imperfection stop you from trying something.

When I hit roadblocks during my journey, I remember to lean on my village, my community. I am inspired by every single woman in my life, each with a different set of skills and knowledge. Together, we empower and mentor each other.

Gandhi said, 'Be the change you wish to see in the world.' All of our actions, small or big, have an impact on the world we live in. Let's try to make this world a better place.

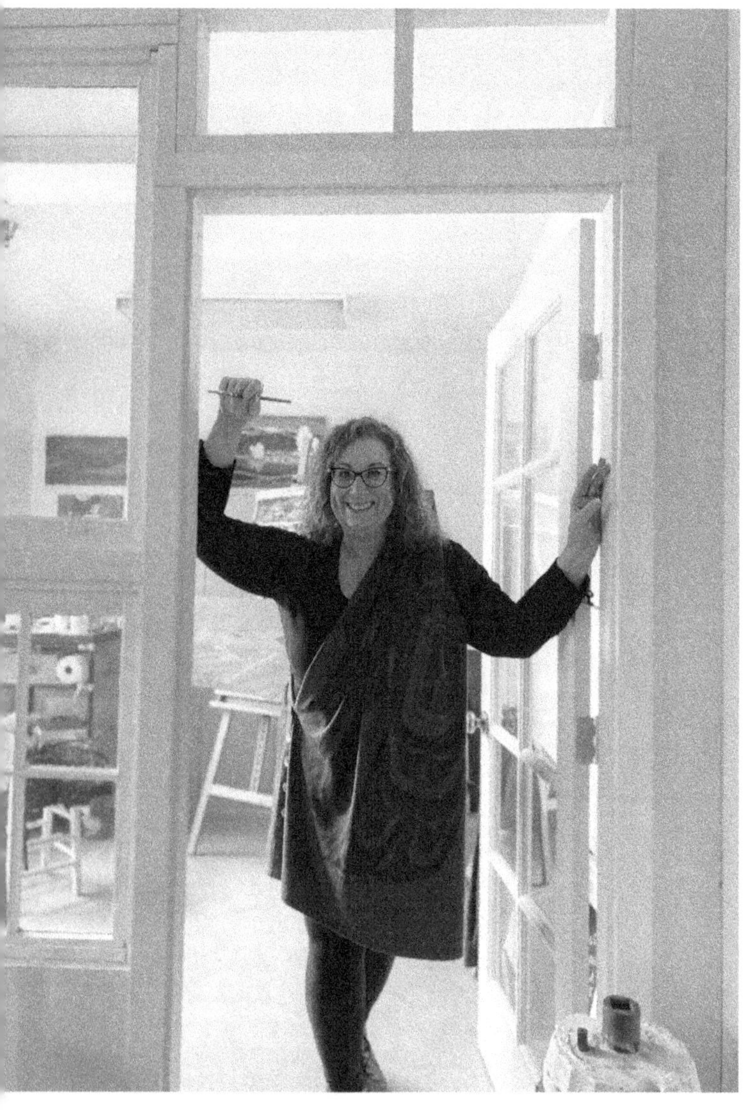

Susan Greig is an indigenous artist and entrepreneur, who finds the silver lining in difficult circumstances.

Susan L. Greig

I walked out of the therapist's office stunned that I'd been diagnosed with PTSD. I'd seen a young girl at my workplace, BC Children's Hospital, that looked like my daughter, who had passed away eight years prior. After three months, it became clear that going back to work in that environment was not going to be possible.

My "bucket list" number 239, "Quit my job to paint and write full time," stared me in the face. It was a long-off retirement goal, but I asked myself, if I wasn't afraid to fail, what would I do? Less than a year later the doors opened on my creation, the largest art studio outside of Vancouver proper, 100 Braid St Art Studios & Gallery.

With expansion over six years, the business grew to occupy 12,000sq feet with 46 art studios, a thriving arts community for the neighbourhood with many events. After five years of running the business, I realized I'd gotten distracted and "busy" with little to no time to paint. Then COVID hit. Then I got notice that the building we were located in would be torn down within six months.

The realization that almost everything physical that I'd built was going to be gone took a few months to absorb. It was not an easy time, but I always remember the quote, "Not every storm comes to destroy... some come to clear a path". In the two months after I walked away from the building, I began to see very clearly how things really were working out for the best-the timing, the logistics, everything. I then had a second opportunity to ask, "what would I do if I wasn't afraid to fail?"

The answer was to continue in business and to be the architect of my own life, a little older and a little bit wiser.

Today I am rebuilding my business but in such a way that I am able to paint every day and do what really feeds my soul.

Life often gives us silver linings in difficult circumstances, but it is up to us to see them, be grateful for the lessons given and move towards the life that is our purpose.

Chelsea Cooper is a lawyer with an entrepreneurial spirit

Chelsea Cooper, J.D.

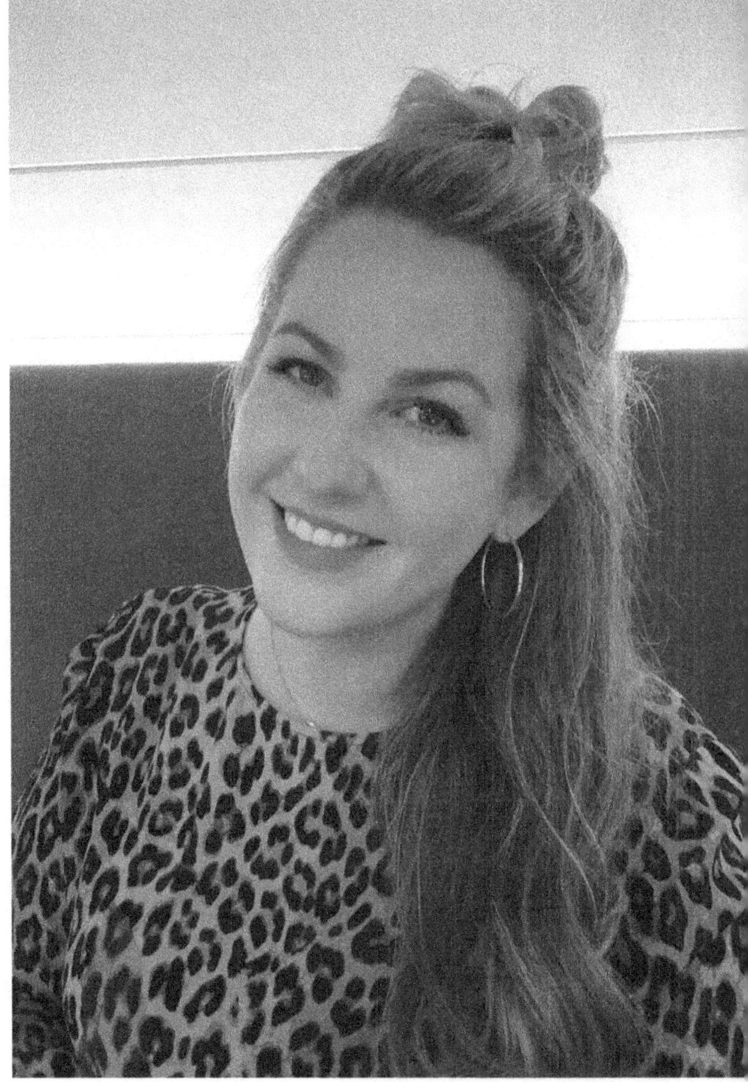

As cliché as it sounds, like a true child of the '90s, the inspiration for my journey to become a lawyer was Reese Witherspoon's portrayal of Elle Woods in Legally Blonde. What I didn't expect, twenty years later, was that my own entrepreneurial journey, and my personal growth as a woman in this world, would be shaped by many of the lessons from the 2000s teen classic.

I didn't expect that now, just as then, people would still judge me by my appearance and/or sex. In my first week of law school, a classmate called our group of friends "the airheads". I spent most of my four years there trying tirelessly to prove my intelligence, my work ethic, and my worth; ultimately learning the only opinion that truly matters is your opinion of yourself.

I didn't expect to constantly struggle with men telling me what I was and wasn't capable of; from the law professor who said he held my future in his hands, to the man who said I couldn't make it without him, to the countless colleagues who said my success was going to be temporary. Though I am lucky to also have wonderful men in my life who support my entrepreneurial side, through all of the resistance, the failures, and the lessons, the one constant has been, "You must always have faith in yourself."

Finally, and perhaps the most pleasantly surprising lesson after all this time, is seeing the power of friendship and community. The entrepreneurial journey can be incredibly challenging, and sometimes, I feel lost in the process. Although I am still at the early stages, I have found that great businesses are not built alone, instead, they are built with the support of those who are there for the good, the bad, and the complicated.

Much has changed in twenty years for women, most particularly recently. It feels fitting to end with a quote from Hillary Clinton, "Women are the largest untapped reservoir of talent in the world." I celebrate those women (both real and imagined) who have paved the way for leaders such as myself and accept the duty to do the same for future generations.

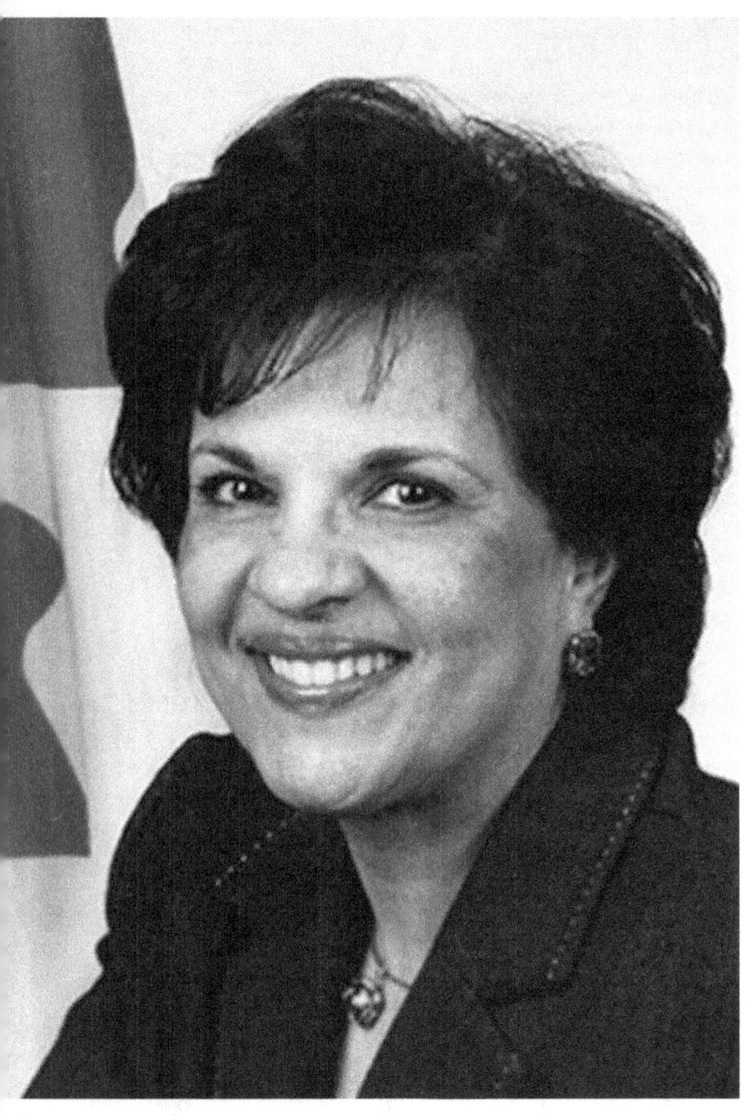

The Honourable Senator Mobina Jaffer is the first Muslim senator, the first African-born senator, and the first senator of South Asian descent. She is also the first woman of South Asian descent to practice law in Canada. Senator Jaffer has dedicated her career, both as a lawyer and a Senator, to fighting for those who are most vulnerable.

Senator Mobina Jaffer

Since I was a young girl I was always taught that the true measure of success is not what I have achieved but what I have helped others to achieve and this continues to motivate me both personally and professionally.

I grew up in a time where women were expected to assume roles within the household. Both of my parents always encouraged me to pursue my dreams. They afforded the same opportunities to their daughters as they did their son and without them I would not bewhere I am today. They built a strong foundation for me.

While I have worked incredibly hard to advance my career, I certainly did not get where I am today without the help of others. When I first started practicing law in British Columbia, many times when I went to court I was mistaken for the interpreter or the accused because at that it was unfathomable that someone who looked like me would be a lawyer. I remember how grateful I was to my mentor The Honourable Thomas Dohm for coming to court with me to sit there and support me so I knew I was not alone. He removed many barriers for me.

The Right Honorable Jean Chretien former Prime Minister of Canada appointed me to the Senate Canada. I was the first Muslim Senator and I arrived to the Senate just one week after 9/11. This was an incredibly difficult time for Muslims in Canada but Prime Minister Chretien and many of my honourable colleagues went out of their way to welcome me to the role. He removed many barriers for me.

As a Canadian Parliamentarian and legislator, I remain focused on eliminating barriers that still exist for women and racialized people in Canada the same way so many individuals did for me throughout my career.

Linda Mackie is an award-winning brand and lifestyle photographer, makeup artist, creative producer, and vlog series host of The Eloquent Entrepreneur, highlighting inspiring entrepreneurs and changemakers. Linda's journey as a visual artist began with her profound love of all living things, passion for the creative arts, and lifelong desire to make a difference in the world and inspire others to do the same.

Linda Mackie

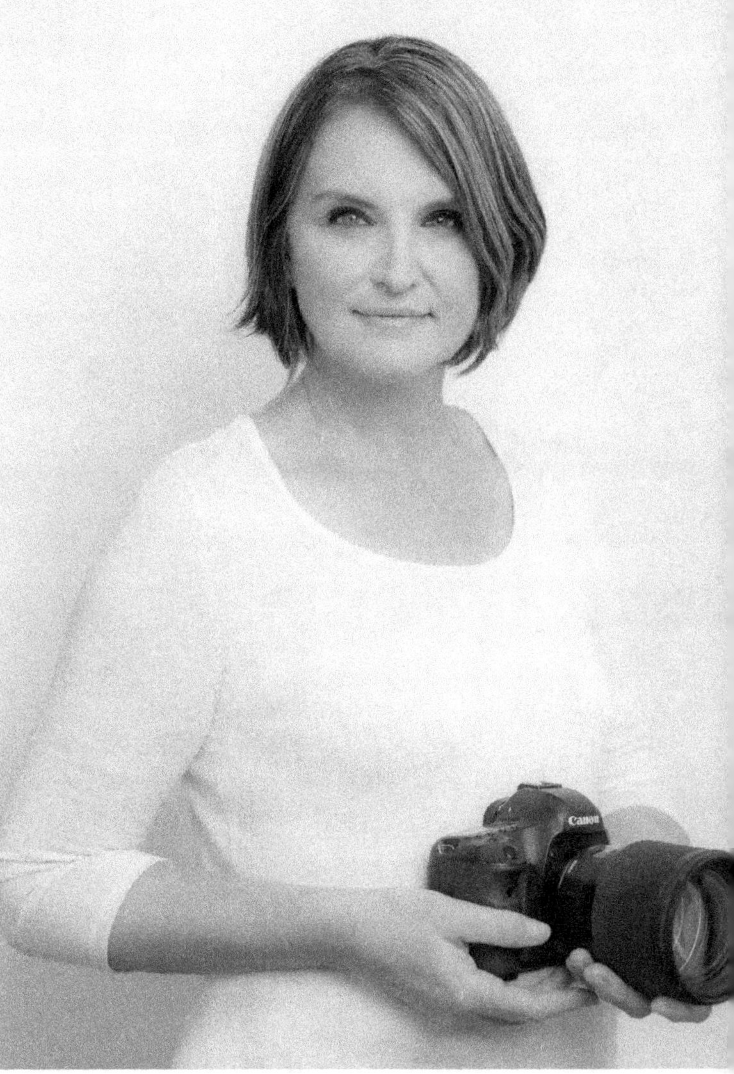

Photo Credit: Linda Mackie Creative

It was a subtle yet pivotal moment that would set me on my quest for purpose and self-expression. I watched intently as a herd of antelopes leaped gracefully across the huge screen at Expo '86. Already a sensitive teen, I wept in awe at the vastness of the universe and the incredible beauty that lies in the mystery of our little blue planet. It dawned on me just how tiny we are in the grand scheme of things and how everything is so interconnected. One thing became clear: I would somehow make a difference for animals, and this moment of wonder was the spark that ignited the creative fire in me.

Becoming a photographer was the next major step in my journey. I discovered I had a gift that allowed my subjects to shine through in their portraits. Watching them blossom in front of my lens as I captured their spirit and personality, was empowering and enlightening. This crazy symbiotic connection of energy between us became the magical ingredient that allowed me to express myself as an artist and, in turn, help my clients stand out in their own passions.

As my business grew, I realized I needed to come out from behind my camera and share my voice with more clarity and conviction without dampening my compassionate heart. I discovered my gentle and empathic nature is actually my superpower and I can not only use it to create my art, but also empower other highly sensitive creative entrepreneurs.

My "why" and ultimate purpose has strengthened since becoming a mom with an ever-evolving ability to embrace my power, express myself more fully and share my knowledge and expertise with other creatives like me in their journeys while continuing to create work I'm proud of and inspire others along the way.

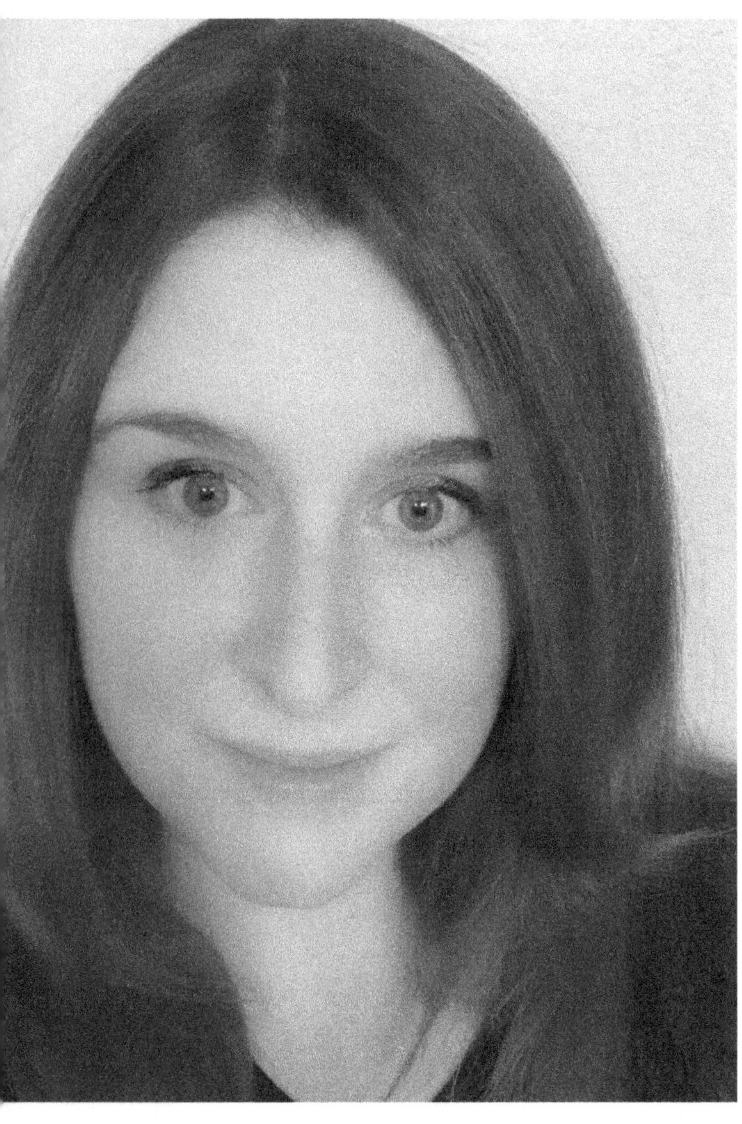

Alisha Schilbe reflects on the village, the scale, and the pandemic.

Alisha Schilbe

Long-held wisdom has stated that it takes a village to raise a child, but what happens when you lose the village? When COVID hit, I had a three-month-old and a four-year-old. I was also in the middle of what was supposed to be the final semester of my bachelor's degree. Just when I needed my village the most, I lost it, just like hundreds of millions of women around the world. As moms, we put so much pressure on ourselves to be everything, be everywhere, and do everything. Even on the best day, the balancing act that is our lives is precarious, and one small misstep can knock the entire thing askew for days or even weeks.

So, can you imagine how it has felt for us, as mothers, to not just have the balance tipped, but to have the entire scale tossed into the air; pieces of our carefully organized lives scattering as we frantically try to keep it all together. Every mother I know has this feeling right now. Some of us just let the less important things fall and focused on those that really mattered. For nearly a year now, we have been in what so many of the other mothers that I know have described as "survival mode," one more minute, one more hour, one more day. Some of us were able to move out of survival mode over the summer as cases dropped. We could go to parks or beaches, see some family and friends safely again, we got a small bit of normalcy. Now we are back in lockdown, back to the scale being tossed in the air, and once again we are all in survival mode.

Now we have to be everything for everyone, all at once, and every single day, we feel like we are failing. Last March, we dropped everything we could to be with our children, and to keep them safe. We put careers, school, hobbies, and everything else on hold to be there. We worked while trying to be teachers and parents because that's what moms do. With, or without our village, we just keep going, but we are exhausted, and we ask that anyone reading this just please remember that.

Maria Velve is a makeup artist, green beauty expert, and mom of two with a service-based and product-based business. She focuses on helping women transition to green, non-toxic beauty products while supporting clean, Canadian, female-owned brands. Maria is passionate about teaching women not only how to look good but also how to feel good about what they put on their skin.

Maria Velve

I have pushed boundaries my whole life. Whether it was my curfew when I was a teen or crossing Russia with a backpack by train in the middle of winter, I have quite a list of interesting experiences from around the world. My belief about life has always been that it should be experienced to its fullest. I truly believe that there are no limits, except the limits I set for myself.

From surviving the Thailand tsunami floating in a ferry boat to going back to university at nine months pregnant to start my master's program, I took all challenges head-on, never faltering. But of all the challenges, nothing could have prepared me for motherhood. It is hands-down the toughest experience I've ever had to live through.

The hardest part of it all and one that no one prepares you for is breaking up with yourself. Ending the long-term relationship with the person that you have become up to the point when you decide to become a mother. If you are an adventurous free-spirit like me, you know what I'm talking about. The free bird that was me had to be caged. Life wasn't about her anymore. After my first son was born, I sat idly on the sofa for months counting the minutes when he would wake from his nap. I went days without showering. I lived on coffee and chocolate. If I was depressed, I didn't know it. But a little spark inside me told me I wanted more than feedings and diapers. That this wasn't it for me. I loved my baby, but it became apparent that I had to save myself first in order to be a good mom to him.

The last eight years have been about finding balance and I continue to grow both as a mother and a woman. My boys are now eight and six, and I dream of the day that they'll be able to carry their own big packs and join their adventurous mom on a trip to Southeast Asia.

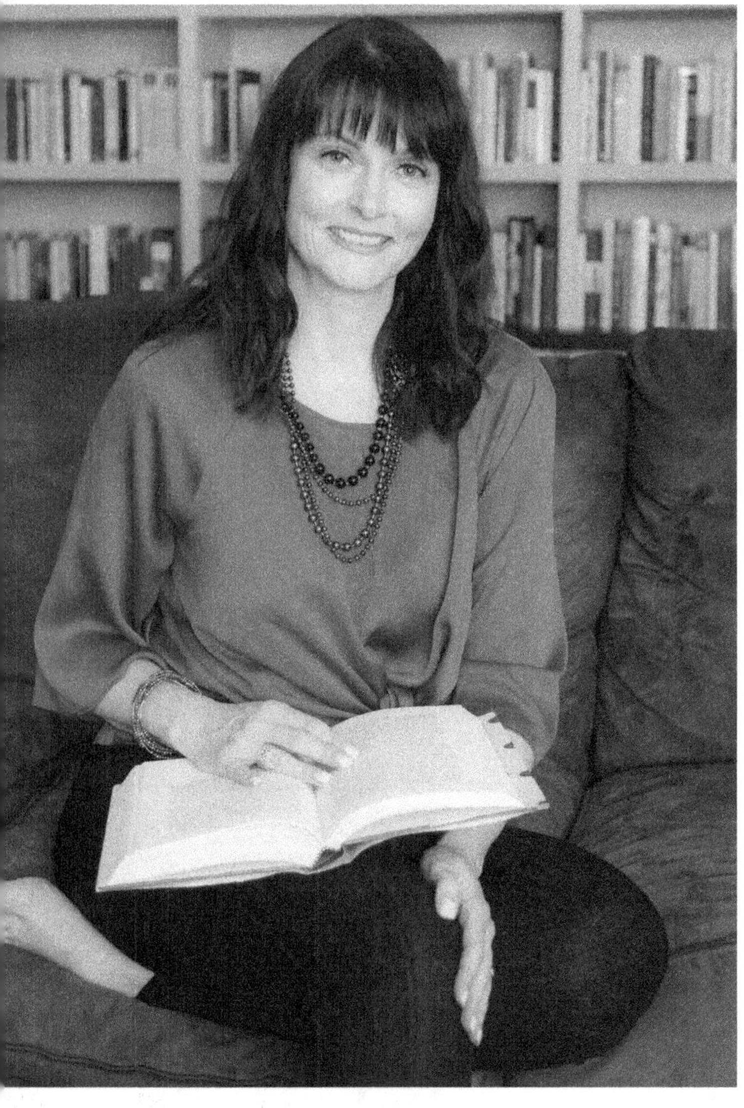

Victoria Theriault helps individuals and teams find their strengths through the conduit of behavioural profiling.

Victoria Theriault

I love what I do. I haven't always been able to say that though. While I've spent most of my life intrigued with what motivates human behaviour, I didn't listen closely to my inner voice and I took a rather circuitous route along my career path.

"It is never too late to be what you might have been" - George Eliot.

There are several reasons why the quote above is one of my favourites. First, the independent female perspective. George Eliot was a pen name for Mary Ann Evans, a writer in the Victorian era. She wanted her work to be measured on its own merits rather than be judged for her gender.

Second, George Eliot is credited with being the first writer to apply psychological analysis to her characters. I share a kinship with her in exploring what makes people tick!

Third, of course, is the statement itself. It resonates strongly as it took me almost twenty years to hone in on what I wanted to do and chart my own course for happiness and success.

The best part about my work is helping others find their strengths and identifying obstacles that restrict them from achieving their goals. We are all inherently talented at something; the rub is that finding it may require us to step out of our comfort zones.

Some people find their passion early in life. For others, like me, it takes time to reveal itself. As George Eliot imparted, it's never too late! Wouldn't spending twenty, ten, or even five years of your life doing fulfilling work be better than spending a lifetime of mediocrity and wondering what if?

I'm not a risk-taker, so launching my own business was a terrifying prospect. However, my inner voice was no longer whispering to me, it was screaming! What began as a spark of interest was fully ignited and when I recognized that the feeling wasn't complete fear, but mostly exhilaration, I knew what I had to do. It hasn't always been easy, but it has been intentional, purposeful, and incredibly rewarding. I've never looked back.

Curiosity about the human body drives Karen Angelucci's passion to embolden herself and clients to live, move and feel better in their body.

Karen Angelucci

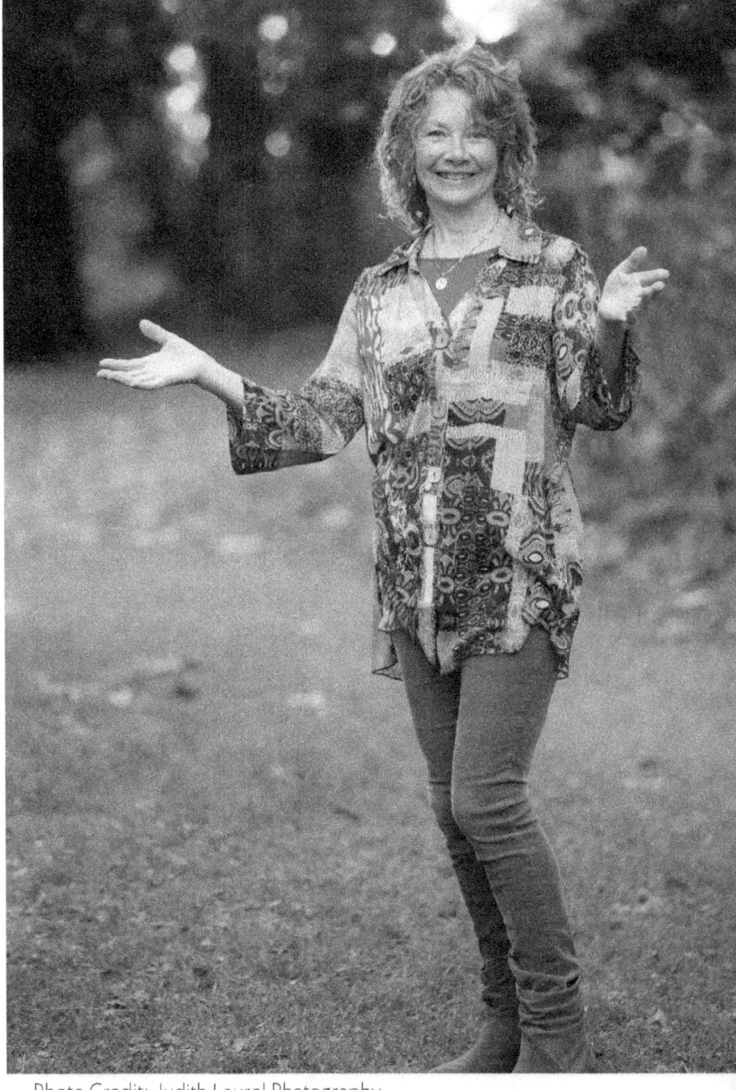
Photo Credit: Judith Laurel Photography

Control of my life, my feelings, and my sense of direction was a muddle when I was in my thirties. I pushed all the wrong buttons attempting to access my internal drive while the constant malware program of not feeling good enough ran in the background draining my energies. Adrenal fatigue and emotional eating were my habituated operating system as a single working Mom in an average paying desk job with big dreams to be my own boss.

An earlier injury along with emotional distress smacked me into conscious awareness with the four-letter word that streamed into my head, RISK. Making changes meant, I needed to risk doing things differently and I had no clue where to begin, so I thought. In fact, my body was giving me clear indicators for my direction, my health recovery, and my evolving life career, even though I didn't know it at the time because understanding my body was like interpreting a new language.

Speaking the language my body was teaching me meant starting down the path of self-discovery exploring physical pains, being curious about pent-up emotional overwhelm, and learning what my specific nutritional needs are, not eating food because someone said it was good for me.

I tend to be a DIY gal but realized my body has more to tell me than I know how to interpret. Asking for help from practitioners to open the **P**hysical, **E**motional, and **N**utritional **(PEN)** doors to my wellbeing when I need it is one of the keys I use and teach as a Health Creation Coach. The other two keys are having specific self-care skills to keep me moving and knowing personal health care requirements from various tests I've had.

At age sixty-six, I honor my body as the magical motor home that takes me on this amazing adventure of life, the navigators are the **PEN** choices I make that guide me daily. I invite you to invest in your body **PEN** health to enjoy fulfilled living at any age, you're worth it!

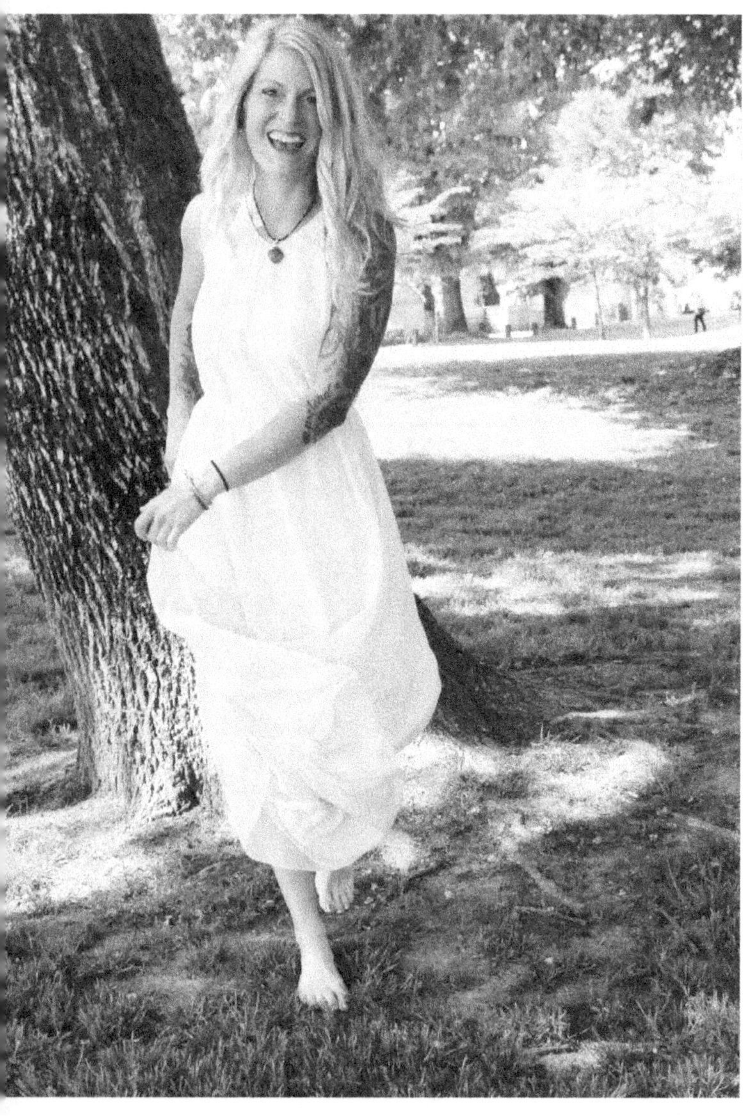

Danielle Arsenault is a Raw Food Chef and Plant-Based Educator whose deep desire is to empower women to revolutionize their health through a living, whole foods lifestyle.

Danielle Arsenault

A journey of a thousand miles starts with one step. Throughout my journey towards becoming a raw food chef and plant-based nutrition educator, I have taken many steps that have brought me to experience life-altering realizations. The one constant has been inevitable change and, as a result, immense personal growth. From a near-death rock-climbing accident to the creation of a ukulele album, learning to speak Spanish fluently, and birthing a baby, I have done the work. All from the ground up. I truly believe that the evolution of the soul through the expression of life on Earth is through change. When we resist change, we stifle our growth, our evolution. A keystone to this growth is failure. Failure is an opportunity for change. It is the portal for great transformation and ultimately awakening. Consciousness comes from the creator, from the light. I have run, walked, crawled, and dragged myself through failure towards that light. Sometimes it may look like a small dot in the distance, but eventually, that small dot becomes a sun of possibilities. Walking the entrepreneurial path, the path I chose for myself, has not been easy. In fact, it's very familiar with "failure." Time and again, it has pushed me out of my comfort zone. And it is through this discomfort, I have overcome the struggle and arrived at the most rewarding and fulfilling experiences I never thought possible. A life lesson of which I am always reminding myself - do not resist or fear failure, but rather welcome it as a teacher. Learn to roll with the punches and flow like water. Lean into it. Never give up, no matter what, and eventually, you'll arrive, feet sore yet with the ability to heal. I am worthy as I am, even amid so-called failure. Because even when you think no one is listening, you've just inspired someone immeasurably, and that makes the hustle worth it. You are worthy as you are. You are successful beyond measure already. The pursuit of happiness is letting go of the pursuit and learning to feel full in the present moment, the true wealth of life, failure, and all.

Sherry Sobey is living a fearless life that she orchestrates, with endless possibilities.

Sherry Sobey

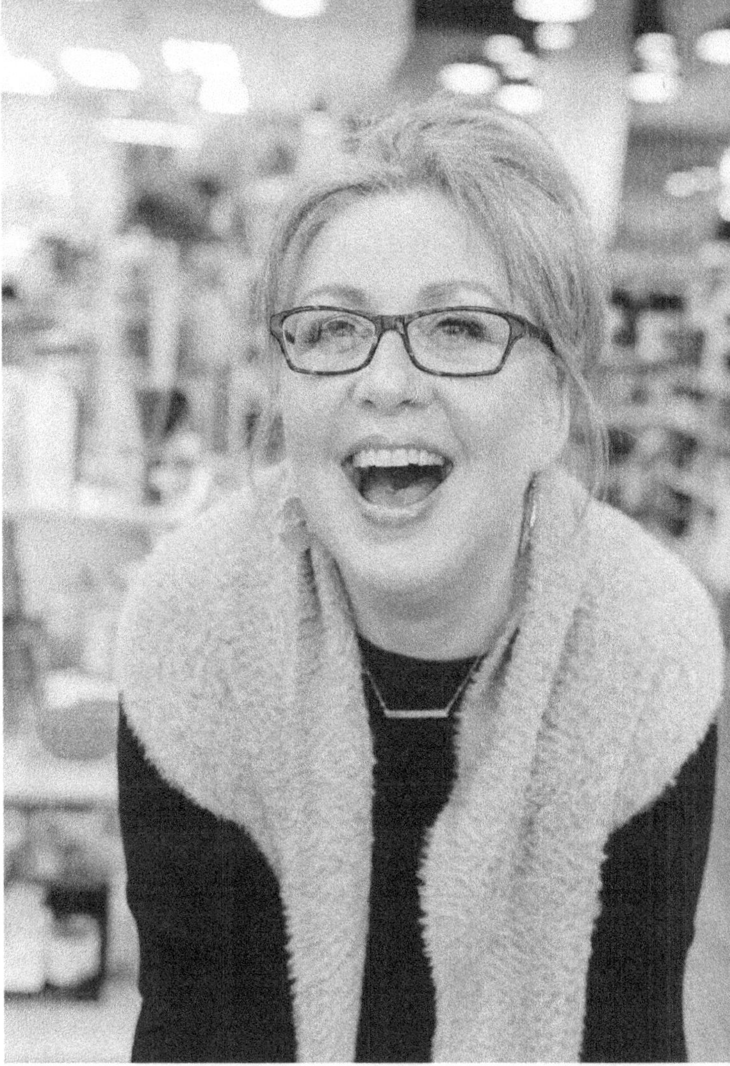
Photo Credit: lynette.photographer

I'm not that remarkable.

That was the very first thought that entered my mind when asked to participate in this project. Then I reflected on the topic, "the pursuit of happiness," and I connected there.

If you had asked me growing up what I wanted to be, I would have simply replied, "happy." It was never about a certain career, an accomplishment, or anything tangible, really. Simply to be happy was all I dreamed of. I believe having that as my focus, combined with the gift to lose myself in a meditative type of drawing from the age of seven, was what helped me survive nine years of physical, mental, and sexual abuse as a child. I was able to leave my body and find safety in that dream. It truly saved me.

I knew I was going to survive, and once I had the opportunity, I would find happiness. Asking to be taken from my family home and placing myself in care at the age of thirteen was when my real life began. It was then I experienced safety, encouragement, and genuine care from others. My confidence and belief that I was deserving started to settle inward. I never wanted to look back for fear I might hear the voices that told me I was stupid and made me feel worthless. Eventually, I became stronger than the voice, was able to face it head-on, and release the shame I held deep within, along with all the dirty secrets.

I will forever carry those bags, but the difference is, I repacked that suitcase myself and got rid of the things that didn't serve me in my pursuit. Every day I look for the good and practice gratitude for the journey thus far. I know life is not always going to be rosy, but I also know I can overcome anything!

I will rise to the challenge whenever the threat to take that happiness away appears, and most of all I know my purpose, I know myself, and I am living a fearless life that I orchestrate and believe the possibilities are endless. My head and my heart are in sync, and in that I trust.

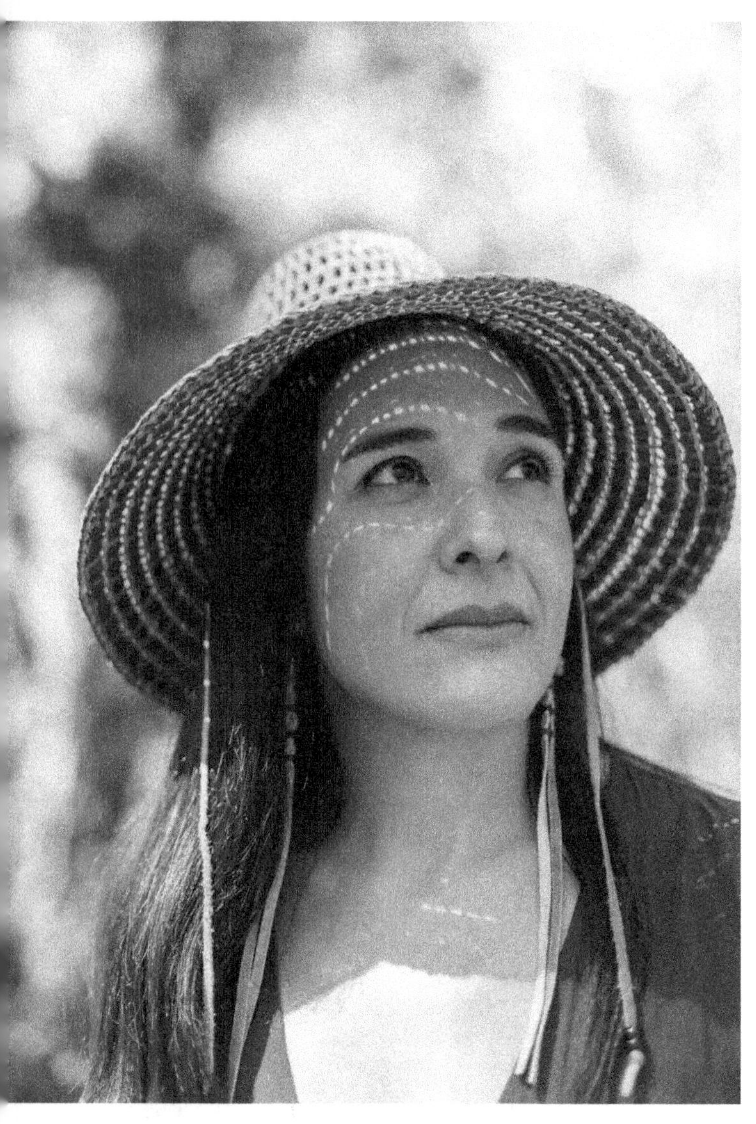

Styawat / Leigh Joseph is an ethnobotanist and the founder of skincare brand Sḵwálwen Botanicals. As a heart-centered person, she feels things deeply. This has led her to contemplate both the traumas that her Indigenous family and community have lived through as well as the resilience embodied by her ancestors. It is this awareness that inspires her work with healing and her dedication to Indigenous teachings.

Styawat Leigh Joseph

From the time I was small, I have felt most at home in the natural world. Whether playing for hours in the garden building tiny worlds amongst the flowers as a child, sitting at the edge of the ocean contemplating life as a teenager, or finding my way home to the traditional territory of my Squamish ancestors as an adult, I have always sought ways to connect to a place.

Nature inspires me, and time spent harvesting with family feeds my spirit. I feel nourished when I care for myself through plant foods and medicines. I am also a plant nerd. I love learning about plant life cycles, habitat, and identification, and my spring and summer seasons are guided by when certain plants grow leaves, bloom, or provide fruit.

This love of botany inadvertently led me on a path of cultural connection, deepening my identity as an Indigenous woman. As I grow into myself, understanding that my relationship to plants and to the land is integral to who I am, I am moved to share this knowledge in creative ways. By contributing my voice and perspectives as an Indigenous woman, I am finding ways to lean into my authority and occupy spaces where Indigenous women are still not present in large numbers such as academia and business.

Harvesting kw'enikwáy (kwa-in-i-kway), or cottonwood, each spring with my children, I can hear them quietly whisper thank you to the trees as they pick the fragrant leaf buds. This is one of my favorite experiences. Knowing that my ancestors took part in this exact harvest for thousands of years, and honoring the knowledge that these practices were stripped from my grandmother and great-grandmother's generations, it is essential to me to support the process of cultural reclamation and healing through my life's work.

It's never too late to change your path in life.

Kelly Arsenault

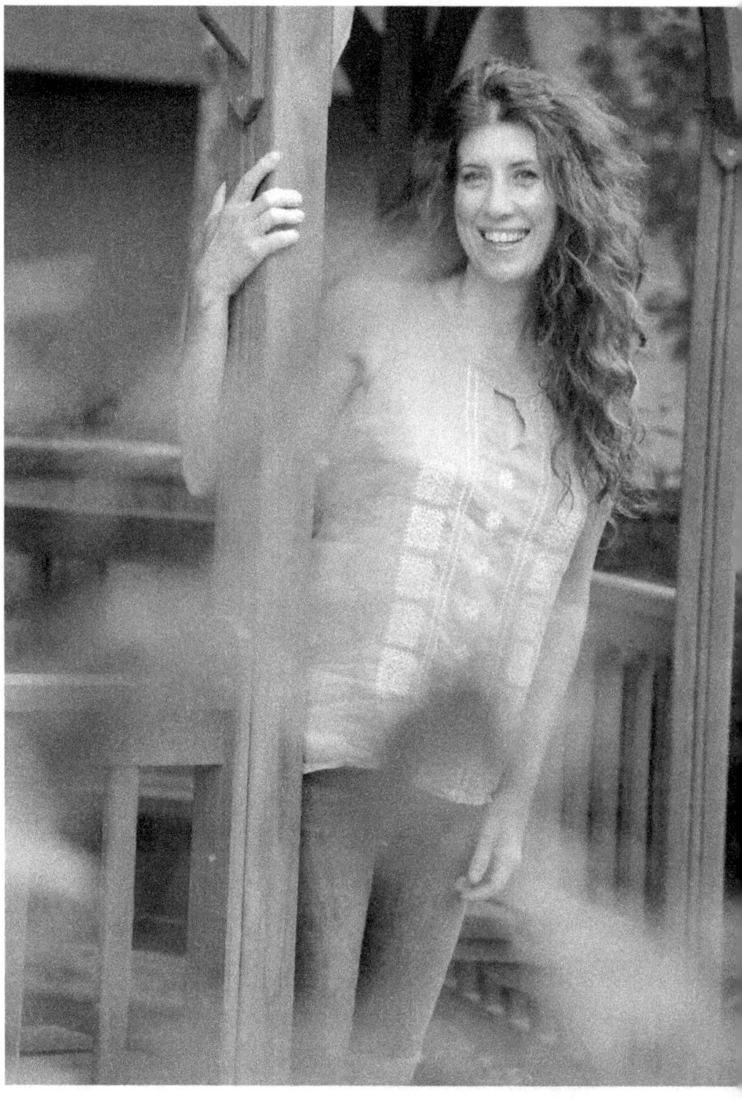

It's a theory that sounds so simple, but for me, it's taken half a lifetime to truly process. Growing up as an only child in a small town during the '70s and '80s, I never felt like I fit the typical mold as to what I "should be." We are taught as children and young adults to "go to university, get a job, have stability, save money for the future." But for me, meeting the right partner, having the perfect home, or living a life that was considered ideal was not necessarily a simple destiny. I had a desire for travel and romantic visions of how I wanted my life to be that superseded my need for stability. I established myself in a successful, exciting career that spanned two decades. I pushed away feelings of doubt and worry when I processed that I may live life alone.

In time, my career in television was on fire. I had purchased a home, and I had met someone who I thought was my forever love. It felt "normal." In time though, I realized my partner and I had very different visions of how our futures would look together, and my old childhood fear came back. Would I be alone in my later years? I didn't have children, brothers, or sisters. I had many friends, some, who are like family, to this day, but each and every one of them had someone just a little bit closer, be it a child, a sibling, or a partner. But then, my miracle happened at age forty-two. I unexpectedly became pregnant. I was going to be a mother.

The journey as a single mom hasn't always been easy, but it has been the most joyful love I have ever experienced. The growth, change, and evolution in me had beauty and inspiration to it that I sometimes struggled to see. I learned that what once felt like fear could, in fact, become a source of motivation and strength to find new paths. I'm proud to say, others around me have also fed from that growth. In middle age, I am embarking on a new career path and have found joy once again in my personal life. Life has been a journey of perfect and imperfect moments but I'm eternally grateful and excited for what is to come.

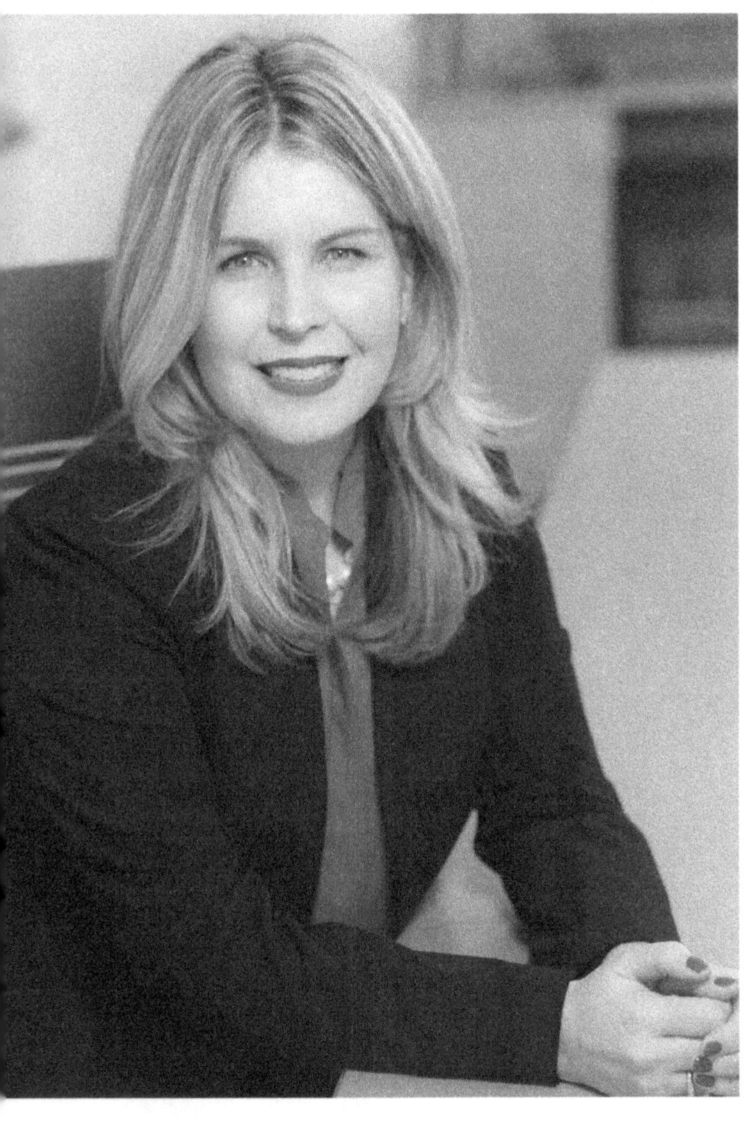

Alana Walker Carpenter is a trailblazer. She has redefined what it means to lead, what success looks like, and the gift that love, compassion, and empathy can bring to the boardroom.

Alana Walker Carpenter

There is nothing that brings happiness like the fragrance of a freshly picked bouquet – even the very first bouquet of dandelions our toddler son once picked for me. There is the happiness of getting a win at work and equally, if not more so, in seeing someone else you've mentored get that win. And, then there is the sheer bliss of connecting with an old friend.

All of these moments are beautiful.

Yet, I have found I am the happiest when I have entered into someone else's deep pain and suffering. When I'm able to sit at the bedside of someone who is terminally ill, when I am able to listen on the phone when someone can barely catch their breath through the tears of devastation from their partner's affair, or when I am able to go for a walk and listen to a heartbroken parent whose child has derailed – these experiences of offering the profound gift of friendship are where I find happiness because this is where I am able to offer hope.

I recently saw a commercial with two young guys sharing investment strategies – one had secured his first home with the other friend longingly admiring the new digs. The one friend who achieved success stated, "hope is not a strategy," but I would beg to differ. Hope is a strategy for happiness. It simply depends on where your hope comes from and if you freely offer it to others.

For me, hope comes from my Christian faith, and that is the very reason I chose to abandon my career in Corporate Canada almost twenty years ago. Consultant to Chaplain is not a typical career move. But I saw it as a solution to the masquerade of pretend happiness – one I was all too familiar with on Bay St.

During the pandemic, a number of people have been soul searching, asking life's new questions, taking the pause they have never been able to take. There is a common theme of restlessness from wanting to find where one's purpose and hope comes from – essentially where one's happiness comes from.

No matter what one's circumstance there is always hope.

Where is your hope?

Nahla Hopfe has impacted the lives of many! She is an entrepreneur, people connector and leader who creates and builds community. She served as a board member on many committees, including being a Vice President and Youth Chair for many years at Douglas Park community centre. Nahla is also a recipient of the City of Vancouver Volunteer of the Year award.

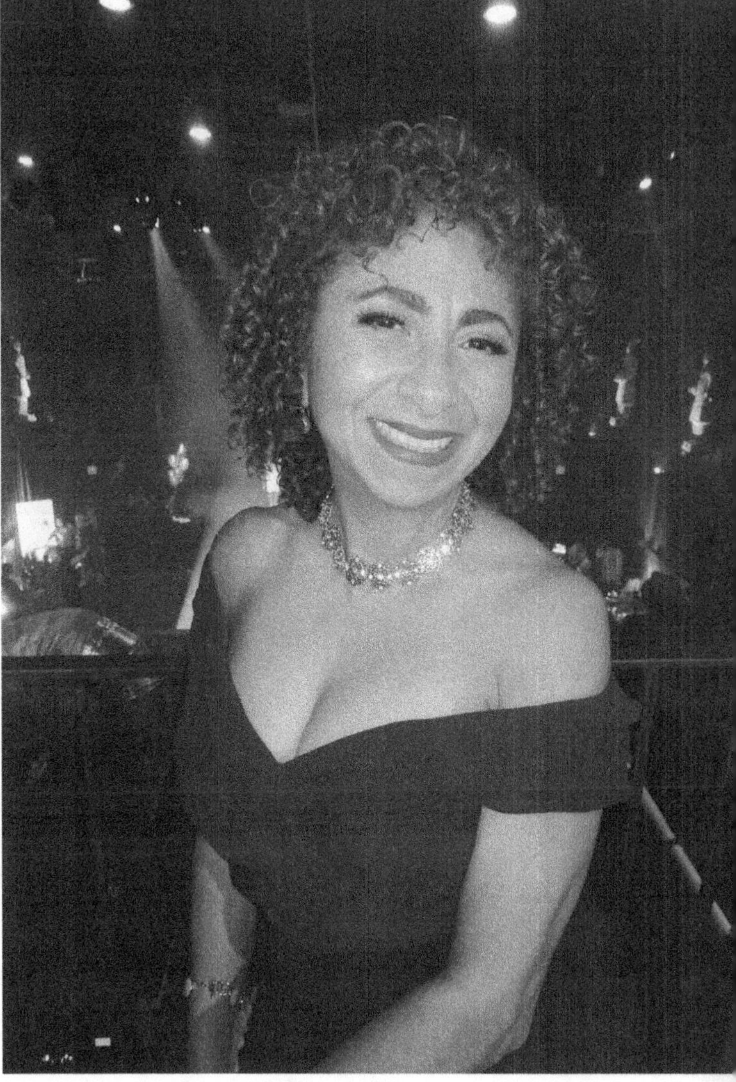

Nahla Hopfe

After earning my business degree, and finding success in the corporate world, my heart led me to a different path. With my passion for building community and advocacy for equality and multicultural diversity, I found incredible joy in supporting children and empowering youths. To achieve these endeavors, I was passionately drawn to the fulfillment of coordinating community, art, and fashion events as well as successfully fundraising for many causes.

As a firm believer in continuous learning, I returned to school to study education. This ultimately led me to my current career as a behavioural interventionist supporting children, youths, and families dealing with autism. I learn so much from every student and have taken the approach of building on their strengths. This validates my philosophy in life - turn adversity and challenges into opportunities and strengths. As Helen Keller said, "Optimism is the faith that leads to achievement." I am presently writing a children's book about autism.

Working with children has taught me to slow down and view the world from their eyes with genuine curiosity and enthusiasm and finding wonder in the smallest things. Children and youth are our future, and mentoring, coaching, and empowering them is building our communities and a better world. As a youth coach, the feeling is beyond magical when I empower and involve youths in an event or a project, and they, in turn, become confident to become leaders and engage others to do the same. The ripple effect is immense!

I believe in living life to the fullest and cherishing every moment where the power of nature recharges me and feeds my soul. I don't let the rain stop me, instead, I'll dance in the rain and encourage others to join me. I smile at strangers and always aim to have a positive impact on people's lives on a daily basis. I don't wait for solutions or change to happen, I create change.

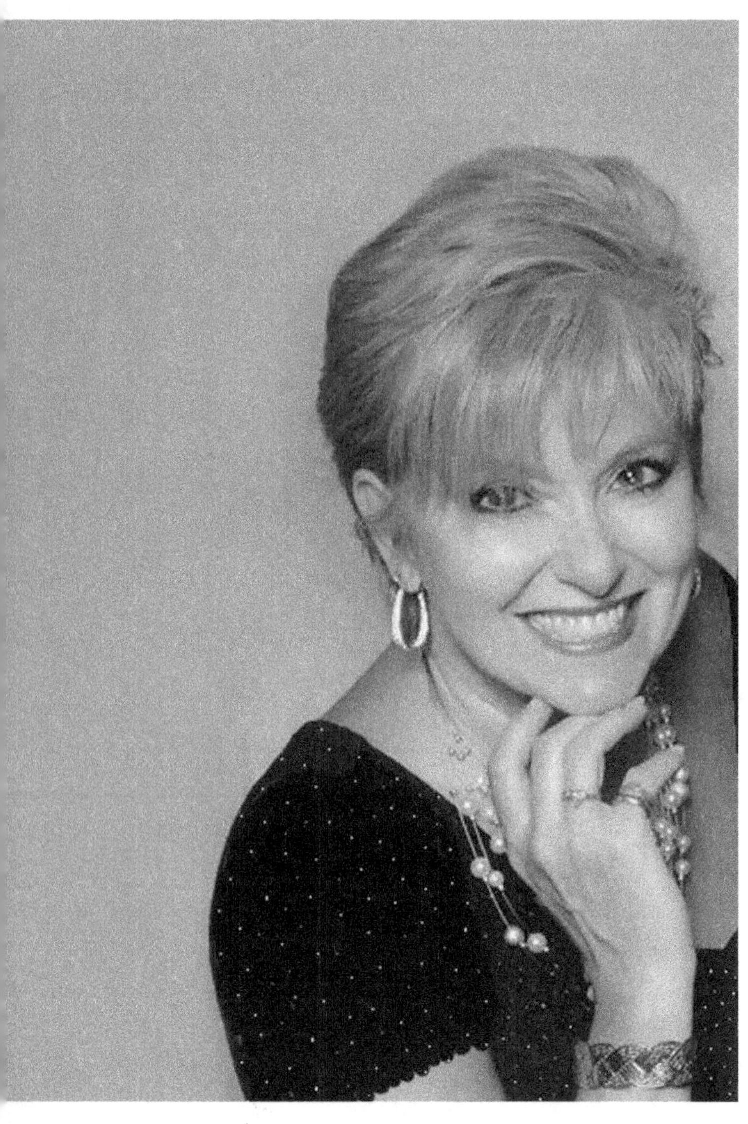

Deborah Lohrenz is the owner of 2Motiv8U, and an entrepreneur working as a Life/Career Coach, Human Resources Professional, and Professional Trainer/ Facilitator.

Deb Lohrenz

For years, I struggled with the meaning of success and my purpose in life. When I look back, my life ended before my teenage years; and I began living in my mid-40s. Abuse, in its many forms, happens, and when I became the object of my father's sickness, my life became one of survival – a different form of living. Not only my day-to-day but also my moment-to-moment was figuring out how to stop this monster from "having his way" with me or destroying me, as he put it. I didn't want this life, but when my father handed me a bottle of pills and said to me, "take these, the world would be better off without you because you are stupid, ugly, and a waste of a human," I did – I was 16. Fortunately, my mom walked in and rushed me to the Emergency Room. After pumping my stomach, I heard a voice saying I was worth something and I needed to be strong! Although it took several more years, I finally moved out of that situation and house and moved on.

Well, that is what I thought. But I was wrong. I became obsessed with doing the "right thing" and "being good," and still, I felt I was not living. I began working with victims and became a life coach, and still, I struggled. I listened to people telling me to move on and that I needed to forgive and forget and even write a letter to my dad saying I forgave him. I did write a letter! It didn't work! When I realized forgetting would never happen, and forgiving didn't take away the pain and memories, I decided to embrace who I was now and who I have become – on my terms!

I realized I like who I am and am proud of the person I became. My purpose in life is to help people - including myself. Even though the emotions still overwhelm me from time to time, I take a step back and take a hard look in the mirror and realize I survived! I achieved my success, living and loving my life, and I am proud of my accomplishments – personally, emotionally, and professionally!

It's not the path of resistance, rather the path of true fulfillment within your own identity, no matter what arises in life, creating a steady balance between tranquility and expansion daily in my new existence.

Stephanie Barnes

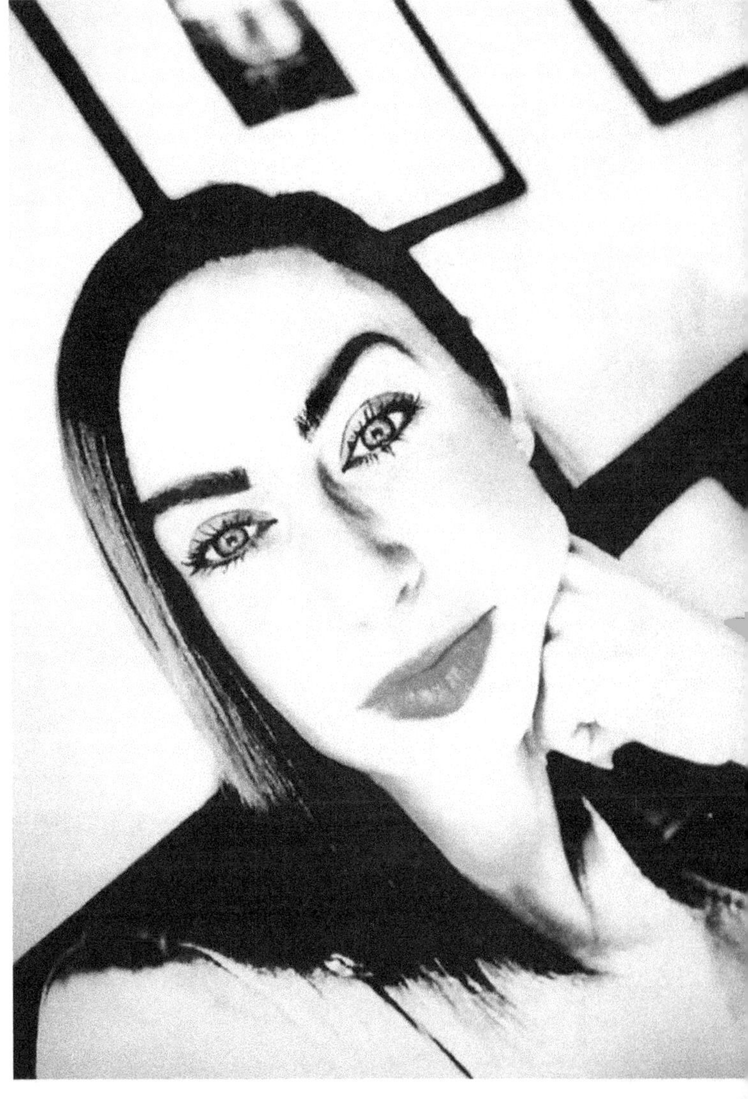

I awoke out of ICU at thirty-three; a true gift of a "life - after death." My marriage had been over for years to me, my interior design business office staff were now working without me there, down to 93 lbs, hair falling out, and the list goes on. I felt that I was a shadow, standing there alone, that no one else understood, as hard as they tried.

Working with the top neurologists and epileptologists in Canada, they found three intertwined brain tumors in areas of the temporal lobe. That area of the brain where they are located operates cognitive functions speech, reading, thinking words, and memory.

I had a rushed craniotomy brain surgery. During this process, I had three strokes. I remember they asked me to move my right leg and I wasn't moving anything on that side of my body. I came out of ICU with a partially shaved head, areas of my brain removed, the right side of my face drooping, hardly any mobility, memory, or speech. I didn't even know my dogs' names anymore. I knew something had changed while lying in the hospital wondering if I would recover. But I believed.

It was a spiritual awakening. Five and a half years of recovery learning to walk, talk, write, and basic functionality in a new way I never could have imagined even if I saw it. I have newfound gratitude in my life. Today I am healed in a new light. Running, training hard, incredible international design work, and I do remember the dog's name now! From the minute my feet touch the ground in the morning, I thank the Universe for my presence. I never gave up. It is possible that I still forget things or take moments to grasp a word; years of memories are probably gone for good, but I am here, and I have no sadness on that front. None.

Today I am single, spiritually grounded, and happier than I ever imagined. I work on incredible design projects around the world, train daily, eat clean and live minimally. This is my path and mine alone. I know my worth, my boundaries, and I'm making it all happen.

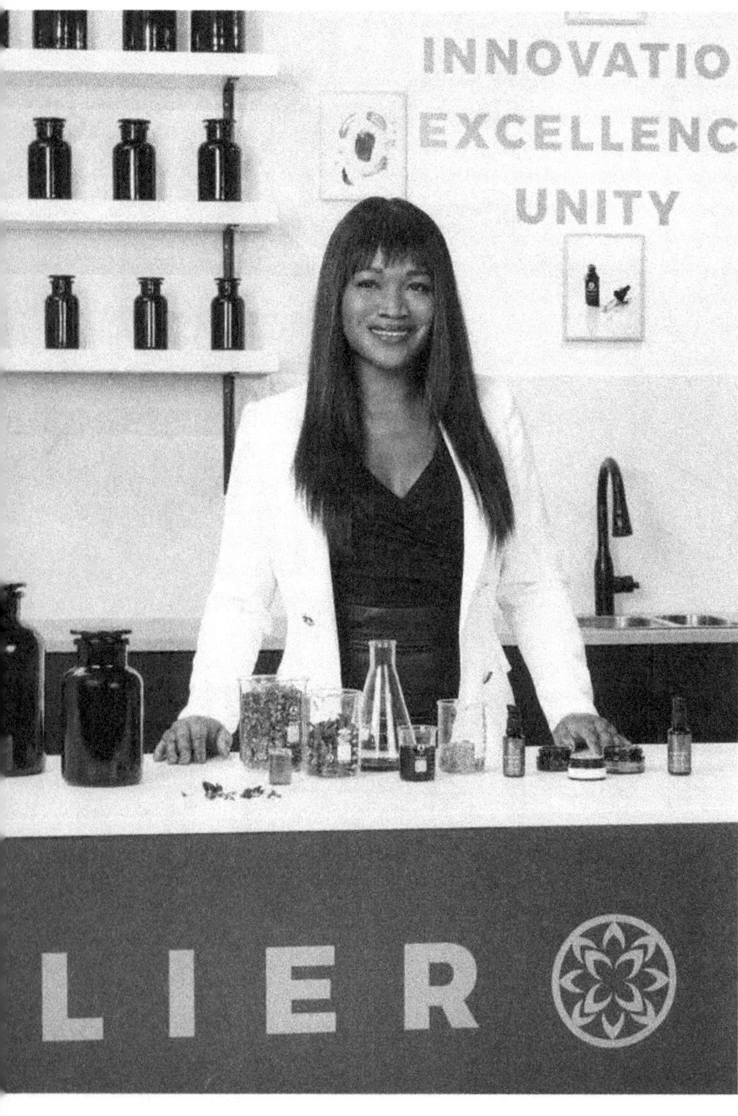

Oyéta Kokoroko is the founder of OKOKO Cosmétiques

Oyéta Kokoroko

Dreams and challenges go hand-in-hand: it's when you learn to embrace the challenges that your dreams blossom. Since I was a young girl, my dream was to become an entrepreneur. After watching the sacrifices my parents made to immigrate to Canada, I was motivated to create a positive impact. Being an immigrant came with many challenges, but eventually, those challenges turned into lessons of resilience, determination, and perseverance. Turns out, sometimes our struggles are the key ingredients we need to make our dreams come true.

For me, being an entrepreneur was about independence and freedom: and also, an opportunity to positively impact people's lives. When I discovered my passion for formulating natural skin care products, I finally found the path to channel my dreams into to continue the legacy of my parents' sacrifices.

Beauty is more than skin deep: it's about everyday self-care and confidence. Seeing testimonials of how we've helped people build better self-care habits or achieve clear skin after years of frustrating skin problems, always reminds me why I'm still pushing every day. One of our biggest wins was launching our L'Atelier OKOKO in Vancouver's Gastown, where people can get a relaxing moment away from the busyness of life and do something good for them. Celebrating your victories can give you so much joy and motivation to continue onwards.

We all have dreams, but sometimes it can feel like you don't have the support to achieve them. Being a Black female entrepreneur makes me immensely grateful for the opportunities I have, and OKOKO has given back over the years to local charities and championing diversity. Women of colour are underrepresented in the entrepreneurship community, and I want to show them that success is possible for them if they just take the first step. I love receiving notes from aspiring entrepreneurs, saying that my journey has inspired them to pursue their own passions. Uplifting one another helps us cultivate a better community and seeing the positive impact you've made is one of the best rewards you can get.

Wherever you may be on your journey, remember that with the right mindset, every challenge is bringing you closer to achieving what you've been dreaming of.

Heather is the Co-Founder and CEO at WNORTH, a global network of women on the rise to executive leadership. Heather is dedicated to closing the Gender Power Gap by elevating women in the leadership pipeline.

Heather Odendaal

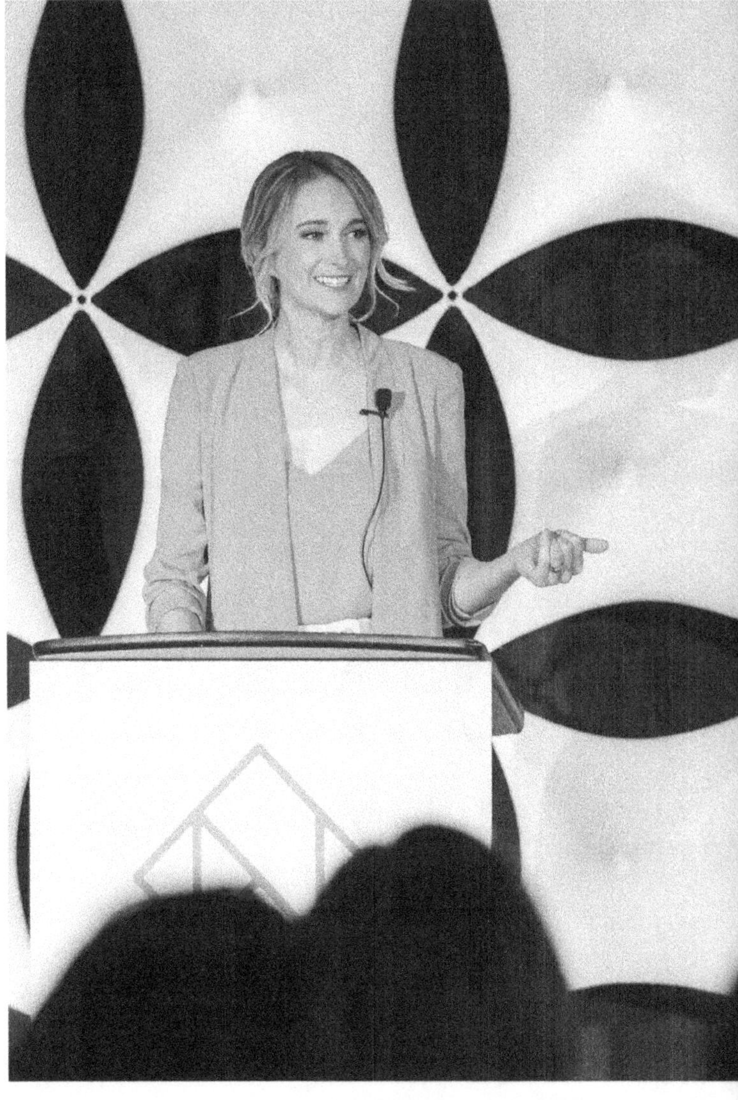

Our ambitions are driven by the big changes that we wish to see, either in the world or in our lives, and as Melinda Gates surmises, "What great changes have not been ambitious?" The great change that I wish to see in the world is more diverse compassionate leadership through the elevation of more women to positions of power, period.

In 2015, while working for a Fortune 500 company, I read that there were more CEOs named John than women CEOs on the S&P 1500 companies. It was very clear to me, from where I sat in my mid-level position, that there was a pipeline issue.

Further fuelling my ambition for change, was my experience of being told that I was not going to be considered for promotion because of my sex, and that I was likely about to have children, so relocating for another senior role wasn't likely. This all contributed to me establishing WNORTH. What's the saying... if you can't find it, build it?

I founded WNORTH as a forum for ambitious women with established careers to connect, learn and grow with each other. The community grew rapidly and organically because, as it turns out, this community was missing for so many. Over the pandemic, our community has tripled in size.

Profoundly impacting women's lives is the fuel to my fire and ambition. In 2021, we are in the midst of a global pandemic. Women are being disproportionately affected by the socio-economic impacts of this moment in time, and one in three women have considered downshifting their careers, risking twenty-five years of equality advancement. I am determined to close the gender power gap, now more than ever.

Over the years, I have read many statistics about the "lack" of women's ambition and it being the reason why so few women occupy the C-suite. Bulls**t!

As women, we set high standards and expectations for ourselves; maybe we don't always feel comfortable sharing that ambition with others. So, here's my ask of you; be bold in your ambition. Be unapologetic about the success that you want for yourself. Create the change that you wish to see in the world.

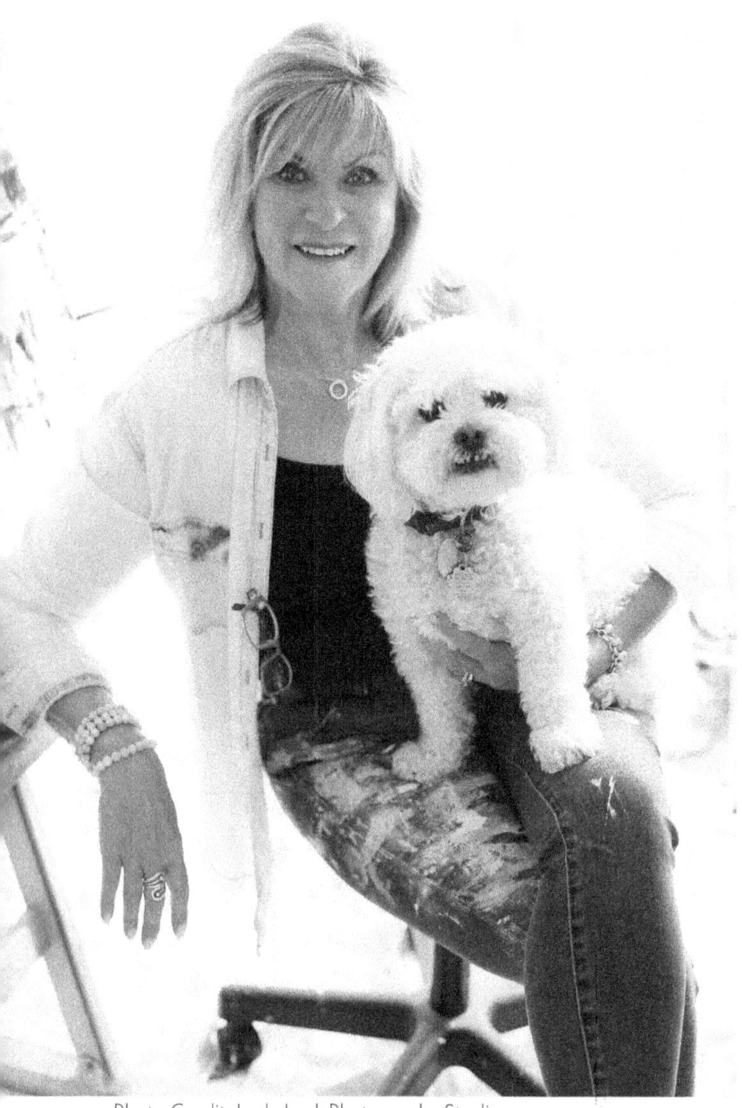
Photo Credit: Lady Luck Photography Studio

Lori Burke is a mother, an intuitive artist, and an authentic collaborator who shares parts of her soul in the form of her art.

Lori Burke

As an intuitive artist, I am intensely in touch with my emotions and the pull of the sensory world around me. I truly believe that my art manifests from a special place in my soul and an inherent need to let the mystical powers of creativity emerge.

Like many in the arts community, I envisioned a life as a full-time artist long before it actually happened. I learned early on to go with the flow and trust that everything would happen in its time. Motherhood beckoned loudly and the joy I felt in building a happy, loving family cannot be overstated.

During these blissful years, I cultivated relationships with family and friends, always appreciating the immeasurable gifts life had to offer.

I put my energy into special projects, collaborating with strong, self-sufficient women, building a community that was empowering and engaging. Together, we struggled, learned a lot, and took care of each other. It was during this trying time that I picked up my paintbrush again. With that first familiar movement of the brush, the colours came alive on the canvas and I knew that this was what I was mean to do.

I am continually grateful that I get to express myself through art and even more, that I can connect to people from around the globe in this unique way. There is a magical quality to the creative process that both grounds and astounds me. I call myself an 'intuitive artist' because I trust my instincts and rely on them to create what is in my heart and mind's eye. Whether as an artist, mother, grandma, soul sister, or BFF, I try to live my life with authenticity, guided by these simple practices—

I am especially thankful for my sweet studio angel Keiko, featured here with me on this page. Keiko, my canine soulmate, you were a guiding force and calming presence in my creative life and will be forever remembered with love.

Give freely and forgive willingly, for that is a gift. Always have gratitude, as without it, you will not find grace.

Faydra Aldridge is the Chief Executive Officer of the BC Schizophrenia Society.

Faydra Aldridge

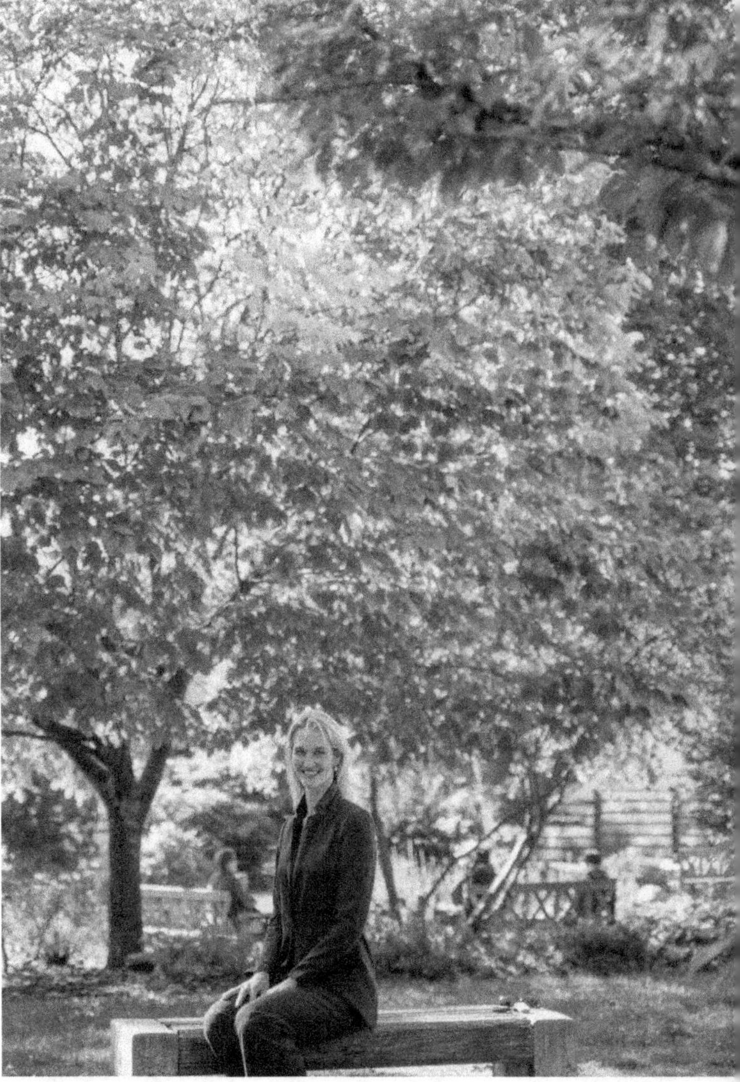

Crazy person. Wacko. Multiple or split personality. Schizo. These are just a few of the adjectives used by some to describe those with schizophrenia. Schizophrenia is a serious mental illness.

It is not pretty in any way. Schizophrenia does not discriminate – it does not care about your gender, education level, the colour of your skin, or the amount of money in your bank. And unfortunately, it is not a rare disease. It affects one in a hundred people and is a leading cause of hospitalization in our country. It strikes people in the prime of their life and there is no cure.

Schizophrenia causes people to interpret reality abnormally and may cause them to see and hear things that are not real (visual and auditory hallucinations). It can lead to cognitive impairment, as well as disordered thinking and behaviours. Schizophrenia is not only a devastating diagnosis for the individual, but also for their family who feels extremely helpless watching their loved one deteriorate and transform into a stranger right before their eyes. It can drastically change the dynamics within a family and cause a tremendous amount of stress and upheaval. I not only have sympathy for these family members but also empathy.

My beloved younger sister, Carissa, has schizophrenia. It is an illness she has; it is not who she is. Carissa is a kind, quiet, trustworthy (probably too much), loving, gentle soul. But sadly, I now have to talk about this beautiful person in the past tense because this illness robbed her of her life in March 2019. Schizophrenia is a devastating illness that makes you feel as though you are walking up a dark, never ending road. But with treatment, there is hope. It is time to come out from the darkness and start shining the biggest light we can find on all mental illnesses. We need to talk about them and take action – through awareness, funding, and working together to find solutions.

The time is now to do a better job of helping those dealing with the illness, as well as supporting those that care for them. Schizophrenia - a 'crazy disorder' that is anything but pretty, but one we cannot forget.

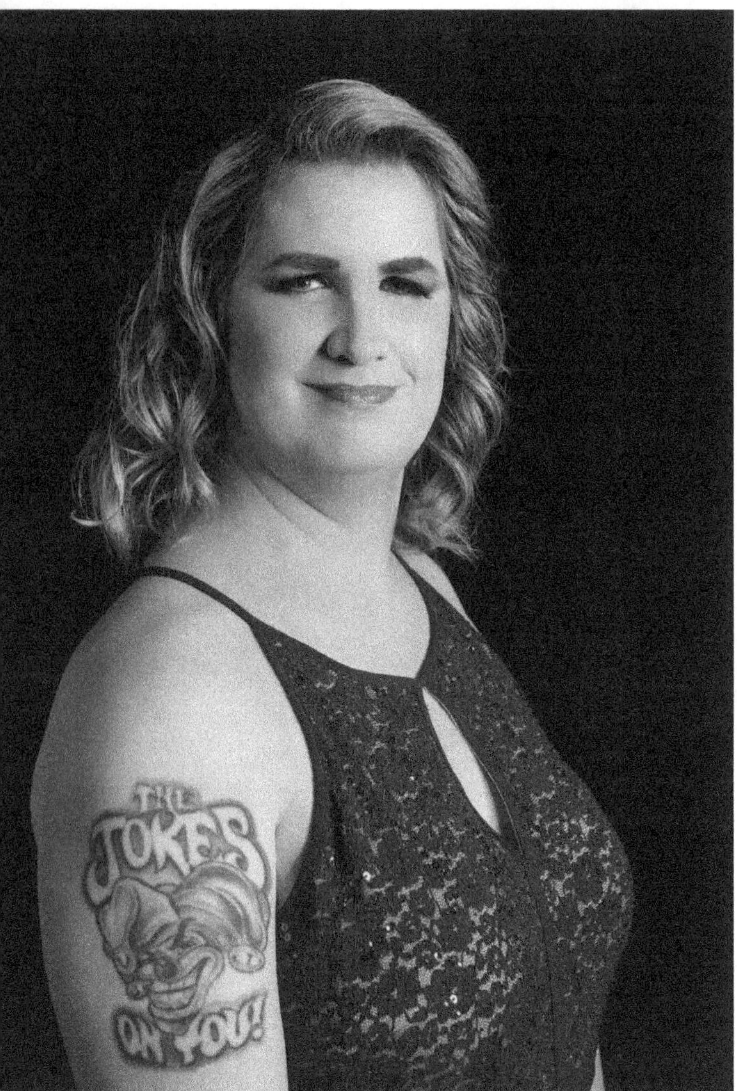

Photo Credit: Riz Herbosa

Alexis Ellis is a co-author, podcaster, speaker, and pageant girl, who is not stopping there.

Alexis Ellis

I was born in the wrong body. I knew it when I was young, and I wasn't happy.

I didn't like being a boy, so I would sneak into my parents' room and try on my mom's clothes. It was a comfort. I would steal clothes from her and hide in my room and wear them. Around the year 2000, I saw ads for being a model, and I tried drag makeup model couple times. It awakened my gender change again. I wasn't too serious until 2013, when I went to a transgender clinic to discuss options, and in July of 2014, I started on hormones in low dosages. When I told my family I was transgender, my mom told me I was supposed to be her daughter when I was born, and she happy she finally got a daughter.

With their support, in 2016, I made the decision to schedule my surgery and on November 19th, 2017, I flew to Montreal to have my vaginoplasty surgery. It was first time that far away from home. The staff at the hospital and recovery house were amazing. While staying in the recovery house, I saw butterflies, and I never knew anything was that beautiful.

I lost two jobs because of my change; a clear human rights violation that I am still battling today.

I have since entered an empowering fitness makeover challenge for women. I didn't know I was the first transgender participant. In 2019, I joined the pageant world to advocate for leadership, and confidence. I didn't know I was the first transgender participant. I went to a national pageant, and I will keep learning and growing, and advocating for confidence and leadership in this space.

I am now co-author of three chapters, a podcaster, a speaker and a pageant girl, and I believe no one should stop there. Dream and you can grow.

I want to inspire others to enjoy their life and reduce the suicide rate of transgender people. I want society to know we have feelings and rights and are just born in the wrong body, but we are just like anyone else. The best part of my journey has been all the people who support me and give me the courage to keep being me.

Khadija, also known as Kat, is an experienced businesswoman and a founder of a venture called Simply Office.

Khadija Jiwani

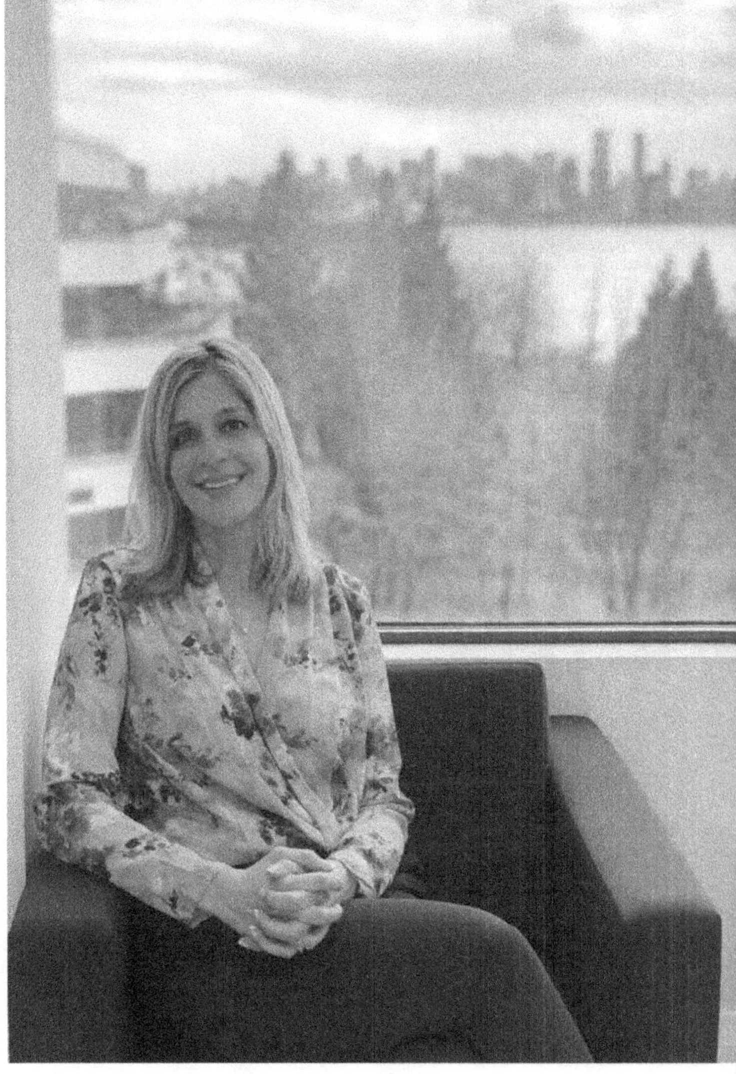

I established Simply Office 8 years ago to fulfil a demand for existing small and medium size businesses that require flexible office space without being tied into long term leases.

Simply Office has now grown to three locations across the Lower Mainland with over 150 private offices that share common amenities such as boardrooms, kitchen and reception areas.

Being a true Aries, I thrive on challenges and novel situations. I am highly motivated with drive and enthusiasm and committed to success. I base that success on being able to help each of my clients' vision come to reality.

Born in Kenya, raised in Ivory Coast and England, I live with my husband, my two teenage boys and my rescue puppy in North Vancouver. Having completed a Masters degree in Human Resources and a Bachelors degree in International Hotel Management, I feel I am well equipped to handle the trials and tribulations with owning your own business.

In my spare time, I love to exercise and attend Bar Method classes regularly and spending time with my growing family. I am an active member of the Ismaili community where I volunteer my time and donate to numerous charities to benefit the wellbeing of counterparts all around the world.

Finally, I believe it is important that my boys see equality at home, in terms of my husband and I both working hard to provide for our family as a whole unit.

The only way to achieve success is to love what you do!

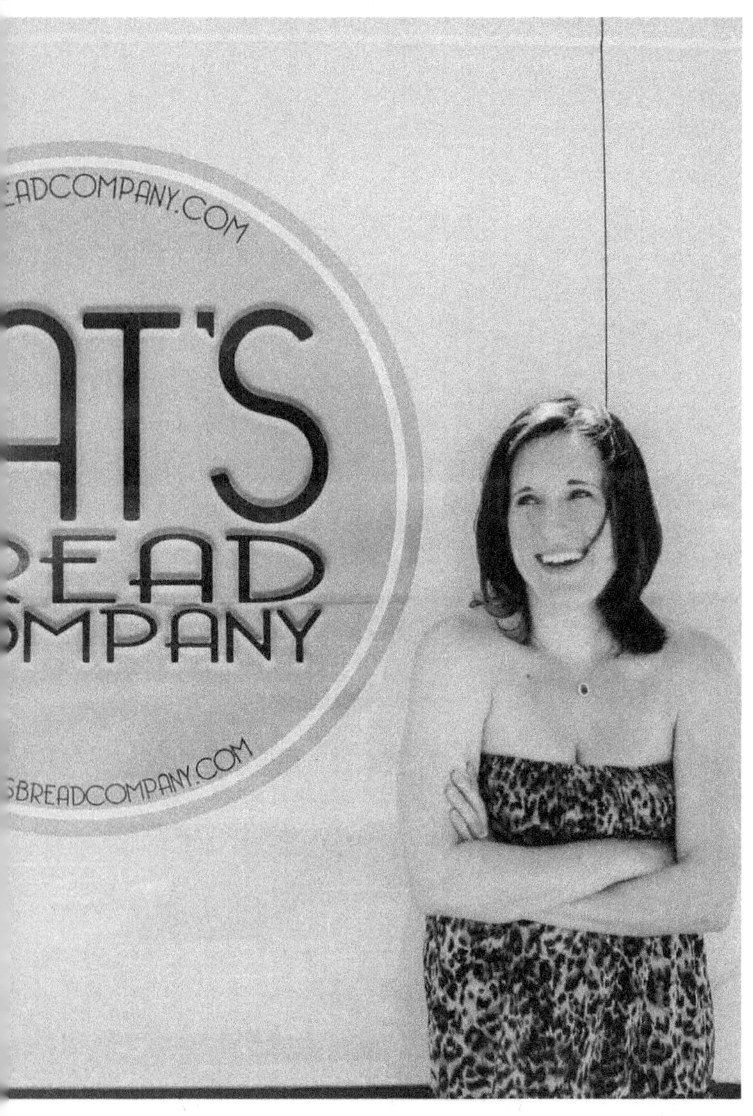

Natali Harea is a bread baker, entrepreneur, mother, and wife.

Natali Harea

I started my business – Nat's Bread Company – in January of 2013, when I was twenty-eight years old. Nat's Bread Company is a wholesale bread bakery in Ottawa, which focuses on providing high-quality bread products to the wonderful restaurants, hotels, caterers, and retailers located in our nation's capital.

I am a graduate of the Algonquin College culinary management program. Before opening Nat's Bread Company, I worked as a chef in many great kitchens across Ottawa. Since taking the plunge into entrepreneurship in 2013, both my business and personal life have gone through waves of change. I married my then-boyfriend of eight years, James, in April 2015. We had to close down the bakery so I could have the Saturday off!

"Nat's Bread" started very small. We rented restaurant kitchens overnight, when they weren't in use, and delivered our goods in the morning. In 2017, we finally signed the lease on our very own commercial kitchen space! It was such a big business milestone for me, it had been my biggest long-term goal since the start of the business, and I was so proud of myself for achieving it. I had another big life change in 2017: my first son, Clifford, was born. He joined in on all financing, leasing, and construction meetings for the new "Nat's Bread" space. I don't think I know another baby that was as comfortable as he was toddling around our local bank branch.

When the lockdown was initiated in mid-March 2020, we lost 90% of our business in the course of a day. We quickly learned the meaning of "pivot," and started offering fresh bread, delivered to private homes, safely and without contact. I have never been so challenged and felt so anxious as an entrepreneur. I'm proud that I, and my wonderful team, have been able to keep Nat's Bread Company afloat, and even help the business thrive through this crazy year. 2020 also brought me more change personally. My second son, Roger, was born in July. A true pandemic baby! Surely to be raised eating sourdough, waiting for mom at the bank.

Amanda Cox is the founder of Rock Candy, a luxury gemstone bead jewelry company. She designs and handcrafts bespoke pieces using precious and semi-precious gemstone beads. Amanda lives with her husband in Vancouver, where she continues to grow her burgeoning business and take advantage of her big backyard – Whistler and Wine Country.

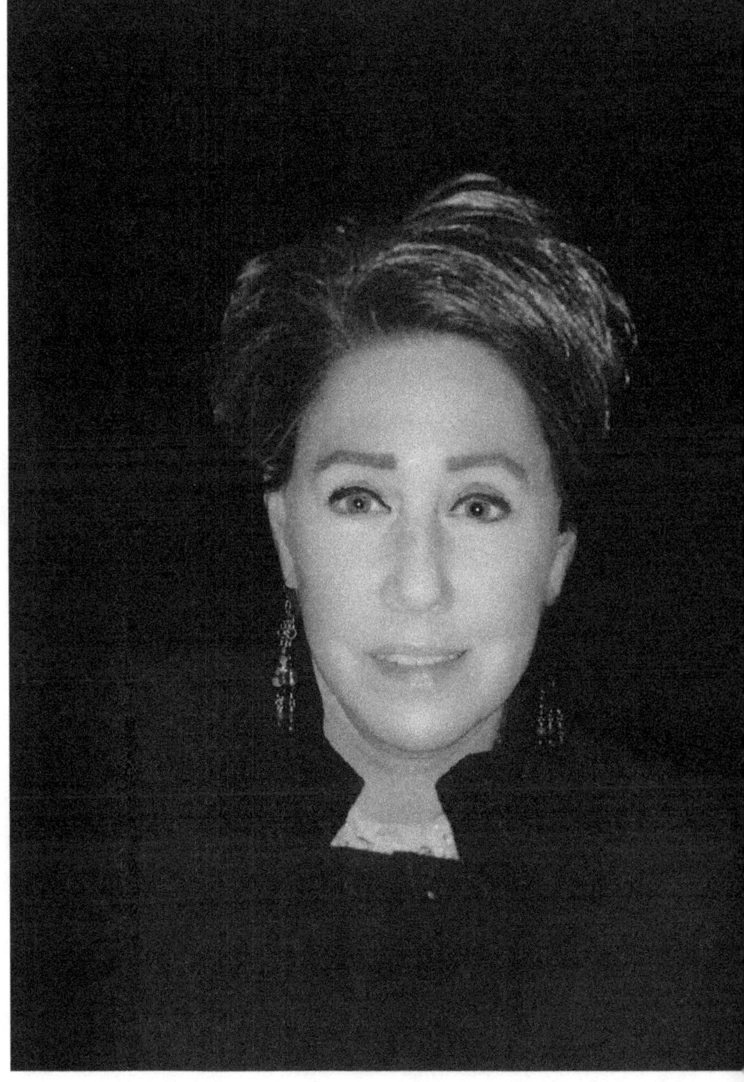

Amanda Cox

I was inspired at an early age by ancient beads and art, and cultivated a broad-based knowledge of art, architecture, and design through academia and travel. I studied Art History at Columbia University in NYC before earning my Masters in American Indian Studies at the University of Arizona, and then my Law Degree from the University of San Diego. I returned to my passion in 2019 after a successful 15-year career as a Senior Executive in Finance, leading global operations at such firms as JP Morgan in New York and Scotiabank in Toronto. My business acumen, entrepreneurial nature, and passion for and knowledge of art and design serve me well in my creative endeavors.

My work is characterized by asymmetry, non-uniformity, and juxtapositions of color and texture. Basically, how I live my life. My approach to life is reflected in every piece: accentuate the unique, espouse strengths, be generous, take risks, be fearless and bold. Create your own way, and be true to yourself. Some say my animal spirit is the honey badger. I call it tenacity. Fearless, irreverent, generous, kind, funny. Genuine, outspoken, accomplished, polished, wry. I have found the greater the challenge, the stronger you become. I feel exceptionally strong.

In my pursuit of success and happiness, I am cognizant that challenges create a full and fulfilling life, one which requires resilience, intelligence, and a huge sense of humor. Know your capabilities. Don't let others dictate the terms of your success and happiness (you'll likely never measure up to their paradigm).

I am thankful for the support of my sister and husband as I build my first creative venture. While in all other parts of my career I have taken risks and consistently challenged myself and the status quo, I would not have had the fortitude to forge a path of my own without their instrumental support and encouragement.

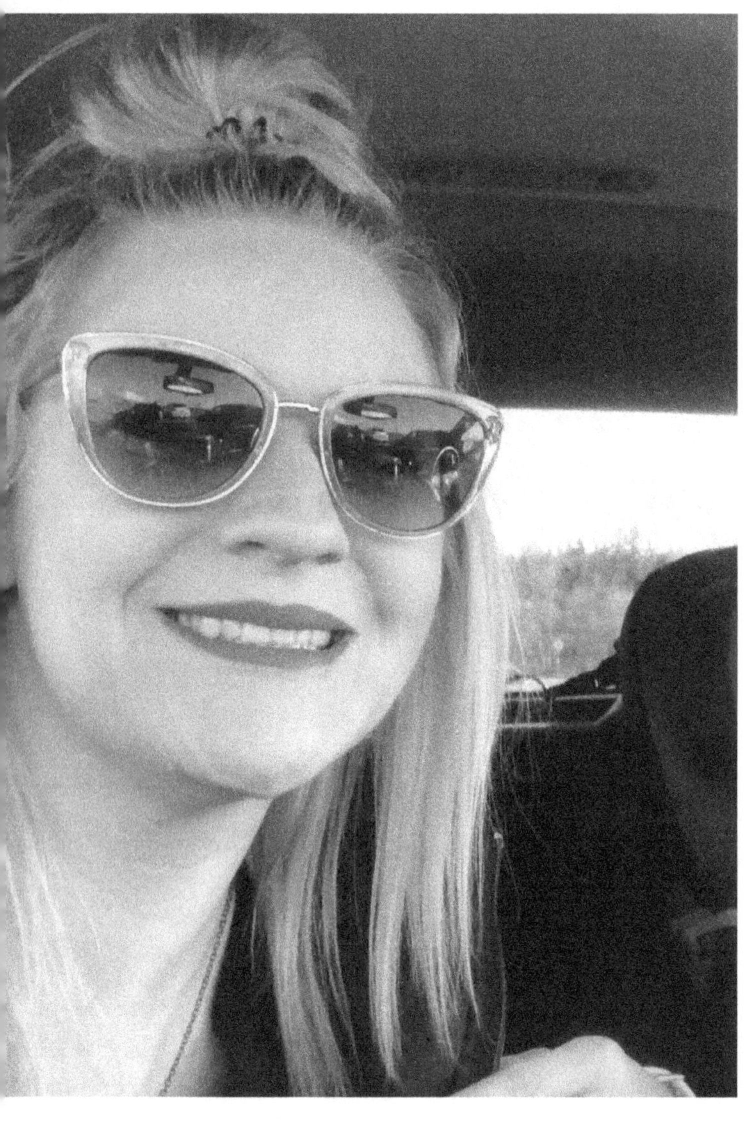

Teresa Simmonds is creative, entrepreneurial, and gets to play with makeup for a living – and that is perfect.

Teresa Simmonds

"Stop comparing yourself to others, and happiness will follow you. I am proud of you."

June 28th, 2017 - those were the last words my best friend, my Mom, said to me privately before she passed from cancer.

For thirty-four years, I compared myself to everyone and anyone; I was never pretty enough, small enough, smart enough, strong enough, or good enough. I grew up in a house with four strong, brilliant, and vivacious women, and an intelligent father who believed finding your path involved family, God, university, and a high paying job. After receiving my degree, I told my parents I wanted to go to makeup school. Let me tell you, the shock was there. Although supportive, there was a little cajoling, "What about becoming a teacher?" I always felt that I was not as good as my sisters who are teachers, accountants, and pharmacists. I would joke about how I was the black sheep of the family because I played with makeup for a living. When I would tell people what my profession was, I would get a look of amusement or disbelief.

I started doubting myself and the career I chose. Unhappiness set in.

Why was I unhappy? It was because I looked at my family, friends, and people I did not even know, and I would compare myself to them. I started to lose control of my life. It was not until my Mom said those words to me that I knew I had to make a change. It has not been easy. With the help of my counselor, I have slowly started to move past a lot of self-doubt and damage done by bullies growing up.

I went back to school again to obtain a diploma in a career I am so passionate about.
Graduating with my Esthetics Diploma and working in the industry, I can finally say I am happy. I am on the way to owning my own business. The most important thing I have done is stop comparing myself to others.

I am me, and I am perfect.

Moderation does not exist in Courtney Powell's vocabulary.

Courtney Powell

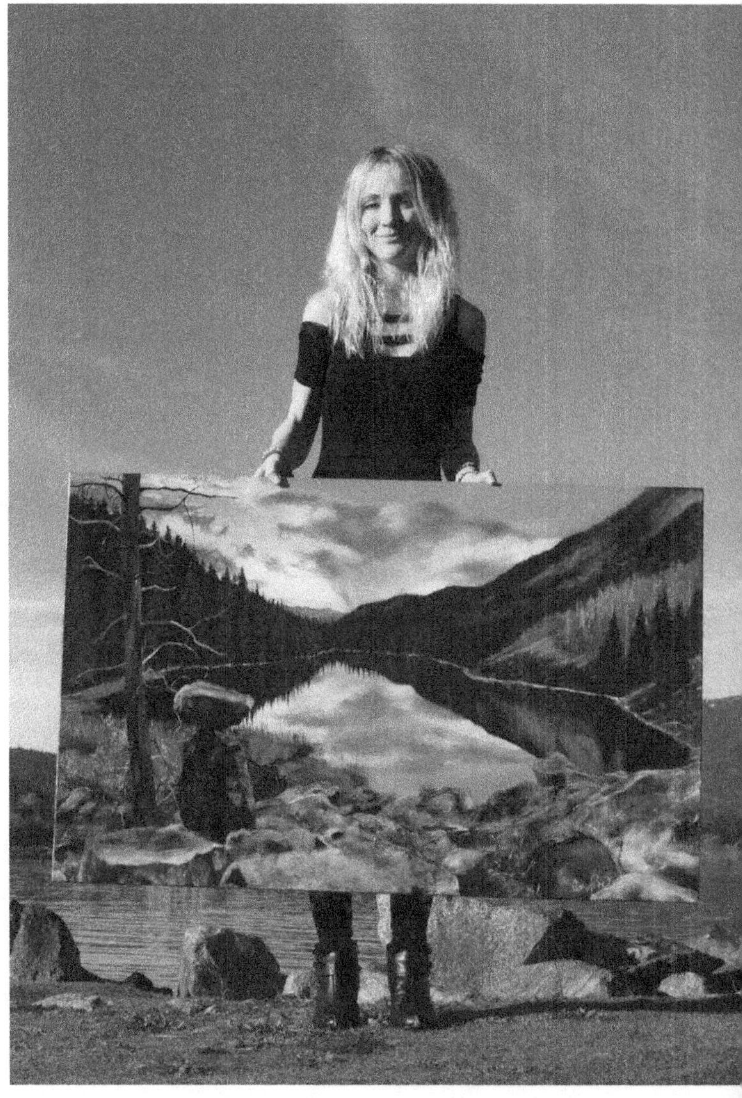

For as long as I can remember, my life has been colourful. My moods, energy levels, and enthusiasm have been described as "intense" or "extreme." I remember sitting on the gym floor for an assembly, and suddenly standing up and shouting to the entire school, "I DECLARE TODAY CRAZY DAY!". I remember spending four hours on homework in grade four when others would spend ten minutes. I remember staying up all night and working on a project worth 5% of my grade.

I can remember the shame and embarrassment of feeling like a misfit because I could not control my emotions. I remember locking myself in the school's bathroom and crying for hours. I remember excusing myself from class and hiding in the hallway until the tears stopped flowing. This depth of emotions and intensity continued into adulthood. After having my heart broken, I strapped on my running shoes and ran two hours in the snow at midnight, running for the first time in five years. For the next two years, I woke before the sun rose and trained until sundown. I then ran the Boston Marathon in under three hours.

My highs and abundance of energy felt like a gift until my lows kicked in. I did not know why I was crying all the time. I could not get out of bed. I felt like a failure and a burden to my friends and family. And yet, it did not occur to me that I could be bipolar. After being diagnosed with bipolar II, my world has changed. Everything makes a bit more sense, and I have found ways to regulate my moods.

The high highs and low lows have helped me as an artist. I can translate these emotions onto the canvas. My paintings range from extremely happy landscapes to sad black and white depictions of ladies floating in the water. When my energy strikes, I can paint the night away, sometimes twenty hours in a row.

Yes, my life may be colourful, and doing things in moderation may be difficult, but in the end...

I would not have it any other way.

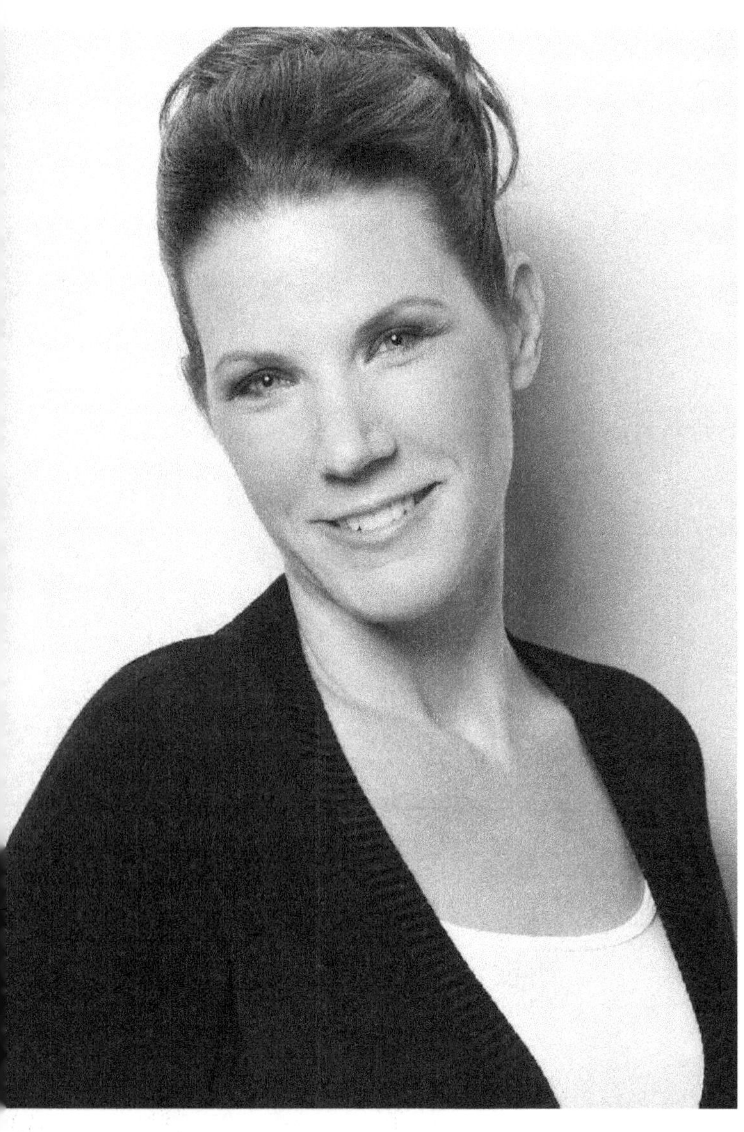

Joanne Turnbull is a fighter, an activist, a philanthropist, an artist, and a confident woman who loves to inspire.

Joanne Turnbull

My younger years began with me as a spunky and curious young girl. I came from loving parents, a large family, and a built-in best friend because I am a twin.

My fondest childhood lesson was every Christmas, volunteering at local hospitals or Hospices. We didn't have the big Christmas that many children know today, including my own. This fueled my passion for wanting to make a difference throughout my life.

One of my first stints with making a difference was when I was in high school and elected as VP of Student Council. When I was in the full swing of things, about halfway through my term, I found out that I was pregnant, at eighteen. This could have been a defining moment, but I refused to be a statistic. I was determined to have my baby, complete the VP term and graduate high school. I graduated post-secondary school with my class, and my motivation was my beautiful daughter.

I met a charismatic man who made my daughter and me his priority. We married and had two beautiful children. It wasn't long into the marriage before drinking became a daily thing, and he became emotionally and physically abusive. I never thought the words domestic violence would ever come out of my mouth.

When I planned our escape, I knew I needed to work on myself. I needed my confidence back. I have been working on myself every day since. I made my personal life my priority and focused on slowing things down and enjoying the things that are important to me; my family and friends. I am finally living my dreams by making a difference in helping our planet through farming and bringing more natural ways to produce goods.

I was able to be part of the fight against COVID. I was responsible for ensuring frontline and essential staff were safe with adequate and appropriate protective equipment while responding to our first global pandemic. I worked alongside the most inspiring women who constantly empowered and taught me.

Today I am a fighter, an activist, a philanthropist, an artist, and a confident woman who loves to inspire.

Shirley Weir is the fifty-four-year-old founder of Menopause Chicks, and the author of Mokita: How to navigate perimenopause with confidence and ease.

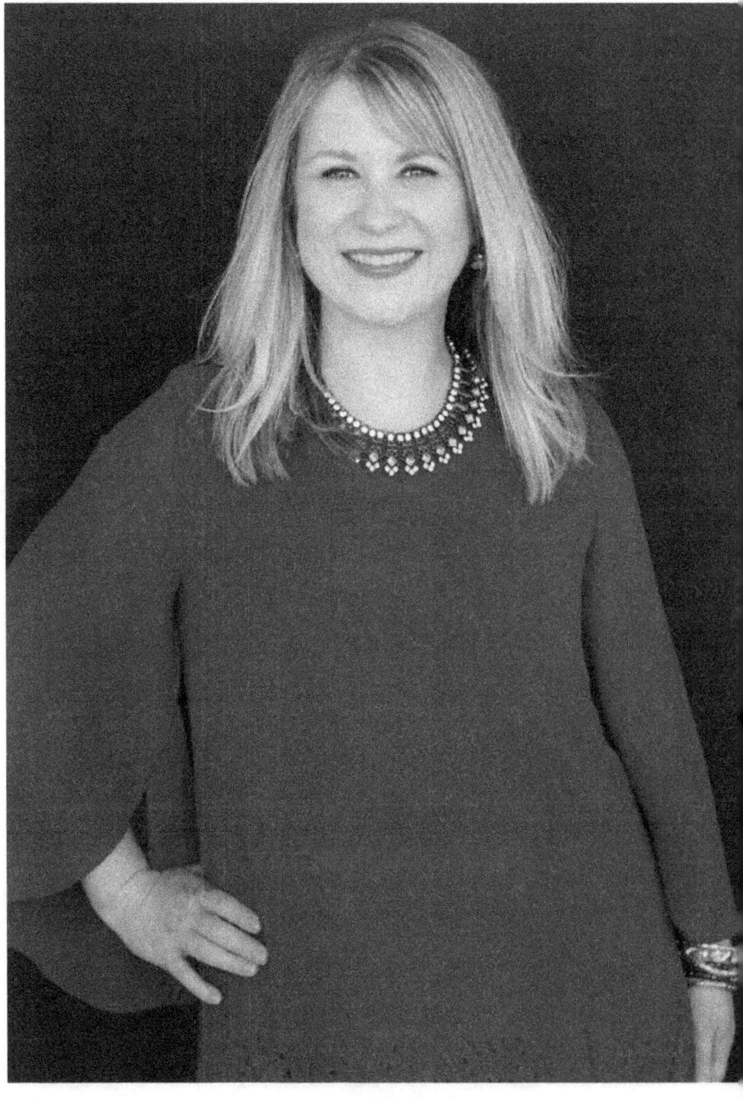

Shirley Weir

I was forty-eight when I did this for the very first time. It was New Year's Eve 2015. I was lying in my bathtub—and I looked down at my body, and I said, "THANK YOU." I thanked it for giving me two amazing children. And for carrying me this far on my journey. It seemed rather insignificant at the time—but reflecting back, I realize it was a pivotal line-in-the-sand I drew between, "this sucks," and, **"I've got this!"**

Although it was impossible to know that night, I was a year away from reaching menopause (the twelve-month anniversary of my final period). My journey through perimenopause (hormone shifts, sleep challenges, debilitating brain fog, mood changes), plus stress-induced burnout, had been at the forefront of my busy mom and entrepreneurial life for the past ten years. The bathtub is my sacred place. But it had also become the place I frequented to curl up and rock back-and-forth after losing my temper with one of my kids, or my place to try to escape feelings of depression, anxiety, and overwhelm.

Now, you must know, I am the ultimate cup-half-full girl. "Change is good," "Be the change you want to see in the world," and Maya Angelou's, "We delight in the beauty of the butterfly, but rarely admit to the changes it has gone through to achieve that beauty." Those are my go-to mantras. But in my tub, surrounded by my favourite magazines, I noticed the headlines were all negative. It felt as though someone was trying to convince me I wasn't good enough, that I was broken. Even with a career in marketing, that message didn't resonate with me.

I didn't need fixing. But I was changing. I prayed that meant for the better. So, I decided to replace words like "hot" with "whole." And "bitchy" with "beautiful." I bounced out of that tub because I had a family to care for, a business to run... and fifty more years to embrace! I convinced myself to put my own health at the top of the to-do list, take on the job of meeting other women where they are, and become their "concierge" for quality midlife health information and trusted health professionals.

I was being called to crack open the conversation about perimenopause and menopause; then disrupt it.

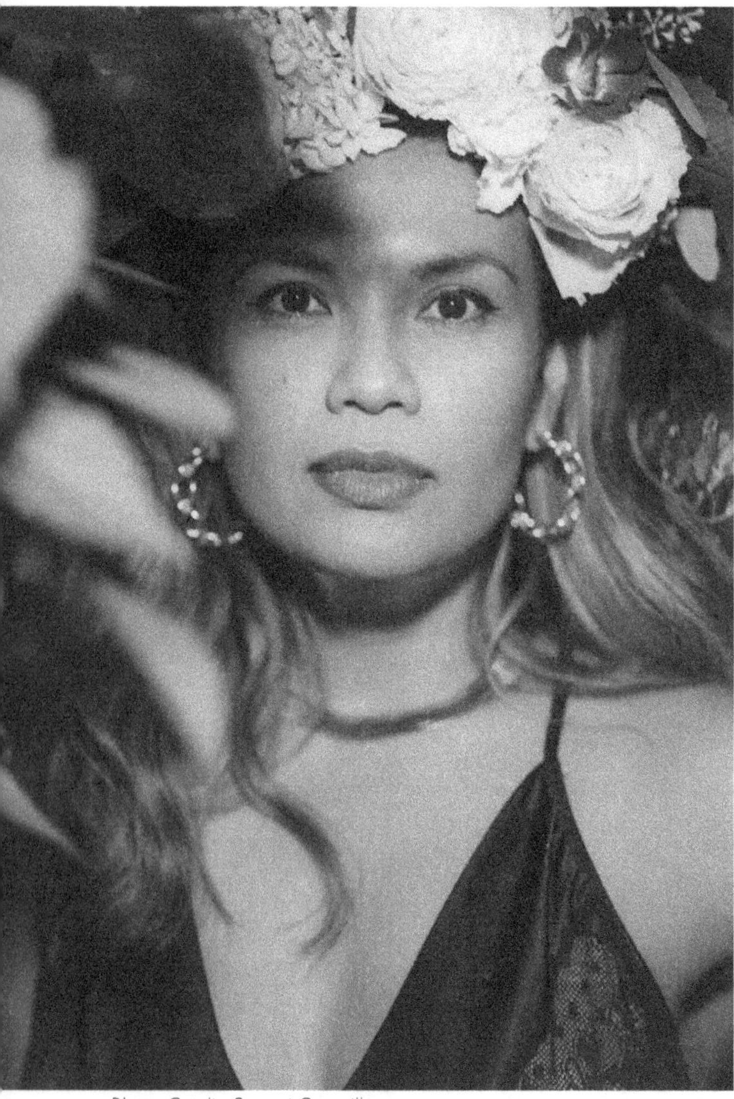
Photo Credit: Sewari Campillo

Kim Chhay is an enthusiastic funny girl, unofficial life coach, wife, and mom.

Kim Chhay

"All is well in my world," I whisper, repeatedly, under my breath as tears stream down my face. I am pulled over on Lougheed Highway in Coquitlam, about five minutes away from my house. I am driving to visit my sister, and suddenly my heart starts beating so quickly it feels like it's going to jump out of my chest.

I call my sister teary-eyed, "I'm gonna bail. I just don't feel 100%. Sorry." I hang up before I have to tell her I'm having a panic attack.

Four-year-old Eloise and six-month-old Rosalie are in their car seats quietly studying me. They have seen this before. "Mommy, I love you," Eloise offers in the sweetest, softest voice. This is not the version of powerful femininity that I want to be for them.

I planned to have a career shift that maternity leave. As much as I loved my boss, I felt like my opportunities for growth had peaked with my current role. I was either going to start my own e-commerce business or transition to a new company.

However, while I was crying in my car, I realized that I was not strong enough to do either. I would go back to my comfortable old role. It wasn't that bad.

Weeks later, an acquaintance replied to an email about a job inquiry that I sent months prior. The role was in my area of expertise, and the hiring manager was interested in connecting with me. The company was a renowned Vancouver-based yoga apparel company. It was the perfect opportunity to merge my education in fashion design and technology with the career I developed in supply chain.

I would not let my panic attacks block this incredible opportunity. I reframed them in my mind. Despite panic attacks, I would thrive. I got the role.

That experience taught me to listen to my body, to breathe deeply, and even deeper when necessary. I learned to be vulnerable in front of my children. I allowed myself to be taken care of and to be waited on by my husband.

This is powerful femininity.

Randi Winter Co-Founded *The P2P Life*, amalgamating travel, events, philanthropy, and media. She's also a social entrepreneur in health and wellness technology.

Randi Winter

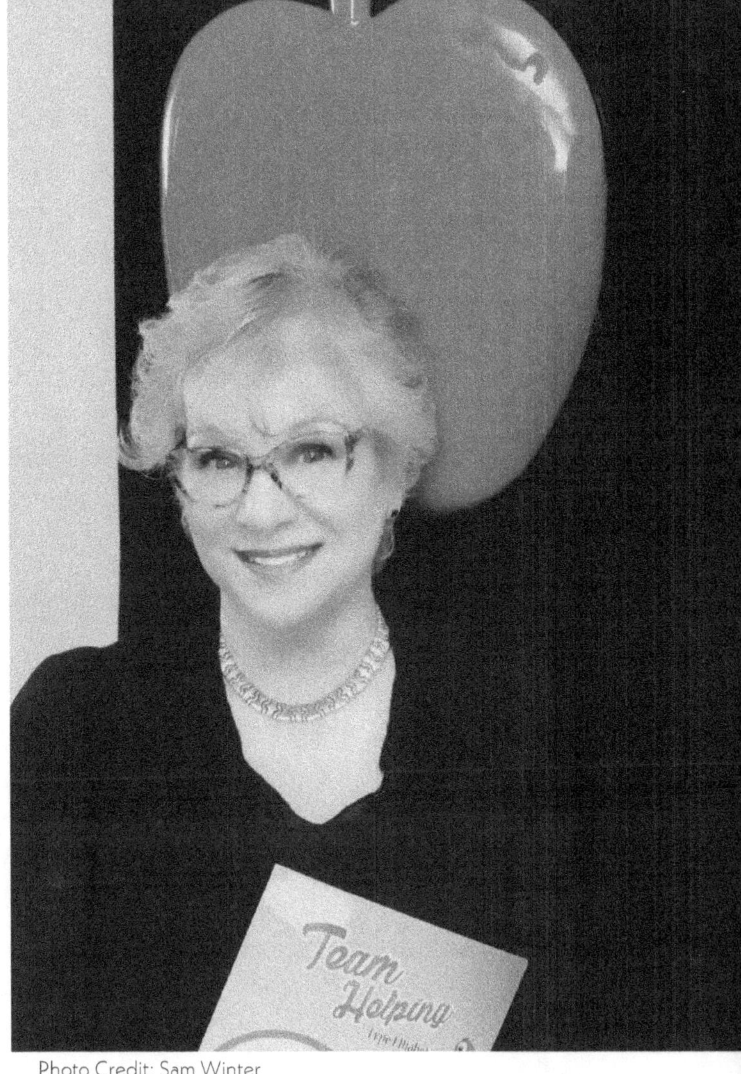

Photo Credit: Sam Winter

A Promise with Pizazz!

My mother made me promise to never lose my ***"NY Pizazz".*** She could never imagine how far from NY my Pizazz would travel. First living in Israel for my junior year at Hebrew University, finding my true love-at-first-sight in the Sinai Desert on a tour bus, returning home to plan a wedding in six weeks, and move to Canada. Fifty years, several careers, two children, and four grandchildren later, I keep that promise every day. For me, ***"NY Pizzaz"*** computes into two equations:

the right 1 + the right 1 = infinite possibility

passion + purpose = making a difference in the world

I broke barriers as a teacher, then owned sporting-goods stores employing Canada's top athletes. Each journey towards personal excellence, inspired me. I had an epiphany and traded my physical inventory investment for something more valuable and self-fulfilling. As a facilitator, I could share how travel transforms both traveller and destination. Then, interests and passions become life-changing experiences. As a social entrepreneur, I strive to inspire people to combine philanthropy, health, and personal transformation to make the world a better place now and for future generations. I created Passionate Travel, Travel with a Cause, and co-created ***The P2P Life*** because travel is the only thing that we spend money on that makes our lives richer. The value of our lives doesn't come from cash in the bank, but time well spent.

My writing and global community involvement organically flow from my family and an understanding that if you make a difference in the life of just one person a day, you've made a difference in the world, every day. I found my "daily quota" in the streets of New York, in Israeli society, Canada's multicultural landscape, in Albania and Kosovo with Muslims who saved Jews during WWII, co-founding a US non-profit called Diabetes and Me, for newly diagnosed kids with type 1 diabetes, like two of my grandchildren. We wrote a book ***Team Helping: Type 1 Diabetes***, have a 24/7 online support for parents/caregivers, and a T1 Summit for ongoing learning that you are not alone. I support new technologies.

COVID-19 grounded me, but genealogy took me back in time, reuniting my husband's long-lost Holocaust family. ***PIZAZZ!***

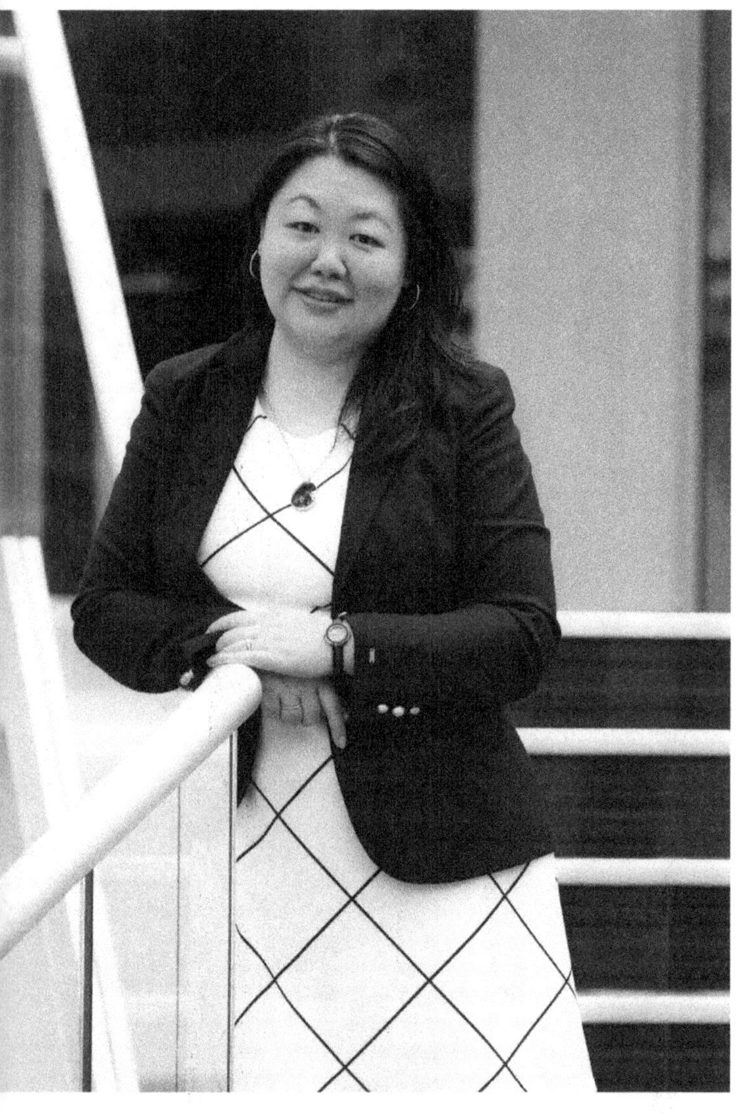

Denise Wong, CPA CA, is the Managing Director and Lead Consultant at D-Squared Consulting, Chartered Professional Accountants.

Denise Wong

Have you noticed just how many sports analogies are made to describe how business owners, entrepreneurs, professionals should behave? Do we really need to "go for gold," "sacrifice the body," and just "go flat out"? Is it any surprise that many business leaders burn out?

I am an avid and fanatical tennis player, aspiring to be a professional tennis player at one point in my youth. The game of tennis evolved from the wooden racquets that required tennis players to have finesse and skill to guide the ball across the net to the more modern power game, where the make of the racquet head and the strings can impact your game significantly.

I started the game like most people do, picking up a racquet and playing at a local court. Without an official coach, I would learn through observation and trial and error, thinking, if I just hit the ball hard enough every time, I would get the win. In the beginning, when you are playing with other beginners, sheer muscle can get you the win, but as I progressed to intermediate levels, I noticed smacking the ball with all my might was not getting me the wins, and if anything was just rendering me gassed and demotivated. Tennis is known as a mental sport, and once the element of doubt sets in, sometimes it is enough to sink your game and spirit. One day, while feeling deflated and hating on my game, I realized something pivotal that changed my game (and business life) forever. I do not need to pummel the ball every chance I get. My perspective changed. My goal is to keep the ball in play and wait for the right moment to make my move, and "put the ball away" for the win.

Translated to my everyday life, as a professional accountant turned small business owner, I am trained to go all in all the time. However, I have learned, it is not about sacrificing the body and trying to operate at full capacity all the time. Slow and steady wins the race. When aligned, the right opportunity will present itself for you to put away the winner. Game. Set. Match.

Karen Lee has advice for start-up female entrepreneurs.

Karen Lee

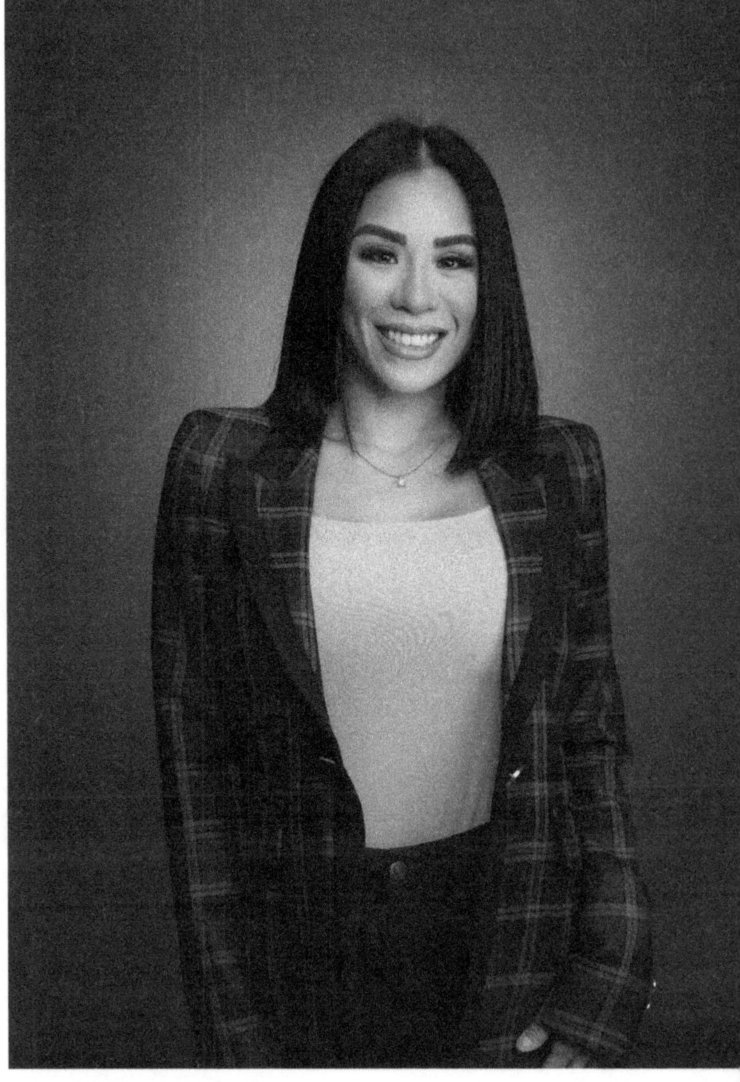

My advice to start-up female entrepreneurs:
You are not just a woman. You are an entrepreneur! That supersedes any other identity you have.
The minute you put another identity above that, it becomes a limitation for yourself and in your own perception of your abilities. If this is what you want to do, think of yourself as an entrepreneur first and foremost, not as your gender or your nationality, nothing. Be brave, go out, make connections, talk to people.

One. Be confident, not confrontational in asking for what you deserve. Women entrepreneurs have unique and powerful perspectives to offer every industry and walking in that power means walking with confidence – not arrogance or fear.

Two. Be sure to ASK.

Three. Be willing to walk away from things that cease to align with your values and mission. One of the most challenging things to do is saying NO.

Four. There is no such thing as making a good deal with bad people.

Five. Compromises of character are not worth any cost.

Six. In general, be steadfast in your principles, and trust yourself. There are so many books on strategy, fundraising, product development etc. The most important, and in my opinion least emphasized, is preserving a positive, value-based sense of self.

Resort, guests, cabins, restaurant, marina, boats, we had it all at Saratoga Resort and Marina!

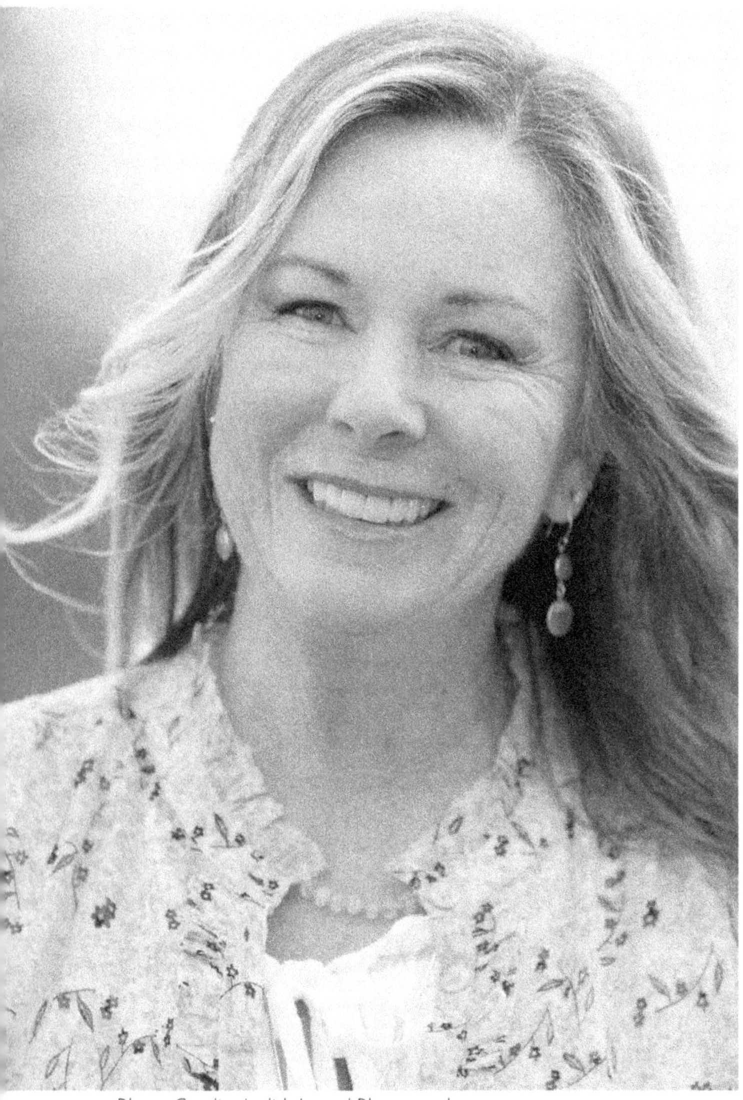
Photo Credit: Judith Laurel Photography

Lynda Honing

I was eleven years old when my adventurous, hardworking, visionary parents decided to buy a resort at sunny Shuswap Lake. My summers would never be the same.

The bell rang, and school was out. I hurried home with excitement. We were on our way to "The Lake" for the whole summer. The anticipation for this Gemini was overwhelming as adventure and spontaneity are my middle name. The next eighteen years would shape my whole world.

I learned to cook, clean cabins, landscape, pump gas, and create an epic holiday place for guests worldwide. We were known for our outstanding homemade food and our bustling resort playground. I loved it beyond words. I was never afraid of hard work or challenges, so this was a dream lived. We had all the water play toys including canoes, paddleboards, parasailing, beach volleyball, and more. I learned that play was as important as work, and we played hard. Our nightly campfires proved community and conversations were essential to human existence with songs and stories shared.

This incredible experience inspired me to recreate the resort I grew up in. Presently, on our 60 by 120 lot we have created our own resort, **"The Urban Oasis." Gathering people and making a difference has been my life's mission.** My busy Reiki and massage practice is nestled in the tranquil surrounding gardens with private patios that create a peaceful setting. It's a sacred space to work and play, allowing every day to be magical, meaningful, and productive.

My life at Saratoga taught me to be resourceful, resilient, grounded, determined, and to challenge myself to live each day with urgency! To be inspired and be of service. To not wait, there may not be time! To leave a legacy worthy of attention. To live passionately with a brave heart and a desire for greatness. I learned that life is not a dress rehearsal and stepping out of my comfort zone is where I thrive and grow. To heal, risk, instill curiosity, and to burst with passion like a rose intent to BLOOM!

Angela Campagnoni has been a well-known leader in the fashion industry for over thirty years. She is the founder of Atlantic Fashion Week, and currently the North American Brand Director for Elita Intimates, the ladies' division for the Canadian Iconic brand Stanfield's

Angela Campagnoni

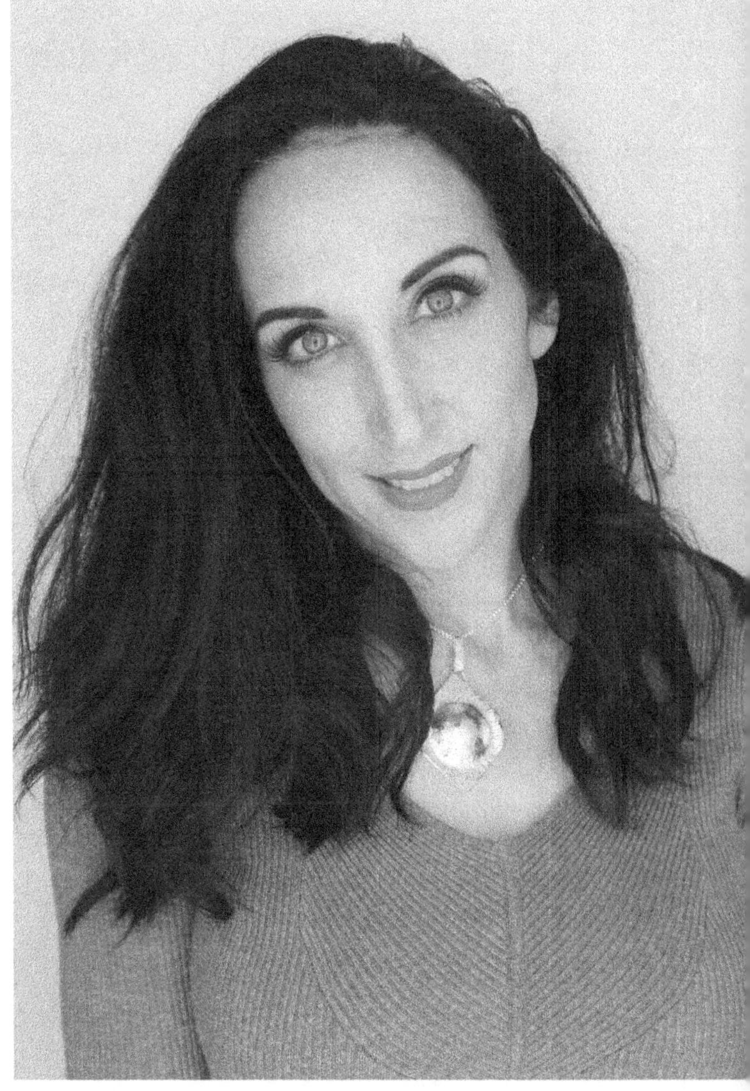

In life, I try to live by one simple rule... that I am not in competition with anyone but myself. When you can truly live by this rule, you open the door to help those around you and to help yourself live a life free of comparison.

Let's face it, we live in a culture obsessed with measuring talent and ability, against a set of ideals that are often curated in someone else's social media feed. We spend hours scrolling through the pieces of someone else's life that they have chosen to share, and we somehow begin to think they have things so much better than what you may have happening in your life; when in fact if you had not seen it, you would not have even thought something was missing. When you do not see the full picture of someone's life, it seems silly to compare yourself to it.

Gratitude, integrity, honesty, and personal drive are the things that fuel me, along with the genuine desire to see others succeed. If I can leave a person feeling inspired, whether it's from the encouragement I give or an idea for their business, then I cannot ask for a greater gift to myself. I feel today that we often overlook the important role of inspiration. To me, it means leaving someone feeling limitless, letting someone else truly see their unlimited possibilities. Inspiration to me takes our ordinary experiences and excites a person to be better than they thought they could be. It's about transforming the way someone perceives their own capabilities.

I hope that my life inspires my three daughters to go after whatever they may dream in their own life. I hope that I can teach them that they have no limits other than those they place on themselves. And if I was to give one piece of advice, it would be to remember that we are blessed with the ability every day to make the choice to believe in ourselves. No one can take that away from you except you, I choose gratitude above all else.

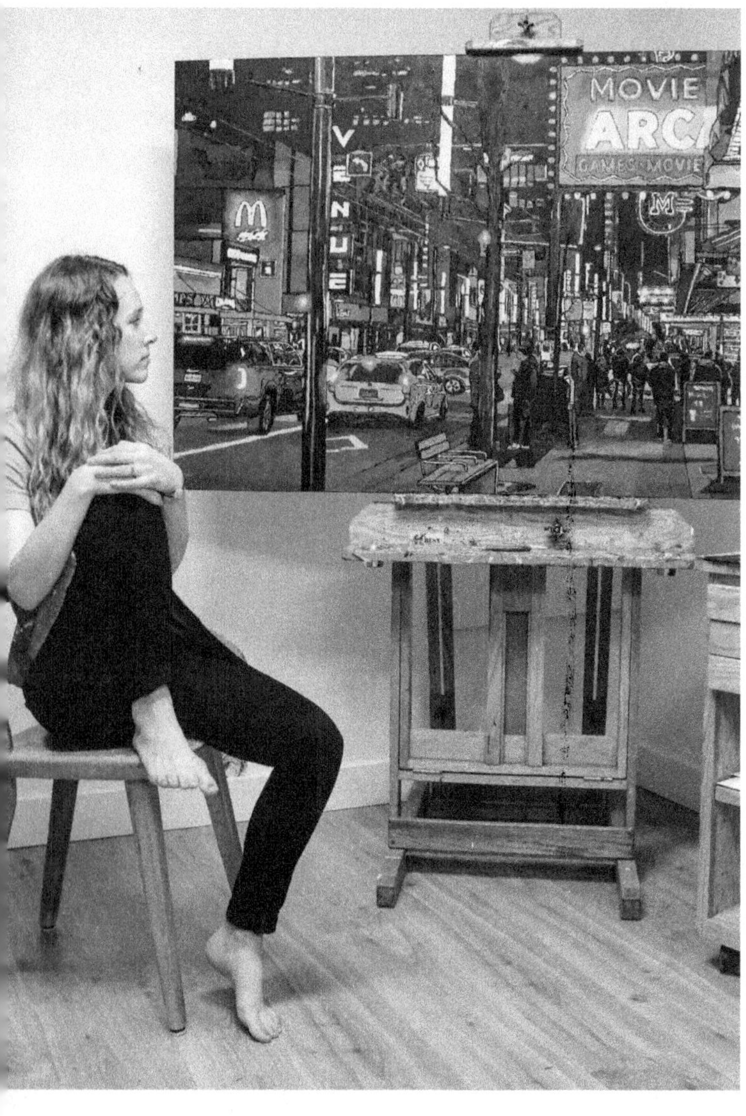

Emilie Fantuz is a Vancouver-based artist who embraces life's adventures.

Emilie Fantuz

From her Vancouver studio, artist Emilie Fantuz hones the practice that's built her the life she loves—pursuing growth and adventure at every chance. Before she moved to Vancouver, Emilie lived in Hawaii, where she began the artistic method of using palette knives, a change that would ultimately deepen her passion for creating art. Throughout her life, it's been her willingness to take chances with exploring the unknown and pushing her own limits that has brought her happiness and growth. Whether it's running a marathon or climbing Mount Kilimanjaro, Emilie's love for the journey, not just the destination, is what has guided her and culminated in a rewarding career and a fulfilling life.

Our lives are full of twists and turns that offer us the chance to step out of our comfort zone. Some of those chances might seem small, like trying out a new method for creating art, but they often pave the way for other life-changing opportunities, such as a vibrant new style of art, as in Emilie's case. It was her willingness to take on any change, big or small, that prepared her for one of her life's most significant adventures - driving cross-country to leave her home in the United States and forge a new life in Canada. The challenge of quitting her job, selling her house, and packing up a van with only what she needed most was daunting, but just like traversing a mountain, you must be willing to step into new territory to reach new heights.

As in art, life too offers unlimited space for growth and exploration. The unknown can be unnerving, but few adventures take place within our comfort zone. Emilie sees the parallel between learning to love the process over the destination within her artwork and within her life as well. Whether it's packing a van with her paints and palette knives to move to a new country or exploring a new technique in her art, it's the pursuit of life's endless possibilities that has taught Emilie to love the journey and embrace the adventures along the way.

Mary Painter is grateful.

Mary Painter

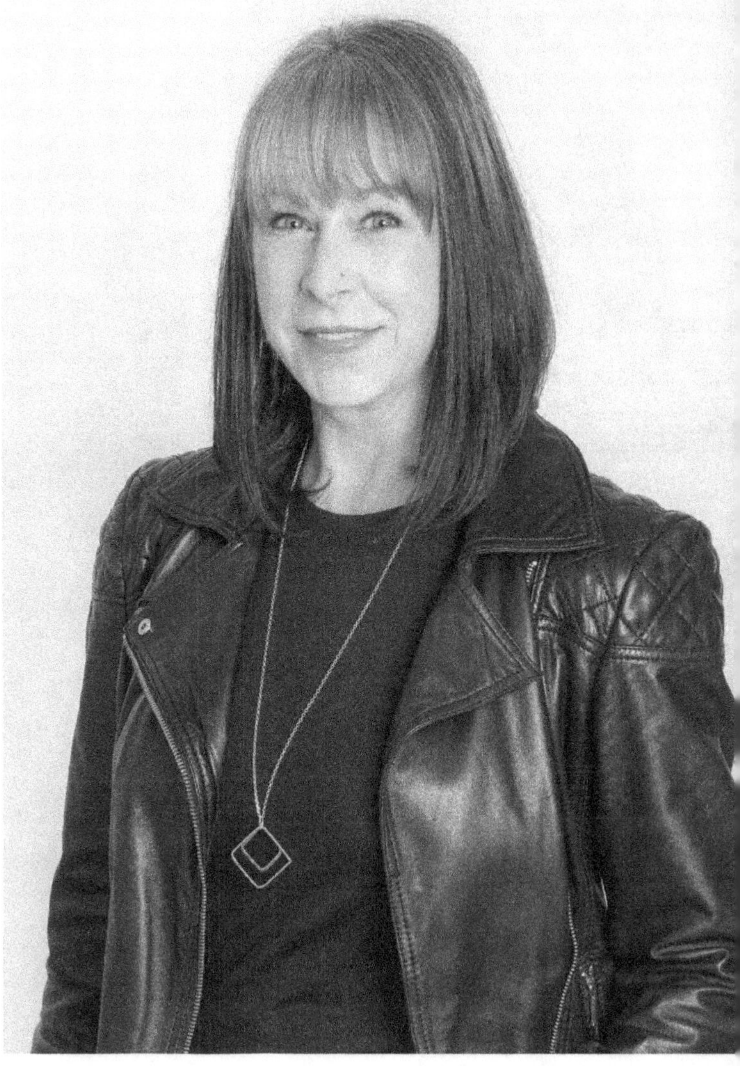

How do I tell my story without it sounding like a laundry list of comedies and tragedies minus the comedies?
I've always been awestruck by those who rise to every challenge they meet, kick-ass, and stand victorious. I often ponder what sorcery it is that fuels them.
Me, I get through the best I can. I drag myself out of bed each morning with my pillow wrinkled face and nest of hair and think, gawd, I just want to go back to bed. I am exhausted, but I am grateful.

Grateful for my loving husband, who holds me up and wipes away my tears in my less than fine moments, and in all my moments. He's my hero, he knows exactly who I am deep down, and he hasn't divorced me yet, bless him!
I am grateful for my son, who gives his all and more every day while living with Autism. His intelligence and capacity for knowledge are inspiring. I confess I'm slightly confused as to where he got his brains from - it wasn't me.
I am grateful for my ex-husband - no, not a typo! - who supports my son unconditionally and remains a dear friend to me and my husband.
I am grateful for the medical technology that allows me to live more comfortably with autoimmune disease. Plus, I love my bionic hips!
I am grateful for my brothers; for lightening my dark early years with their music and friendship, and for trying to tutor me in math -likely receiving a lesson in frustration instead! This one is not an easy statement for me but...
I am grateful for my Dad. I learned a few things inadvertently from him; to try to be kind because you never know what someone is going through or what tragedies they have seen that have shaped them. I only wish we could have known each other outside of his addiction.
I am forever grateful for my Mum, Daphne Mavis. I miss her every day. She is the inspiration for who I am today and what I do. She is the reason you're reading this page right now because, without her, there is no me.

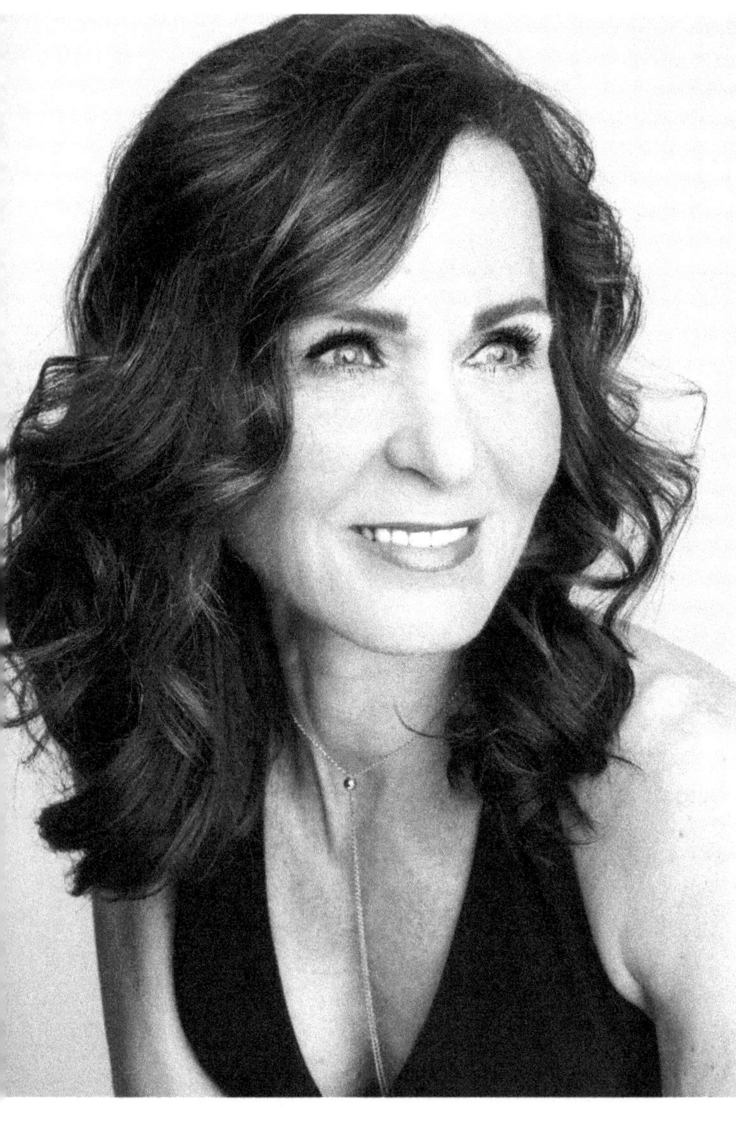

Katherine Taylor has been on a strange and wonderful journey.

Katherine Taylor

1968. The tanks rolled in, and we rolled out. At four years old, the prospect of a communist revolution in, then, Czechoslovakia, was lost on me, but not my parents. Leaving everything behind - a great home, solid jobs, and all our friends and family - was impossibly difficult, but we did it anyway. My mother always said they wanted a better life for me in Canada, and with little more than a suitcase and a few dollars, we headed for Vancouver.

Before leaving, I caught the attention of a figure skating coach who encouraged my parents to put me into lessons. Arriving in Vancouver, my parents did just that, and in the blink of an eye, I went from being four years old to standing on the ice representing Canada at the Sarajevo Olympics in 1984, in Pairs Figure Skating.

It came with a price. Leaving home at sixteen, being alone without my family, it was easy to fall into the traps that were waiting for many young athletes. Yet to all the world, I was a happy and accomplished Olympian without a care in the world. "Lucky" is what I often heard.

On the world stage, with millions of people watching, the music started, I shut my eyes and did what I had trained a lifetime to do. Behind those closed eyes, I also had to block out years of insecurity, depression, loneliness, and injury. The pressure of making my parents' decision worthwhile was sometimes unbearable and all while being judged on how I looked, my weight, and a million other things that come with public life. The constant attention and criticism were impossible to keep out of my private life.

Today, with the support of my beautiful family, I better appreciate all that competitive sports has given me, yet I sometimes still struggle to re-enter the world of "normal" - something much harder to do than most realize. In my quiet moments though, I can't always escape the darkness and need to fight hard to hear the music again. A strange and wonderful journey indeed.

Rycarda Smith is a crocheting nomad.

Rycarda Smith

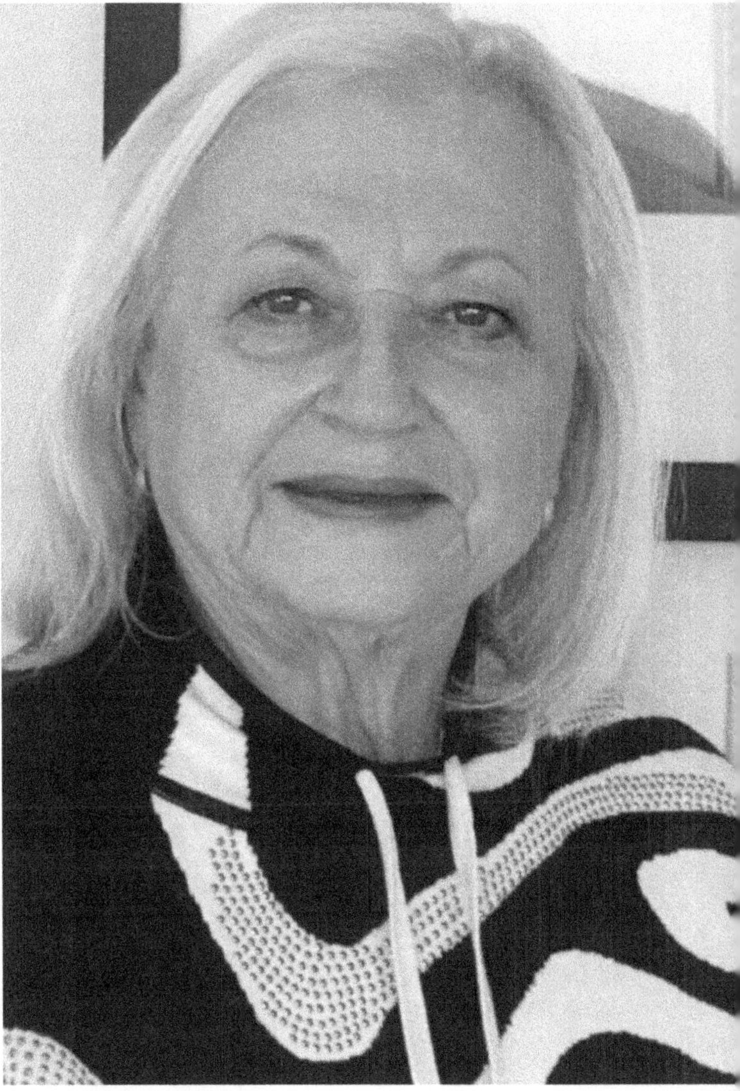

I like to sit down with my crochet hook and begin another prayer shawl. I know that someday soon someone will be comforted by my efforts of this evening.

Crocheting has gotten me through many trials of life that have come my way. My sorrows started with the shock of my brother's unexpected death at the age of forty-six while working in Nigeria. I think that this was the time when I first become angry with the challenges of life. Zbyszek's death meant that I was left to care for our elderly parents who lived 1047km away in Exshaw, Alberta while I lived in White Rock, BC. My father was diagnosed with dementia soon after my brother died. Dad couldn't understand why Zbyszek died so young when he, himself, had survived WWII. My dad died in 2006, leaving my independent mother living alone in the family home. Still 1047 km away from me and a ten-hour drive. My days as a nomad began.

From then on, every six weeks, between April and September I would get in the car and drive ten hours to be with mom,

spend two weeks at a time, helping her with her chores in the house and around the garden, taking her to her doctor appointments in Canmore and shopping to Calgary. In August, although I would spend three weeks with her, she would say, "Can't you stay longer?" During the winter months, I would fly into Calgary, rent a car, drive the 65 km to Exshaw. Sometimes I would be driving in a fierce blizzard. My life was on hold, no crocheting prayer shawls during this time, but I kept myself busy with my Real Estate career, my many community and church organizations, as well as being an entrepreneur.

I started a Prayer Shawl Ministry in 2015 when several other crocheting ladies joined me. Our shawls have been delivered worldwide to comfort folks in their times of need. Satisfaction in helping others has helped me dispel the heavy loneliness of carrying my family's burdens. Mum passed away in 2013 and I thought I could get back to my busy life. For a few years, things seemed to settle down until my husband was diagnosed with dementia in 2017. So, the question, "Why me Lord"? came back to the surface. My husband died in the middle of this 2020 pandemic craziness from renal failure. During this lonely time of isolation, it is my strong faith in God that has sustained me, just like a cozy comfortable crocheted shawl.

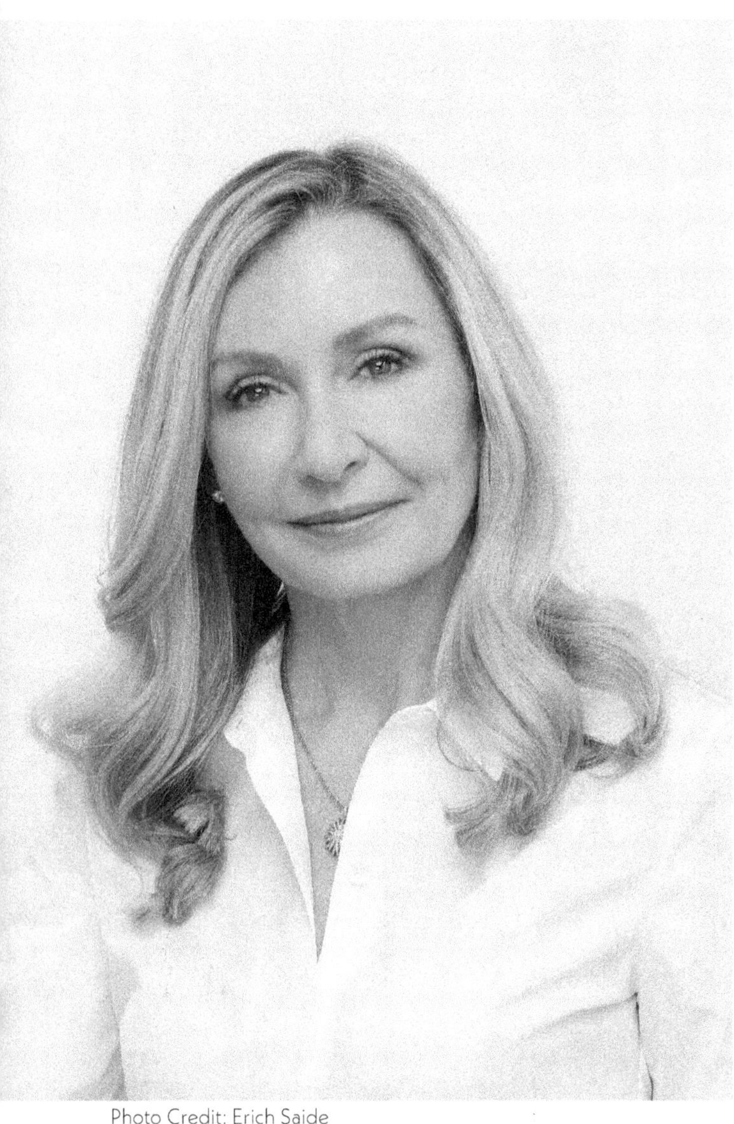
Photo Credit: Erich Saide

Lorna Vanderhaeghe, mother of four and grandmother of ten, has been voted one of Canada's Top 100 Female Entrepreneurs several years in a row, and knows what it takes to create a business that helps people.

Lorna Vanderhaeghe

Anyone can do it - build a business in four years and sell it to the largest nutritional supplement company in the country. It comes with knowing what you want to create, not listening to the naysayers, surrounding yourself with talented, hardworking people, and never giving up.

There is no luck involved in becoming successful. It takes focus and commitment. My motto is, do what you are passionate about first and the rewards will follow. I want to inspire women to be brave.

Maybe not as fearless as I was. I maxed out way too many credit cards and mortgaged the family home several times to fund my business venture. I had a big family to feed so failure was never an option.

Nothing should hold you back. I left high school before I was finished and had four children. When my oldest daughter developed head to toe eczema, I visited many doctors, but none had a solution. A health food store owner came to our rescue, and not only healed my daughter's eczema, but also changed my life. I discovered the exciting world of nutritional medicine and decided to return to school to get a degree in sciences, all while working full time. Now a single mother, I became a prolific writer to help pay the bills. My writing led to lectures, radio shows, television appearances, and eventually a product line of nutritional supplements. The books and supplements allowed me to do what I love, which is to educate people on how to prevent and treat disease and ultimately feel fabulous. And, of course, there were amazing mentors who encouraged and supported me along the way. Those mentors shared their failures, successes, and things they wished they had done differently – and I listened intently and applied their recommendations. Every day I help women with their health issues through my website www.lornahealth.com and social media. Family and children are important to me. The next phase of my career is going to be dedicated to children. Think of what the future will hold if our children get everything they need to be emotionally, mentally, and physically healthy. There is so much exciting work to do.

Hoai Dang-Lachance is a business professional and contemporary abstract artist, with creatives reflecting ebb and flow of colour sought from past and present journeys.

Hoai Dang-Lachance

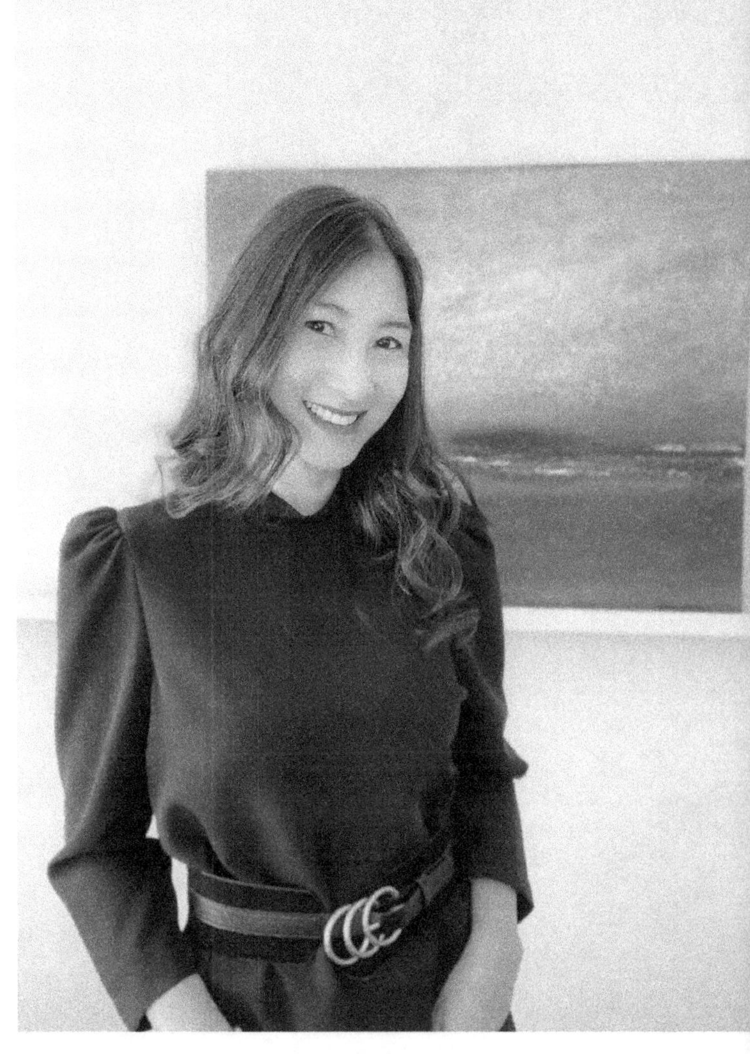

At a young age, I discovered my happy place was simply to create, which paved a path to designing ladies' accessories for retail. Having set aside my creativity for years to immerse myself in the corporate world, it is with much irony my journey has led me back to creatives once again.

I had read about other women experiencing burnout within the corporate world; I never imagined it would happen to me. The thought of having a work-life balance was something that existed in a land of rainbows and unicorns.

Perhaps my hustle train of thought and work ethic comes from being raised by a single mum, whose selfless and unconditional love for her children, strong will and courage, enabled her to live through colliding worlds of fortune to poverty as a result of war.

Having traveled through unthinkable journeys and surpassing truly dire circumstances, I was provided with a new life and a fighting chance. Embracing my roots, I had built my life around actioning sacrifice in order to succeed at any cost. Let's say "sacrifice" won for a moment in time. It's as though I had run into a brick wall, with absolute mind and body exhaustion. The feeling of shame, sense of failure wrapped with anxiety took a toll on my mental and physical well-being.

Looking back, there are certain life lessons that hold close. The action of loving you, putting yourself first without guilt is freeing. Who knew, self-care and the fact you cannot be everything to everyone is indeed acceptable?

Surround yourself with humans who will lift you up and inspire you, as you're never alone.

Never forget you are capable of change, embrace the possibility of self-improvement.

Let go, embrace the feeling of being comfortable with uncomfortable and learn that you can truly create your own life balances.

As my path evolves, so will my desire to create art that will bring joy and enable those who embrace it the opportunity to conjure up inspiration through their own journeys as experienced.

(With a grateful and empathic heart, I dedicate my journey to my mum and all those who have turned their own lives from impossible to possible.)

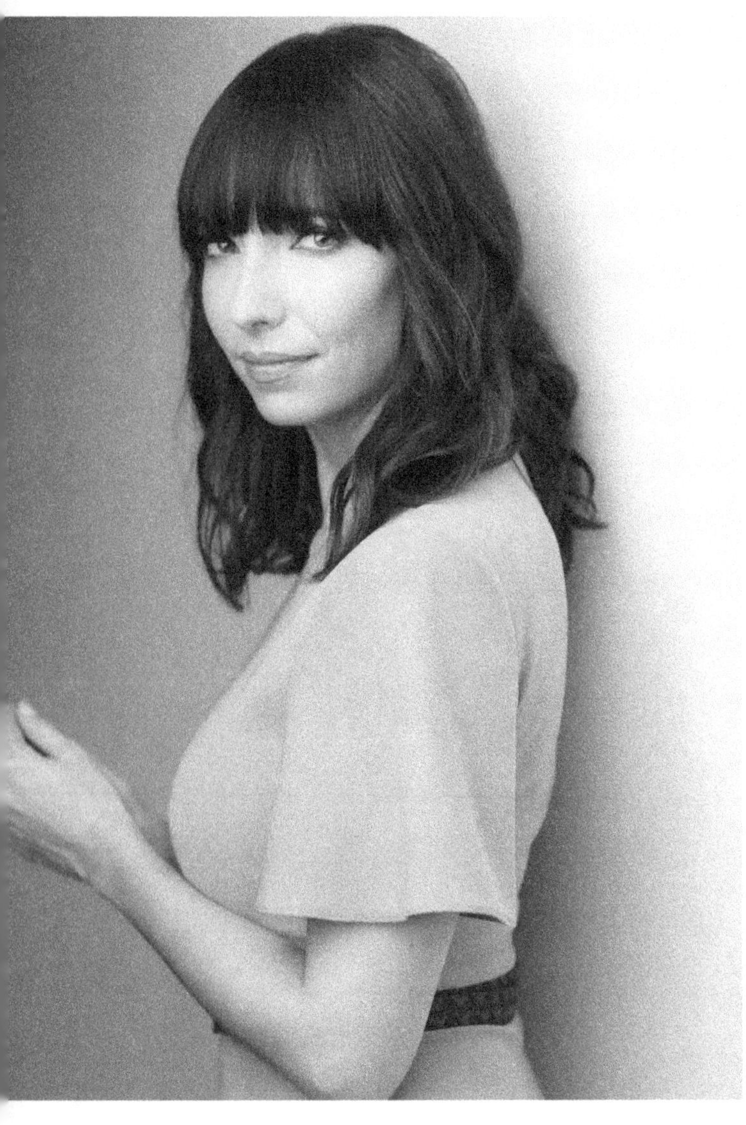

Jodie Emery is a long-time high-profile cannabis advocate who owns and operates Cannabis Culture, Pot TV, and Jodie's Joint. She has run for office, engaged with various governments, practiced peaceful civil disobedience, and continues to campaign for drug policy reform, human rights, and true cannabis freedom.

Jodie Emery

One of the greatest gifts in this world is the gift of inspiration. When someone inspires other people, they spread sparks of enlightenment through their words and actions.

I have been so deeply blessed, for so many long years, to receive countless messages in which people thank me sincerely for inspiring them. They have seen my speeches and watched my interviews; they have witnessed my devastating losses and my enduring strength. They have seen the bold risks I have taken, and the peaceful and essential activism I have engaged in, and they tell me that I inspire them.

They share with me the work they have done, the projects they have launched, the laws they have changed. I hear beautiful stories of people from around the world — some imprisoned, some in political office, some in business, some among the many millions in our global rallies and protests against inhumane and unjust anti-cannabis laws — and they tell me of the way I inspired them. They took lessons from my countless appearances, they educated officials with the knowledge I have shared, and they took brave steps to implement change and help make the world a better place.

Beyond becoming inspired and enlightened themselves, they have in turn inspired others. And that is one of the greatest gifts of all: to hear from fellow human beings that they have had their lives improved and uplifted through the simple magic of inspiration. The spark of passion, the blooming of compassion, the drive that ignites an engine within our hearts and minds — that is inspiration. The courage to carry on when others step back, the quiet pride and honour of being strong when others need support, the creativity and ingenuity that comes bursting forth from within — that is inspiration.

When I am inspired by others it feels like I've been touched by a bright light that ignites a fire within me. And when I am told that I have inspired someone else, it is like feeling the warmth of that growing and eternal light. To know that you can change the world just by being someone who inspires... that in itself is inspirational too. Keep sparking up those fires!

Grace Lanuza is a mom, CEO, and business partner.

Grace Lanuza

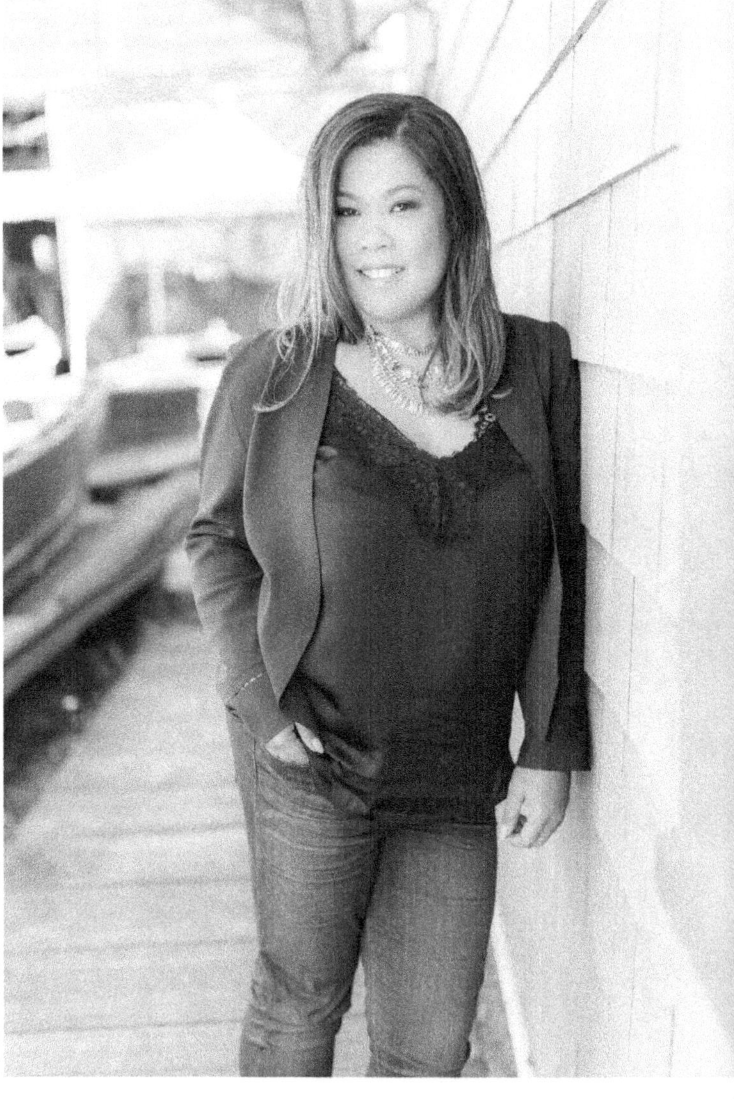

"And the day came when the risk to remain tight in a bud was more painful than the risk it took to blossom." ~Anais Nin

What does it mean for anyone to take a risk they're fearful of? Some say I'm a risk-taker, which usually gets me in trouble. It's true - I'm risky, but not reckless (aside from getting bangs in grade nine, a regret to this day)! On a more serious note, what do entrepreneurs risk every day of their lives? Everything. When it comes to entrepreneurship, I'm what East Van folks call: "ride or die."

As a serial entrepreneur, single mom, and abusive relationship survivor, risk and failure isn't something I shy away from.

Why? Because with options, there is no scarcity mindset.
Taking a risk not tied to an outcome creates an abundance of opportunities. In business, I'm often asked if I feel women have a long way to go regarding entrepreneurship. Definitely. Do women perpetuate the cycle of being seen as "less than," and are they pushed to "acting like a man" in the boardroom? Absolutely. I've seen this happen repeatedly.

For the purpose of this piece, I'll call out the gender of my male assistant. Whenever I say to a male client, "My assistant Joshua will follow up with a meeting placeholder," it's business as usual. When it's a female client, the response is, "Oh, you have a male assistant? Is he cute/single?" Excuse me? Highly inappropriate and the very thing that perpetuates the cycle. If it was the other way around, there'd be an uproar.

Why the need to validate roles with "cutesy" labels. Real empowerment comes when we go toe-to-toe with anyone regardless of gender, and as equal business allies. Instead of "gender-ising" labels, invite men who can handle women in their full feminine self to join the conversation.

Today, I choose global impact in business and work alongside my partner and biggest supporter, Jonathan Parsons, because he fully believes in the power of women in business, and me as a mom, CEO, and business partner.

No cutesy labels needed.

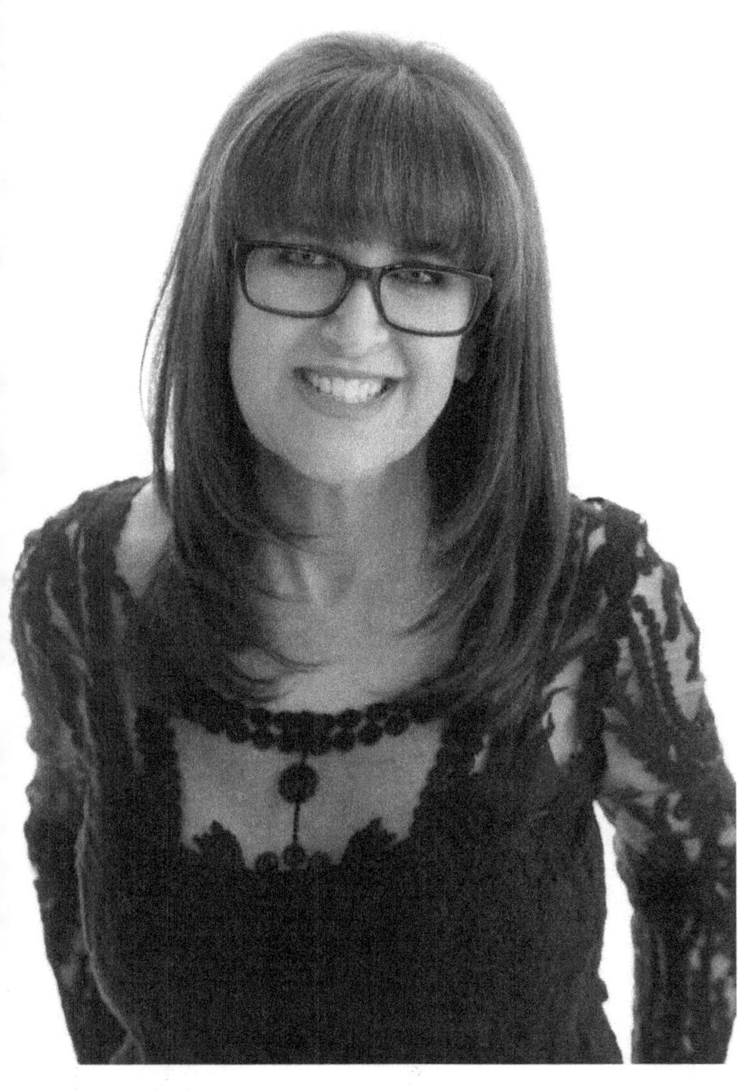

Judy embraces the joy of the "little moments," both professionally and personally. It could be a client's hug or a smile from a much-loved grandchild; both are cherished.

Judy Doduk

Can you relate to my personal experience where I had a, "what am I going to do with the rest of my life?" moment?

After decades of working in the beauty industry as a trusted makeup artist and skin care specialist, my mission is to help maturing women feel more beautiful both inside and outside. I created my blog for women gearing up for the second stage of life and are eager to explore the pursuit of beauty inside and out while discovering the possibilities that lie ahead.
As women, there are a multitude of changes and challenges that come our way as we mature.

We face physical changes that occur not only to our skin but to our bodies, and not all are welcome. I have found that practicing self-care daily is crucial for finding the balance for our spiritual/emotional and physical health. It is by embracing these changes together that we empower each other. Sharing our reality has been incredibly powerful. I have experienced some physical and emotional setbacks. The expression that goes something like, "it's not how many times you get knocked down, it's how many times you get back up that matters", is certainly true in my case.

By sharing my journey, I hope that I can be the spark that ignites and inspires a woman to be who she was born to be. After taking a deep dive into my why and what now, I have re-evaluated, re-calibrated and recharged! My mantra:

I am strong
I am resilient
I am progressing
I am beautiful

Many of us have faced adversity and come back victorious. It is time for us to rise and embrace this season in our lives with enthusiasm and joy! Indeed, this can be the most extraordinary time of our lives! Let's do this together, delighting in our precious moments with head held high, a little lipstick on, and have some fun along the way!

Sharon Sloane is an artist and a mother who has found empowerment through independence.

Sharon Sloane

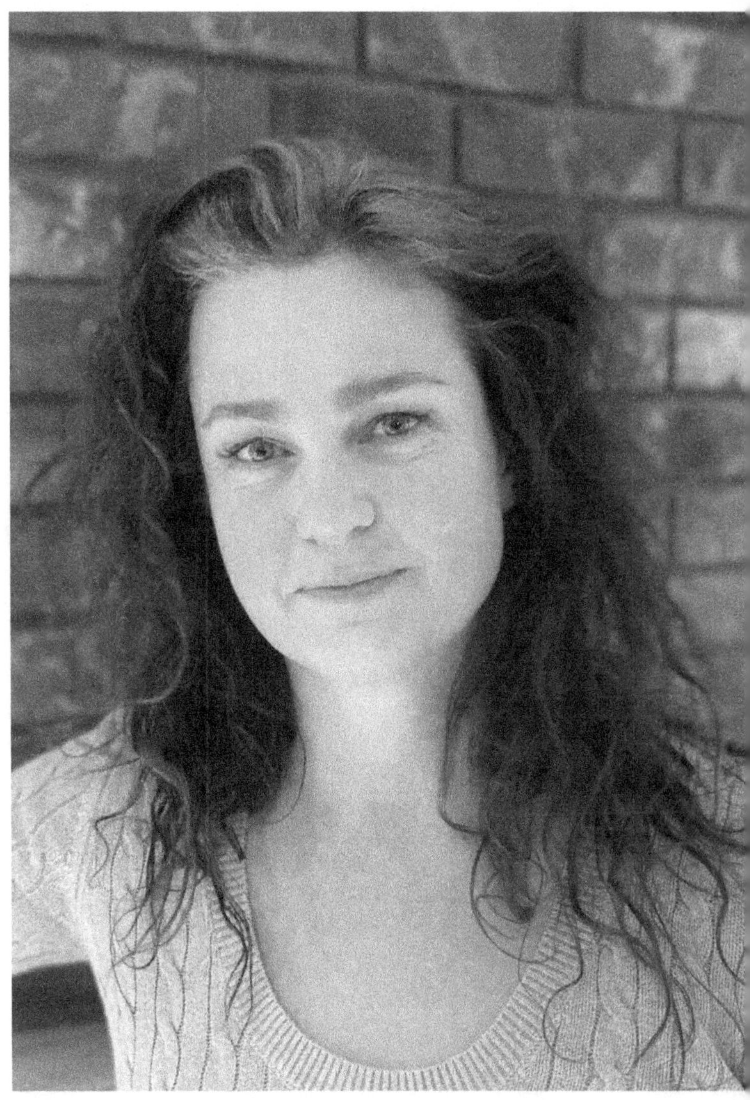

My life, like many, has been a series of choices pasted together. Some of these choices were intentionally made, and others less so. Starting over in my forties was terrifying. There were many days I truly wished I could just disappear. It took everything I had to find independence and create a new life for myself. So, I fought. I fought not only for my independence, but also for the life I wanted for myself and my children. The fight was both exhausting and exhilarating.

The fight began with the end of my twenty-year marriage. I used to be a stay-at-home mom on a farm, working with horses and drawing or painting every day. Having declared bankruptcy, I found myself on the opposite end of the spectrum in many ways. Thankfully with my art background, I was able to find a good job that fit my skill set. I went from painting animals and children to painting film sets. I don't think I ever saw this being my life.

My daughter lives with me now, and my family has supported us in many ways, however, it has always felt like us against the world. We survived and have found more happiness and clarity than we have had in a long time. With my own independence came the independence of my daughter. She has grown from a young country girl taking transit for the first time to someone that organizes all aspects of her life. Thank goodness one of us has their shit together.

It's such a mental challenge to take life one day at a time, but life becomes so incredibly overwhelming otherwise. There is an inner voice that is always there, trying to enhance the feelings of inadequacy, self-pity, and hate. Beating it back is harder some days than others. I found that being single was an emotionally positive experience for me. I was able to put myself first without guilt. I've found that being in a relationship and feeling alone is far worse than actually being single. I do believe that there is someone out there for me, right time, right place. I am proud to say that I'm feeling closer to the path I believe I'm meant to be on, or at least the path that will hopefully lead me to my best life with balance and happiness.

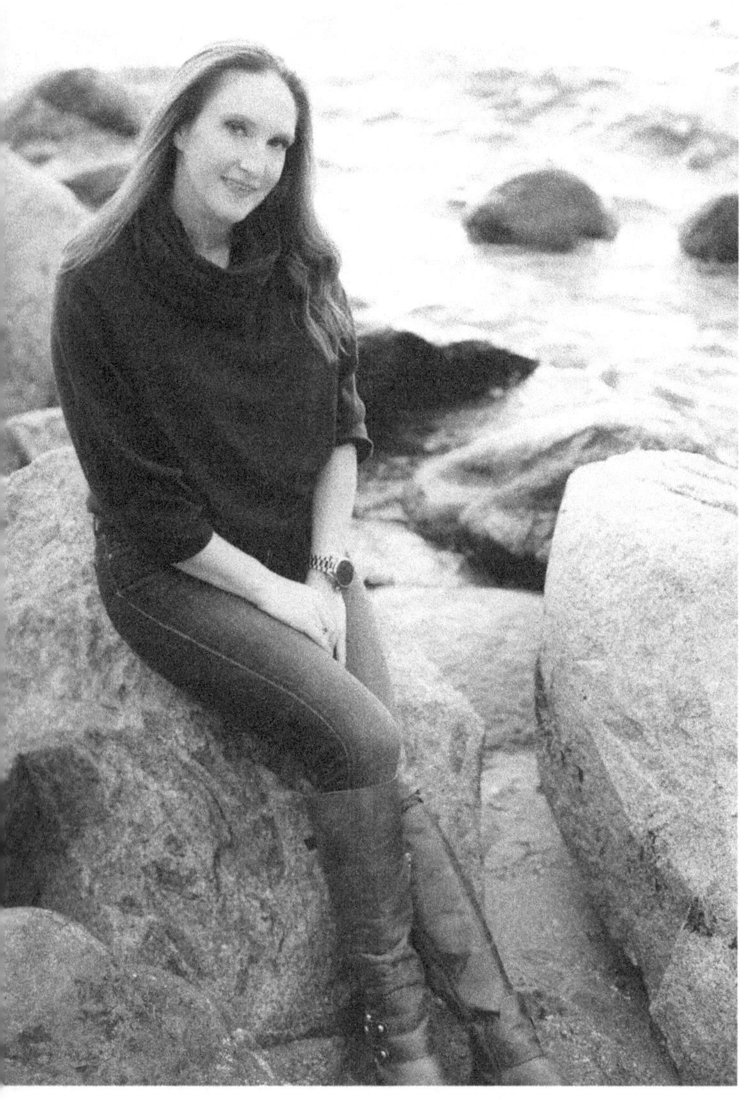

Rebekkah Stainton is a Registered Clinical Counsellor and the Founder of WestCoast Vitality Inc.

Rebekkah Stainton

I never planned to be a therapist and yet, I know I'm doing exactly what I'm supposed to. I was drawn to learning about people and helping them to bring out the hero within. Working with sexual trauma called to me right from the start and through this lens I began to expand into other areas of specialization, including anxiety and working with high performers (i.e. those of us who look like we have everything together yet are still subject to the same human frailties as everyone else). I once heard a client describe therapy as "uncomfortable wellness." How incredibly accurate! I believe it takes a lot of courage to be completely open about your struggles, to allow yourself to expose those difficult emotions that we all feel at certain moments in our lives. For many people, sitting in the counselling space is the first time they have allowed themselves to be completely honest, perhaps even with themselves. It is an incredible honour to know that my clients trust me with their stories.

A passion for my career doesn't mean that it's been easy or there haven't been setbacks. Holding space for others, sitting with their trauma, their hurt, their anxiety takes a toll. I've spent a lot of time struggling with finding a balance that allowed me to show up fully for my clients while still ensuring there was something left for my partner, my friends, my family... myself. I get overwhelmed and it's easy to get pulled into self-doubt. There have been many times that I've questioned "am I enough?" This is my signal that it's time to slow things down, take a moment to reflect, and figure out what's really going on. Paying attention to this signal and responding is what allows me to continue to develop both as a person and as a professional. Psychology is an area of continual growth and I truly believe that the day I think I know everything is the day I need to retire!

When things feel hard and there is the natural urge to deny or avoid, I would encourage you to consider this quote by Sarah Dessen "Anyone can hide. Facing up to things, working through them, that's what makes you strong."

Zahra is a business coach who helps healers, coaches and holistic practitioners market their businesses and heal their relationship with money so they can charge handsomely for their gifts.

Zahra Efan

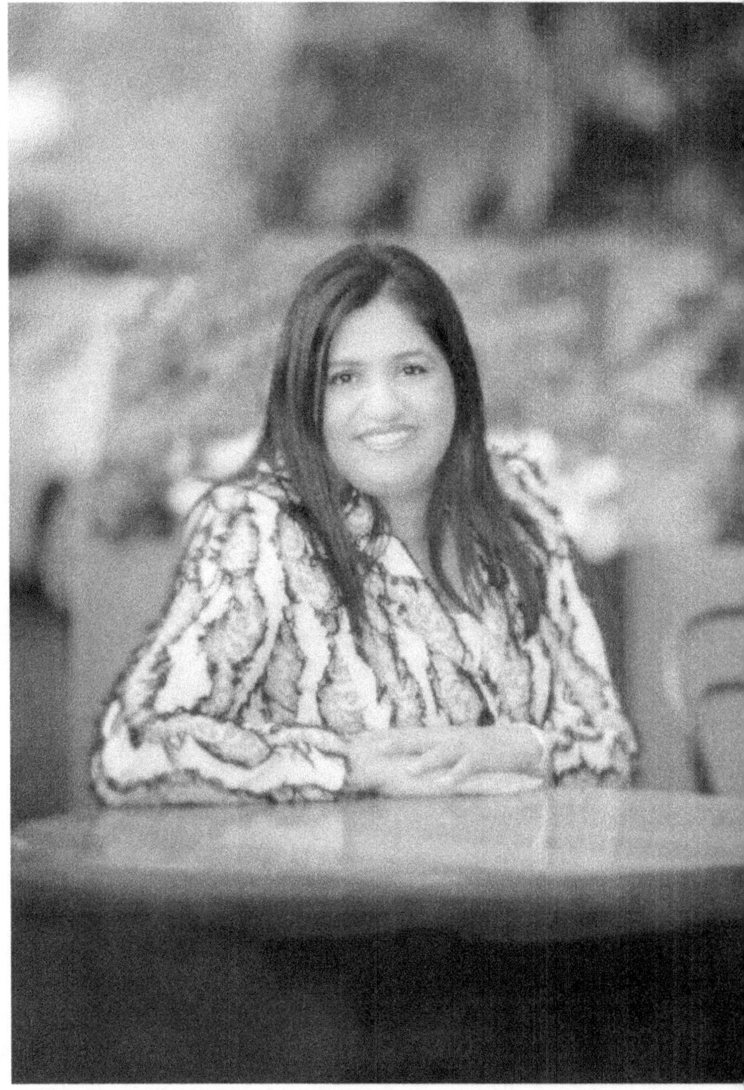

As a business coach for women for over a decade, I saw a pattern in my client's lives that made me add money healing work to my practice. What I noticed was that when it came to stepping into the next level of success in their business, my clients needed to change their relationship with money from the inside before they were able to charge more for their gifts and grow their business.

Our basic survival and safety depend on money. If we experienced traumas around money, it isn't possible to make more money unless we heal the money traumas we grew up with. Our instinctive response to money traumas can show up when we ask our clients to pay us for our gifts. We can either go to the "fight" response and come across as pushy or working too hard to make money, or we can go into a "freeze" response, that disables us from asking for the money or from taking the money-making actions altogether. Alternatively, we can also go into the "flight" response by escaping or denying the situation with money.

The reason for all of this is because women, in particular, have been unfairly treated over the years, either in our families or in our culture at large. The unfairness and injustices we experienced affect our relationship with money as the trauma around money happen in relationships with other people. And in business, we need to have relationships with people, including our customers.

Money also represents power. People with money make decisions in business and politics, unless we are comfortable with stepping into our personal power, we will not be able to make money. We need to heal the split between money and power. If we have had a painful relationship with people in power, we will have a difficult time asking for money unless we heal the gap between money, wealthy people, and power. Our wounds gave us sensitivity to help others heal, and stepping into our power will give us the courage to ask for money for our gifts.

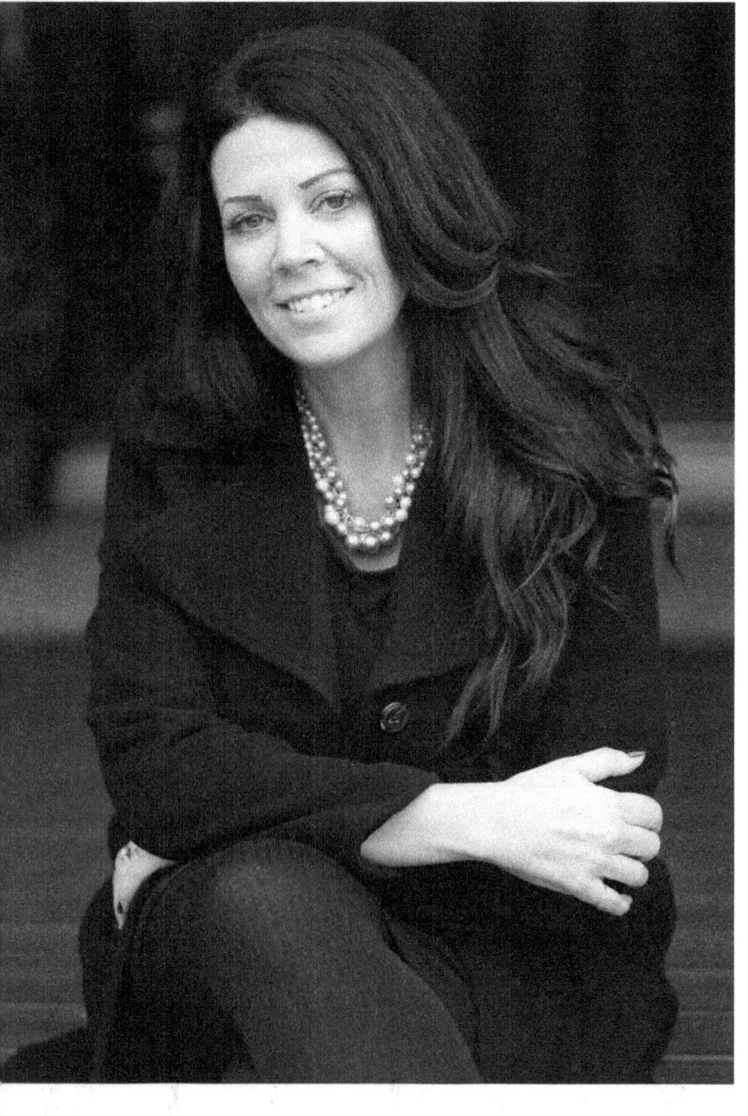

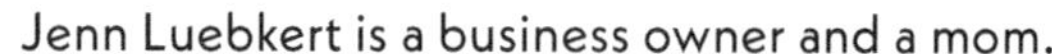

Jenn Luebkert is a business owner and a mom.

Jenn Luebkert

I dreamed of being a businesswoman since I was a little girl. I didn't play with Barbies or dolls, instead had a cash register and receipt books to sell items to my parents in my pretend store, autographing each sales receipt with a well-practiced signature.

My dad was a major influence in developing my entrepreneurial spirit. Always nurturing my smarts, brainstorming with me on my thoughts on different business ideas. Spending time out on the road with my dad, visiting clients, and listening to him on phone calls, I noticed that being genuine and not "sales-y" was his natural style, and it worked. Connecting with people and really, truly wanting to provide a solution to their problem. This is how I intuitively operate as an entrepreneur. Being genuine is something that people sense, and you build trust and loyalty from that and success follows.

Divorced by my mid-twenties, a single mom with two daughters and two jobs, I still dreamed of being my own boss. In 2003 I made the leap and started my first serious business and never looked back. I still run that business to this day. I am also involved in real estate with my husband and own a beauty salon that my youngest daughter Talia manages and together we run the day-to-day. From the outside, it all looks wonderful, but my path has been extremely challenging.

My oldest daughter, Brittany, got on the wrong track in her early teens and has been battling addiction since. She is thirty-two years old now and addicted to heroin. Everything I did revolved around her battle and how I could help get her on track. Nothing ever lasted. You find out the hard way that nobody is coming to save you and that no matter what, the world doesn't stop for your problems. The bills still need to get paid, so you have to dig really deep.

When your child is out there suffering, it consumes you. You question everything you have ever done and find yourself paralyzed in your own goals and dreams. It requires an incredible amount of strength and positivity to push through some days.

It breaks my heart every day, but I stay hopeful. With the emotional support of my amazing family and friends, I do my best to live my life and find joy in it now. Practicing gratitude is key for me, and every morning when my feet hit the ground, I find a list of things to be grateful for, get my mindset straight and get ready to tackle the day!

Ellen Bradley Cheung is a mother, artist, yogi, comedian, and student.

Ellen Bradley Cheung

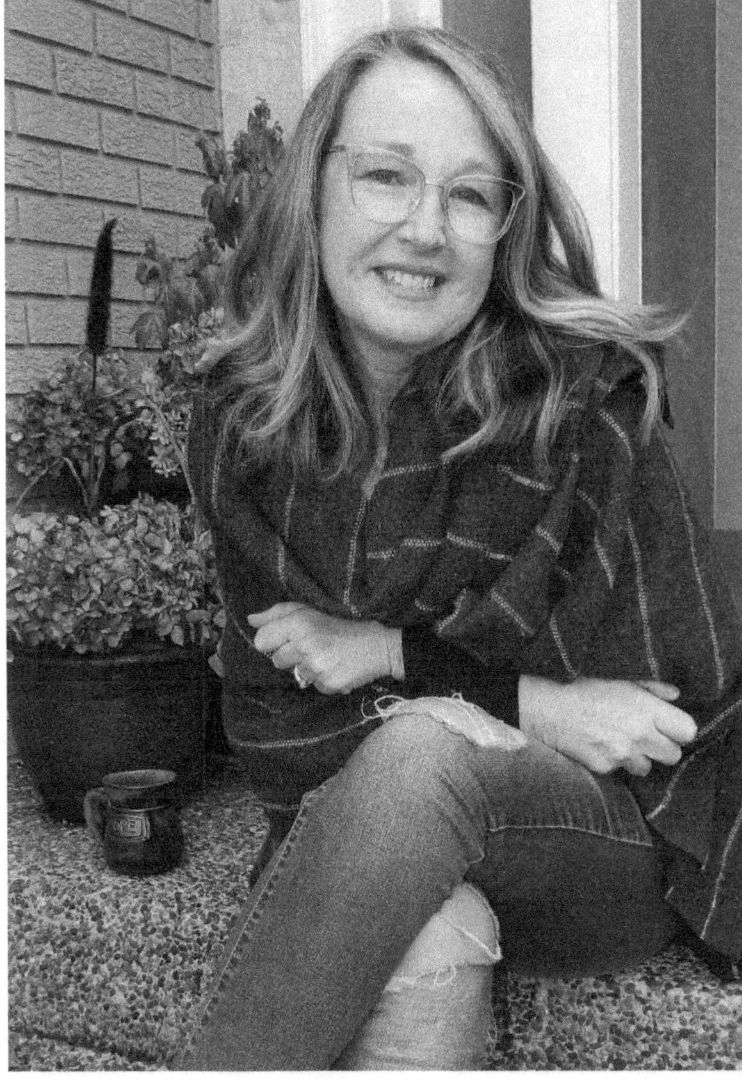

I am from Nova Scotia, and my maritime roots are very dear to me. I was always shy and socially awkward as a kid. Growing up, I was involved in sports and music; however, I often felt I did not fit in. I left for Vancouver after I received my B.A., and attended nursing school, which was more aligned with my true nature, and with my passion for caring for others. After my second daughter was born, I started upon a new full-time career, raising a family, and instilling in my two daughters my love, values, and sense of respect for all.

My love for art and painting also flourished over the years. I hosted painting parties and displayed my art. Throughout this time however, my mental health was declining. I had always secretly suffered from depression and loneliness, and it became difficult to manage and keep hidden. I used alcohol to numb the pain and suffering yet living in unbearable pain and shame. I had so much to be happy about, but the dark pit of depression was getting deeper.

I have done much work on myself, connecting with who I am, taking off the mask, and showing up as me. My mind is now clear, and amazing opportunities have since presented themselves. Thankfully, I found my way to recovery. I started displaying my art in Roam Gallery. My self-confidence and self-worth have brought me on stage as a stand-up comedian with Hilarapy, sharing my story vulnerably, with humour, to give hope and shed light on mental health struggles. At fifty-two, my journey as a yoga instructor began, and now I offer yoga, sound baths, and meditation. Meditation has been one of the key modalities in my recovery. I am enrolled in a transpersonal counselling program where I continue to learn about myself and look forward to using these new skills to support others. My experiences are continuous, expansive, and amazing; I can now connect with myself and celebrate what I have achieved. I can show up vulnerably and admit, "I am struggling today," knowing I will be ok. I have the deepest of gratitude for who I am today!

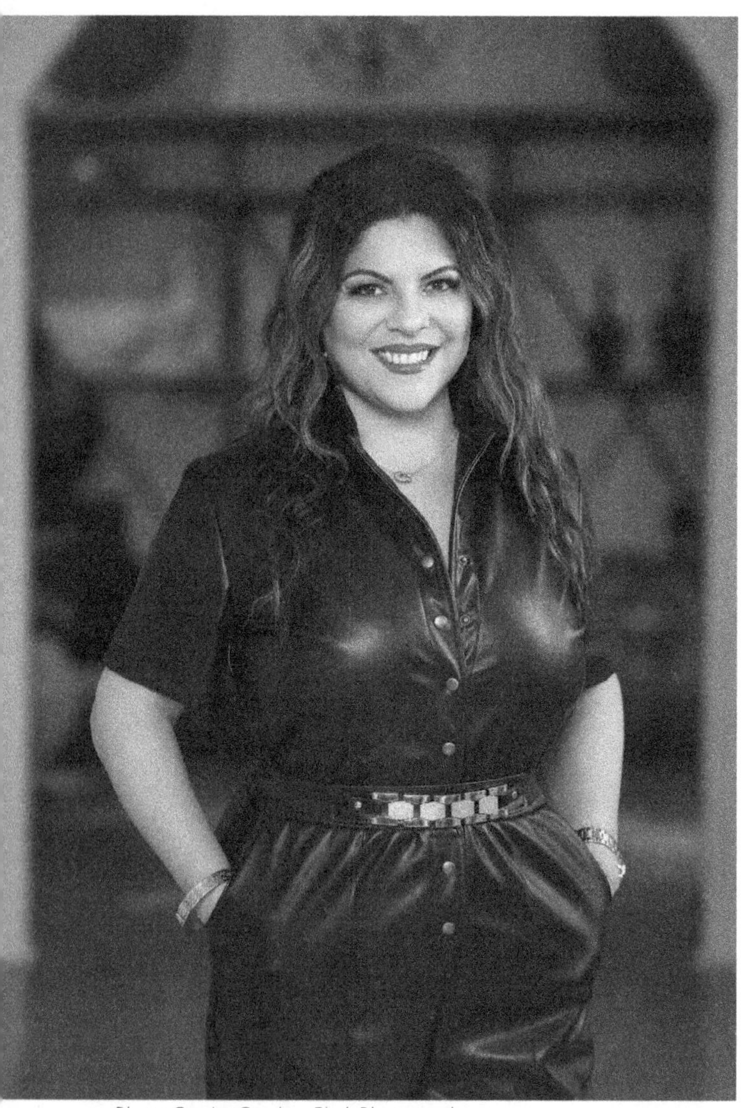

Photo Credit: Gordon Clark Photography

Cathy Cena is a Managing Partner at FDT Academy, an Entrepreneur, a People Connector, a MOM, Wife and a local Media Personality, who loves Life!

Cathy Cena

I was born in a small town in Italy called Taurianova, Province of Reggio Calabria. I landed in Vancouver, BC, Canada in 1972. As the eldest of three, I embrace life and always try new things, and am full of energy.

I started volunteering at the age of twelve which marked the beginning of me giving back to my community. Now at the age of fifty, I continue to give back and volunteer while contributing to my community... a place I call home. I had two children by the age of twenty-three. As a young mother, I was determined to teach my children the following - love yourself, love each other and try to give a hand where you can. I feel I have instilled these traits in both my children.

As a long-time Port Moody resident, I am an active community member and advocate and have established a great reputation among my peers and colleagues. I currently work alongside my son and daughter as we run our family business FDT Academy Inc., where we focus on teaching hundreds of students the art of Debate and Public Speaking. In my spare time I created Catching up with Cathy, a radio show, The Chat TV, a women-led talk show, and I am currently the President of Port Moody's Arts Center and the Optimists Club of Coquitlam. As busy as I am I love it when a connection is made between companies and people. Some call me the "People Connector". When I am not around town networking, I enjoy spending time with my children, Frankie and Tonya, and my husband, Dave. I was proud to have been nominated for the Tri-Cities Chamber of Commerce "Community Spirit" Award and as a Woman Influencer in the Community Steward category. I have always had a passion for politics and decided to run in the election in 2017. I feel more women are needed in politics and more gender equality is necessary. Although unsuccessful, that has never stopped me from pushing forward and pushing through my comfort zone to achieve more.

My Favorite Quote is, "We may encounter many defeats, but we must not be defeated" - Maya Angelou.

Farzana Jaffer Jeraj is a best-selling author and motivational speaker with a focus on mindset, neuroscience, and meditation.

Farzana Jaffer Jeraj

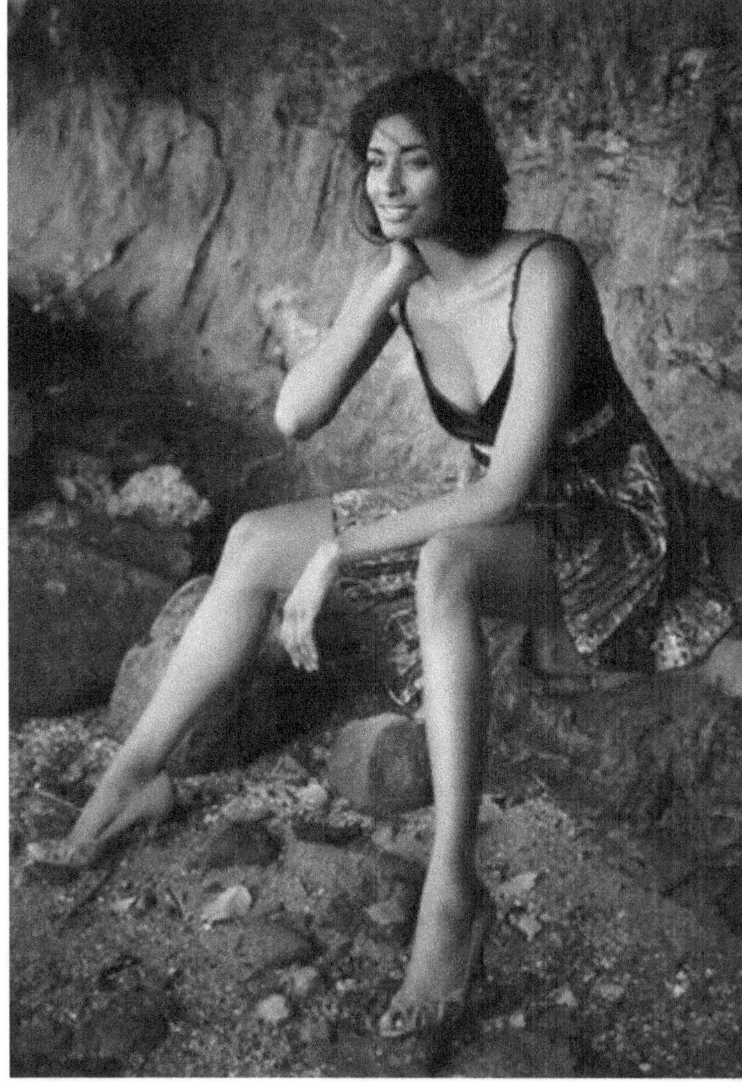

Photo Credit: David Fierro

It has taken so much work to get to where I am today. Not just business-wise, but deep gritty self-work. After years of bullying, I never believed anyone would ever care to hear what I had to say. Every time I'm asked to speak my truth, I have to muster up courage, give myself a pep talk, and remember that ultimately it is being of service is all that matters. I worked to cultivate my personality, and then to cultivate a strength of self so that I don't feel a need to be anything but myself. I have worked to define my values and beliefs to be in alignment with who I truly am. Not what my experiences and others might have told me I am.

...and yet it is in the moments of mindfulness where I sit in silence and listen to myself that I truly sense who I am.

Who are we as individuals? Are we a collection of the events of our lives? Are we our jobs? Are we a reflection of our social circle? Our daily habits? Our beliefs, thoughts, and emotions? Our challenges?

I don't believe any of these things really make us who we are. Our challenges are as real as we perceive them to be, our emotions so powerful they warp our sense of time and reality. Challenges pass, thoughts come and go, and your beliefs and values can be changed by you in a heartbeat. Emotions are just chemicals and they truly can't remain forever.

We exist beyond these things. It is the self that chooses. When you don't feel like yourself, that is your self that reminds you of who you truly are. It is the same self that decides to wiggle your big toe that can choose what you believe and value at any given moment in your life.

Is there work involved. A thousand percent. Ultimately, I love my high heels and I love nature. I love meditation, the spiritual conversations around consciousness and existence; and I also love science and the material physical gifts of this world. None of those things are truly who I am.

You are not your past actions; you are the choices you make today. Events pass, emotions don't last, you are always.

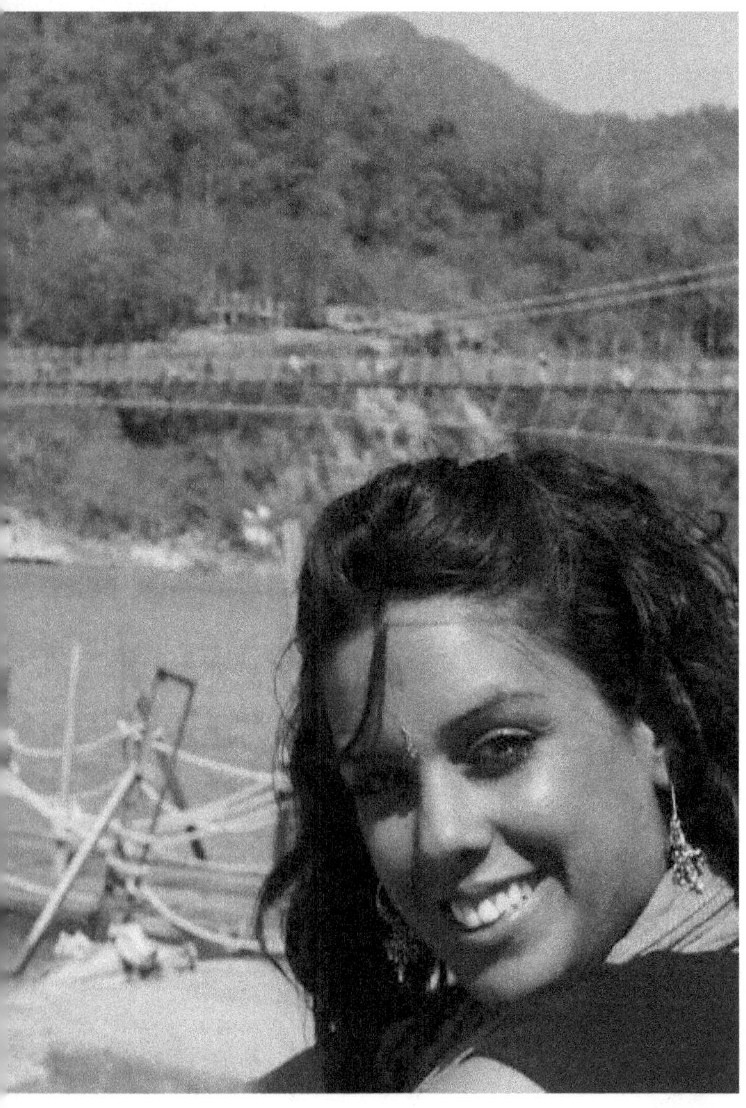

Nina Bains is a mother, a filmmaker, a traveller, who blazes her own trail.

Nina Bains

What did I want to do when I grew up? This question my mother asked on our daily walk during one cold winter afternoon. Without thinking, I responded, " I want to make movies and travel around the world." I was only eleven years old.

I was not sure how I would make it happen; I just knew that I would find a way. I was destined for an extraordinary life, and I was not entertaining any thoughts to the contrary. You see, the odds were stacked against me. I was born the daughter of two Indian farmers. Both barely out of their teenage years, they were shipped off to Canada in hopes they could escape the remnants of the bloody Partition of 1947. They became engaged via a photograph of each other, plucked from their villages, and met for the first time at the Lester B Pearson Airport in Toronto. Shortly after, I came along. I grew up in Toronto, the oldest of five children. The responsibility of setting a good example was heavy. A career in the arts was not a responsible choice, according to my Indian parents. The more they pushed me towards a responsible career, the closer I moved towards Bollywood and Hollywood. I spent more time than ever thinking about creating and getting lost in the beautiful, rich, and colourful on-screen worlds. Despite the challenges that presented themselves, I have taken advantage of every single opportunity that aligned itself with me. I have been consistent with my dedication to turn my daydreams into my reality.

I now live a beautiful and adventurous life working in film and television, and I am invited as a guest to film festivals around the world. I started The Ottawa International Film Festival before moving into the world of production.

I laugh out loud. I do not sugar coat anything. I am bold, daring, and outrageous, and I like to sing out loud in the car with the windows rolled all the way down.
I am a mother. A filmmaker. A traveller. I blaze my own trail and dance to the beat of my own drum. In this way, my story is like no other.

Kelly Mallinson takes a holistic approach to her business, incorporating intuitive energy healing work to help others experience the power of essential oils, and their capacity for physical and emotional healing.

Kelly Mallinson

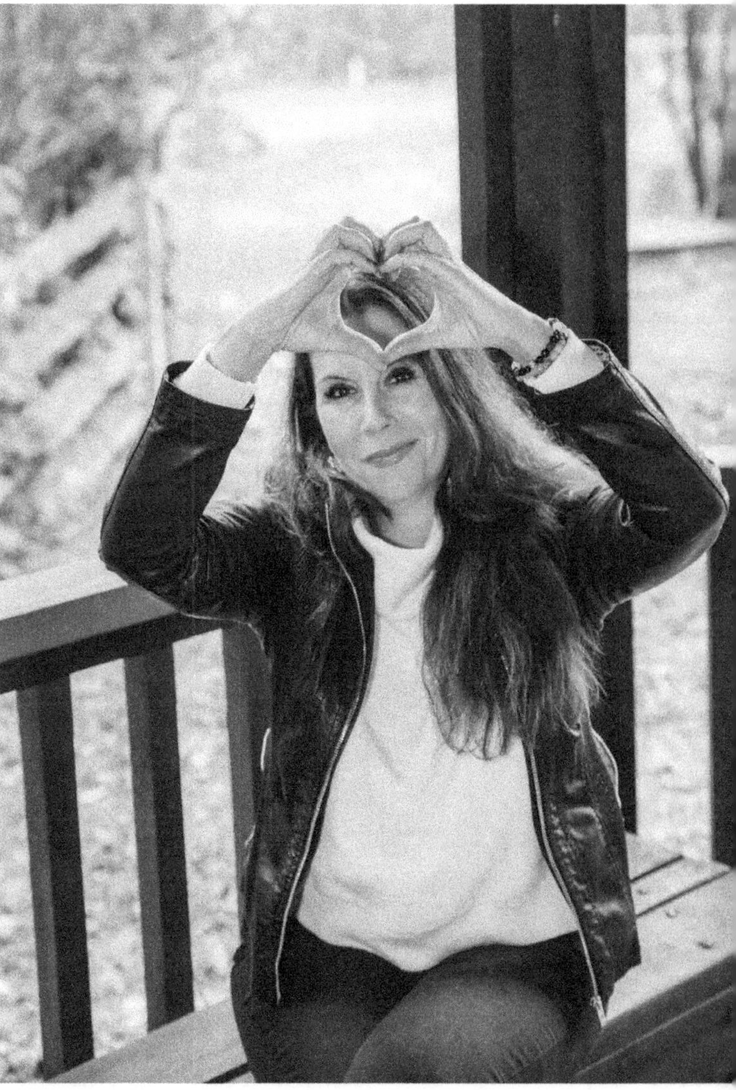

I want to spread as much happiness, healing, and positivity as I possibly can in my lifetime. I have learned that when you make people feel good, you feel good too. Being a bright light for people and spreading positivity, especially now when there is so much negativity, is something I am inspired to do every day. I recognize the good in everyone because opening yourself up to accepting all versions of people leads to wonderful friendships and experiences. I love people, and I love including everyone in anything I'm doing. Being in situations where I am surrounded by people energizes me.

I love helping people tap into what will heal them as they break through personal roadblocks that convince them they cannot do what they really want to do or be who they really want to be. Everyone deserves support and kindness from others; nobody should ever feel alone. My "aha moment" happened last year at a conference in Prague that aligned my love for helping people with a profound realization that I myself was not alone, that I didn't have to figure out how to succeed in my business on my own. The moment I realized that I couldn't do this alone was the minute my career changed and elevated me to the next level of my life and my business.

I am surrounded with kindness, love, and support from so many sources; my children, my business, my friendships, and it makes me excited to live my life. On days when I don't feel great, I get myself back on track by using the resources I've gathered that have taught my mind and healed my heart. Listening to meditations, inspirational speakers, and songs I love, journaling, exercising, and most of all, using my beautiful essential oils every single day to help me be the best version of myself. I see the possibilities in every person I meet and I believe that anything is achievable through kindness, acceptance, positivity, and essential oils.

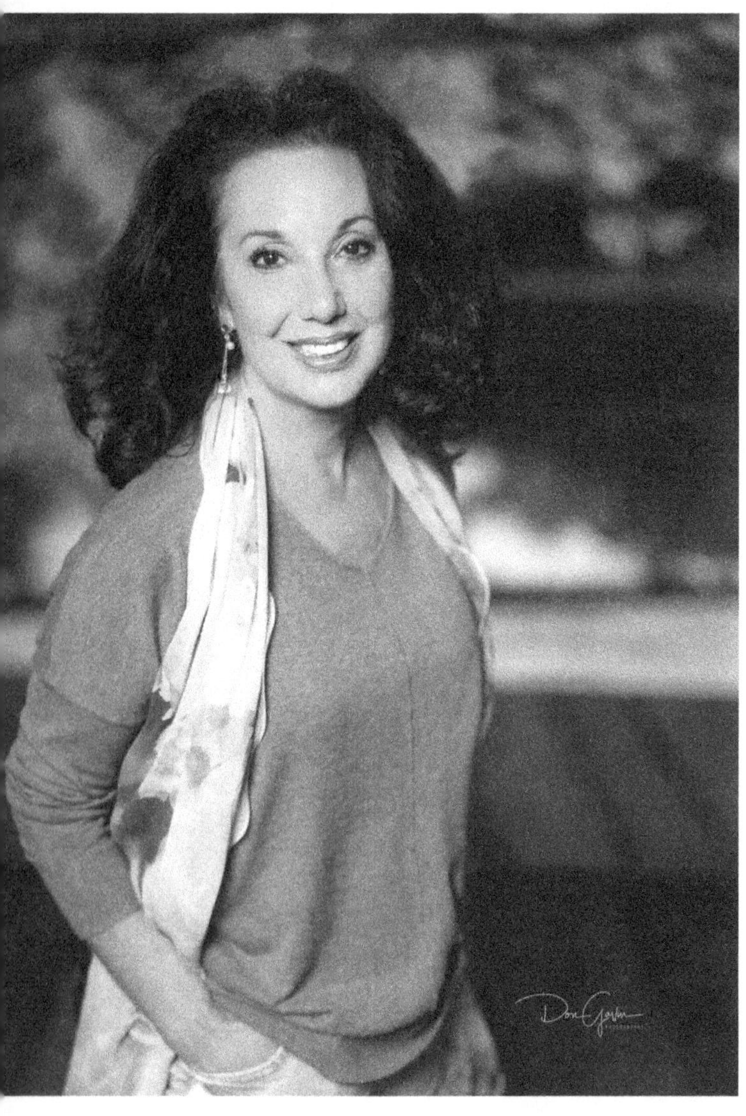

Charlene Luedke is a country girl from Kamloops, B.C., a lover of horses, especially my Appaloosa Hiawatha along with many other animals, and am an animal advocate across this planet.

Charlene Luedke

My purpose in life is to help people see the world's beauty, enhancing their well-being using my acquired skills in the arts, social networking, and animal connections.

I started my acting career early in life. A penchant since childhood. Moving to the big city of Vancouver in 1982 I started out with Ramona Beauchamp's Modelling and Acting Agency while working in the Food Industry. This would lead me on a fulfilling journey embracing changes and opportunities as they presented. Next through being a showroom model for Neto Leather, I would join this family for almost seven years and become a traveled junior designer for leather garments, as well as working the wholesale sales end of the fashion industry. Next, I was married to my long-time life partner of thirty-one years. We have two children, a daughter, and a son, both of whom we are immensely proud of. Before jumping back into my actor shoes, I would spend almost seven years selling Real Estate, taking us into the new millennium, where I was met with my mother fighting for her life with lung cancer. It was upon her death that I had to stop, catch my breath, and discover my path back to my true passion. Back to acting, I went.

Fast forward to today. Six talent agents later. My journey, having many fulfilling moments, would also be riddled with extreme challenges. Suffering years of postpartum depression, a cancer scare, losing parents, family relationship struggles. Being bounced from one agent to the next, as though I could not even get arrested in this town. Yes, talk about a dark horse.

"A dark horse; a person the emergence often to prominence through the rival of many challenges." That is what I do; I find my pathway through. I may not have prominence, but I have persistence and many wins. We all have stories; they are all worthy of being told. Thanks, pursuit:365, for providing this space. From this Entrepreneurial Actress with love.

Lorraine Zander is an entrepreneur, mentor, speaker, and dreamer – igniting a generation of powerful young women!

Lorraine Zander

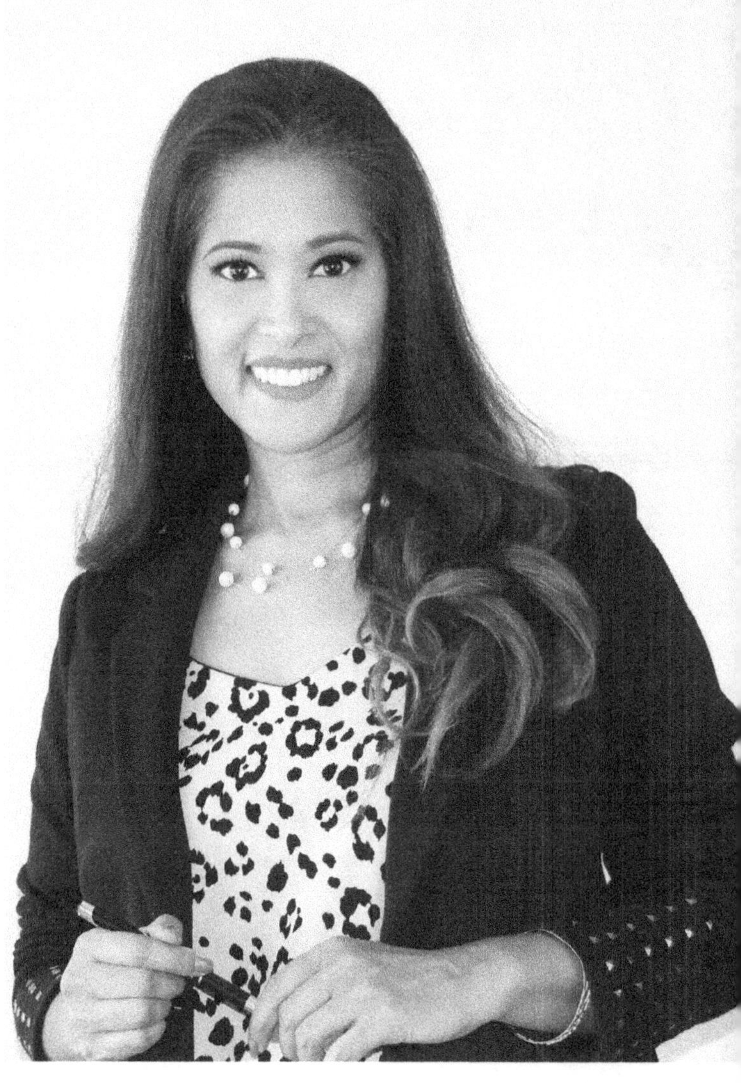

I'm often asked what it was like to start my own magazine. Simply put, I was ignorance on fire. I had no experience in publishing, no formal writing background, and truthfully, I wasn't even an avid magazine reader. But I had a strong desire to try to make a difference. That was it. But it was enough.I remember in the early stages when I was in the midst of doing background research in my industry, I was lucky enough to get a one-on-one meeting with a magazine owner and publisher of a very well-known national publication. He kicked off the meeting by leaning forward, looking me in the eyes, and asking, "How do you become a millionaire?" Before I could blink twice, he said, "Start with a billion dollars and then start a magazine." I kind of laughed, and dismissed his funny-not-funny message, because like any self-respecting, unstoppable, newbie boss lady entrepreneur, I was certain my magazine would be successful, and everyone would love it (unshakeable certainty is always helpful when starting a business).

My magazine's mission was simple: to inspire and empower young women. Over the twenty years since that meeting, I have worked many twenty-hour days, sometimes consecutively and including weekends. I have experienced devastating and deflating defeats, thankfully tempered by pinch-myself and shout-from-the-rooftop motivating wins. I have laughed and cried, sometimes at the same time.

But most importantly, I have been fulfilling my mission. I have been privileged to meet some of the most inspiring change-makers on the planet, like Melati Wijsen, who by the age of twenty, led the charge to ban plastic bags on her home island of Bali. Maureen Muketha is helping to end hunger and fights every day for gender equality in Kenya. In Nepal, Dipika Badal is tackling environmental policy change. I have shared their stories, which light the path for others to make our world a kinder more compassionate place. And knowing that in some small way I am helping to make a difference, I feel richer every day. I'm not saying you shouldn't make becoming a billionaire your mission. But please don't make it your only one, because you'll never find real wealth in your bank account.

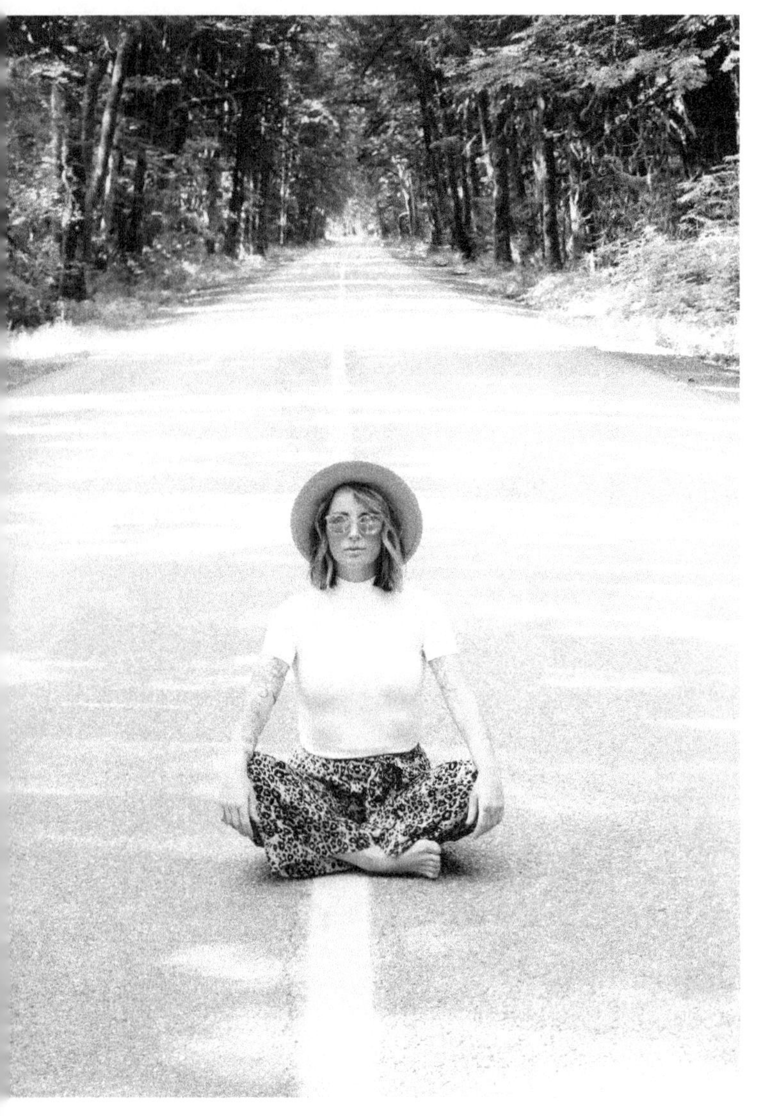

Amber Spence is a dedicated and proud woman in business, hustling entrepreneur, and mom to her daughter Nixon. Amber's knowledge and determination in creative strategy and visual design turn information into action which leads to her success as a social media marketing and brand expert with experience managing multi-level teams and projects in magazines, fashion, health, and wellness. She continues to grow her business and is always looking for new opportunities to challenge herself further

Amber Spence

Hey, I am Amber! I am a social media manager specializing in marketing, branding, and content creation. I started my business over ten years ago, helping small business owners show up on social media and build an authentic community through done-for-you content strategies and customized training. I am proud to be me.

Being proud of myself is another way of saying I have a strong sense of self-worth. And people who are proud of themselves tend to have a great passion for life, feel content and grateful, and are excellent at motivating others. To me, believing in your greatness is what inspires us to find solutions and make things better. So here are a few reasons I am proud of myself right now...

I am proud of making difficult decisions and challenging myself. My ability to get through hard times and my achievements, both in my everyday life and the huge steps I have been able to climb the last xx years. I am also proud that I know myself well.

I am proud of the goals I set. I am proud that every time I set goals, I do my best to achieve them. And when I fail, of course, I get upset, but it drives me to work harder by analyzing and working on my mistakes.

I am proud of the passion and dedication I have. I am not exactly where I want to be — but I am getting closer. I am taking steps toward my destination each and every day. I have made mistakes, but I have also made achievements. I have rediscovered myself. I have found out what I really want from this world and am working towards grabbing it.

I am ME; I am proud to be ME. I am proud that I love fiercely. And proud that I'm living my life for myself and for unapologetically being who I am.

Janviere Mukama is a Learning & Development Facilitator, and a founder of UWI Marketing & Media.

Janviere Mukama

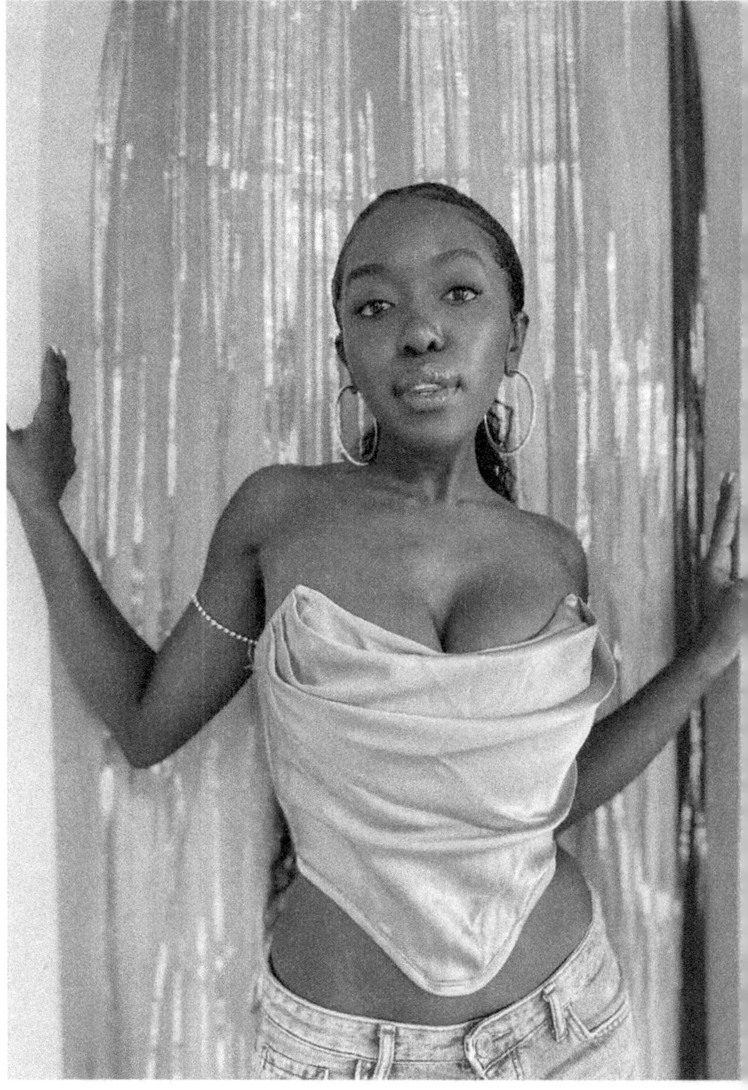

In my pursuit of happiness and success, my greatest lesson has been balance. Whether it's a balanced diet, relationship, or spending habits, balance has held a key role in my journey.

Many facets of our lives are centred around this theme. Anatomically, at the core of who we are as humans, balance gives us the ability to maintain control over our bodies. Biologically, a balanced ecosystem allows us to sustain life on earth. Emotionally, balance gives us the ability to form meaningful interpersonal and intrapersonal connections. Mentally, balance allows us to freely navigate through the ups and downs of life. I seek to inspire and empower the people around me to live their life as authentically and as bravely as possible by fully embracing new experiences, most of which I owe to my travels abroad. Travel has become an integral part of my journey to fulfillment and with it, comes excitement and sometimes fear. One of my favourite motivational quotes by Susan Jeffers is, "Feel the fear and do it anyway."

Sometimes I find fear to be paralyzing, which can lead to things like creative block, perfectionism, and stagnation. My secret sauce to overcoming these crippling feelings consists of three things: self-awareness, self-care, and self-improvement. Collectively, these encapsulate my favourite mantra, give yourself grace.

I've learned that this can show up in many forms. Grace can look like journaling my introspective thoughts. Grace can look like curling up with my favourite cup of tea. Grace can also look like getting my body moving through disciplined workouts. I've learned along the way that being kind to myself isn't always the easiest thing to do, it means doing what's necessary to foster growth.

I have stumbled at least once in all aspects of my life. Each adversity has led me to a deeper understanding of my strengths: empathy, intellect, relationship building, the pursuit of excellence, and harmony. I've been able to flex these skills having dabbled in various professional roles including shift management in a high-paced restaurant, Style Advisor in evolving retail environments, and currently working in a tech start-up as a Learning & Development Facilitator.

As rewarding as this professional growth has been, it has been accompanied by personal growth patterns in both my modelling career and as a new small business owner. After all, it's all about balance.

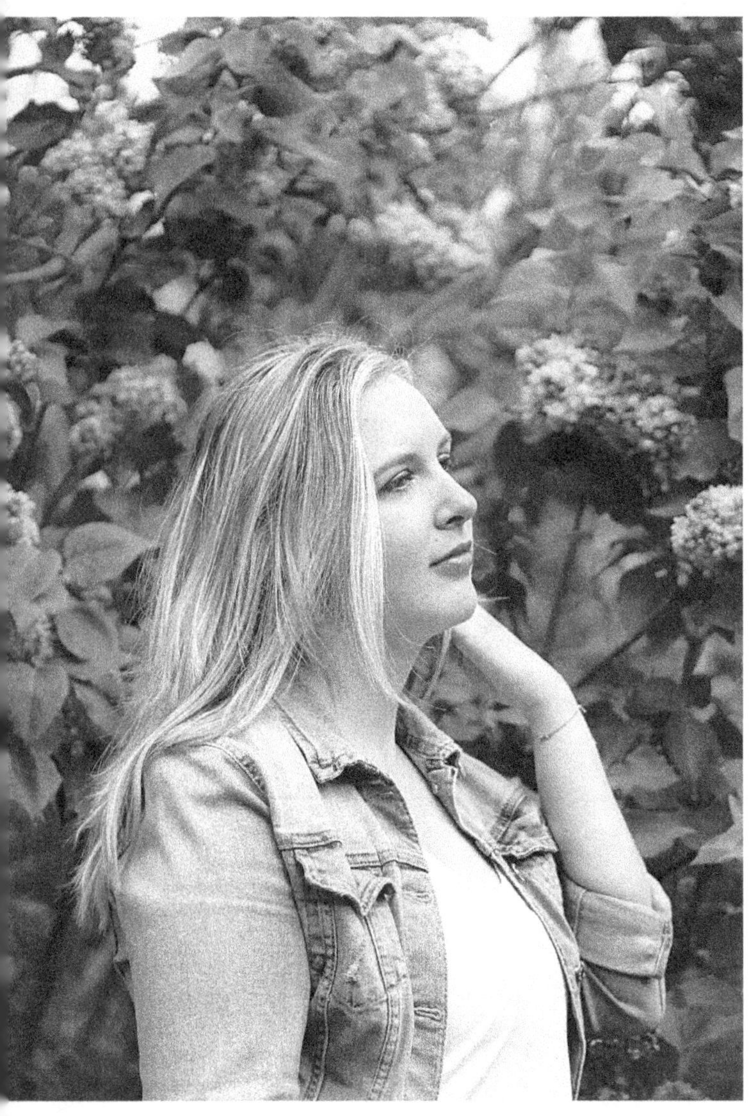

Sarah Zoschke is a student in the Master of Teaching program at the University of Toronto. A woman of many passions Sarah also energetically consults on destination weddings as an accredited Destination Wedding Planner.

Sarah Zoschke

Since I can remember I have always been a dreamer. I was that girl in class, staring out the window, thinking about my next steps. That was me, the daydreamer. My grandmother always loved hearing my dreams, the stories I created, and most of all, my passions. She always encouraged my dreams, however, she had one dream in particular for me – and it's in the works right now. Even at the tender age of seven, when most kids don't even know what they want for breakfast in the morning, I already had a career in sight; books. I wanted to work with books. As I grew older and my dreams were slowly clouded with reality, I pushed through.

The important thing about dreams is they do come true in some capacity, maybe not today, but with perseverance, they eventually do. The other thing about dreams is once you achieve them, it opens up room for you to create more. With this knowledge, and the support of my family, I moved to Toronto to pursue a career in publishing; a small-town girl embarking on the big city. I found myself bouncing around, first from contract publishing position to contract positions, then through various industries. But every time I found my fit, it was as though the sheet was pulled aside and all these issues came to light. I kept working hard at it, picking a new dream, a new destination.

To know me is to know my resume, although it might look like an undesirable narrative of multiple jobs, I look at it as a dream checklist, an achievement list. Without it and the inspiration from my mom, I would have never found the courage to go back to school and pursue the dream my grandmother held for me. To become a teacher and guidance counsellor. Even though she isn't here today, I like to think about her smiling, thinking, "she did it!"

Following the path of kindness and curiosity, founder and creative, Caroline MacGillivray experienced adventures that have led to friendship, career opportunities, and bringing hope and healing to women and youth!

Caroline MacGillivray

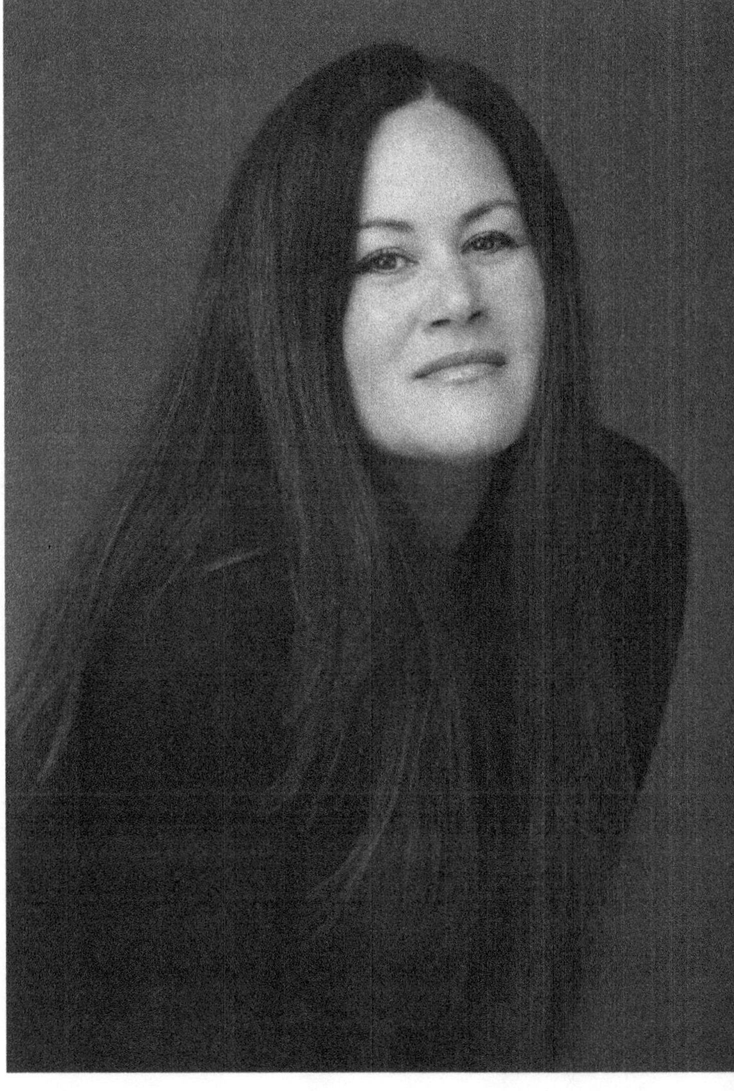

"Oooooh, I love your lipstick! What shade is that?" are words that I have spoken and received vastly different results. Once I got sucker-punched by someone who thought I was hitting on her. Another time, I booked my first voice-over gig and writing assignment. Thankfully, most of the time when I compliment someone, it makes them smile. We can't control someone's reaction to us. There will be times we get kicked in the teeth and other times when it forges friendships. I've found approaching the world through the lens of curiosity and wonderment has brought success and joy to myself and others.

My curiosity and love for beauty have led me to meet like-minded people. Some adventures I've experienced include screaming into a microphone as the sound engineer winces pulling the headphones away from their ears as they capture a sound bite for a project for film and television, getting flown up to a recording studio in Haida Gwai to record backup vocals for bands recording albums, and picking chanterelle mushrooms amidst the forest to prep for dinner. This has also led to writing lifestyle segments for tourism publications, hosting a sexual health and relationship radio show, teaching pole dancing, raising money for charity teaching bunny yoga, becoming a medical Qi Gong therapist, and creating projects that build community and healing in marginalized communities.

Once I volunteered at a shelter and offered to help someone struggling to curl her hair. The woman that I helped thanked me and told me that I made her feel "human." That act of service led to founding the charity, Beauty Night Society. The past two decades have provided opportunities to create hope and healing for women and youth in Vancouver's Downtown Eastside.

By being kind and curious to myself, I am able to create a ripple effect of hope and healing for others. Surrounding myself with people who make me laugh, love, and give me hope lets me continue to share kindness and curiosity.

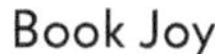

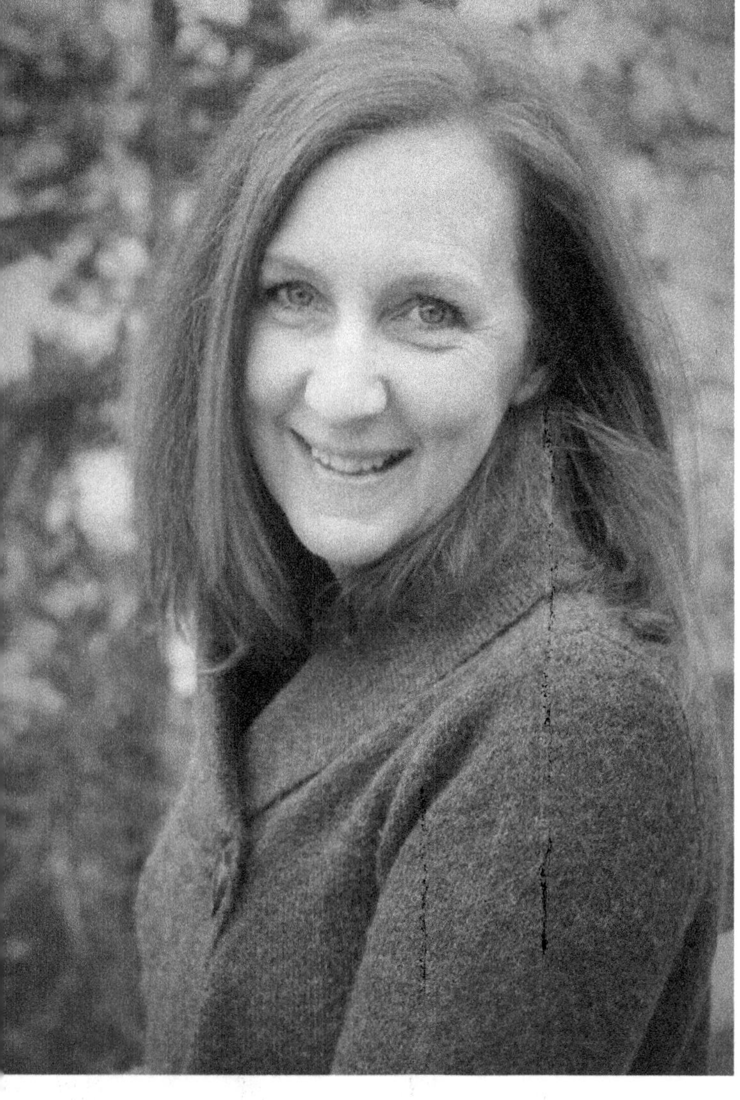

Adrienne Gear

When I was eight years old, my dad bought me my first book: **Little House in the Big Woods** by Laura Ingalls Wilder. I had been reading books from school and the public library for years but there was something magical about having a book that was my very own. I read it over and over again. Looking back, I believe that was the moment I felt my first burst of "book joy." Anyone who knows me personally knows how much I love books. I don't feel just a small affinity for them. I'm talking heart-racing, book-sniffing, trembling-fingers love that knows no bounds.

My career path has grown out of this deeply rooted love of books. When I became a teacher, I brought my passion for books and my love of reading into the classroom. Anyone who knows me professionally knows how essential children's literature is to all aspects of my teaching practice. Picture books are woven through the fabric of almost every lesson I teach and become the undeniable link to my students. Books have a way of inviting the connections, conversations, and deep learning that I am convinced are not possible through any other means. These are not literal conversations about content: "What's the boy's name" or "What color is the car?" (Imagine the women in a book club answering twenty-five multiple-choice questions about their books and handing them to the host to mark!) They are the conversations about our lives: our families, feelings, friendships; conversations about bullies, basketball, worries, and dreams. This is where "book joy" comes from.

Toni Morrison says, "The words on the page are only half the story; the rest is what you bring to the party." By teaching children that reading is not simply about words on a page, but what they bring of themselves to those words, we are helping them to find their own "book joy." Reading is not about "getting the right answer;" reading is knowing that the thinking we have in our heads and the feelings we have in our hearts are equally as powerful as the book we hold in our hands. And that, my friends, is book joy.

Amelie Nguyen

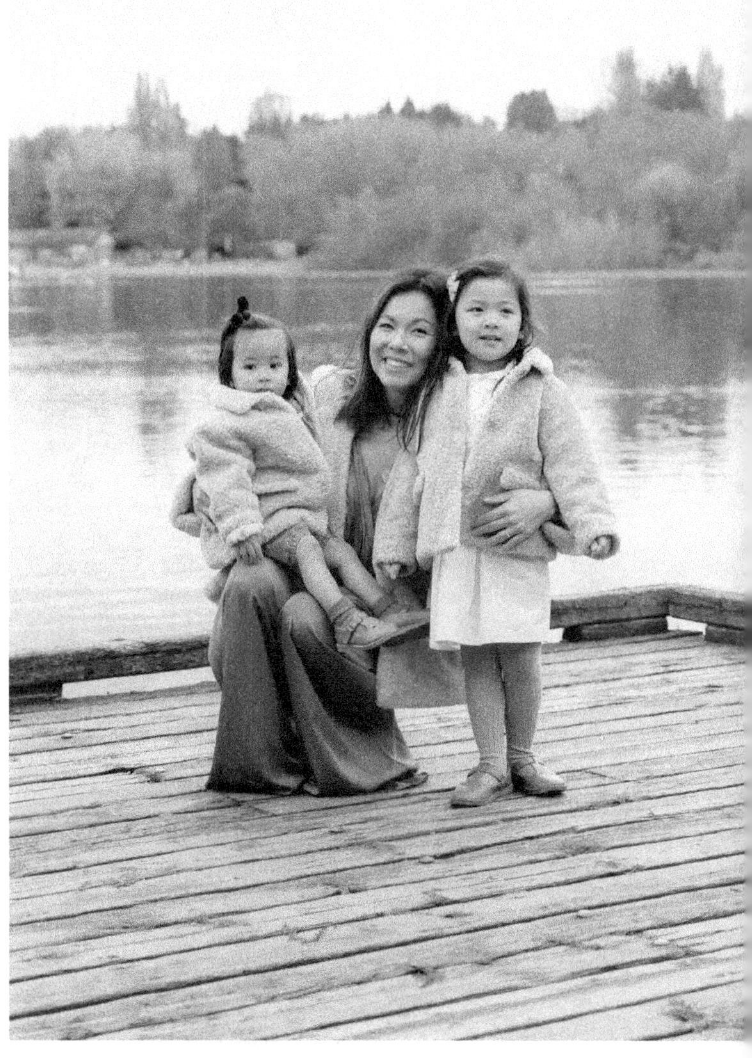

Like other young people, I believed in happily ever after. I believed that love conquers all and that if we set out to follow our passion, everything would naturally fall into place.

I had a picture-perfect life by forty: married with two daughters, worked for the World Health Organization, created a film about my family, and founded one of the best restaurants in Vancouver. Twenty-twenty saw the global pandemic, our hospitality industry took a huge hit, and my marriage came to an end.

I hid my struggles while doing everything to save it. Counselling, cooking, cleaning, hiding my achievements, you name it. The more I tried, the more I failed miserably. I held onto my fairy tale so tightly - afraid of what people would think, afraid of disappointing our families, afraid that I would no longer be a role model for the most important humans in my life - my daughters. I had three choices: accept the status quo, leave with resentment, or stay with a different mindset.

If you really know me, you'll know I thrive on challenging the status quo. I am also so joyful that I would not let drama or hate weigh me down. The only thing left was to pivot. I reached out for guidance and, in turn, gained light-years of wisdom and courage. I began trusting that things happen for me, not to me. I accepted this failure as a learning opportunity. I let go of perfection and dismissed fairy tale myths and cultural norms. I welcomed a new way of being. This shift freed my spirit. For the first time in a long time, I connected with my partner on a far deeper level. We experienced how we can redefine our family.

Today we are consciously uncoupling. We are committed to raising our daughters together with love, respect, generosity, and compassion. I have never been more excited to reinvent our family's story.

It is not what happens to us, but how we respond that defines us. I learned that I cannot always get what I want, but all I need to do is shift my mind, and the rest will follow.

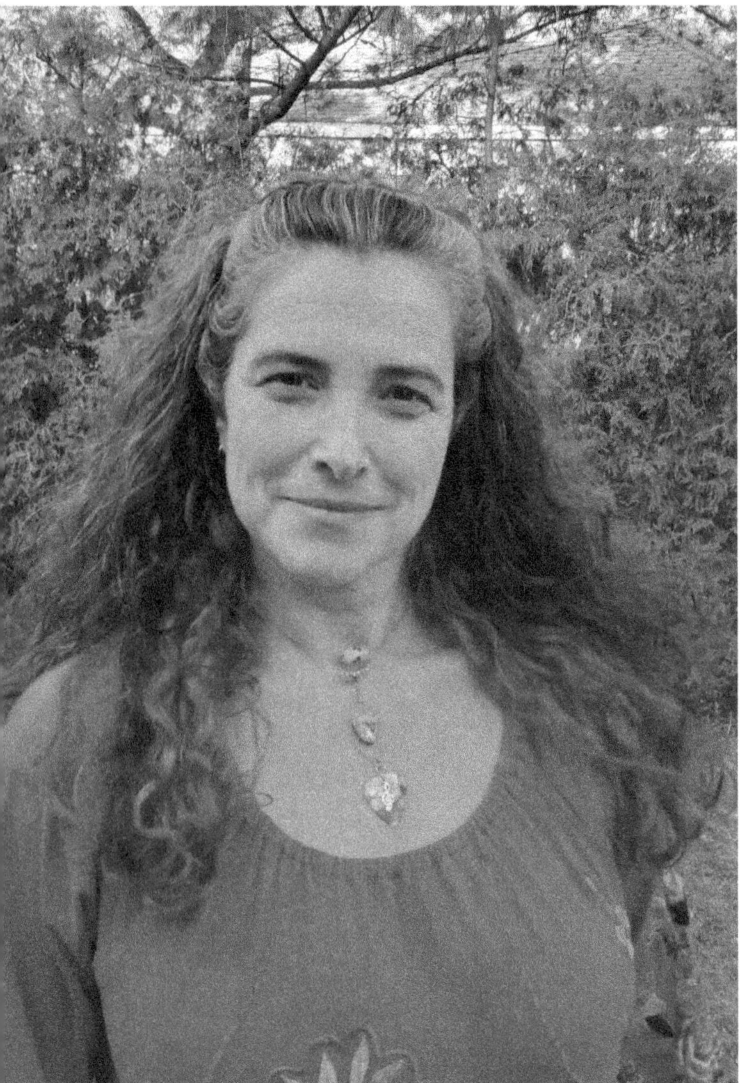
Photo Credit: Rémi Sauvé

Anik Thibaudeau, M.A., RP is a psychotherapist and small business owner at Do Re Mi Bracelets etc.

Anik Thibaudeau

All of my life, I have been the kind of person who stands out. I have a very big personality. I am an extreme extrovert and have a very A-type personality (outgoing, ambitious, impatient, proactive, etc.). Though these can be wonderful qualities, they definitely did not win me any popularity contests when I was younger.

My mother told me that people would appreciate these traits when I was older. Thankfully she was right. But more importantly, she did not suggest that I change who I was in order to fit in. I was given permission to be who I was. This was only one of the many gifts of wisdom that my mother gave me.

Today, the people in my life are those who don't just "put up with me" but who embrace my intensity and my authenticity. This is a two-way street, however. I give as fiercely as I take in relationships. I will support and inspire those around me (including in my practice as a psychotherapist), but I will not do so at my own expense. Through good times and bad times, my philosophy in life has been to create a sense of well-being, happiness, and beauty for myself.

When I am doing well, then I can offer those same gifts to others. But, like any human, I am perfectly imperfect, and I have on occasion let my well (my well-being) run dry. This is a mistake. A dry well is good for no one. I do not however fault myself for my imperfections. They are a part of me and what make me human. I find it important to recognize them and care of myself when I am not at my best.

The ability to find beauty in life's and people's imperfections has not only made me a better psychotherapist but has also been the basis of my small business. I take the broken pieces and discarded strings from various instruments and transform them into objects and jewelry that will once again be loved and appreciated and that bring beauty to people's lives.
If you look for beauty, you have a much better chance of finding it, in yourself and elsewhere.

Janey Ganson is the founder of My Daughter Fragrances.

Janey Ganson

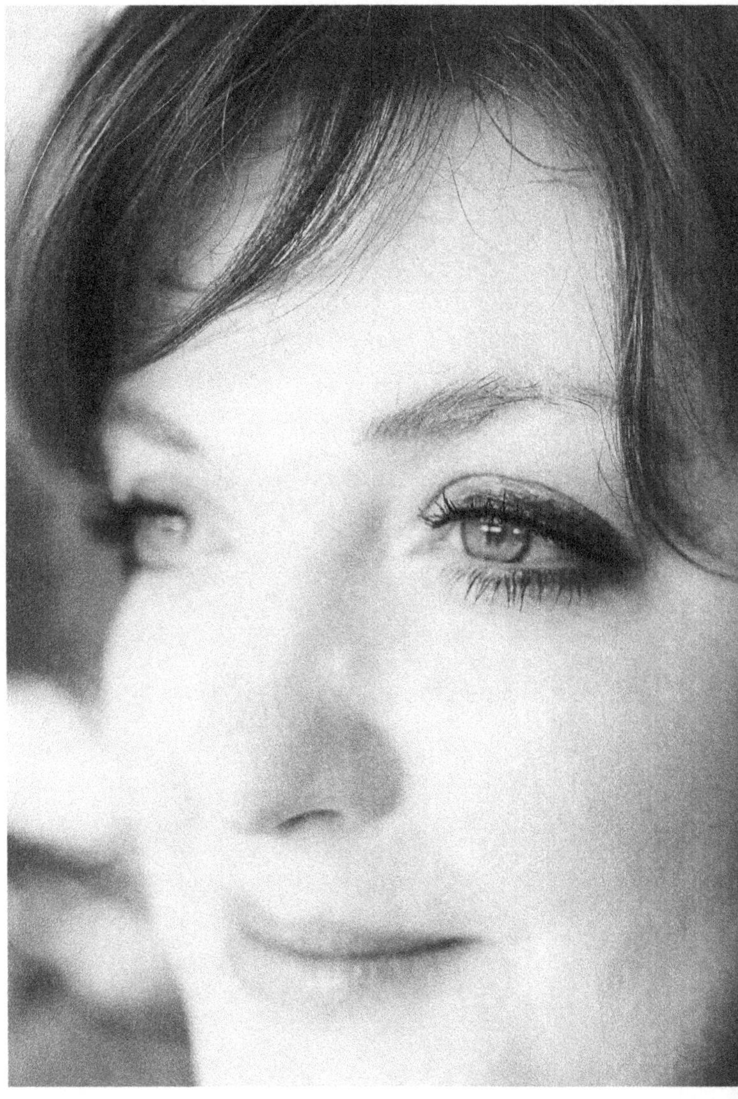

Joy, where are you?
Joy, we seek it, chase it, long for it.
Where are you joy? Are you here, or are you out there? It's always there... joy, somehow squished in the cosmic sandwich. A ray of light hovering above us, even when sadness shows up like she runs the show. What we feel comes from what we believe.

Growing up in the prairies of Alberta, imagination was everything for me. Playing Laura Ingalls was a pastime for me. In my imagination I was her, creating my latest adventures in my head. Creativity was a literal pastime. It didn't matter if it was glorious mud pies with fresh Alberta wild roses on top or making collections of sticks and leaves and shoving them in containers to make up magical tinctures for made-up ailments. It was fun! But most importantly, I believed I was her, and what that did for me is allow my girl-child feelings to be those of adventure and happiness. It allowed me to embrace a sense of curiosity and discovery that I still hold to this day.

Right now, it's barely 2021, and all I can think of is the year 2020, a literal poop on a cracker of a year. The meme of "if 2020 was a potato chip flavour, it would be toothpaste and orange juice" - now that is hilarious! My business, family, and day-to-day life look completely different. Even the contents of my fridge look different. My ability to transform, adapt, and change are being put to the test. That's really all life is. I am just being pushed to reshape it and do it quicker than ever before. Finding that creative juice, and business fortitude when the world is upside down has been life-changing, but you know what? I am figuring it out. I don't even want to use the "C" word, but I used it as a creative adventure, a time to ponder, but most importantly, a time to FEEL differently about everything! And what I discovered after months of this, is that joy is actually right here with us, literally sitting just above. She can be kind of hazy, but she's right here.

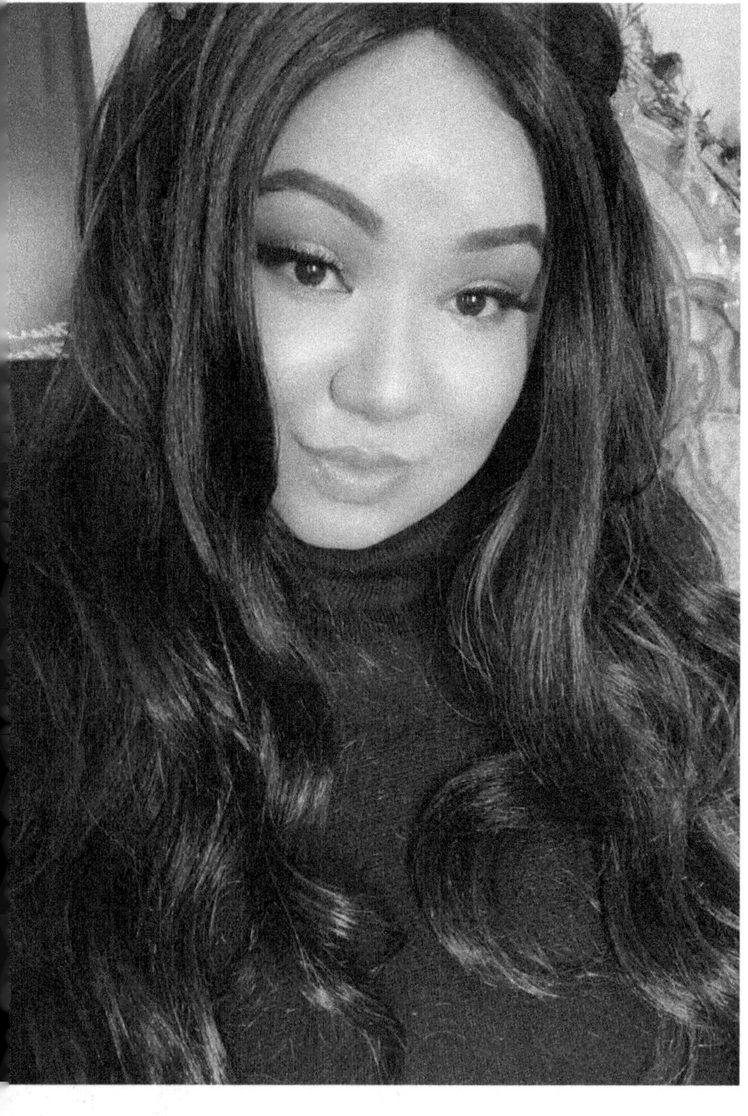

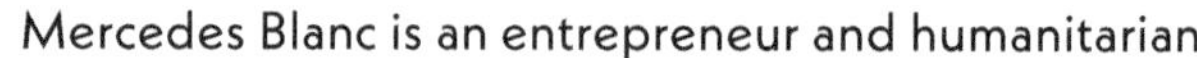

Mercedes Blanc is an entrepreneur and humanitarian.

Mercedes Blanc

As the daughter of immigrant parents, I knew from a very young age that I wanted to help as many people as possible, I grew up seeing my mother help any and every person she could, and I wanted to be just like her. I wanted so much to do even more than my mother had done, and she has done so much. I knew I had set the bar very high for myself in order to make her proud of me. This shaped what would become my vision of success and happiness. I have always been the unconventional, spirited woman with an unbridled passion for fashion, art, and a desire to change the world, one person at a time. Many people see me as just a black woman; I feel like I'm always aware of the fact that I will have to work harder than many of my peers to be seen as an equal, or simply to be seen at all. Because of this, I work that much harder on every project I put my hands on, and it has pushed me to be the very best. I want to break so many barriers for future generations that I do this with a willing heart.

My picture of success has changed a lot over the years, but how I view and feel about happiness and fulfillment has not changed because it's a daily achievement; it's in the small things I accomplish daily. If you had asked me prior to 2020 what my definition was, I would have had a very different answer. However, during the beginning stages of the pandemic, success would have been just getting out of bed before 11 pm. It took me a while and a lot of prayer and soul searching to find my balance and motivation, adjusting to everything. I had to readjust my goals and set new limits for myself. Sometimes we set limits for ourselves based on our comfort zones, and if 2020 has taught me anything, it's that I needed to re-evaluate what I consider my comfort zone and step outside of it. As a result, I have found creative ways to give back.

No matter what comes my way, I will continue to push forward, projecting love and light on everyone who crosses my path.

Jana Maclagan is a boy-mom, wife, teacher, makeup artist, entrepreneur, skincare advocate, charity volunteer, and an empty-nester. She is passionate about helping people improve their skincare and makeup routines while learning to love their own skin.

Jana Lee Maclagan

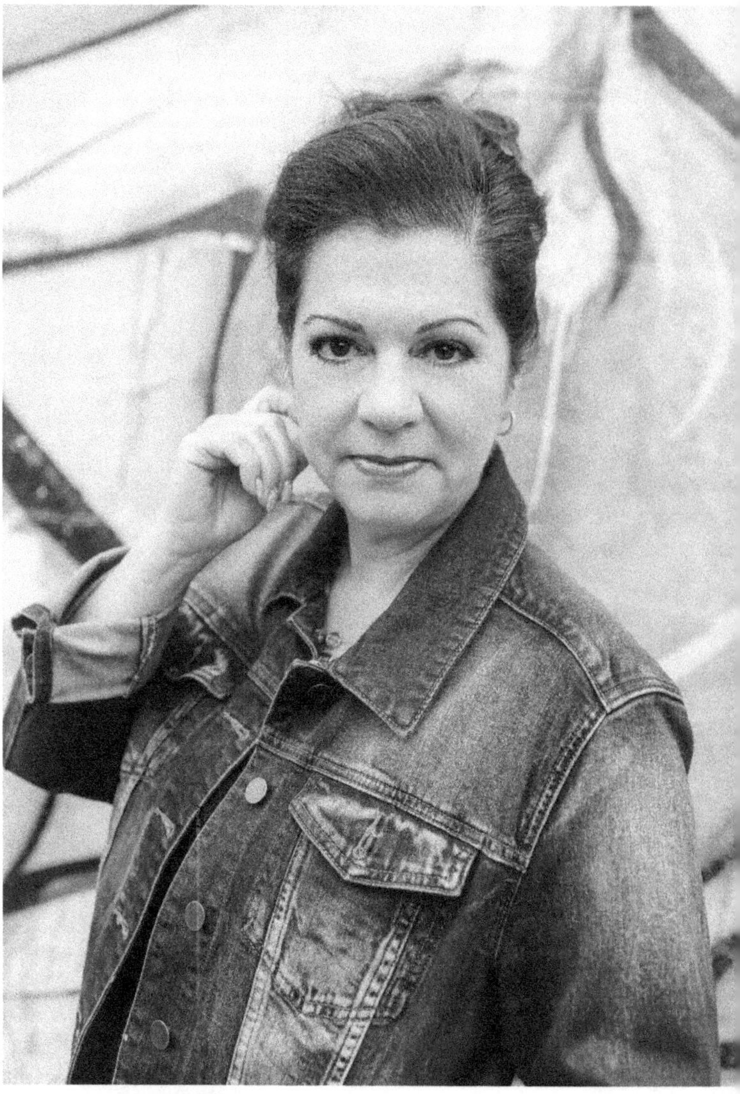

After devoting twenty-two years of my life to raising children, I was suddenly unemployed. This occurred much earlier than I had anticipated. Both my boys moved out when they were only nineteen years old, and neither of them gave me much notice. Without a doubt, the biggest shock, other than smaller amounts of laundry and fewer groceries consumed, was the amount of extra time I had on my hands. I hadn't held a paying job outside the home in fifteen years. Could I find something else that was fun for me while making a little money without doing a traditional nine-to-five job? More importantly, how could I make new friends as an adult? As your children leave home, your social circle can get smaller, and mine did. My involvement in multiple charities allowed me to contribute to some very good causes, raise awareness and also raise a lot of money, but with one exception, it has not built my circle of friends. It filled time but wasn't completely satisfying me.

I joined a company on a whim because I wanted magic lipstick. What I didn't expect was a group of amazing mentors, cheerleaders, and friends that I didn't even know I needed or wanted. I learned I was a hugely competitive person that thrived on recognition and providing value to people was very important to me. Consequently, I have actually discovered the kind of "girl power" that I didn't believe was real. I am a Boss Babe.

I get a million wonderful things from this new venture. It feeds my soul, my brain, and my heart. For the first time in a long time, I feel independent, recognized, valued, and beautiful. Unexpectedly it has allowed me to expand my charitable contributions, alone and with the assistance of my customers. I have found a place to belong, a crossroads of service and sales, and of personal growth and learning.

The secret shoe money?
That is my bonus.

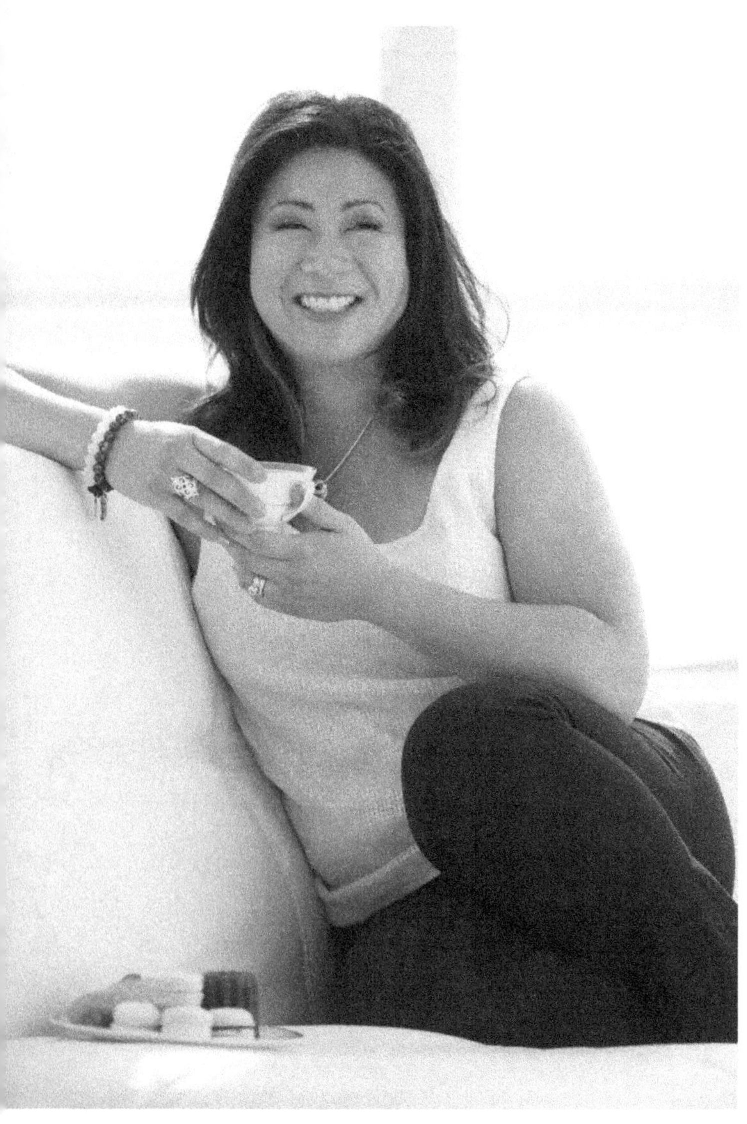

April May Bellia is an intuitive life purpose coach and spiritual guide. She is a lover of life and a seeker of truth.

April May Bellia

I used to be that girl whose name you might forget. It started with my favourite high school teacher in grade nine Socials Class. As a result, I subconsciously set out to be the girl that people would remember. I learned to bake delicious pies, cheesecakes, and chocolate cake, which was an easy way to be liked and remembered. For ten years, I was known as AprilCakes, a home-based wedding cake business. For the next ten years, people called me Granola Girl, after a cereal company I founded and later sold in 2020. Who sells and exits a business in 2020? I did!

My social media name was changed to April May Bellia. That would surely be memorable! In between my titles of cake queen and granola goddess, I was also an event producer, networking maven, speaker, facilitator, mentor, wife, and mom of three kids. I worked very hard to be seen, acknowledged, and remembered.

I created all these roles I thought I needed to be. I overcompensated. I felt drained. I crashed. I hit rock bottom -a few times! My marriage suffered. I tried so hard to be more, do more, have more. After taking the long scenic route from my head to my heart (it never really is a straight line!), I finally discovered that I AM ENOUGH.

As long as I remember who I am and what my gifts are, this is enough. I am enough. Feeling solid and connected in who I am, means there is no need to be more, do more, prove anything, nor defend. In my defencelessness, I am free.

So, who is April May Bellia, version 2021? I got a glimpse of my future self when I first hosted Serendipity Tea Party networking events for heart-based entrepreneurs, healers, intuitives, and coaches. A group of wonderfully unexpected people showed me a preview of who I was to become. I had no clue then that today, I would be jumping out of bed each morning as an intuitive life purpose coach and spiritual guide. Finally, I am living my purpose by helping other creative visionaries reignite their passions, live out their Sacred Gifts, and feel on purpose.
Finally, I am me.

Michelle Kam is a Toronto-based broker, specializing in high-volume downtown condo properties, who fell in love with the real estate landscape once she had all the chips in place.

Michelle Kam

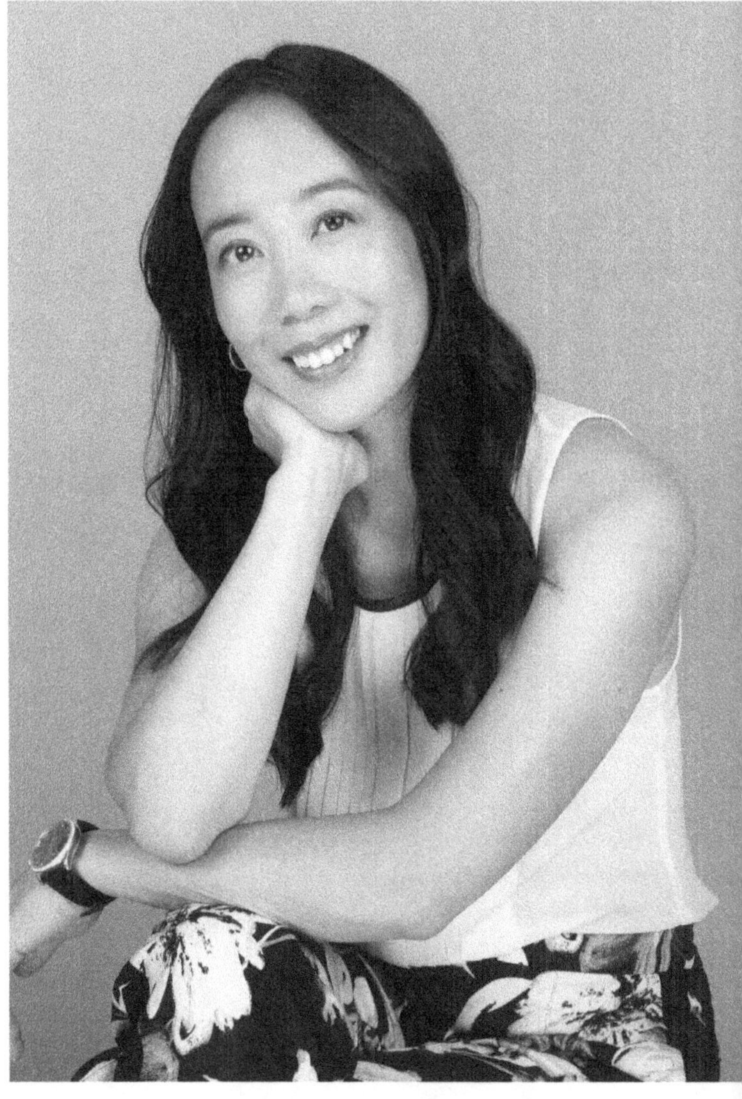

As a child, I was obsessed with putting puzzle pieces together. "Where's Waldo?" 1,000-piece dinosaurs were a revelation. Learning to match the patterns and pieces to look like the image on the front of the box thrilled me. I began to imagine how I might assemble my life in a similar manner. Only, life doesn't always come with all the right pieces, or with a clear picture of what the whole thing should look like when it's completed.

When starting my career, I signed with one of the best-known brokers in the business, imagining all there was to learn from this "mentor." Within months, as more of the pieces I was given seemed never to click into place, my mentor became my tor-mentor.

Instead of support and empowerment, he would sabotage deals I was working hard to accomplish. One night I cried myself asleep on the floor. When I awoke and dried my eyes, I began to make out the pattern. Whenever I was close to finishing a deal, he would withhold pieces until the whole thing was about to collapse. Then he'd step in at the eleventh hour and snap the right piece into place to complete the picture I'd put together. Casting himself as savior, he was the one who was paid the commission.

It took a while before I realized it wasn't me or the profession itself that was the problem. So, I quit my tormentor and set out to build my own picture puzzle, with all of the pieces I needed to become sole proprietor of my own career. The result was that more of the pieces then fell into place. I was moving ahead with success at a pace that surpassed expectations, watching my tormentor's anguished face fade in my rear-view mirrors.

My career is one part of the puzzle, as are my personal happiness and family-life ambitions. The pieces you're given in a neat box with pretty pictures aren't the only pieces you need to complete the whole picture.

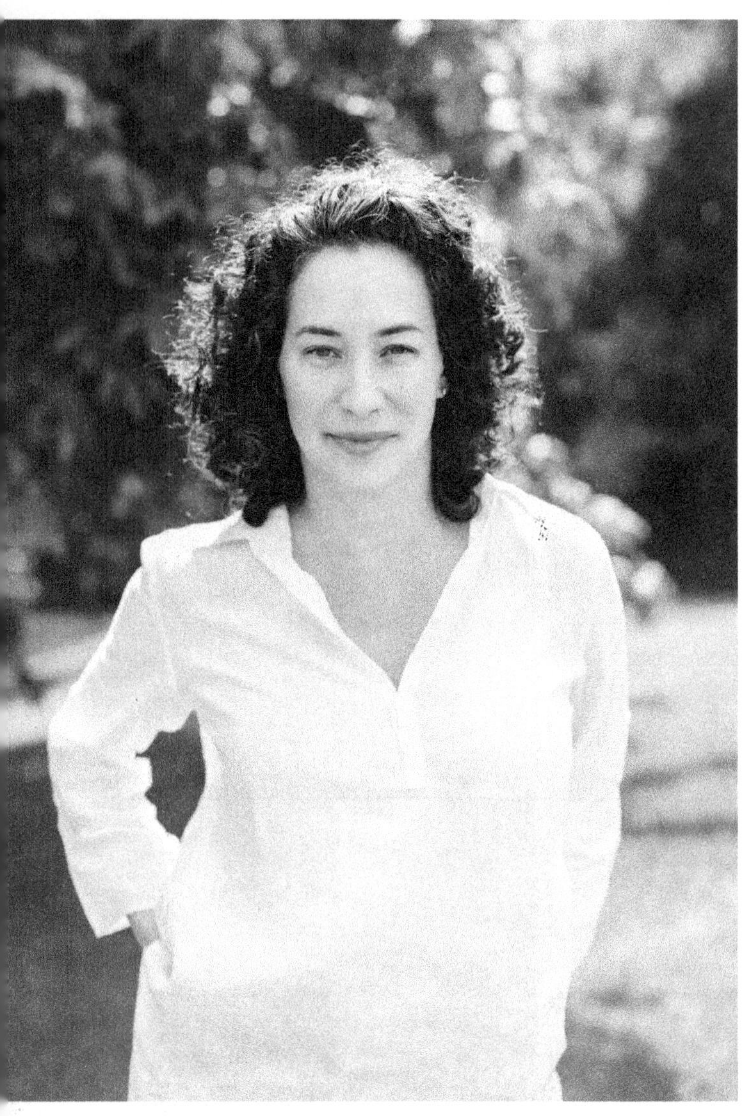

Lori Joyce is the founder and CEO of Vancouver-based premium ice cream brand Betterwith Ice Cream. She also co-founded the bakery franchise Cupcakes.

Lori Joyce

A couple of years back, I was running out of money and fast. Living in Vancouver, well technically West Vancouver, and despite a very successful launch of my premium ice cream Betterwith Ice Cream into grocery, I was unable to attract any investment capital for my startup. Being new to the CPG (consumer packaged goods) space, I was starting to feel the harsh reality of how difficult it was going to be to go up against the Nationals in the frozen space. It was me against the Goliath(s), and quickly I was beginning to understand why most were so eager to convince me to stop rather than push on.

But no one ever told me it was impossible. And for this, I kept pushing on. It also meant that I was going to have to make some sacrifices and make a few difficult decisions. The first one was made for me. It was the Spring of 2018; I was coming home from school with the kids in tow and found an Eviction Notice taped to the front door. In the same week, a prominent potential investor told me he assumed I must have been supported by a husband that was 'backing me'. He said, "How else could I have done what I was doing." So little did he actually know.

In 2018, many people still remembered me from my reality TV Show called The Cupcake Girls. Yes, it was a huge success - a Gemini-award winning success that was sold into over 90 countries worldwide. But what most didn't know was that my husband and in-laws shamed me for doing the show. They absolutely resented me for it. My successful reality TV Show embarrassed them.

So, once the school year finished, I moved with my youngest son back to Victoria and back in with my parents on a five-acre self-sustaining, organic farm. And in regard to my business, well, I have even better news to share – I have found success with growth and production. And I am deliberately and proudly sharing my past with the present.

I will forever be a Cupcakes Girl, and with conviction, I am going to shout it out loud!

Jacquie Stebbings is a Personal Life Coach and Facilitator.

Jacquie Stebbings

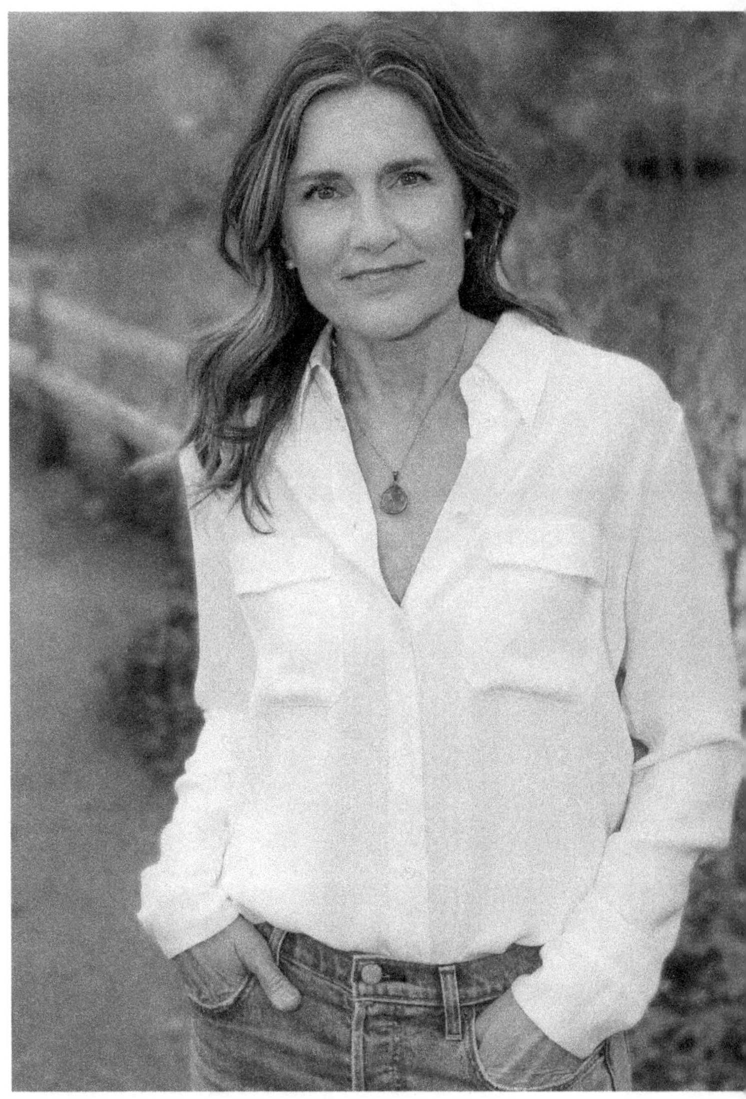

"We don't need you anymore." When first hearing those five words, I unknowingly folded them into my self-identity.

I was thirty-six and my baby nine weeks. I had trained one of my staff. She would help during the new-born phase until I could return to the helm, running the day-to-day operations and guiding my team. My business partner and friend of ten years had a different vision. He hit me in the gut with those five words.

Full-time-at-home-mothering was never my plan. I had always imagined some version of running my company and motherhood. But with no longer a company to run, and a spouse who travelled for weeks at a time, our three young children pointed me to the obvious. So, I got busy mothering but with a wounded sense of my value whispering in my ear and the feeling niggling in the background that there was something more.

Moms know that while there are endless tasks and to-do's, there are just as many hours of idle brain time. My brain looped around the question of self-worth. Looking back, I see earnest volunteer hours as an effort to prove I could do more than just meal-plan.

There's a black and white baby photo of me lying in a pram, lifting my head to catch the eyes of the photographer. That baby would grow into a woman committed to knowing her inherent value beyond what she does for others or the income she creates. That baby would one day start teasing apart the gnarly knot of the value of being from the value of doing. Motherhood would trigger that quest.

Today I champion and coach women ready to take bold action for their own lives and happiness. Alongside all their doing for others is a sincere call for something else. For some, the focus is what's next? For others, it's life purpose or their need to fill their own cup and create strong, balanced relationships. Regardless of the pursuit, self-care supports their vision of what life could be. When a woman is freed from self-imposed boundaries and she moves to achievements only imagined, we all get to draw from her inspiration and power.

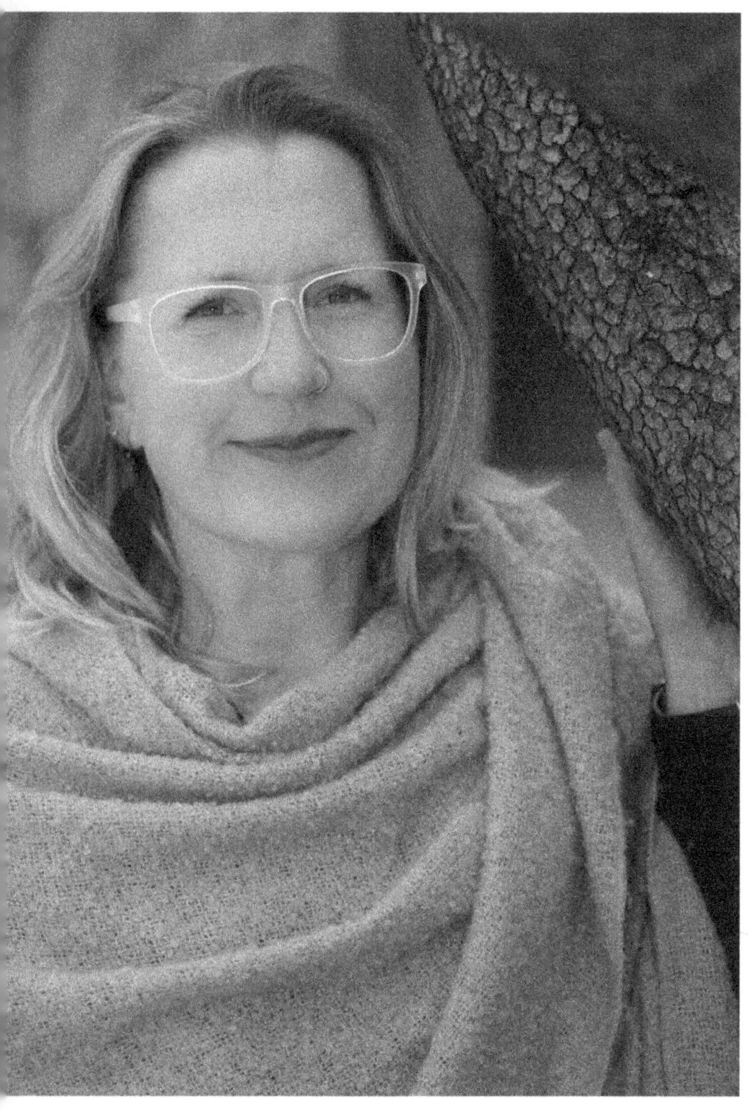

With every last ounce of will, Marika pressed on. For months, this became the agonizing norm: the sleepless nights, the tearful walks to work, her husband coaching her by phone, just so she could walk through the doors. Hitting rock bottom was necessary and opening herself up was vital to begin healing. Marika is learning to find peace within by focussing on her journey, not the destination.

Marika Houston

Happiness comes from within. Your career, your relationships, your appearance, your finances, none of it matters.

On the outside, my life was great! I had a wonderful husband, a successful career, took fabulous vacations, and so on. However, I loathed myself. I always felt I was not enough. I felt like a walking, talking imposter in my own life. I was depressed and extremely anxious. My whole body ached. I recognize now that my soul, my inner voice, was crying out for me to take-care. And so, I listened. I left work to work on myself.

In this time, I have met with doctors, with therapists, and gratefully discovered the transformative power of yoga. Despite doing "all the right things," my mental health still suffered, and I contemplated suicide. I took a hard look at myself, and I decided one more step I must take was to stop drinking. I reached out for support; this shifted everything.

Cutting out alcohol was hard, but it is not impossible. In fact, it is THE best thing I have done for myself! I feel so much better, not only physically, but emotionally. I am discovering a lot about myself and uncovering the sources of my depression and anxiety.

I have learned the only way past this darkness is going through it, my work continues daily. I am on a whole-body journey of healing, from inside out.

It is okay to feel. Being vulnerable is not easy for me, but to heal, I need to let others in. Isolation is dangerous. Vulnerability is not a sign of my weakness but is a sign of my humanity. I am learning to love myself by honouring my needs and nurturing myself, physically, emotionally, and spiritually.

Trust your inner voice; it will always guide you.

Hannah Fletcher is an award-winning fitness leader who has devoted her life to helping others reach their health, fitness, and body composition goals in a self-compassionate, loving way.

Hannah Fletcher

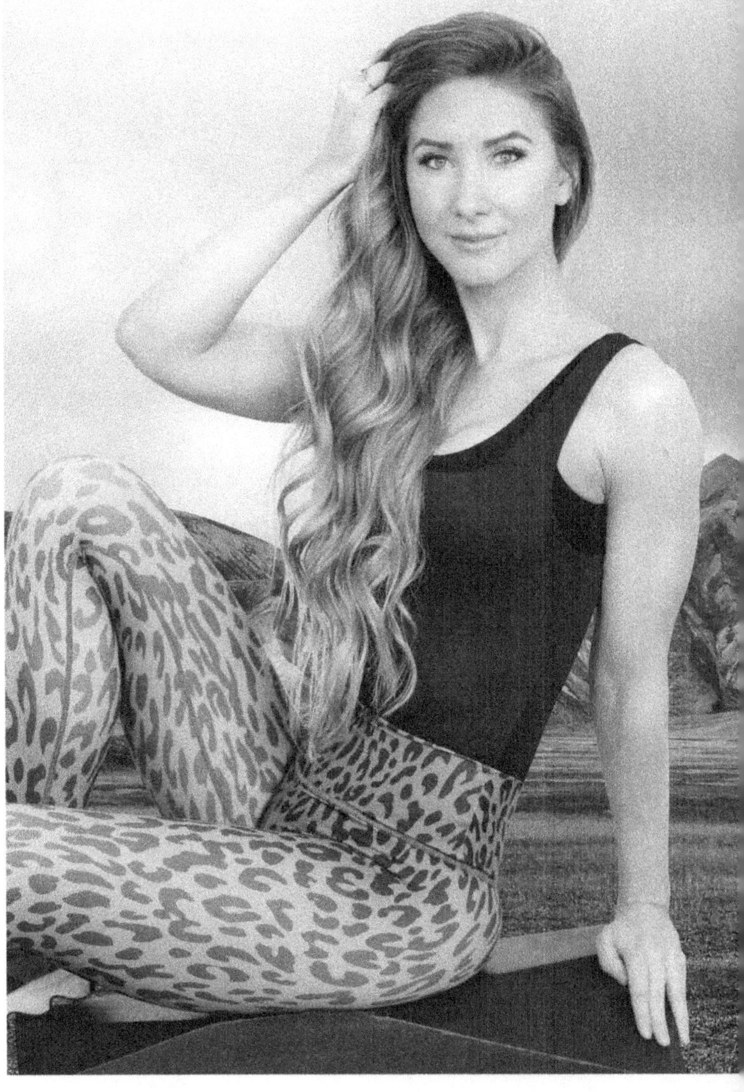

Foggy, depleted, and in the early stages of separation from my then-husband, I found myself alone in Iceland. Out of habit, I was still wearing my diamond ring.

Not a soul knew where I was. My cell phone didn't work --no WiFi, no reception -- not even to dial 112 (Iceland's emergency services). There were dangerous wind warnings of 90+ km/h, but I had planned my road trip to Diamond Beach carefully so that I would arrive back at my cabin before the storm hit. After hours of driving, I felt I was on autopilot until a rainbow appeared. I pulled off the road into the endless dirt fields to take a photo. As I walked from the car, I suddenly felt the strangest energy and intuitively knew something was wrong. I looked back at my rental car and saw that the front tires had sunk in the lava-ash dirt-like quicksand.

Only five cars drove by that hour. I jumped in front of all of them. Fifteen strangers from all over the world pushed, pulled, and dug with their bare hands to help me. I was so moved, but we were unsuccessful. I hitchhiked to the nearest gas station forty-five minutes away where, by luck, I met the farmer that owned the land my car was stuck on. He drove me back and freed my rental car!

Delayed by hours, I carried on.

The glistening iceberg fragments at Diamond Beach were surreal. I felt they were just for me. And I knew that I didn't need the one on my finger anymore.

The winds were getting worse, so I headed back. Road warnings flashed in red: "Cars will fly." It was perhaps the most dangerous drive of my life. While I was in the eye of the storm - alone with my thoughts - I found peace. I began thinking about how much I enjoyed my own company. I realized; I was enough. Everything I was looking for was already inside of me.

A year later I thought back to Diamond Beach. It turns out, life is full of diamonds when you choose to love yourself first.

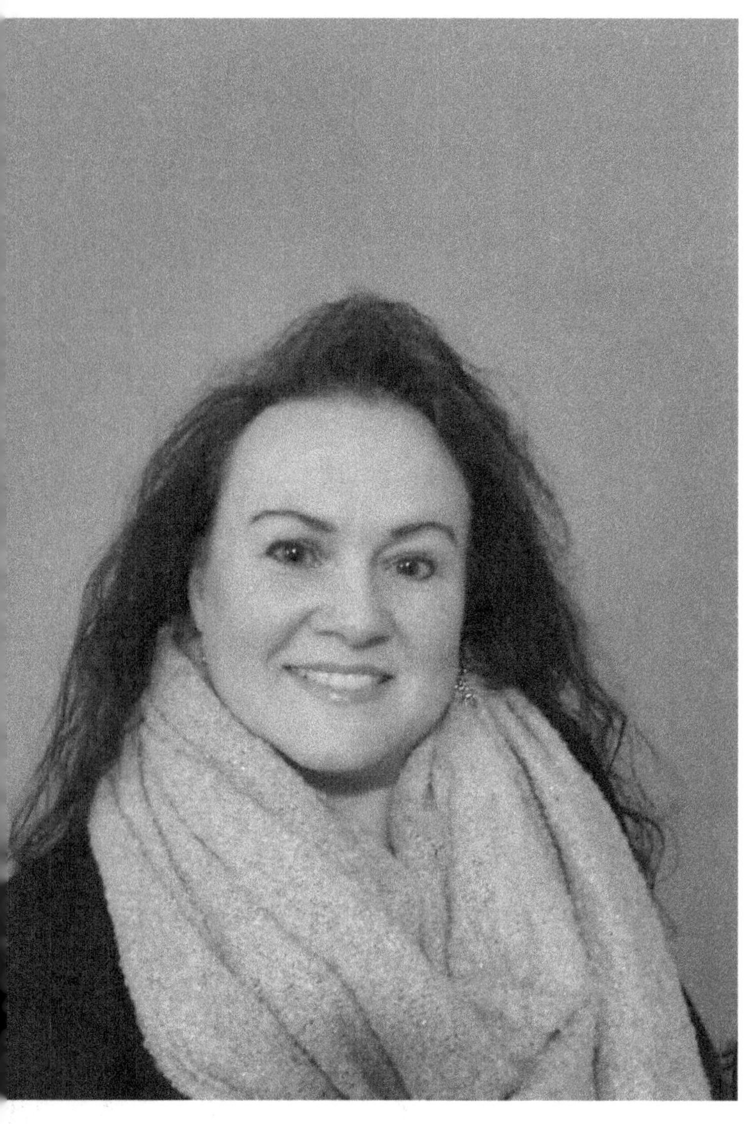

Catherine Trotzuk has been described as a powerhouse of energy and creativity. She is a multi-passionate educator, speaker, author and business owner who relies on her focus and commitment to get the job done.

Catherine Trotzuk

When I was a small girl my father told me I could be whatever I wanted to be and do whatever I wanted to do in this life. I only needed to put my mind to it and not be afraid of hard work. I've been putting my mind to it ever since. Thankful for having this belief instilled in me, I have never been bothered by the 'can't police' or the naysayers of this world, even though they're around every corner. My belief is that 'No' only means 'not yet'.

From building a pool in my backyard at six years old (because that is what I wanted more than anything), I learned the value of trial and error, figuring out a problem, altering a design, and the value of hard work. Long after my friends left to go ride bikes or play on the nearby playground, I continued working on that pool from dawn to dusk every day until it became functional. I did not stop until I was successful.

I also learned that when it comes to hard work you sometimes stand alone, but standing alone often gives you the strength to stand for others. And when I am not actively looking after my own children and family, that is exactly what I am doing. I am standing up for your children, standing up for others, and making changes in business and education. In business, life, and education, I pride myself on imagining the unimagined and carving new paths where others thought not to go. And I still don't stop until I am successful.

I have always been a multi-passionate individual and continue to have several projects on the go at one time. I am adept at juggling all of the balls on whatever court life throws at me. Bringing hard work, passion, and integrity, to my clients, my students, and my business is how I design my happiness.

At six, my dad told me I could be whatever I wanted to be. I believed him.

Take what you've got and run with it. Don't be afraid of hard work. Show this world who you are and what you are capable of. And don't stop until you are successful!

Evelyne Nyairo is the visionary, CEO, and founder of Ellie Bianca, a non-GMO, cruelty-free, and sustainably sourced skincare brand.

Evelyne Nyairo

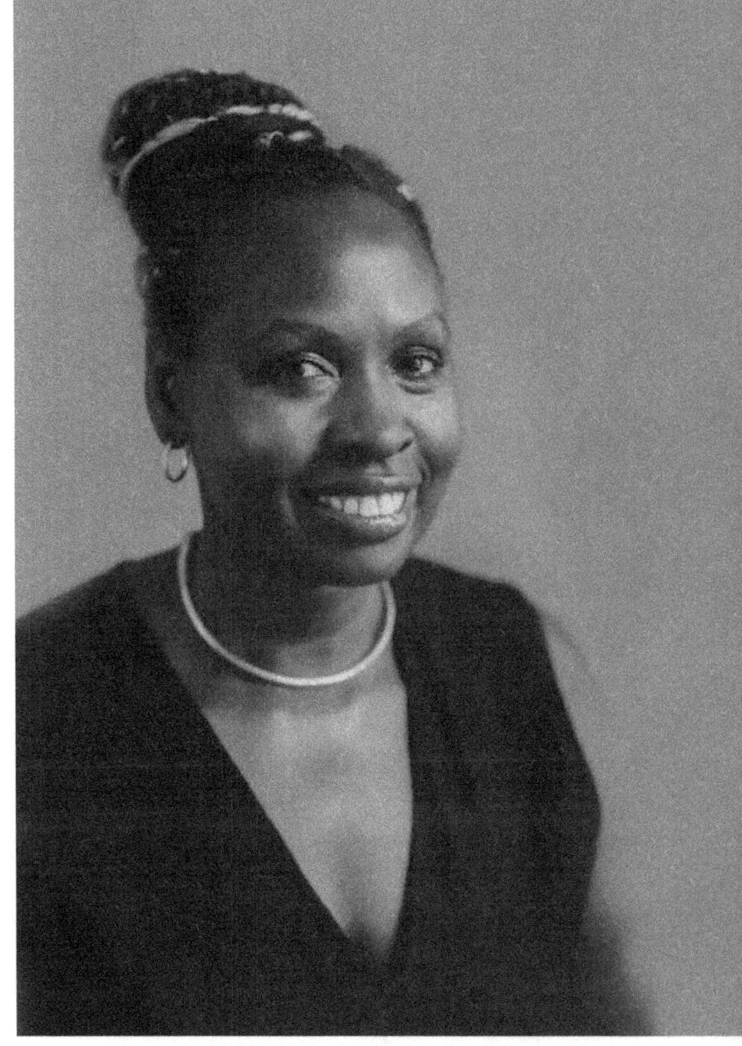

Years ago, I found myself doing fieldwork among the most beautiful wild mango trees in Chad. Not one to waste an opportunity for incredible fresh fruit, I was introduced to a family where the mother and kids proceeded to expertly climb the trees in the hot sun to harvest mangoes for me to eat. Towards the end, I was told to pay the husband when it was the wife that had picked the mangoes. I felt a knot of anger in my heart as I customarily handed the money over to the man. I thought to myself, "This happens everywhere around the world, and it's wrong," and I was motivated to help improve the lives of the women there. That is when I decided to start Ellie Bianca, a natural skincare line built on the pillars 'Kind to Your Skin, Kind to the Earth, Kind to Women.'

Ellie Bianca is a holistic skincare line that cultivates and empowers women through sustainable business practices and fair trade. I moved to Canada from Kenya at the age of 16 and put myself through my Bachelor and a Master of Science degrees while being a single mom. I built Ellie Bianca on my desire to be an example to my daughter of what women are capable of and to empower other women to succeed- from sourcing ingredients from women in Africa and mentoring other women entrepreneurs to running the Ellie Bianca Woman Scholarship for single mothers.

One thing I have learned over the years is not to apologize for who I am. It's important to celebrate you as you are without the obligations you feel about making improvements to yourself. I try not to judge myself too harshly or hold myself to impossibly high standards. Every day when I wake up, I count the little wins, give myself credit where credit is due, and tell myself in the mirror, "Keep being You, unapologetically You, BEAUTIFUL YOU!" To live this out, I aim to be intentional and find that sweet spot when it comes to indulgence and self-control, work and play, improvement, and appreciation.

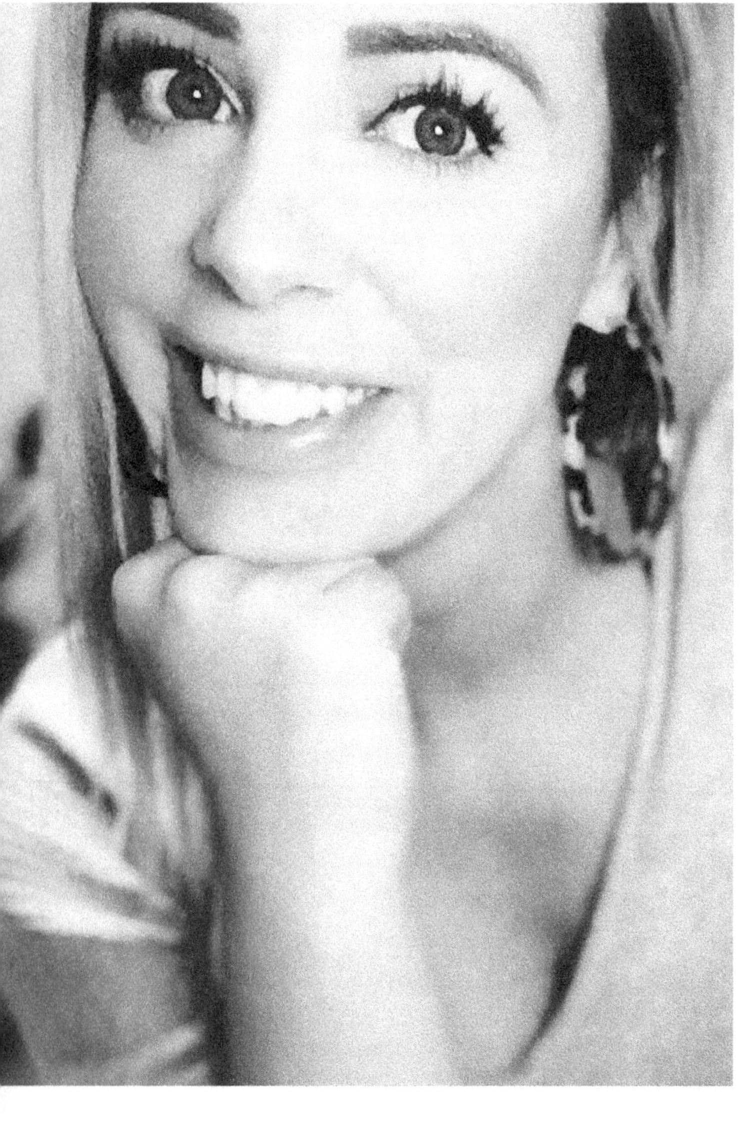

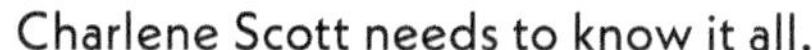

Charlene Scott needs to know it all.

Charlene Scott

"She said she usually cried at least once each day not because she was sad, but because the world was so beautiful, and life was so short." -Brian Andreas

My name is Charlene, and I need to know it all. Everything. I can't stop it either.

tperson in a room or to dominate final Jeopardy in front of millions one day. Instead, I have a strong urge to see and touch everything in this world. I want to look each person in the eye and feel the ground of every single country. I want to make sure I leave this world knowing at least a little bit of something about everything. Simply put, I am fanatical about all of the things I don't know yet, and a lot of my happiness comes from my journey to learn about them. As exhausting as this can be, I am proud to say that this has been one of the biggest elements to my success so far, not only in my career but also in my life. I was raised to always believe in myself and to speak with confidence, but like many other women, somewhere along the way,

I developed a small voice that told me I wasn't quite knowledgeable enough or experienced enough to truly have a seat at the table. I found myself only taking on tasks I knew I could achieve and only contributing to conversations when I was sure I was on the winning side of an argument. Luckily for me, I've had leaders who knew I had muted myself to get by, and because of that, they encouraged my work on things and projects I was curious about and were patient with me when I floundered a bit while learning. They didn't let me box myself in and stop when it got too easy to know just enough. My passion to learn and master things has become a celebrated part of my skillset. I am so grateful to be able to use my curiosity to better myself every day.

Only a few more steps till I can hopefully say I know it all.

Julie Samant is resilient as a businesswoman and celebrated artist.

Julie Samant

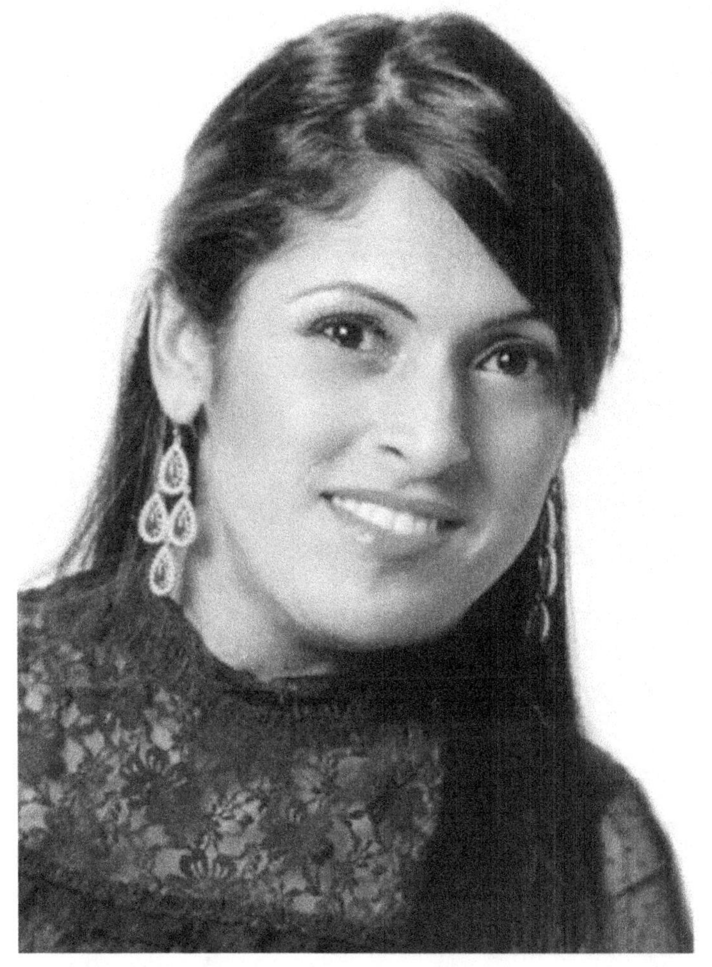

Right after I submitted my offer to purchase my first home, someone told me, "all dreams can come true." I didn't realize it at this point in my life, but I was about to accomplish 60% of my lifelong dream, including travelling solo across Europe. These goals may have seemed attainable to the average woman however, I am definitely not the average woman.

I was born with a rare condition: Cystic Hygroma aka Lymphatic Malformation (benign tumors) resulting in many surgeries and hospital visits throughout my life. I realized as a young adult that I wasn't like the majority of young women - until I realized how I was.

I was very protected as a child and given limitations by society. I felt like I was put in a box and told this is all I was capable of handling in life. My automatic response was to jump out of that box and run as far away from it as possible.

As I started to fulfill my dreams, I immersed myself in the healthcare field, my chosen career path. Healthcare was my passion from a young age. I did part of a nursing program with no backup plan because I was so determined to complete it. Soon after, I hit a roadblock. I didn't pass a semester, and I realized it was going to be a physically demanding career. I was devastated. Surprisingly however, this setback led me to a rewarding and amazing career as a medical secretary at several hospitals in the lower mainland, including Vancouver General Hospital.

Alongside my work at the hospital, I unleashed my creative and business sides. My new passion became painting landscapes and contemporary abstract artwork to share with the world. I have painted for several years and have been featured in places such as Roam Gallery, and the Cardiovascular Clinic in the Gordon and Leslie Diamond Building. I have always accomplished my successes with great determination. My upcoming venture will be to establish myself as a Vancouver-based artist where I can continue to inspire.

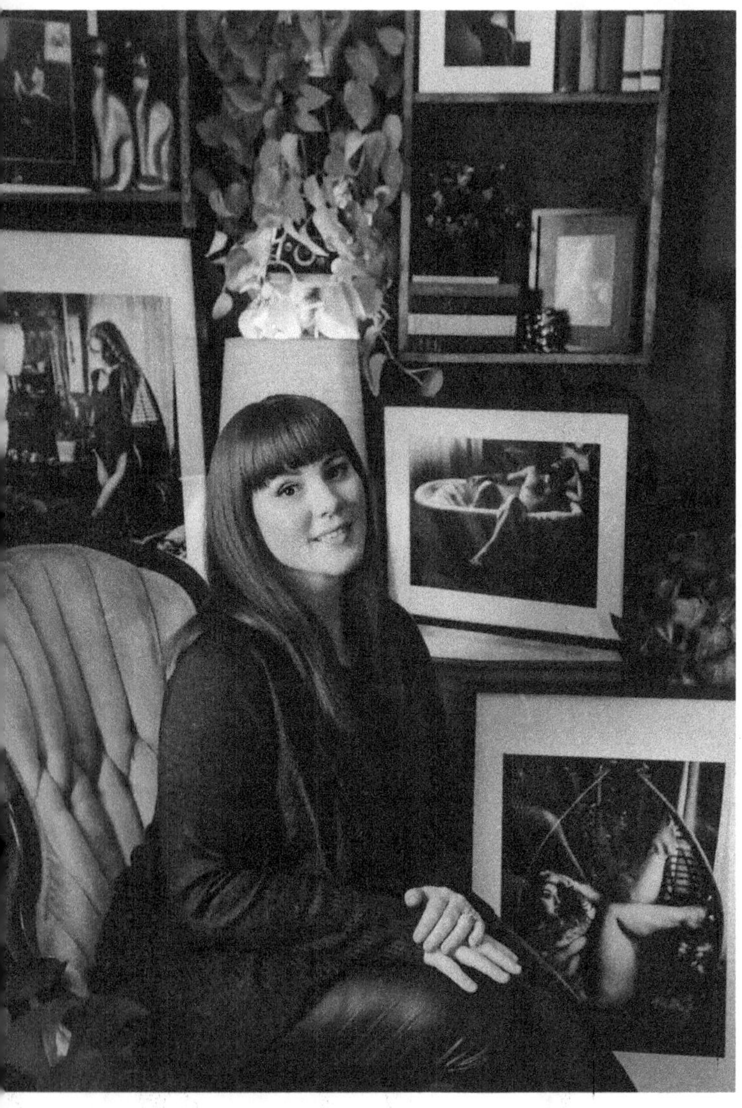

Jessica Rae is an artist and entrepreneur who empowers the people around her to tell their stories.

Jessica Rae

It's funny how when you are young and the world is at your fingertips, that you could feel so powerless. So much so that you let society take the reins and make life-altering choices on your behalf because anxiety and self-doubt are deep in your bones.

I took the nine-to-five job. I bought the house, I got married, I had the kids. I did all the things you're "supposed to do." Over the years, I began to box away my heart, my dreams, and everything that made me... me. I look back now, and it feels like a hazy dream. That's what living in survival mode can do. As a single mother with three young boys, no solid career path to fall back on, and struggling to overcome crippling self-doubt and low self-esteem due to an emotionally toxic relationship; I was scared and alone. There was only me. One would think that this would be the time to be practical. Go back to the nine-to-five, predictable, consistent, expected. And I did for a moment.

It was safe. It was smart. It was killing me.

I recall sitting in my car one afternoon, while out making sales calls for the aforementioned nine-to-five job. I had opened the car door, but I couldn't move. I felt paralyzed. I managed to pick up my phone.

"I can't move." I texted a friend.
"You're having a panic attack!" she replied.

What?! I thought panic attacks were hyperventilating, heart racing, etc.
This was silent and still. FIGHT, FLIGHT, or FREEZE. For so long I was FIGHT. I didn't know how to deal with FREEZE.

So, I quit. Despite all the responsibilities that were heavy on my shoulders, I felt a weight lift.
I could breathe. I could move. I was free. No more nine-to-five for me. I couldn't do it anymore, it was quite frankly, going to kill me. So, I did the unthinkable. Something society tells us from day one to avoid at all costs.

I followed my heart and went after my dream.
I would be a full-time artist and entrepreneur.

Kathy Swift found her voice through art and harnesses the power of art to break generational cycles.

Kathy Swift

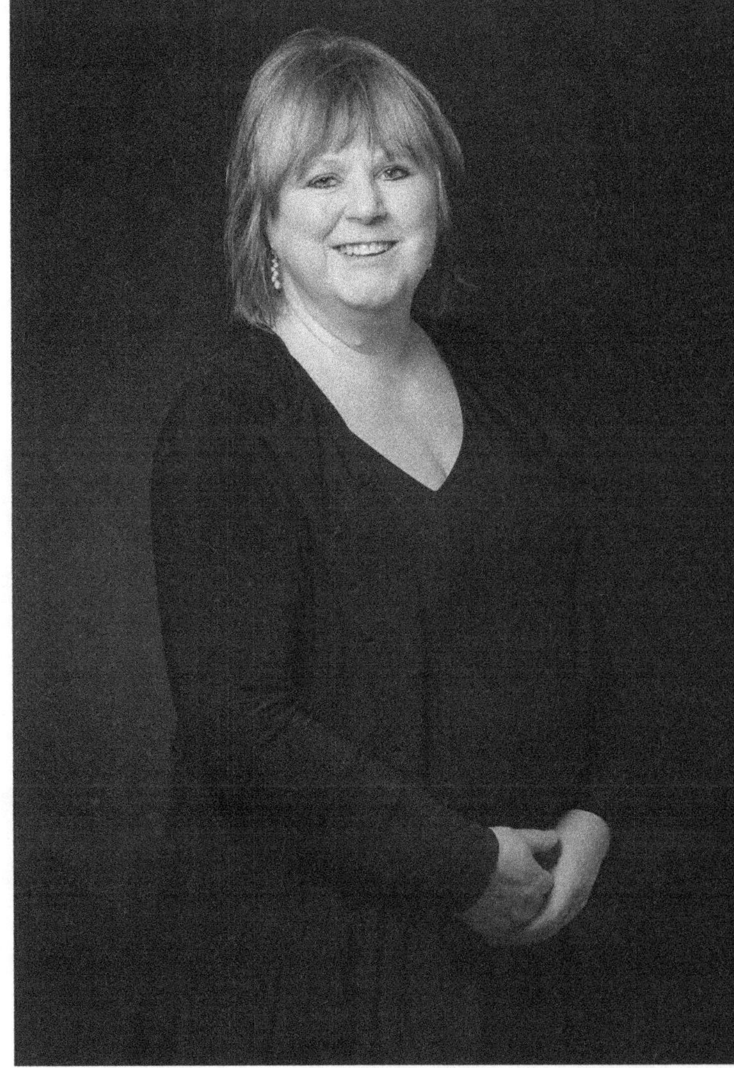

Ours was a family admired and envied, for we appeared on the outside to be the ideal family, having what others wanted.

Inside the walls, however, the family was rife with struggles and loss. The pain was unspoken and buried, but the scars were very palpable to me as a young child. I did not understand the pattern of abandonment that my perfect family had bequeathed me, but I felt it deeply as my own, in silence. Always in silence, the family's coda.

My great-grandmother died in childbirth and my grandmother, who was raised in an English orphanage, was sent to Canada as a young girl to care for other children. After marrying a philandering husband, the birth of her daughter, and years of abuse, she escaped her marriage to fend for herself. In doing so, she left my mother behind, herself a young girl. As an adult, my mother became secretive and distant, conducting many affairs while my father locked his emotions inside, safe from us all, he thought.

During my early years, the legacy continued. I was abandoned to the daily care of neighbours who kept me in a dank cellar, lit by a single light bulb. I was cold and so very alone in the dark. And silent. Often, I was accused of doing things I did not do, but because I remained quiet, a powerless young child without a voice, I absorbed the blame just to stop the crazy stories. This childhood pattern of "misbehaving" labeled me for life; Kathy could not be trusted.

Not surprisingly, I sought solace in substances as a teenager to escape the chaos in my life and my self-destructive beliefs. But I chose not to abandon myself on that path...

In the face of burning pain and confusion, I found my inner voice deep in the creative processes and dialogue with my art. When I sense the energy in a room, I know what is truth and what is not. I trust my knowing. I have learned to feel it and let it out. My voice is silent no more as I embrace the grist of life's lessons and express them with artistic abandon.

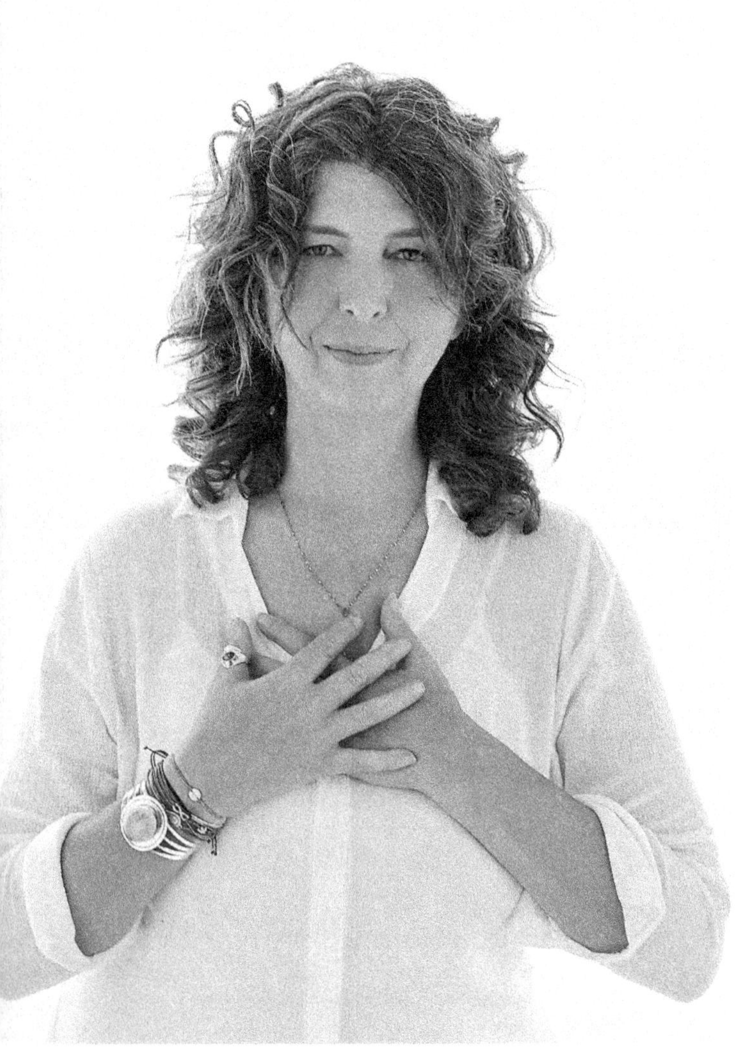

Patricia Clum is a life coach, spiritual guide, and the owner of Evolution of the Heart, and Wild Heart Sisterhood.

Patricia Clum

I lost my father twice; once at four years old and then at forty-six. My father's accidental brain injury forever changed our family's life.
My mum, a nurse, and mother of five, at the hospital, was told my father might not make it.
With the road to recovery slow, he healed enough to come home. Even at four, without language to articulate my feelings or observations, I knew he was different and so was my world. Our exchanges were often reactionary as his injury affected his patience, compassion, and ability to empathize.

On my voyage from childhood to adulthood, I concerned myself with my heart's journey. Opening to my soul's healing, birthing compassion, and forgiveness. My relationship with my father was limited time, only at family gatherings and pancake breakfasts. Years passed as I jumped into personal and spiritual growth through travel, working with horses, a film career, marriage, motherhood, divorce, and remarriage. Funnelling all my pain into the curiosity of the human capacity to love. Overtime letting go of viewing my father through the lens of childhood pain, letting go of childhood expectations that my father, might change.

On a summer day in 2012, I got the call and volunteered to support my father by dropping by his home for a ten-day period. Checking on him twice daily and bringing his favourite meals while navigating his ever-changing temperament. The man underneath the injury revealed his heart to me. Through a series of brief moments at a time, he communicated his love and wished me a good life. Love, forgiveness, and healing all shared the same space, transforming decades of pain, hurt and words unsaid into enlightenment. The power of the heart-soul connection and the depth of willingness to choose love over being right or over being afraid was right in the moment a living demonstration.

"Handing the Impossible Over to God" created the momentum that cleared the past and created the ability to appreciate the present. On the tenth day, I said, "see you later." Early the next morning, he died peacefully in his sleep. My father gave me the key to embracing forgiveness. It's never too late to choose LOVE!

Jessica Di Caprio is intentionally creating her dream life.

Jessica Di Caprio

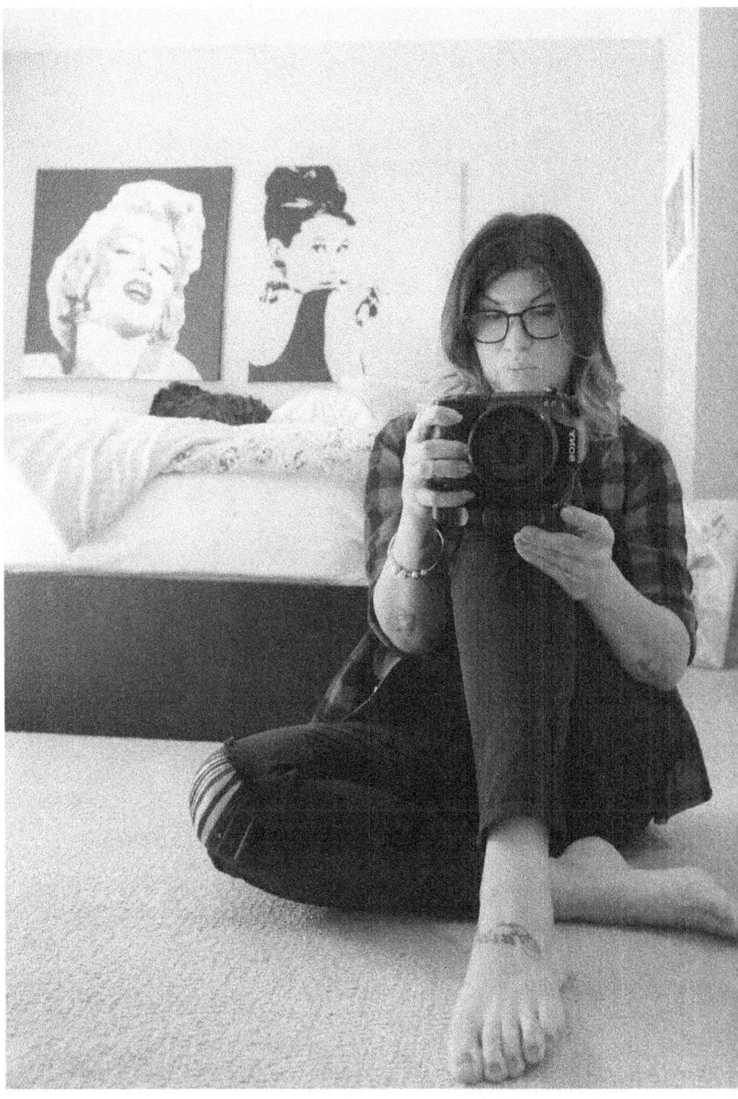

I don't know what your purpose is, what your dream life looks like or how it feels, but I know that you do and within their pursuit and creation lies your happiness.

There was a time when my life wasn't together. It wasn't peaceful, fulfilling, or abundant. I lived in a state of lack and worry. What I never lacked was an inner knowing. I've known since I was a little girl the life that I desired. How it should feel, and the freedom meant for me to experience. I took the longest route possible to arrive where I am today with both beautiful scenic seasons and dark roads travelled. I write this to you, with my twenty-four-year-old self in mind.

We delay the creation of our best life for fear of the unknown, not knowing how it will happen, believing we must earn our happiness instead of creating it. If I'd known then that my recurring thoughts were creating my reality, I would have chosen my thoughts with intention in the direction of my dreams instead of spinning the wheels within my own mind, remaining stuck, repeatedly creating everything I didn't want, delaying my own happiness. If we overstay our welcome in any area of our lives, we tend to create such deep comforts and attachments that it can feel like a life of roadblocks to overcome to get ourselves out of the life that we've created to instead experience the life that we desire.

We are meant to evolve, not revolve. The thoughts we think will create one or the other. The way you perceive, create and experience life is based on what you believe to be true which is based on the thoughts you repeatedly think and the experiences you have created to reinforce your own thoughts.

Get out of your own way. Observe your thoughts like your life depends on it. Begin to think intentionally. Create rituals around the things that bring you happiness and build your foundation on them. Start small. And remember that you don't need to believe everything that you think.

Your dream life is calling. Pick up. This is not your test life.

Denise Mai BA, a TEDx Speaker, entrepreneur, businesswoman, investor, and Realtor, has helped families since 2010 with their real estate goals and dreams. Her passion to help people has led her to win multiple awards as an agent, and she has ranked 32 out of 14,000 realtors putting her in the top 1% of all Realtors in Greater Vancouver.

Denise Mai

Denise Mai truly believes that success is always achievable, but it does require you to push through your fears and limiting beliefs.

Her journey has not always been easy, and Denise has shown that success lies right outside your comfort zone. She credits her unwavering resilience, yearning willpower, and insatiable desire to keep learning as her reasons for her achievements in life. She shares her rags to riches story in her most recent TEDx talk on how resilience was her superpower to her successes.

She grew up in Chinatown, with her single mom who was an immigrant on welfare, located in the downtown east side of Vancouver, known for its high level of homelessness, poverty, crime, mental illness, and drug use-The odds were stacked against her.

There is one thing for certain, Denise Mai has shown that your past or present circumstance does not dictate your future. She's shown you can control your own destiny and create the life you've always wanted and dreamed of-but it first begins with having a desire to want more out of life.

With immense gratitude for everything in life, this has been the key to happiness for Denise. She believes happiness is a choice and she chooses consciously every day to do what makes her happy, especially only surrounding herself with positive, growth-oriented, and like-minded individuals. She continues to lead by example on building up her own real estate portfolio while striving to change lives by helping more families build their investments and net worth through real estate as well. One of her missions is to help families build up their passive income so they can get closer to financial freedom and be able to take back their time.

Denise truly believes everything that has happened in her life, good or bad, has led her to this point, and now her purpose is to make a bigger impact and contribute more to this world. She will expand her contribution by serving others and launching a book and YouTube channel this year.

Christine Awram is the founder of Woman Of Worth WOW Worldwide and is a dynamic speaker, author, visionary, and philanthropist.

Christine Awram

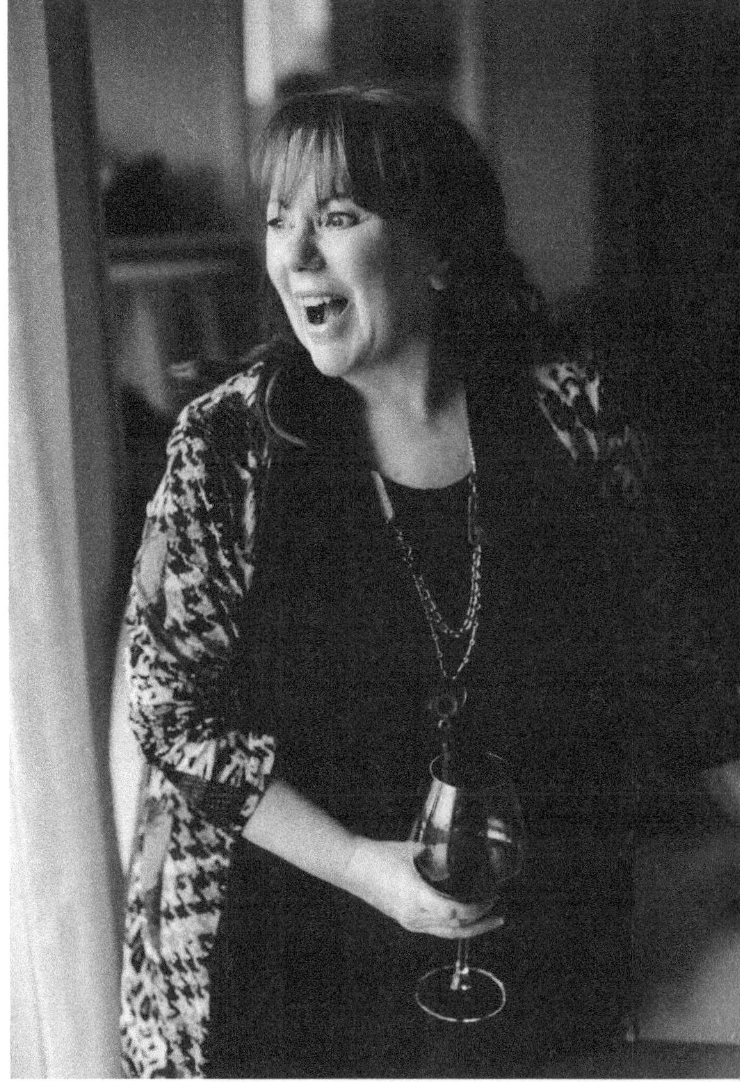
Photo Credit: Kristy Powers

When I was nine years old, my dad beat me on Broadway Street in broad daylight. As I screamed and wept and begged him to stop hitting me, cars drove by and pedestrians crossed to the other side of the road. A belief was anchored into my psyche that day which followed me for decades: "I'm not even worth saving."

Then came years of self-sabotage. I turned into a rebellious adolescent, teenage runaway, and street kid. Miraculously I survived and evolved into a seemingly high-functioning adult, but with a deep hole of inner self-loathing so consuming that I'd disappear for days at a time. Everyone thought I had the flu a lot, but I was actually being eaten alive by a darkness that left me paralyzed. A saviour arrived in my twenties who saw the real me and stuck like glue. He kicked my ass off the road to hell and onto a path of reclaiming my soul. His influence was also the catalyst for forgiving my father, who was a truly good man that temporarily lost his way. This put me on a new journey that led from futility to fulfillment.

One important lesson I embraced was to surround myself with a community of fierce badass ladies who have each other's backs. This led to the creation of WOW Woman Of Worth in 2004, which became an empowerment community for thousands of women. We also started a series of collaborative books, inviting authors to participate and share their 3,000-word real-life stories. Together we've created an ongoing legacy, with royalties donated to charity, and all have become #1 bestsellers.

There is a line from the WOW Credo that particularly speaks to me: "At times I despair and I weep when feeling the pain of a world that has momentarily gone mad. Yet even when I tremble through a dark night of the soul, I renew my faith and my courage in a single heartbeat because my spirit is indomitable."

This personifies courage. We will always have times when we falter, but it's our next steps that define us.
Always remember that you're a Woman Of Worth, and you are absolutely glorious.

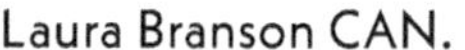

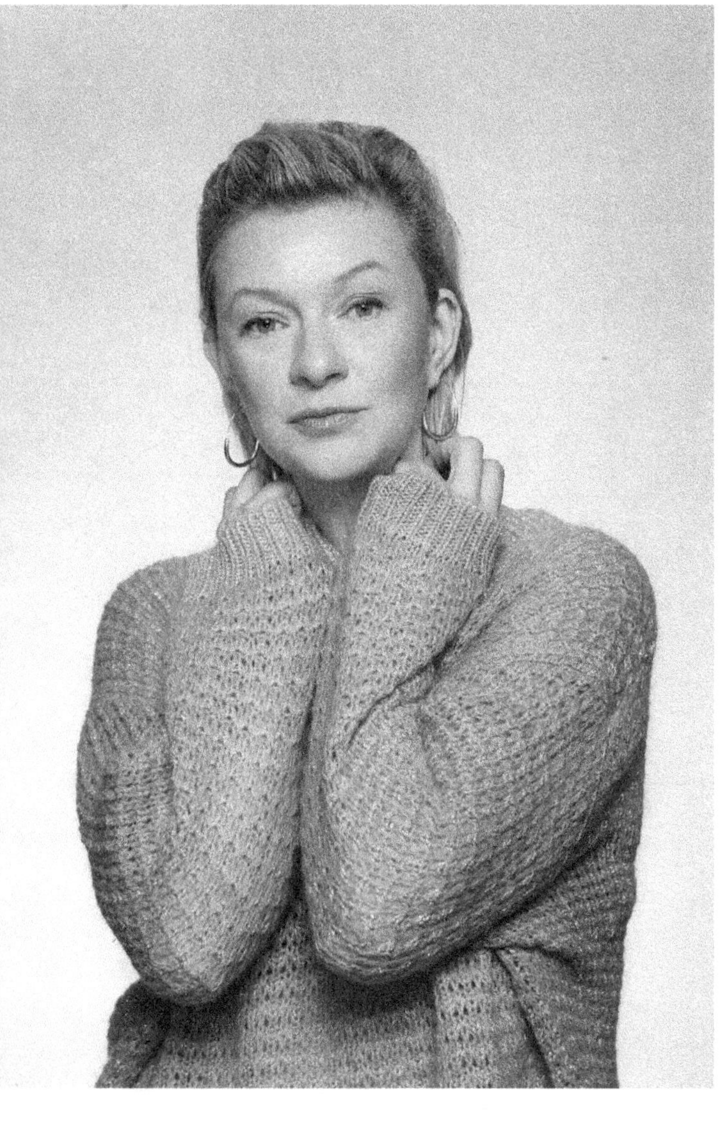

Laura Branson CAN.

Laura Branson

Some spoken words change you forever. In 2017 I competed in a full Ironman competition. A 4km swim, 180km bike, and a 42 km run. Crossing the finish line and hearing Laura Branson, you are an Ironman installed within me the belief that I CAN. Laura Branson, you are an Ironman.

About a month after the Ironman, my father passed away. The date was December 10th, 2017. As I trained for the event, I knew my father's time on earth was narrow, and I poured my grief into five-hour bike rides. One of our last exchanges spoken in his hospital room was, "Dad, I did it. I completed the Ironman." He was proud. A year to the day of his passing, I sat in my doctor's office following a mammogram and biopsy.

I had found a lump a week prior. Cancer. The words "Laura Branson, you have breast cancer" moved me into an entirely new season of my life, and would change me forever. Laura Branson, you have cancer.

I came home and told my husband that I had breast cancer. His response, he was not worried about me but about how we would survive financially. I had been in a physiologically and emotionally abusive marriage for twelve years.

His words were not new.

I am the mother to two young girls, and my time with them was not done. Using my athletic training mindset, I had a mastectomy, eight rounds of the harshest chemo for a breast cancer patient, and twenty-five rounds of radiation.

Despite the emotional strain in my marriage, I had always wanted my kids to grow up in an intact family. I fought so hard to hold together something that had no seams. Perhaps my cancer would show my husband that his family, his wife was precious.

Nearing the end of radiation, he told me we were divorcing.

Then I prayed hard and found strength through faith.

I fought for everything legally owed to me, sheltered my girls, bought a house, kept my business running. I started partnering with a not-for-profit group entitled SheStrong, an all-cancer, all-female athletic community; aimed to inspire and support women with cancer through sport.

Women CAN overcome anything.

Paula Lyons is an award-winning wedding cake designer & chocolatier. She is also a professional pastry chef, a holistic chef and cookbook author.

Paula Lyons

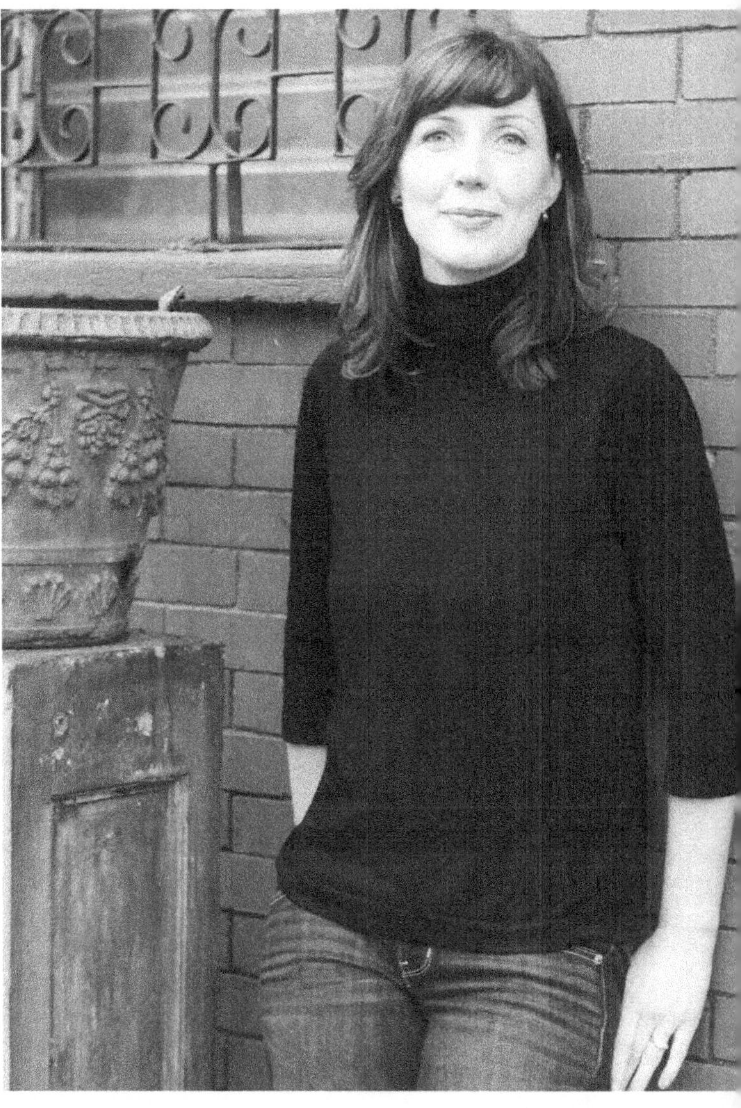

Food has shaped me my entire life, and I don't just mean pant size. It's what makes me tick. It's drawn me to places and invited me to stay.

I've been comfortable in the kitchen since tall enough to drag a chair to the countertop and reach a mixing bowl. My dad liked to reminisce how, at six, I handed him a shopping list so mum – my first pastry instructor – would have cookies on her return from hospital. I innately felt that food was comfort. Food was love.

It was logical to "go professional." My career in pastry began. Professional cooking has been deemed a tough job, but hard days aren't limited to commercial kitchens.

Days when the workplace feels more like a battlefield are the catalyst to pursue goals and seek your real potential. Find those who lift others up and want your success. They're out there.I became an entrepreneur, which can sometimes mean no days off and long hours, and comes with fatigue and failure, but the trials are yours to polish or abandon. It's exhilarating! I created ornate wedding cakes, but then all that changed.

I was thirteen when first introduced to food as healing. My father developed catastrophic arthritis, and his GP abruptly upturned his diet. That word, arthritis, has followed me most of my life. My dad's battle with it ended in June 2014 when he passed away, and weeks later, my son's battle with it began. He was five. It was a time to nourish and learn. I did what I knew; I cooked for him.

Like many who navigate a new diagnosis, I learned we could do more with our diet. Certain foods aggravated his condition, so we bid them farewell. He did better. Surely other families were in the same predicament? I would bake for them! People with food sensitivities deserved birthday cakes and pizza, or gluten-free apple pie. I'm not saving the world with vegan shortcakes, but a smile on a well-fed face is achievement enough. Cooking is an act of love, and feeding others feeds my soul.

"There is no love sincerer than the love of food." George Bernard Shaw.
I couldn't agree more.

Beth Hall is a therapist, high-performance coach, and artist. She is linear, logical, and surgical - highly intuitive and from the heart. Merging these two worlds is where the magic happens. She is a truth-seeker, pattern finder and believes we can build the life of our dreams.

Beth Hall

I am here to discover - truth, depth, what it really means to be human. To give permission to myself and others to architect life experiences beyond our wildest dreams. Transforming loss, failure, mistakes, and fear - all that we push away - into our most valuable assets. Life, being human, is hard - and complicated. And the biggest lie we're sold is that life is supposed to be perfect. Bought into this, we quite literally throw away our greatest gifts - our deepest expression, creativity, and innovation. Our joy. Our love. Connection and belonging.

Through my own pain and losses, I have discovered a deep sense of meaning and a life path far greater than I could have ever anticipated - one that is tapped into aliveness. What I know to be true is that there is beauty and opportunity in the darkest, ugliest places. It is up to us to train our minds and eyes to see it. It's typically not taught, but it is teachable. We aren't taught this because the way through is to lean into discomfort. Collectively, we avoid this. Rather than transforming pain, loss, and suffering, we're taught to numb it.

Transforming our reactive patterns into joy, meaning, connection, and thriving requires us to do hard things. It requires us to relearn how to feel - anger, sadness, rage, irritation, disappointment, fear - and expose the guilt, shame, and not-enoughness that cripple and paralyze us. I also learned to pay attention to the simple things... As I walk, noticing the scent of flowers, the countless shades of green amongst the streets. The shapes, colours, and contrast of the clouds and sky - literally seeing a masterpiece hovering above me every single day. Even on the rainiest of days, noticing the depth of greys, purples, and blues.

The same is within us. In all our supposed flaws, deficiencies, losses, and betrayals - there is beauty and possibility beyond our wildest dreams when we are open to it and courageous enough to feel.

Alice Grey is a health enthusiast who founded iHeart Fat Fudge Foods Inc in 2020 with the goal of providing a healthier alternative to conventional chocolates made with sugar.

Alice Grey

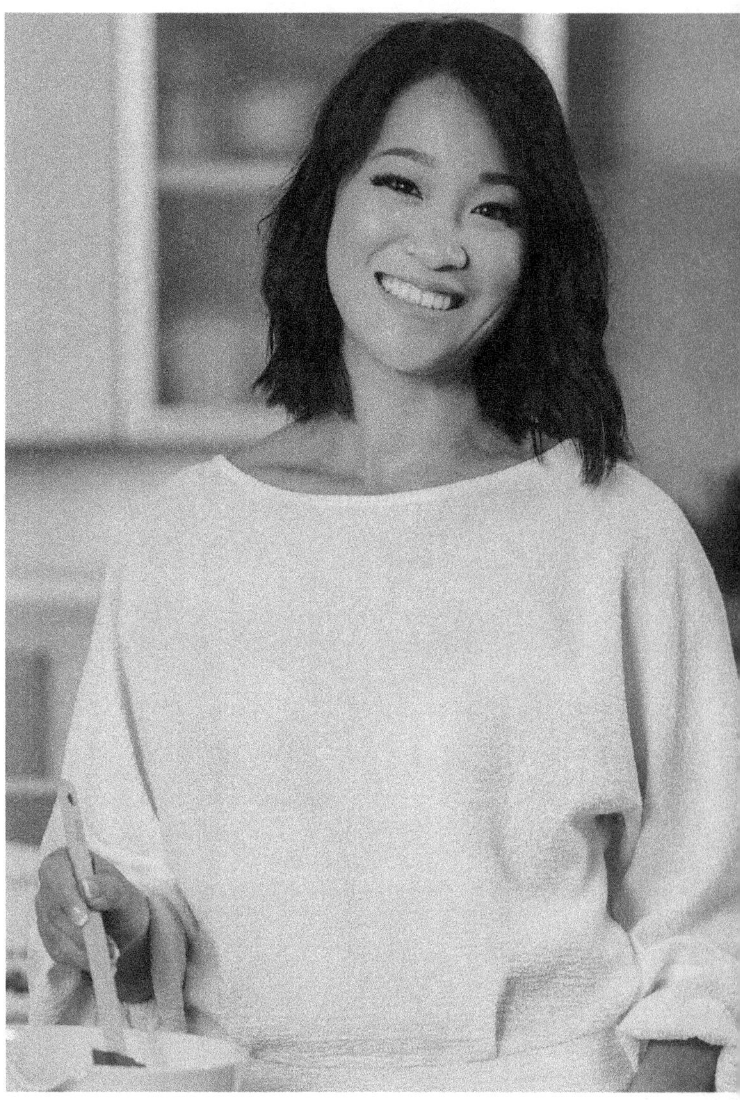

Self-love was something that didn't resonate with me, something I had deeply ignored until I was faced with nearly losing my life. I fought to live, and all the love, hard work, and time I have invested are allowing me to become my best self. It also gave me the drive, courage, and clarity to pursue my dream. But this wasn't always the case...

Growing up the youngest in a large household was lonely. No one was around, and this created an insatiable desire for attention from anyone who noticed me. As I grew older, I was the social butterfly, the outgoing one, the one with a chip on her shoulder who had something to prove. I may have seemed confident to others, but deep down, I lived in fear. Afraid that no one would ever care, love, or accept me for me, I acted like a victim of everyone else's actions; life was unfair. For those who saw through me and genuinely cared, I felt like they were attacking me.

Then my life changed forever. The birth of my second daughter was successful, but immediately after, I knew something was off. I still vividly remember the excruciating pain from multiple hands tugging, scraping, and clawing my placenta from my uterus. Within an hour, I had lost over two litres of blood. I felt cold, I couldn't speak, I couldn't open my eyes, I was alone in my thoughts. I saw visions of my husband alone with our two daughters, and then everything went dark. Four hours later, I woke up. I am forever grateful for the doctor who saved me, but I am most grateful for the fight I had in myself to live.

I always thought the battle to live was for my family, but it was for me. My perspective on life shifted from a place of fear to a place of love. I own all of my actions and live with integrity. I believe everything in life happens for me and am grateful for all of my experiences. I learned that the only love I ever needed to thrive was the love for myself.

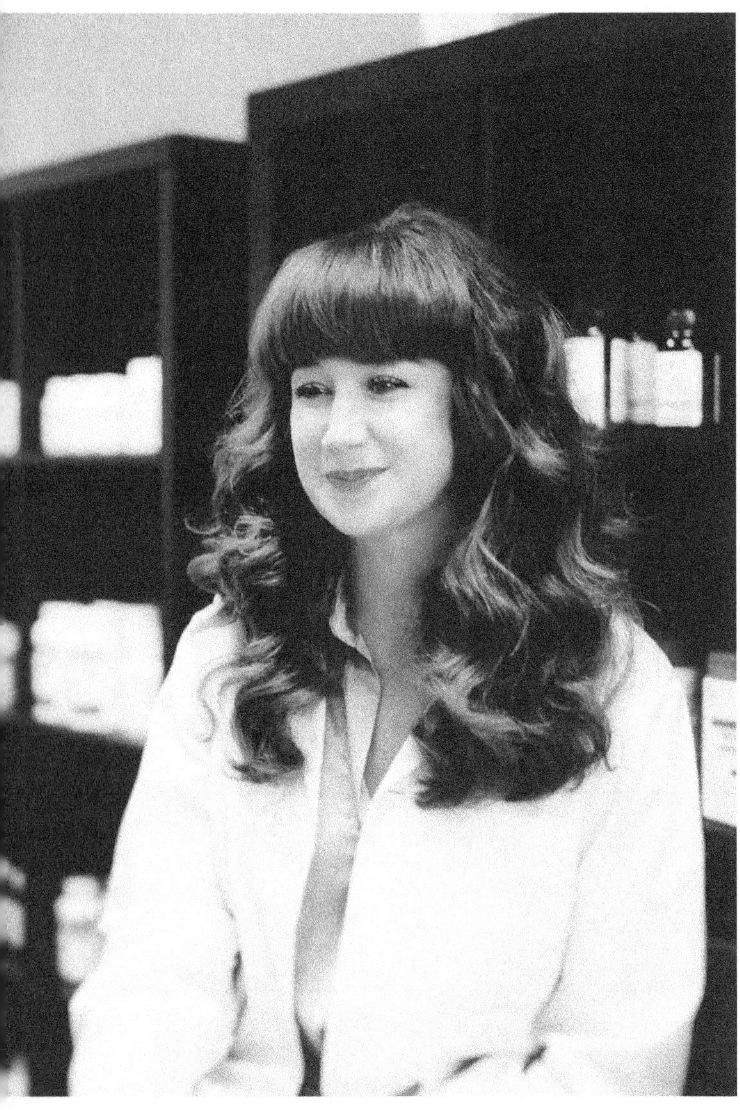

Lisa Blake works with clients and to create natural healing solutions.

Lisa Blake

My family looked well dressed, pristine, and polished from the outside. Inside it was riddled with generations of abuse, addiction, and trauma that, like a family heirloom, we continued to pass on to those we loved. I, too, fell into this endless cycle. I knew deep inside me, even as a very little girl, this was not the life I was meant for, or that I chose. I often found refuge in nature, playing for hours at a time in the forest, picking plants, and making potions. I was also perpetually in trouble for doing this as I loved to mix anything, I could get my hands on!

In the turmoil of my childhood, I found helpers the people like my aunt and uncle who I could truly be myself around. We all have those people the ones who truly show up and shape who we will become. They are those special people you can entrust with your wild ideas or far-fetched pursuits, but most of all, you can trust them with your heart. They teach us to think outside the box and to believe in ourselves. They were my teachers, my realization I had worth and strength in moments that hope didn't look like an option. When happiness just looked like a sunny place across the street I would never live. I knew I had to break this cycle, and with the help, I left home at the age of fifteen.

In that time, I have known hunger, extreme poverty, and in many moments defeat in my pursuits of success, education, relationships, and creating the life I want to live. Like many of us who lead with our hearts, I fall very short, and continue to, but I know amongst the chaos, I can return to nature and to passing on the teachings and good nature of those helpers in my life. My work and who I am today are governed by these principles; that it is important to create a safe loving space for people to freely express themselves, and to use nature as medicine to heal. I have since created my business which encompasses this approach and I work with clients and to create natural healing solutions. My potions have now evolved into healing formulas.

Getting off my high horse and letting go of purpose.

Paula Castellon

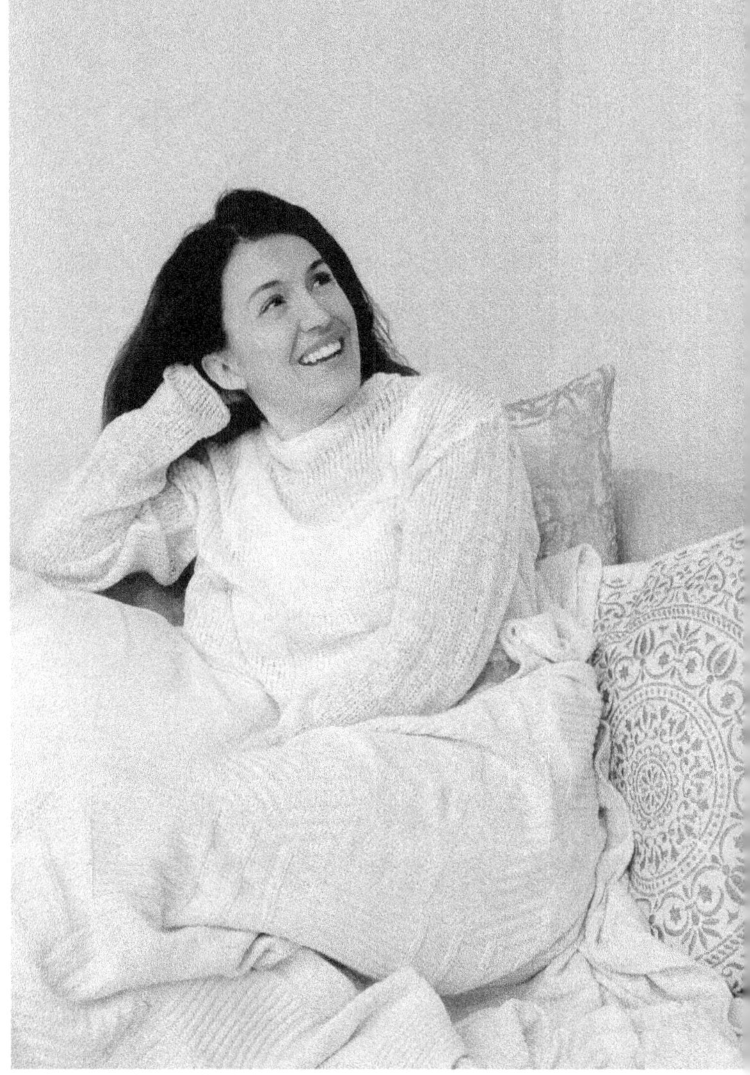

Photo Credit: Eyoälha Baker

Paula has an optimistic worldview and cares deeply about the earth and humanity but is unapologetic when it comes to living life on her own terms.

As a young, educated woman in my twenties, I felt that strong sense of responsibility to protect the world. Social and environmental injustice was impossible to ignore and my problem to solve. Protecting it felt like my purpose and responsibility. As if the world needed me or it would crumble.

Into my thirties, my attention to the big, wide world faded as my purpose shifted towards the role of wife, mother, and entrepreneur. I had to ensure financial and emotional stability in my new, much smaller world. Protecting it felt like my purpose and responsibility. As if this new smaller world needed me, or it would crumble.

In my forties, I finally got off my "high horse" and realized I am actually not so grand after all. If I was gone tomorrow, all these things that "needed me" would figure out how to continue. Turns out the world is resilient and isn't going to crumble without me. Suddenly it seemed I had no purpose.

This may sound sad to some, but to me, it was a beautiful liberation to live a life under my terms, unapologetically. My biggest shift was learning how to support versus worry. Worrying about the world and injustice does not make it better, but our collective actions do. Sleepless nights worrying about my kids was wasted energy, but witnessing their individual growth and supporting them is a meaningful action. As a good wife, for years it was my role to preserve a "fragile" male ego when it came to money, sex, and career. Now I know he was always strong enough and only needed my support, not my protection. And my career shifted from ensuring others are happy to making myself happy, adding deeper satisfaction to my life.

I no longer let the world's needs solely dictate my path. I am finding my true self and know I can nurture and give myself priority while still loving the world and those around me.

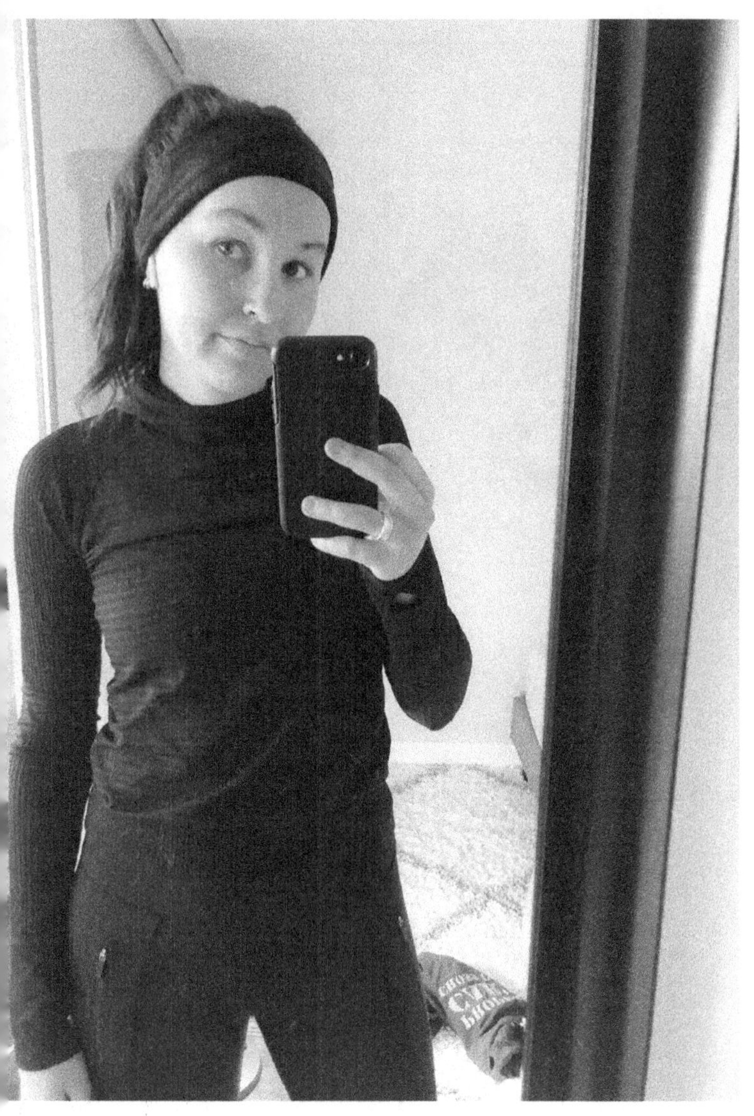

Roz McLean is passionate about the stewardship of long-term institutional capital and spends much of her free time raising funds for charitable Canadian organizations. And running.

Roz McLean

I have always found discipline really hard. Do I have ambition, drive, and curiosity? Yes. But ambition without discipline is chaos.

The pursuit of a more disciplined life has underpinned a lot of my thinking over the past decade. For someone like me who thrives on short feedback loops, working towards long-term goals that bring meaningful fulfillment in life could be frustrating. I would still work towards these goals, of course, but every success I had was quickly replaced with an insecurity, with the question of, "do I have the discipline to sustain this?" I literally felt uncomfortable when people were proud of me – because I thought my lack of discipline would inevitably disappoint them in the end.

Fortunately for me, discipline can be practiced; and while long-term goals still take time, confidence in your capacity for discipline can be improved much more quickly. My trick – my privilege and my pleasure became running. Running is measurable and honest. Your pace tells you how much effort you put in, and your distance shows endurance. Your muscle soreness is a relentless reminder of the work you have done and of the strength you are building. I started off by running a little, and then I ran a lot, but the most important thing was that I followed through on the runs I committed to. It was so empowering to deliver on promises I had made to myself. The promises I made were simple but not easy: just put one foot in front of the other, just keep running, just keep going.

The knowledge that I could do it meant that I could figuratively put one foot in front of the other for a lot of other projects. I began to have confidence in myself. I started to get comfortable with other people having confidence in me; and I began to respect my own capacity and threshold for effort, endurance, and also for rest.

With gratitude for my body and the health that propels me to each next intersection.

Lily Ling is a certified makeup artist, certified hairstylist, and has been published on Wedluxe.

Lily Ling

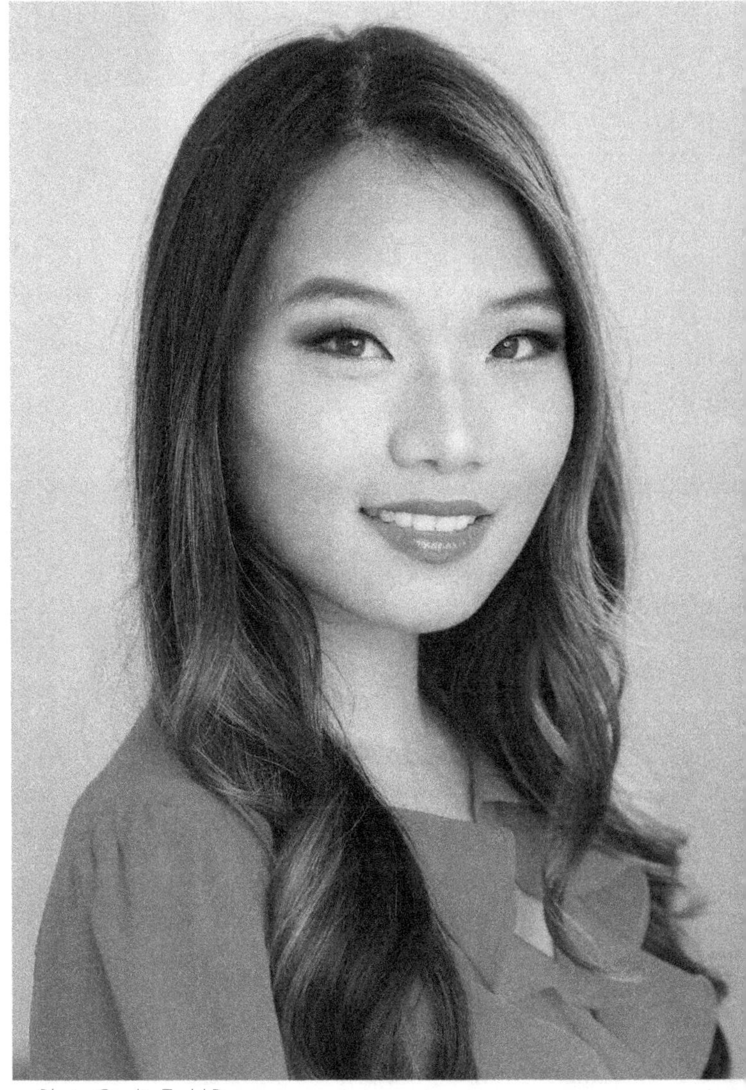

Photo Credit: Todd Duncan

When it comes to beauty, celebrities have a team of professionals to keep them red carpet ready. Having worked with the best photographers in Vancouver, in front of, and behind the scenes in film, who better to consult than Vancouver's very own celebrity makeup artist and hairstylist Lily Ling? Lily, what expert tips do you have for the everyday woman?

One **HUGE** mistake when planning a wedding or event is reserving a makeup artist too late in the game. It is a great compliment to be chosen, but I am saddened when I have to reply that their date and time is no longer available.

PREPARATION IS EVERYTHING: Having planned my own wedding and photo shoots across the world gives me the advantage of working with brides of various skin tones and cultures. It may be their first wedding, but not mine! A photograph is forever, and the more prepared you are, the happier you will be to share your images! Be ready with sample photos. A trial is the best time to discover how your ideas translate on your features.

BE EFFICIENT: Timelines are often severely underestimated. With my experience in front of the camera, and behind as a makeup artist, my vision takes all variables into account. For example, makeup has to be amplified to combat the bright lights of professional photography and a seemingly benign stray hair will destroy an otherwise perfect picture. When time is of the essence, we need to prioritize and optimize what the camera captures. This maximizes the number of photographs to choose from.

SELF-CARE: Use the motivation of your special event to optimize your skin care, diet, and exercise. Too often, brides tell me they didn't take care of themselves before their wedding. Remember to love yourself. Instead of relying on makeup do the heavy lifting, do that at the gym instead! It is heartwarming when women tell me I've been a part of their transformation long after their event is over. One of my treasured clients is a woman who initially sought me out for her LinkedIn picture. She tells me she uses scheduled photoshoots to hold herself accountable!

CONFIDENCE: I am often the last person a performer sees before she goes on stage. She may be nervous during prep, but all her millions of fans see is pure confidence. Remember, when you get in front of the camera, relax and own your beauty because you've prepared for it, emotionally and physically! In fact, why wait for a special event to begin the metamorphosis of being your best? The time to begin is now, and I am honoured to be by your side.

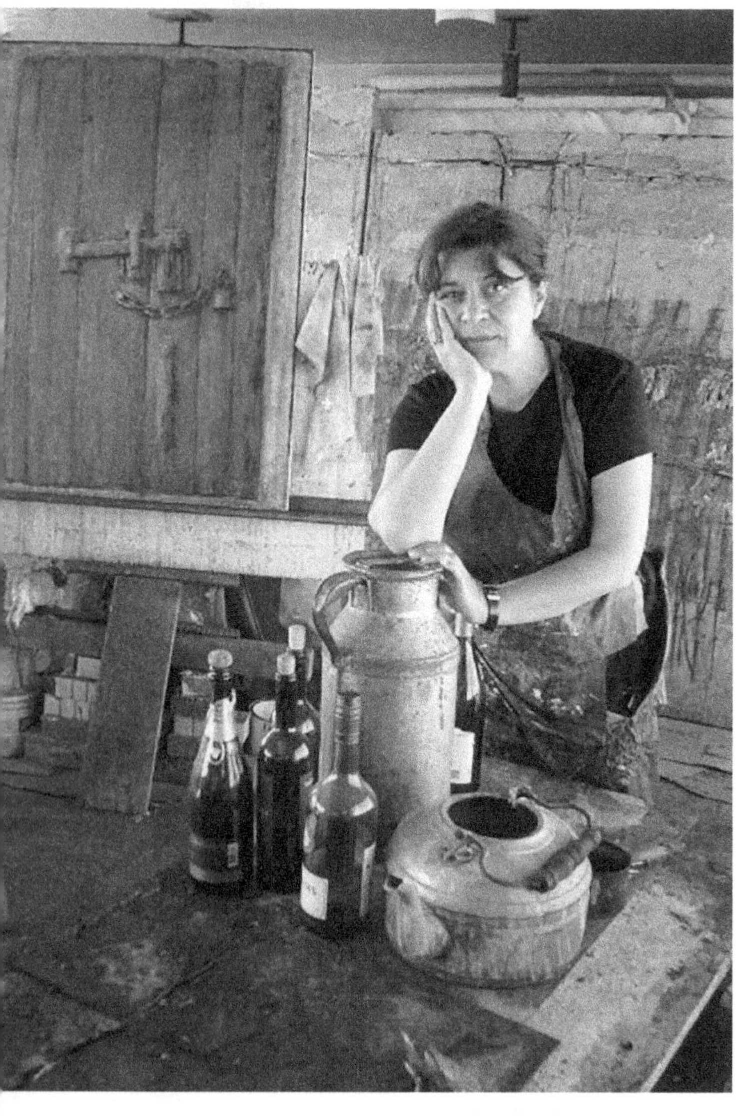

Dina Podolsky is a mom and an artist, who discovers beauty in ordinary objects.

Dina Podolsky

My story is a journey - the journey of being a mom to three beautiful daughters and of being an artist. It's also the story of three cities, three cultures, three chapters of my life.

Born in Moscow, my first childhood memories are tied to art and wanting to follow in my father's footsteps, renowned artist and book illustrator, Lev Podolsky. He worked in the "dark ages" of communist USSR, he struggled and persevered. Immersed in a highly creative bohemian atmosphere, I was so inspired. Influenced by my father's artistic vision, Russian avant-garde, I too wished to find my voice. Years of strictly traditional art education and training followed.

The next chapter starts when I move to Jerusalem – adjusting to a new home, continuing my art studies at Bezalel Academy, feeling inspired, and enjoying the freedom of being, and artistic expression. My personal journey was neither unique nor easy; divorce, being a young single mom, trying to support my daughter through art, taking on numerous teaching jobs, and having my first solo show at the age of twenty-two. Some years later, I find my happiness, I build my family; they are my most devoted fans and enthusiastic supporters of all my artistic endeavors.

The last chapter involves another move, new challenges. I uprooted once again, this time to Montreal. I knocked on many galleries' doors and worked tirelessly to become part of the Montreal artistic community. I was unstoppable and very lucky as well. Today, more than twenty-five solo shows later, having partnered with prestigious galleries worldwide and having my work in meaningful art collections, I am so thankful for the opportunities and people I've met along the way.

For me, the pursuit of happiness means family above all else and, doing what I love, following my bliss. Finding beauty in the ordinary objects of childhood memories, rusty kettles, field flowers, grandfather clocks, and jars with turquoise patina. Bringing these objects to life through mixed media to create multi-layered canvases. I found my voice.

Currently based in Vancouver, Julie operates Julie Heather Photography where she captures large-scale events and intimate moments alike.

Julie Bernard

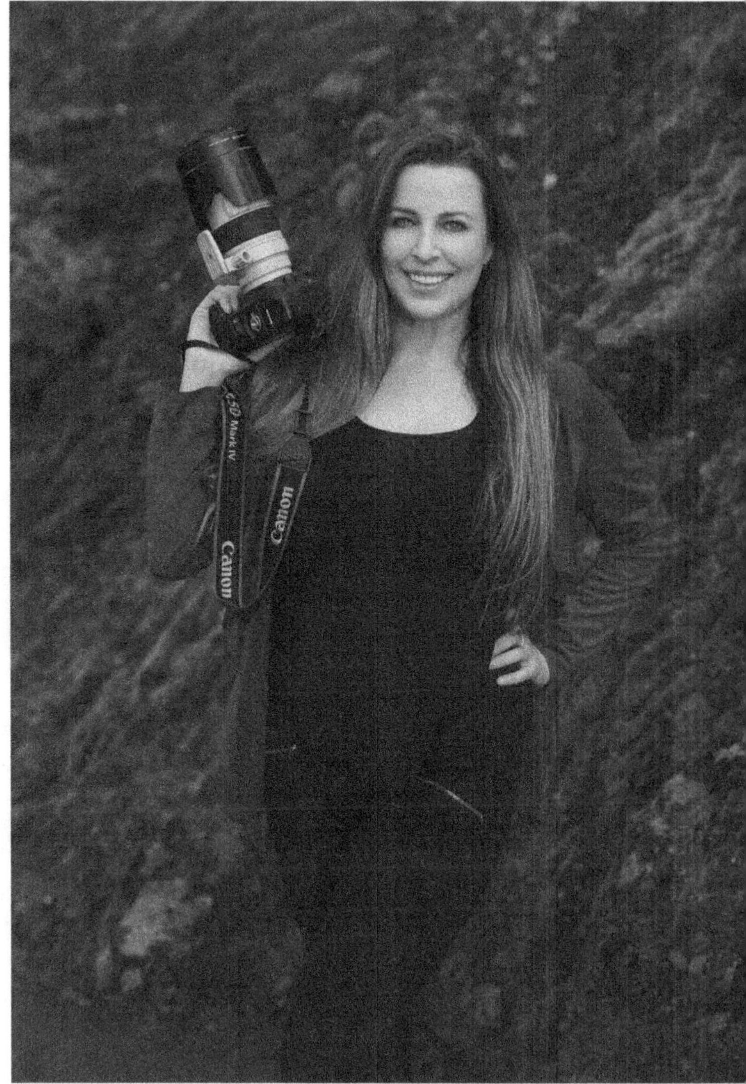

Raised on a farm in a fishing village, and just like a storybook, Prince Edward Island played host to all your childhood dreams. Red sand beaches and a sky so full of stars you'd lose count. I always knew photography was in the plan and while I love "home," I chose to attend college in Ottawa and then relocate to Toronto to focus on building my career.

With additional education and employment in communications and events, sports media, sales, and of course, photography, relationships were created that offered invites to some wonderful celebrations over the years. I've had the pleasure of photographing leaders of companies and countries, celebrities and athletes, cancer warriors, and even an astronaut at events for the Juno's, NBA, CBC Sports, and Golf Canada, to name a few. My work has created opportunities for travel from coast to coast and around the world. As a massive sports fan and lover of the arts, this is an absolute dream.

A favourite part of photography is the honour of being invited to someone's most important day - capturing those special moments with family and loved ones, attending charitable fundraisers and celebrations, playing comedian and cheerleader all at once. Laughter and tears shared with friends and strangers. Oftentimes, you leave a gathering so full of love that you feel like you're floating.

Photography also allows me the opportunity to empower others. Reminding people to be comfortable in loving the skin they're in and witness them rediscover the joy in their smile. I experienced childhood epilepsy, discovered aggressive polyps in my early thirties, and have lived with psoriasis for much of my adult life and these conditions taught me valuable lessons in self-love.

Several work opportunities brought me to BC and, finding myself craving the ocean waves again, I eventually made the move. Though rebuilding business proved laborious, the experience was a humble reminder of why I remain so devoted to my photography career. If you've ever witnessed me working, you know it's not a job - but a passion. When you find the thing that makes you soar, you just need to spread your wings - and fly. And I'll be there to capture it all.

Chrissy McRoberts DDL, PC, is the creator and co-owner of DOG EAT DOG.

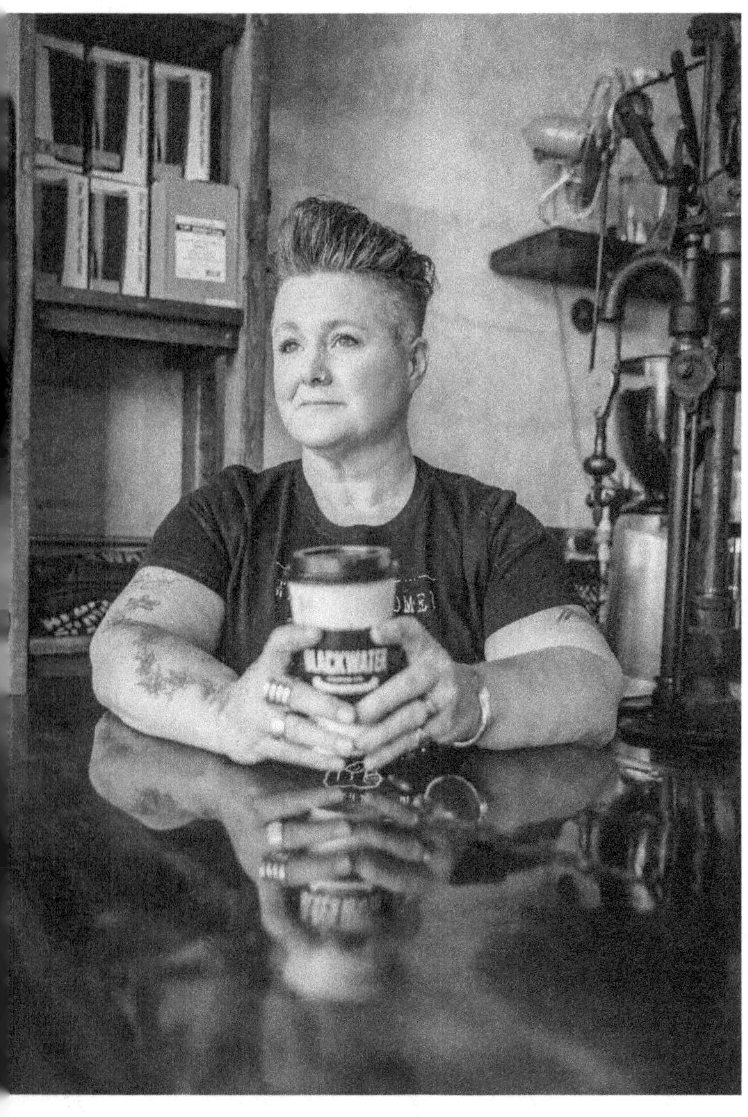

Chrissy McRoberts

I am Chrissy McRoberts DDL, PC (Dedicated Dog Lover), (Proud Canadian). I always wanted credentials to follow my name and now seemed like the perfect opportunity to test them out.

FYI, the unbridled sense of humour that I have unleashed has served me well in all facets of life. I am celebrating a life of fifty years filled with experiences in the Canadian Military, hotel management, self-employment, and divorces (two in fact – what doesn't kill us makes us stronger), two incredible children and dogs.

Without a doubt, I was gifted with the ability to read people, which laid the groundwork for a lifetime career in customer service. It has served me so well, in fact, I felt prompted to share my unorthodox customer service practices in an upcoming Podcast (launch date June 2021) (strong language and brutal honesty).

Imagine a gift store atmosphere filled with a warm yellow glow from rustic-industrial lighting, rusty tin walls, recycled wood slats, and the faint snoring of my two Old English bulldogs, Legend and Fable (that provides necessary character). Above the music and chatter, my colourful vocabulary floats throughout the building like a chorus of angels (Hells Angels version). This store is a replica of my personality which is best described as "Hallmark & Spencer's having a drunken one-night stand." Customers exude laughter, excitement, comfort, and loyalty, which endorses our business plan and behaviours. Every day starts with a shot of Bailey's in my latte, selecting a whimsical t-shirt riddled with dark humour and dog hair followed by a NETMA (Nobody Ever Tells Me Anything) meeting with my business partner. Priorities and routines are the keys to my success!

What is my recipe for strong customer service skills? Transparency is effortless and, comforting the needs of my clients (not that they necessarily care for my bubbly personality) while creating a relaxed atmosphere will assist them with feeling an authentic connection. Finally, in a world of pm's and dm's let's develop stronger customer service skills and leave the texting for after-hours and memes.

Barbara Edie is an intuitive guide, transformational mentor, and best-selling author of Creating the Impossible: What It Takes to Bring your Vision to Life. She also has an unusual superpower—Uncertainty. Not only does she thrive on variety, diversity, and an exciting challenge, but also uses uncertainty as a driving force and potent energy to create the extraordinary. She helps her clients do the same; to live with less fear and more power by tapping into their higher guidance to navigate the unknown.

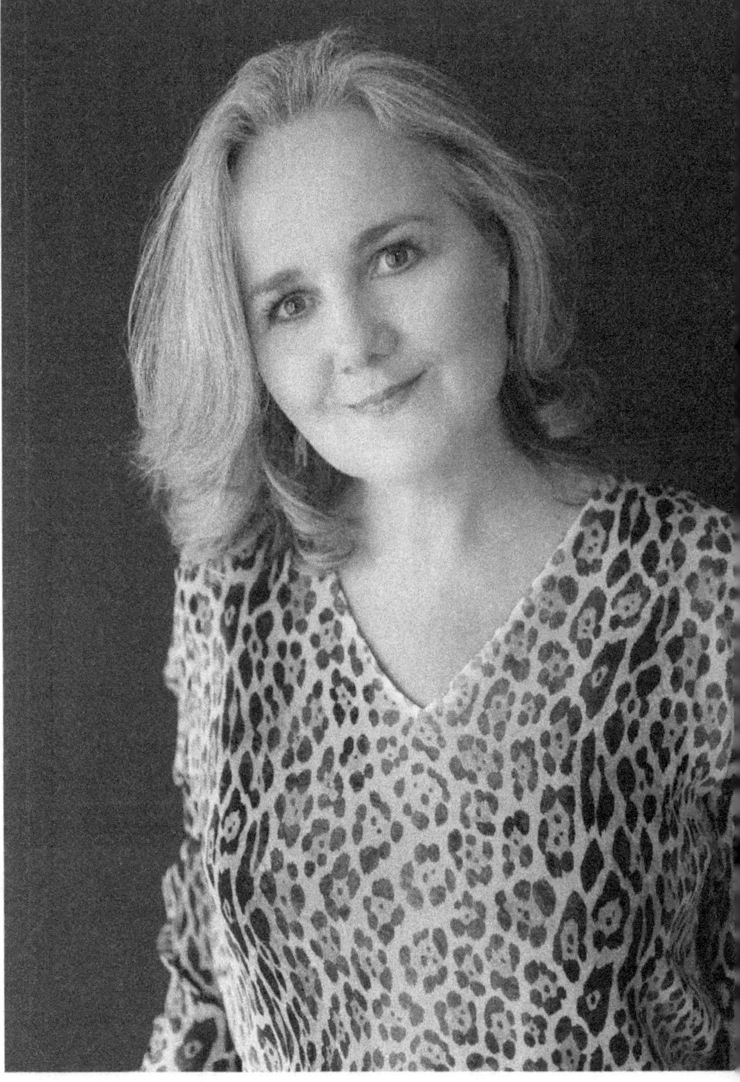

Barbara Edie

In life, work, and the pursuit of true happiness, my mantra is "embrace the mystery." From the space of the unknown, all things are possible. It is only when we have no preconceived idea of what 'should' happen, that anything CAN happen. As Nelson Mandela said, "It always seems impossible until it's done."

Delving into the unknown takes courage and curiosity, but it's also where the magic happens. I believe life is an adventure, not a package tour. Answering our call to adventure requires facing uncertainty and taking risks. "We will only understand the miracle of life fully when we allow the unexpected to happen," as author Paulo Coehlo says.

For example, when I climbed Mt. Kilimanjaro at age fifty-five, I really didn't know if I would reach the summit. No one does, until they are on the mountain. Yet, the uncertainty of the outcome did not sway me; it fuelled me. Each day, grounded in the present moment I embraced the mystery, not the fear, and ultimately reached the 19,340-foot summit feeling "spent," yet exhilarated, and wondering what other big dream I might accomplish next.

Few things bring me greater joy than witnessing my students and clients navigate uncertainty without it stopping them from creating their "wildest dreams," as intuition, higher wisdom, and "Ah-ha moments" show up to guide them. Without needing to know how everything will unfold, uncertainty transforms to clarity. If you always knew how things were going to turn out, you would miss all other possibilities, brilliant innovations, and MAGIC along the way!

Looking to create heartfelt happiness and wild success on your terms?
Here's what works for me: Embrace the mystery (uncertainty). Stay curious. Follow your heart and intuitive guidance.
Allow for magic.

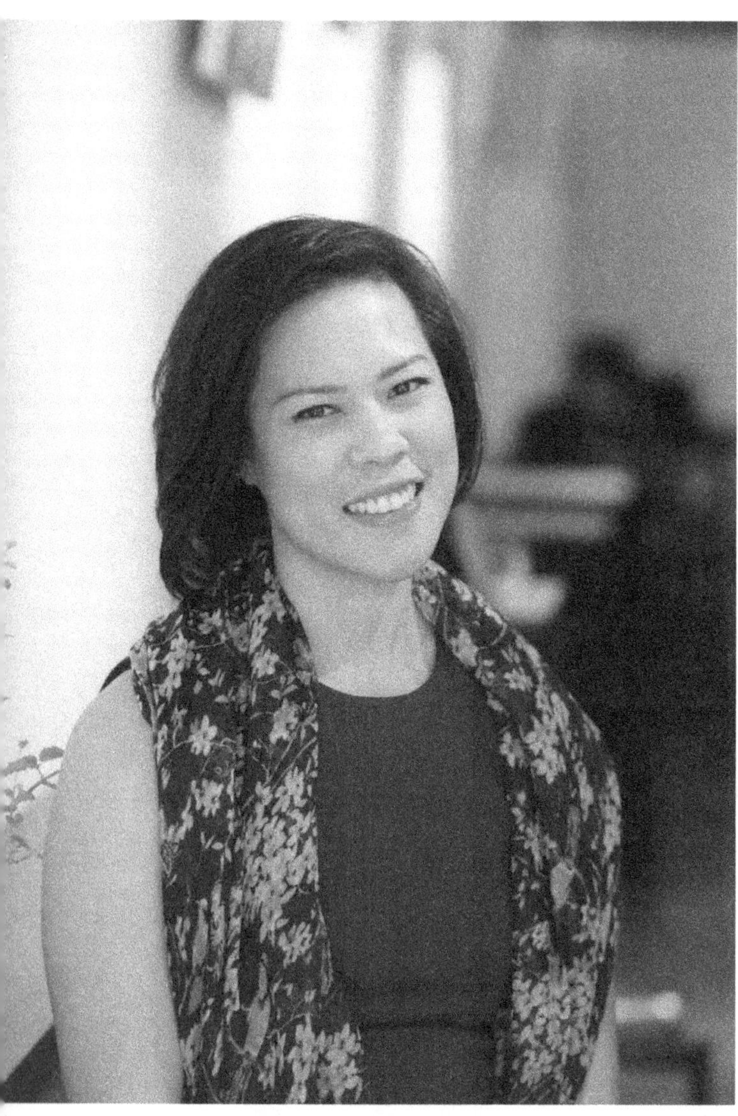

Renée Chan is a registered dietitian and the founder of True NOSH

Renée Chan

Food. My raison d'etre. My father introduced me to love good food, but there was disappointment whenever he gained weight, had high blood sugars and eventually passed away with diabetes complications, Alzheimer's disease, and heart failure. I was born into a very blessed Asian immigrant family in Vancouver with lineages in Hong Kong. My mother made sure I sang, danced, swam, figure skated, did gymnastics, painted, and went to the theatre. My parents never asked anything great of me, but I went to the schools with friends who strived to be doctors, lawyers, and more, so I also wanted more. I believed I was born to be great, so everything I did, was NEVER ENOUGH!

I pursued a master's in clinical nutrition in New York to become a Registered Dietitian, but it was the restaurants that kept me there. Working in restaurants allowed me to express emotions through edible art. Being a dietitian seemed sustainable, but I was missing teaching my patients the significance of disease prevention.

My company merges my culinary passions with the need to invoke change in our food. A kitchen is a place that measures your abilities. You must have thick skin and be courageous to take on roles that may not be ideal for you, but it will help you later. I worked from the bottom up and understood what it takes to run a business, especially what NOT to do!

I don't want anyone to suffer the pain of losing a father so early. I want to be a warrior and not a worrier, but I was one until I found the reason for my legacy through my business, True NOSH. After a few years running True NOSH, I was still unhappy because it was not growing fast enough. I wanted to be financially free of my family's help, I needed to pay my family for things that I received with so much guilt. I became more creative than ever as I realized my worth, and I now remember why I chose True NOSH. I wanted to be strong and free! It represents a healthy Canada embracing all ethnicities. The most important thing for me is the network and friends I made along the way; you never know how they can be there for you.

Lily Zhao is sharing her story and her perspective on finding freedom through responsibility.

Lily Zhao

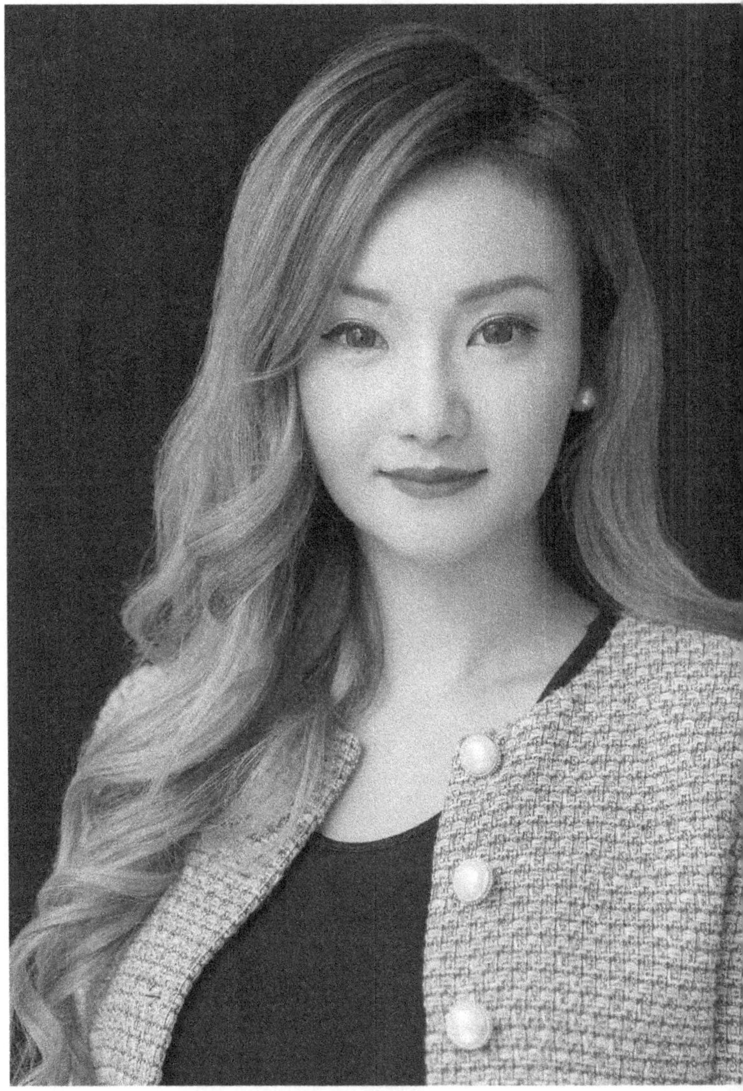

Growing up as the only Chinese kid in Japan, I was constantly bullied and alienated by my classmates. I felt like everywhere I go, I didn't belong; I felt like an outsider. As a result, I had low self-esteem, and I didn't like myself growing up. I thought if I lost the weight, altered my look, I would like myself more. Having low esteem manifested into all areas of life, I was in an unhealthy relationship, and I had difficulty saying no to others.

Since last year, I started to consciously build my self-esteem. I realized the cost of having low self-esteem was too high and made the decision to claim my power back. I started to stand up to my inner critics.

I learned the importance of integrity and making sure my actions match my words. When I compromised my values for acceptance and convenience, I became far more vulnerable to self-attacks. Inner critics love to see these shortcomings, so it is important to think about your core values and principles and act in line with those beliefs.

Note to my younger self:
Do things every day that empower you to like yourself because having high esteem is amazing. It gives you the ability to stay true to who you are and stand for what you believe in, and once we stand for ourselves, we can stand for others.

In pursuit of my happiness, my greatest lesson has been the duality of responsibility and freedom. When I was younger, I thought not being responsible gave me freedom, but I was wrong. My body broke down after neglecting my health. I was controlled in the relationship because I wasn't responsible financially, and my inner critics made me mentally ill. When I learned that you get more freedom by being responsible, it changed my life. I am becoming emotionally free by increasing my emotional literacy; and my ability to love by cultivating positive emotions and compassionately witnessing and transforming negative ones. I am becoming financially free by continuously investing and increasing financial literacy that creates time freedom. With time freedom, I am enjoying living my life by my own design and on my own terms. Lastly, I am working to free my mind by doing meditation daily as my morning routine. Freedom came after responsibility.

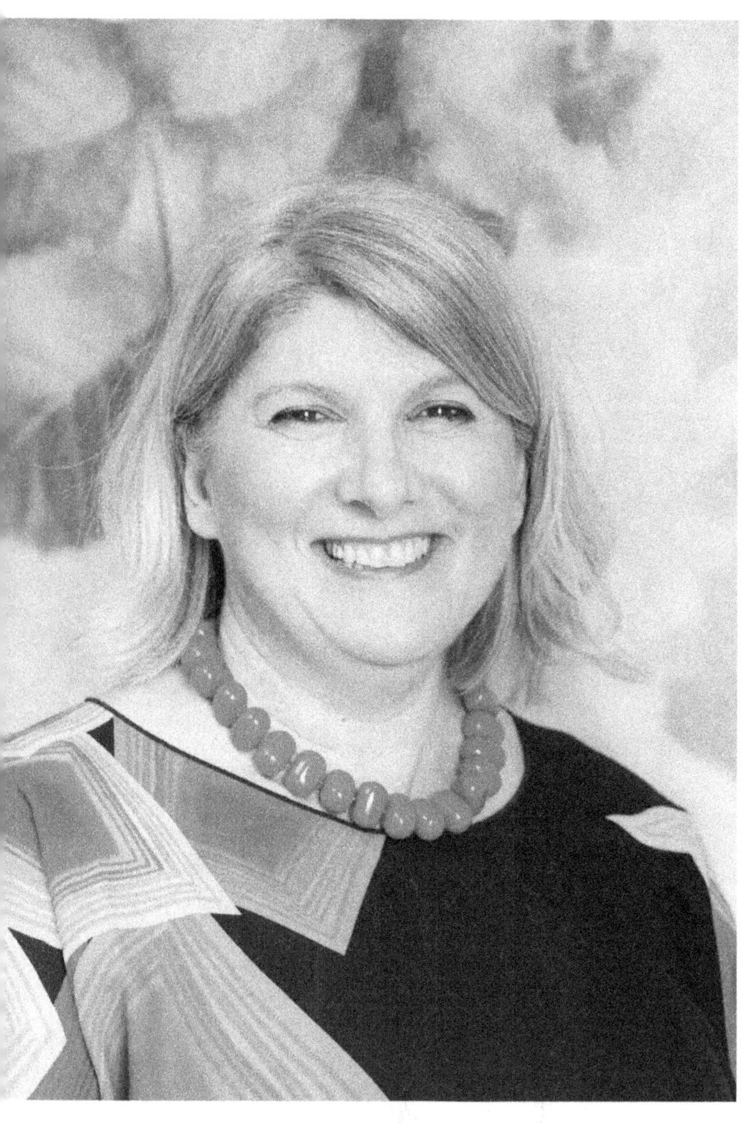

A mother, wife, educator, and a daring woman with a big heart.

Simona Gozner

It is very important for me to pursue a meaningful life in which gratitude, love, faith, and knowledge are essential daily elements. As an Educator, I am dedicated to motivating and supporting students on their learning journey. Being surrounded by caring and talented people is vital in achieving success and building meaningful relationships in life. I created Being 49 on the 49th Parallel Blog to inspire women to read and learn from other women's stories.

Connecting with people from different backgrounds inspires my whole being. It makes me feel alive. Listening to people's stories, journeys, dreams, and hopes have made me realize that we all want the same thing- **to be loved and to love.**

Every connection has taught me valuable lessons about who I am and what is important to me. When I was young, I wanted to change the world, just to realize later that the world transformed me. I was running away from my roots to search for a new meaning, ideals, and to pursue my dreams. People, ideas, and life challenges have put me in situations that have shaped my character and contributed to my transformation from a very shy child to a courageous woman who immigrated to two countries without speaking the languages.

I am a lifelong learner with a thirst for knowledge and a curious mind. I love art, photography, fashion designing, esthetics, holistic nutrition, wellness, education, and the environment. My precious life gift is when I became a mother to Josh on December 24, 1994. Everything changed at that moment. Motherhood has taught me to love unconditionally, be strong in the most challenging life situations, appreciate and accept help when needed, and, most importantly, to surrender have faith in my destiny. I am very proud of the young man Josh has become. His kind heart and strong morals will guide him on his journey. Sophia is the right partner by his side. She is like a daughter to me. My great blessing is the love of my life, My Habibi, my dear husband, Mohamed. After being a single parent for many years, I never thought that I would find true love. He taught me what love, respect, support, and encouragement mean in a real partnership. Every day, I count my blessings and hope to make a difference.

BE YOU BE KIND BE BOLD

Summer Dhillon Giesbrecht has been a storyteller for as long as she can remember.

Summer Dhillon Giesbrecht

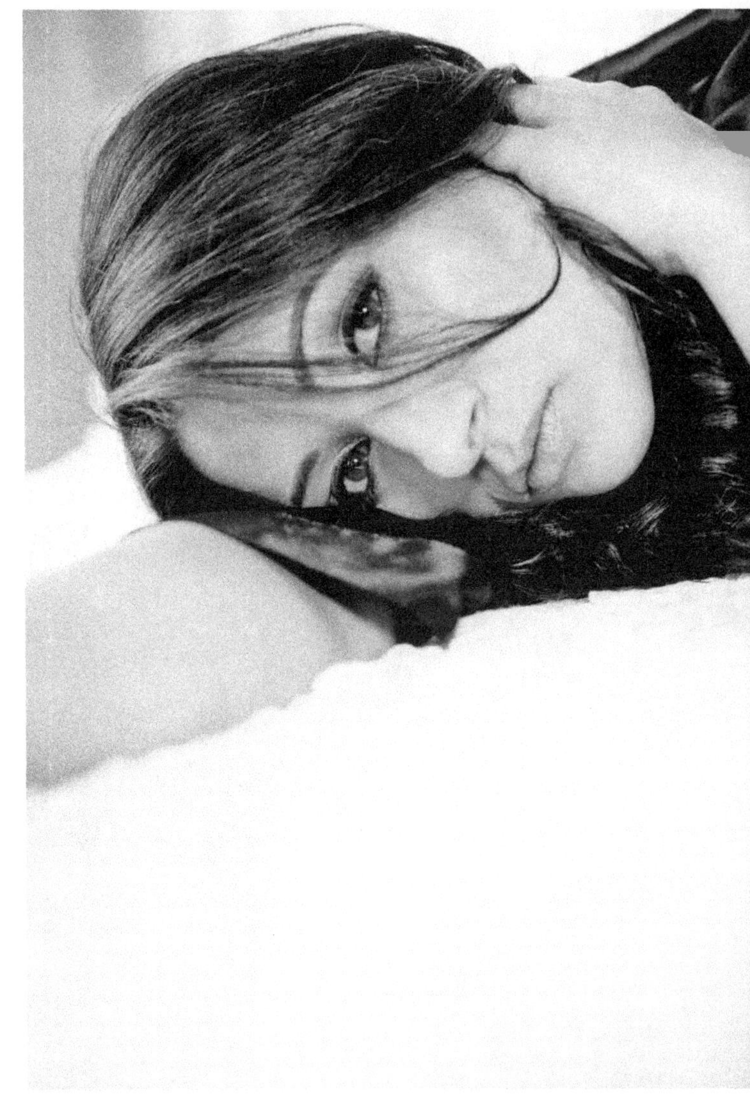

My South Asian background modelled a linear path. The formula meant you excelled in school, went to a top university, pursued a professional career, and then married well. Deviating from this path was viewed as selfish– we are talking very strong cultural conditioning. Our culture is collective in nature and, therefore, the word 'I' is rarely used. Yet, my heart was screaming, "Do you really want to do any of this?"

'Selfishly' the word 'I' was spoken, and I didn't just deviate from my chosen path, I created a whole new one, breaking all the rules. My life story is about my voice. Why is it so important to me and the moments that transpired once I started honouring it?

The journey started with pregnancy and then marrying outside of the 'right mold'. Struggling financially, going to university as a young mother, and then ending this marriage. Then a second relationship was formed, leading to my big tipping point. A culmination of losing my father suddenly, separating again, losing stable employment, and my eldest going to university... all in one year. I couldn't face the world.

Looking back, I was paralyzed with fear but experiencing a breakthrough. I decided to do what was counterintuitive and let go. I visualized a raging river current and allowed it to take me wherever it wanted to. For the first time, and out of pure exhaustion, I allowed the Universe to lead.

SLAP Communications was born out of need, so I could have the flexibility to raise the kids while earning an income, but the name —an acronym for S (success), L (love), A (authenticity), and P (pow) – came from my heart.

I lost my conditioning during this journey. Read daily affirmations like, "Throw me to the wolves, and I'll return leading the pack." I heard myself calling it like it is during client meetings, leaving board meetings to pick up my kids from school, fully expecting to be dismissed. My inability to care was my biggest blessing. Today, I only hear myself and have experienced success on every level. My life. My path. My story.

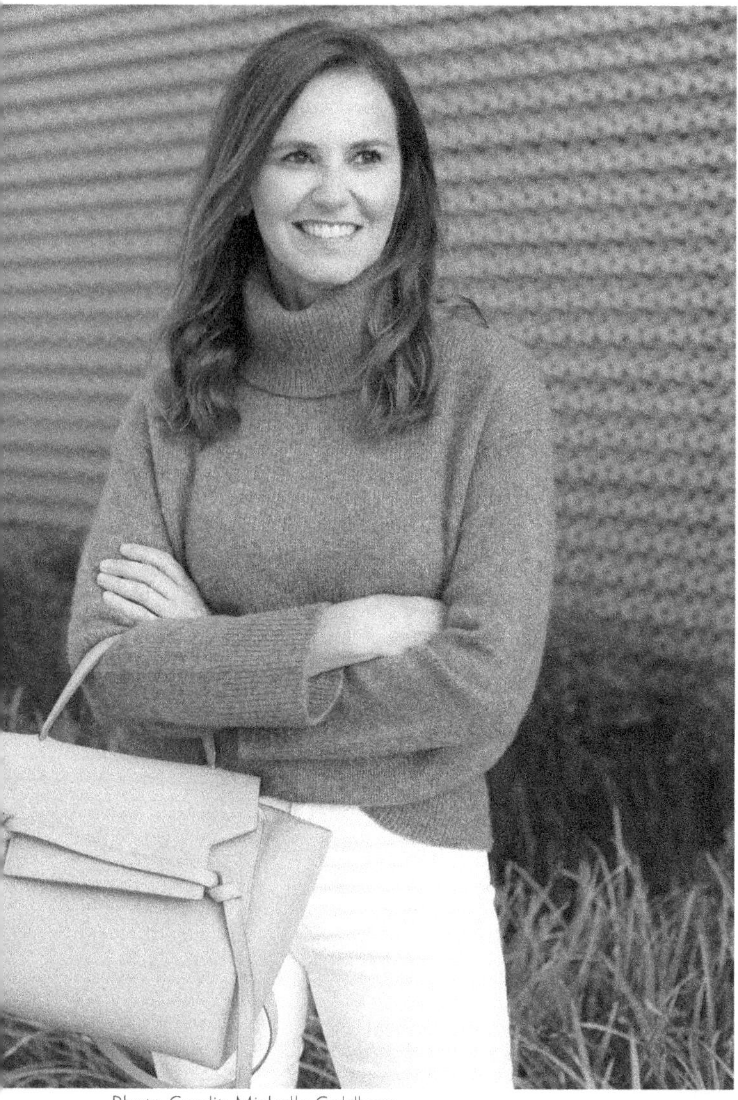
Photo Credit: Michelle Goldberg

Kristina Matisic is the founder of Kristina Matisic Creative, a Vancouver-based public relations and content creation agency.

Kristina Matisic

"Don't complain about the results you don't get with work you didn't do." I'm so grateful for my career success. How did it happen? I can attribute it to four things: hard work, determination, resiliency, and other people.

Upon returning to Vancouver with a master's degree in Journalism from USC, I needed a job but had zero connections in the local industry. After many futile months of resume-dropping, my mom learned that her friend worked for Global TV's news director. (Then called UTV.) She was his house cleaner. We convinced her to give him my demo tape. I was going to find a way into that newsroom, no matter what!

I worked as a reporter/anchor for six years. But news wasn't really my thing. I wasn't a news junkie, and the newsroom environment can be tough - though it was an excellent foundation for the rest of my career. At Global, I met Anna Wallner, and we decided we wanted to have our own TV show. Crazy? Many thought so. But we were fearless and relentless in pursuit of our dream. Our efforts resulted in 12 seasons on W Network with shows like The Shopping Bags and Anna and Kristina's Grocery Bag. The latter aired around the world.

In 2014, it was time to pivot again. Change can be scary, but without it, and without taking risks, good things can't happen either. After countless informational calls, taking classes, and the willingness to take on any small job, I launched a new phase of my career - my own public relations firm where I work with small to medium-sized companies to help them grow their brands and businesses.

I love working for myself because I can decide who I work with and it gives me the flexibility to pursue other passions, including travel, acting, and fashion. I can't underestimate how much our success depends on others. Foster those relationships! From the TV executives who said yes, to my first PR client who took a chance on me, I thank you.

Today, I try to give back my time and knowledge, lifting up the next woman (or person) who needs help achieving her dreams. Pay it forward sisters!

Maria De Cotiis is a fun-loving, high energy woman who knows what she wants, believes that anything is possible, and is always dreaming.

Maria De Cotiis

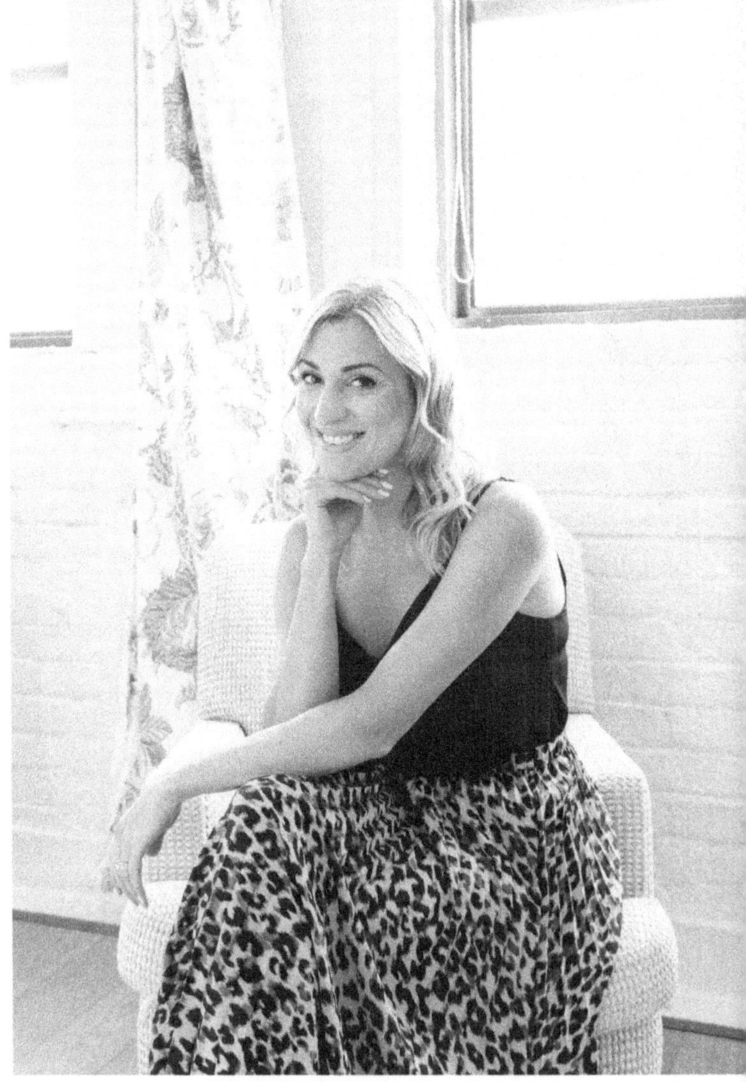

Growing up, I had two visions of my life; to be a successful businesswoman and to have a family. I wasn't sure exactly what "businesswoman" meant – but I knew it would involve great shoes and running a company.

I could feel it and see it so vividly, but I often felt like I was crazy to have such a dream. Maybe it was because there were people throughout my life that told me I wasn't good enough. I was certainly different from others around me; I was louder, I said what I was thinking, and when I wanted something, I figured out a way to get it. As much as I tried to ignore the negative opinions, I allowed the opinions of others to derail my dreams, and the internal light I had was slowly dimming. By the age of twenty-eight, I was married with three beautiful boys. I had the family I had always wanted and chose to put my dreams of running an Interior Design firm aside because it felt easier - what if I failed?

After reading what seems like a million self-help books and consuming endless podcasts, I had enough, and chose to persevere. My positive energy returned, and I started dreaming again. I knew very little about running a company but the desire to realize my vision was enough, I taught myself what I needed to know. Without that time in my life, I would have never gone on a soul-searching journey. I became a better version of myself.

I was taking the time for myself and finding my way again and I continue to do things that I've always wanted to but was too scared of. Other people's opinions of me are none of my business, a simple statement that took me years to understand. I love who I am, I am no longer hiding, I refuse to stop dreaming and while I still have fear I know that we all have fear. The difference is there are those that are willing to do it and those that are too scared to take the leap.

We all lose our way sometimes, and if you do, remember - be true to yourself, ask for what you want, and never stop dreaming.

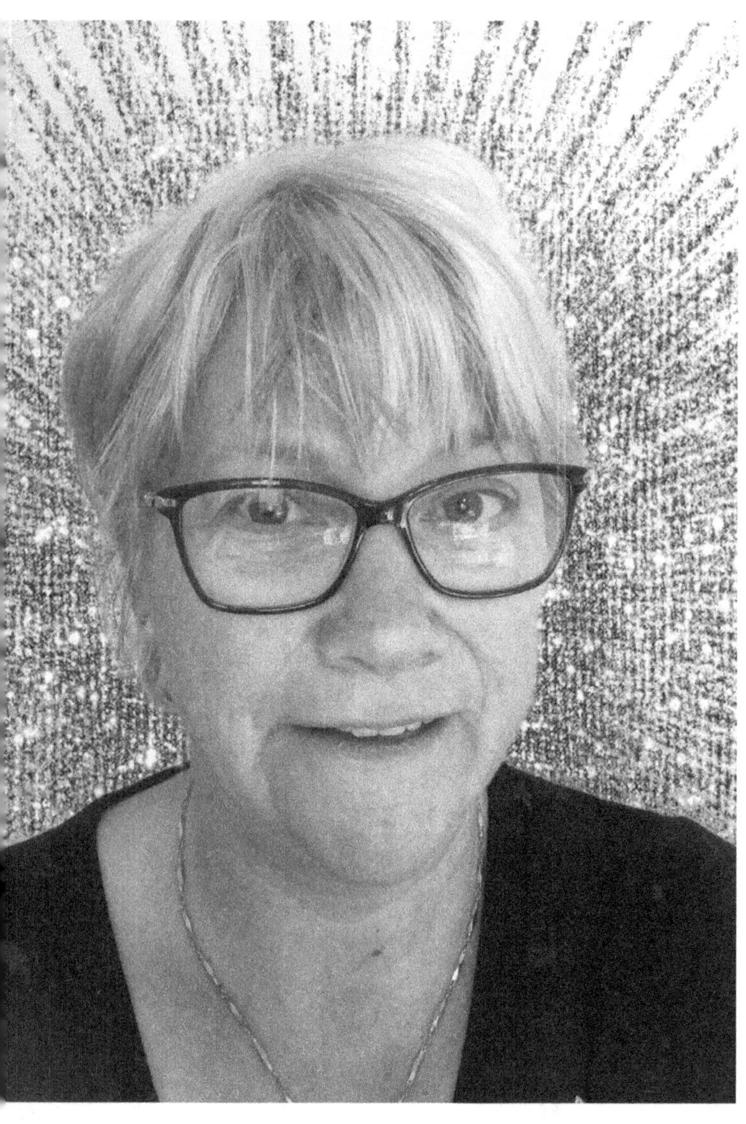

Michelle Fedosoff is a photographer, mother, wife, shoe addict, friend, daughter, sister, wine lover, and creative soul.

Michelle Fedosoff

It is important to note that I have not always described myself this way. Not too long ago, I would never even have thought of myself as a photographer, even though this is something I have been enjoying for more than twenty years. I was too busy being defined by other people.

Over the course of my life, I have had to deal with very difficult circumstances; an abusive father, a highly toxic work environment, anxiety and depression, mental abuse, the death of a loved one, and my husband's cancer diagnosis. I realize that I am not the only one who has ever experienced trauma, but at the time, it sure felt as if I was alone.

What I was not realizing at the time, was that photography was the constant through it all. When I was focused on my subject, it was enough to take my mind off the personal disaster at hand. It was enough to make me proud of myself, even when I did not have the confidence to say it out loud.

I will always remember the day that I finally listened to a good friend who had been pushing me to show my photography. She went with me as moral support as I prepared to be rejected. Guess what? It wasn't.

Since that day, when I finally took a risk, many wonderful opportunities have come my way. Opportunities for my photography; fine art, being published, fashion, and awards. What has been just as rewarding though has been the amount of amazing, supportive women that I have met, just because I took a chance on myself and remain open to opportunities.

Do I still have to deal with the harsh realities of life? Of course. But when I start to feel the heaviness, I pick up my camera and start shooting.

This is what I wish for all women. Recognition. Not by others, but by yourselves. Recognize that you have a talent, even if you think it is too small. Recognize the people in your life that support you and listen to them. Always.

Everything's going to be okay.

Jennifer Angers Daerendinger

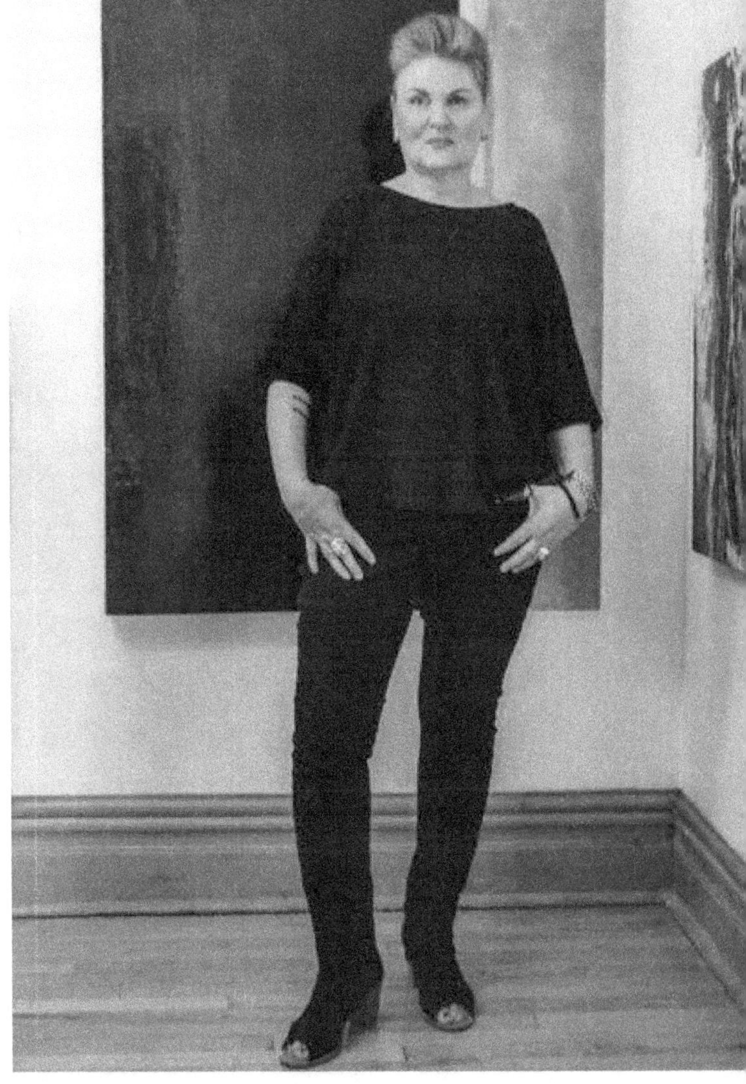

How do I sum up my life in 365 words? I'm not much of a philosopher, but one thing I know for sure is that in this world, your one guarantee is "shit happens." Like many of you, I've had my fair share of it - divorced, fired, overweight, broke. What I've learned in life is that when it does happen, you have two choices: host a pity party or get on with it. Me? I choose to get on with it; put on my big girl pants and figure it out. No excuses. No bullshit. Just do it.

Everything happens for a reason. As corny as that sounds, I believe it. While we might not realize it at the time, there are moments and people in our lives that pivot us. One of those watersheds came in the form of a generous angel who gifted me a space for ROAM Gallery. I was at a crossroads; out of work and out of sorts. Having never owned or run an art gallery in my life, I was uptight about the unknown. However, I moved an old passion for art to the forefront and let it drive my journey. Five years later I put ROAM Gallery on the map. This gift of space created a place for up-and-coming artists and a meaningful turn to my life.

Another game-changer hit me in the summer of 2017. I spent a few years of hard work freelancing without getting ahead. I was running out of money and options. Enter another angel with these simple words, "You know everything's going to be okay, right?" The answer was clear. Sell my Vancouver loft and move back to Ontario. No excuses. Just do it. Eight months later, I was living in my dream house and helping my mom in her senior years. This move was so right. I'm happier and healthier than I've been in a long time.

So, what's my story? My story is this - life is never easy. There are pivots and there are angels, but ultimately, it's up to us. To sum it up: "Mother Teresa didn't walk around complaining about her thighs. She had shit to do."

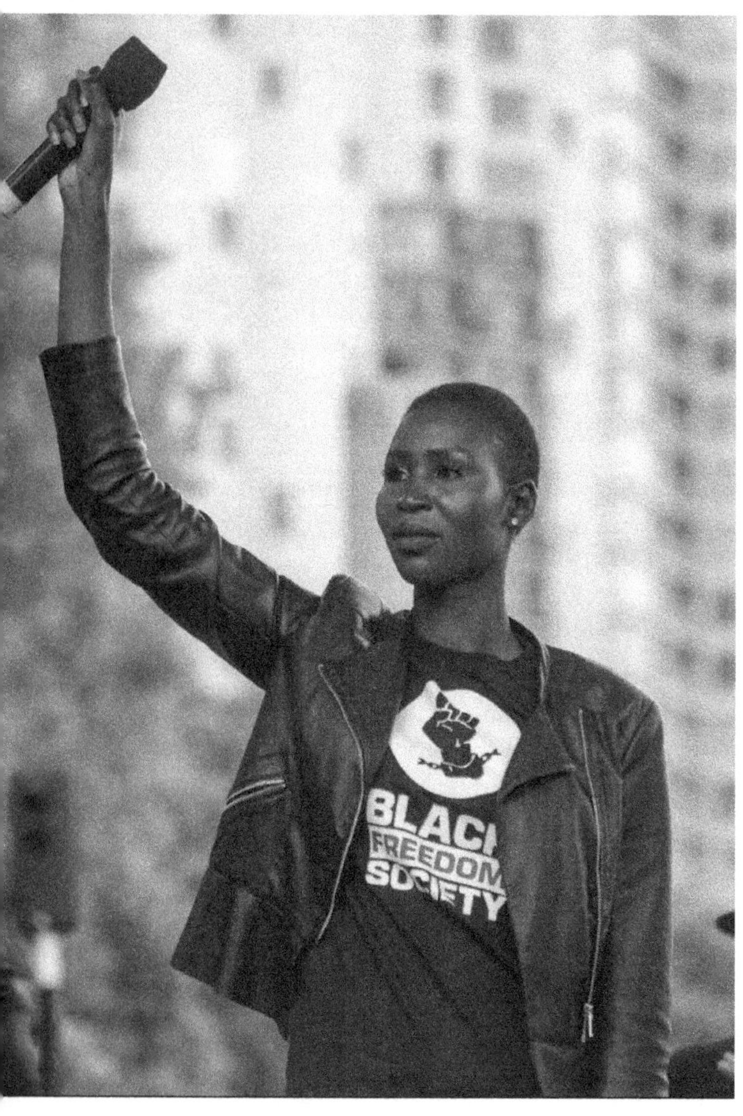

Nova Stevens is a Sudanese Canadian model, actress, activist, and Miss Universe Canada 2020. She will represent Canada at the upcoming Miss Universe competition. Nova is SuperNova!

Nova Stevens

At the tender age of six, my family decided to send me to Canada with my teenage cousin. Growing up without my family I had to learn to navigate life quickly. Life forced me to grow, I had no choice.

Between living alone at fifteen, being a student-athlete, working a job so that I could provide for my family back in Africa, I didn't have time to get into trouble. I guess I have life to thank for that. Experience, in my opinion, has been the best teacher; life has taught me the importance of resilience. I've always known I had to work hard at whatever it is I do, after all, it's through hard work that you find success, they say. As I've gotten older, I've learned that the key to success wasn't only hard work, it was a combination of hard work, perseverance, positive thinking, and faith in oneself. It wasn't until I mixed these ingredients together, that I started to see my goals and dreams come to fruition.

One of the most pivotal moments in my life happened in 2020. With the pandemic, we've experienced drastic changes in the way that we live life. I'm sure we can all agree that 2020 was a difficult year, however, 2020 helped me find my voice. Upon hearing, seeing, and reading about the innocent black people lose their lives to police brutality and hate crimes, I couldn't find it in myself to remain silent. This led to me and Shamika Mitchell co-organizing a black lives matter march in the middle of a pandemic, bringing together 5,000+ people. We all have the ability to invoke change. All you have to do is use the power that you have; your voice. My voice led me to win a beauty pageant I once thought would never happen because I wasn't your stereotypical beauty. My voice taught me the importance of fighting for myself and others. My voice taught me my worth. I encourage you to use your voice because you too are worth fighting for.

Brandy is a seeker, a multipotentialite who loves, lives, and plays hard.

Brandy Kawulka

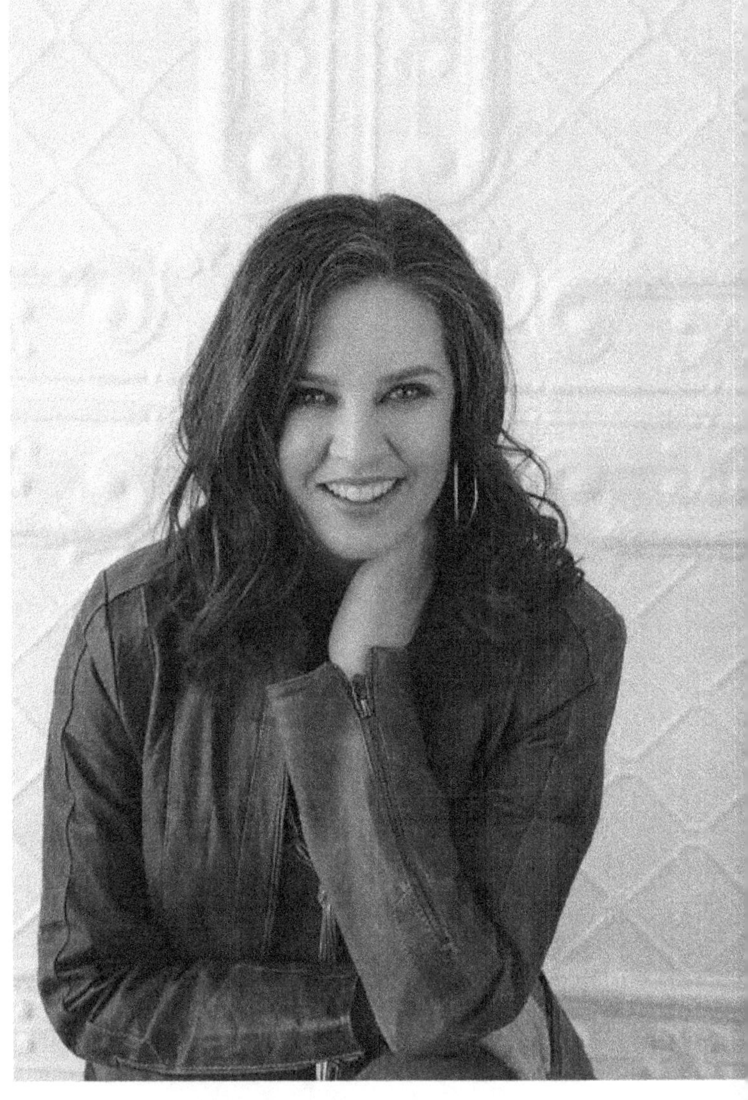

As a fun-loving and hard-working person, I'm fiercely and fearlessly in search of the unique and unusual, and always ready to celebrate life at a drop of a hat. Why accept the mediocre if you don't have to? Why let fear dictate your path? Why not be an instrument of joy and love?

I am many things; a friend, sister, mom, wife. I am also a female general contractor. In this, I know that I'm a rare sight. My path to this role is a Flashdance story in reverse. A ballet dancer turned woodworker (and then entrepreneur). A 180-turn from a feminine to a very masculine field with all the stereotypical trimmings of bullying, misogyny, and offside behaviour that the trades offer along with decency in there too.

As an apprentice, I learned not to take things personally. The BS that goes on even today, was more about "them" than me – it still is, and is so regardless of the color of collar you wear. I discovered that as long as I did my best and maintained a sense of humor, my integrity, and self-worth were intact at the end of the day. What more could a girl ask for?

Today, I love what I do. Owning my own business and helping clients bring their home renovation dreams into reality and seeing the impact the results have on their day-to-day living is the intangible, priceless reward that warms my heart, keeps me rising each day, and striving to provide a renovation experience that clients will love.

I think that switch, that initial loss of my bunhead identity, allowed me to break free of the self-imposed shackles that keep us stuck not claiming our dreams, our voices, or our truth, and trust that I'd always find the way forward be it through success or failure.

On this day, the last of the year, I would encourage us all to embrace the things that we want to do and achieve, the audacious dreams that we dare not speak of aloud. We are not only what we do but the choices we make.

Be Bold Beautiful

Co-Author Directory

Except where indicated, all contact information listed are website and instagram addresses.

A

Adera Angelucci	aderaangelucci.com	@aderaangelucci
Adina Neufeld	adinaneufeld.com	@adinasocial
Adrienne Gear	readingpowergear.com	@readingpowergear
Alana Collins	alanacollinsfitnesscoach.com	@agingfearless
Alana Walker Carpenter	intriciti.ca	@intriciti
Alanna Falys	primetuitive.com	@primetuitive
Alexis Gail Ellis	alexisgailellis.com	@alexis777cdn
Alice Grey	iheartfatfudge.ca	@iheartfatfudge
Alisha Schilbe	Enquire with Book Publisher	
Allana Polo	polohealth.com	@polohealth
Allison Patton	ardourwellness.ca	@allisonleepatton
Alyson Jones	alysonjones.ca	@alysonjonesassociates
Amaal Ebrahim	amaal4real.com	@amaal4real
Amanda Asta	transcendwithbreath.com	@transcend.breathwork
Amanda Cox	Enquire with Book Publisher	
Amanda Da Silva	Amanda-DaSilva.com	@amanda.da_silva
Amanda Doucette	shtb-law.com	@tax.chick
Amanda Lavery	cocabee.com	@cocabeeinc
Amber Spence		@amberlynnspence
Amélie Thuy Nguyen	anhandchi.com	@anhandchi
Ami McKay	purebyamimckay.com	@puredesigninc
Amy Spadafora	ueinc.ca	@ueinc
Andrea Fehsenfeld	andreafehsenfeld.com	@acf_creative
Andrea Ross	andreamross.com	@andrea.m.ross
Angela Calla	countoncalla.ca	@angelacallamortgageteam
Angela Campagnoni		@angelacampagnoni
Angela Feser	socialblissblueprint.com	@socialblissblueprint.com
Anik Thibaudeau		@doremibraceletsetc
Anna Wynn	unapologeticstories.com	@unapologeticanna
April May Bellia	aprilmaybellia.com	@aprilmaybellia
Ashley Hassard	drawbox.ca	@TheHassard
Asiza Demetrian	asiza.ca	@asizart
Ava Lee Millman Fisher	creatavalee.net	fb: Creatavalee

B

Barbara Edie	barbaraedie.com	@barbaraedie
Barbara Wallick	barbwallick.com	@barbaraswallic
Beth Hall	lionsgatecounselling.com	
Betty Lam	@Betty_Glam_Boutique	@Itsbettylam
Beverley Boone	bevboone.com	@bevboone.realtor
Bif Naked	bifnaked.com	@bifnakedofficial
Blair Kaplan Venables	blairkaplan.ca	@blairfromblairland
Brandy Kawulka	woodbeart.com	@wood.be.art
Brenda Wong	mvmagency.ca	@mvmagency

C

Caitlyn Vanderhaeghe	kidstarnutrients.com	@kidstarnutrients
Cara Thien	aaxll.com	@carathien
Carmel Ecker	speaknowcoaching.com	@carmelecker
Carmelia Rey	carmeliaray.com	@CarmeliaRay
Caroline MacGillivray	carolinemacgillivray.com	@caroline_macgillivray
Cate Giannousopoulos		@cate.giannousopoulos
Catherine St Germain		@catherine.stgermain.33
Catherine Trotzuk	Enquire with Book Publisher	
Cathy Cena	fdtacademy.com	@cathycena
Cathy Derksen	inspiredtenacity.com	
Cathy Kuzel	cathykuzel.com	@cathykuzeltcw
Charlene Luedke	twitter: shebuffoon	
Charlene Scott	Enquire with Book Publisher	
Charlotte Espeth Hill		@elsieannevintage
Chelsea Cooper	greatlakeslaw.ca	
Cheryl Bodnar	cherylspaint.com	@cherylspaint
Cheryl Brewster	theintuitivelife.com	Facebook:TheIntuitiveLife
Cheryl Hughes	Enquire with Book Publisher	
Chloe Angus	chloeangus.com	@chloeangusdesign
Chrissie Bettencourt	chrissiebettencourt.com	@chrissiebettencourt
Chrissy McRoberts	dogeatdog.ca	@dogeatdogsarnia
Christina Rose	christinarose.co	@christinarose

Christina Weizman	pivotalconcepts.com	
Christine Awram	aWomanOfWorth.com	twitter: womanofworthwow
Christine Monaghan	christinemonaghan.com	@stress_is_optional
Cindy Van Arnam	cindyvanarnam.com	@cindyvanarnam
Colleen Kirk	kirkgroupmedia.com	@kirkgroupmedia
Connie Peters	helloconniepeters.com	@xoconniepeters
Corinne DiPietro	corinne-dipietro.squarespace.com	@corinnekdipietro
Courtney Powell		@courtneylaurap
Crystal Bonnet	crystaldawnculinary.com	@crystal_dawn_culinary
Crystal Carson	crystalcarson.ca	@crystalcarson.ca

D

Dale-Lynn Desabrais	fraserfinancial.com	
Daniella Fisher	naturallygiven.com	@naturallygiven
Danielle Arsenault	pachavega.com	@pachavega
Danielle MacLean	dcllaw.org	@dcllaw
Danielle Menzel	realestatepemberton.com	@pembertonbcrealestate
Dannica Lamoureux		@dannicadots
Daria Bunting	idare-yadesigns.ca	
Dawn Chubai	dawnchubai.com	@dawnchubai
Dawn Reid	zenwand.com	@mala.zenwand
Dawn Williams	Enquire with Book Publisher	
Dayo Alabi	fb: fashionavenueNW	@daahyoo_bc @bivdancechallenge
Deanna Rose	deannawrose.com	@deannawrose
Deb Lohrenz	2motiv8u.com	
Debbie Bromley	extraeffortlandscaping.com	
Debra Schubert	sabr33n.le-vel.ca	
DeeAnn Lensen	deeannlensen.com	@dlensen
Denise Dupre	roamgallery.com/denise-dupre	
Denise Mai	denisemai.com	@denisemai_realestate
Denise Wong	dsquaredgroup.ca	@dsquaredconsulting
Diane Lacaille	arthritisresearch.ca	
Diane Rolston	dianerolston.com	@CoachDianeRolston
Diane Webster	cuervoboutique.ca	@cuervoboutique
Dianne Watts		@diannelwatts
Dina Podolsky	dinapodolsky.com	@dina.podolsky
Divi Chandna	drdivi.com	@drdivi
Donelle Clarke	silverfinchjewelrydesign.com	@donelle.clarke

Donica Canova	DonicaCanova.com	@donicacanova
Donna Giraud	donnagiraudart.com	@donnagiraudart
Donna West	yoyomama.ca	@yoyomama

E

Elaine Tan Comeau	easydaysies.com	@elainetancomeau
Elisa Kurylowicz	elisaunfiltered.com	@elisakurylowicz
Elise MacDonald	tebua-macrame.myshopify.com	@tebua
Ellen Bradley-Cheung		@ellenart
Emilie Fantuz	emiliefantuz.com	@emiliefantuz
Esther Topaz	esthertopaz.com	
Estrellita Gonzalez	estrellitagonzalez.com	@dermabright
Evelyne Nyairo	elliebianca.com	@elliebiancabeauty

F

Farzana Jaffer Jeraj	farzanajafferjeraj.com	@farzanajj
Faydra Aldridge	bcss.org	@bcschizophrenia
Fiona Forbes	fionaforbes.com	@fionaforbes

Gabriela Trujillo	fb: byspeakyourtru	@speak.your.tru
Genicca Whitney	globalgoddess.co	
Gladys Loewen	Enquire with Book Publisher	
Golfo Tsakumis	golfoart.com	@golfoart_
Grace Lanuza	thegracefiles.com	@itsmegracel

H

Hannah Fletcher		@hannahfitness
Heather Haslam	www.truespirithealingarts.org	@heather haslam
Heather Haynes	heatherhaynes.com	@heather_haynes_artist

Heather Nightengale		@hnightingale1
Heather Odendaal	wnorthconnect.com	@wnorthconnect
Henrietta Devine	tagulan.com	@tagulan
Hillary Samson	samsonconsulting.ca	
Hoai Dang-Lachance	hoainotart.com	@hoainotart
Holly Decker	hollydecker.com	@hollydeckermakeupartist
Holly Skyy		@holly_skyy

Inez Cook	salmonandbannock.net	@Salmonnbannockbistro
Iris Mes-Low	irismes-low.com	@iris.mes.low.art
Isabelle Mercier	leapzonestrategies.com	@leapzone.strategies

J

Jacinta Sarpkaya		@farrahkayaartwork
Jackie Diy	everiathing.com	@everiathing
Jacqueline Fowler	@guerajacquelina	
Jacqueline Woywitka	healthyheartcoachjakki.org	@healthyheartcoachjakki
Jacquie Stebbings	jacquiestebbings.com	@northvan.mom
Jan Rankin	janrankin.com	@jan_rankin
Jana Lee Maclagan	jana4faces.com	@jana4faces
Jane Stoller	organizedjane.com	@organizedjane
Janet Pliszka-Hughes	visualhues.com	@janet_pliszka
Janey Ganson	mydaughterfragrance.com	@mydaughterfragrances
Janice Skoreyko	rawfoodfoundation.org	@janiceskoreyko
Janine Jones	janinejones.ca	@jjonesart
Jann Arden	jannarden.com	@jannarden
Jannette Salvador		@enhancing.simplicity
Jen Govier	myhux.ca	@livein_themoment_
Jenn Luebkert	encoreoffice.ca	
Jennifer Daerendinger	roamgallery.com	@roamgallery
Jennifer Harper	cheekbonebeauty.com	@cheekbonebeauty
Jennifer Henczel	inspiredinfluencers.com	@jennifer.henczel

Jennifer Italiano	liveorganicfood.ca	@liveorganicfood
Jennifer Podemski	jenniferpodemski.com	@jenniferpodemski
Jenny Gough	jennygough.com	@jenny.a.gough
Jenny Wun	jennywun.com	@wunhaus
Jessica Buchanan	1000flowers.ca	@1000flowersperfumer
Jessica DiCaprio	sudioninety9.ca	
Jessica Marola-Hugh	wearecatalyst.ca	@wearecatalystmarketing
Jessica Rae	artistjessicarae.com	@ArtistJessicaRae
Jessica Séguin	jessicadawncoaching.com	@jessicadawncoaching
Jessie Lyon	pokoloko.com	@pokolokoltd
Jiali Kimoto		@jialikimotoessentials
Jill Earthy	womensenterprise.ca	
Jill Ganton	addyandcoedesigns.ca	@addyandcoedesigns
JoAnn Fowler	mysappho.ca	@my_sappho
Joanne Patenaude	etsy.me/2P1rfe8	@joanne_f_patenaude
Joanne Turnball		@joannatmojo
Jodi Takhar	familiesdorecover.com	@familiesdorecover
Jodie Emery		@jodieemery
Jonica van Rikxoort	teritalesproductions.com	@teritalesproductions
Joy Peirson	joypeirsonart.com	@joypeirsonart
Judy Doduk	judydbeauty.com	@judydbeauty
Julia Oosterman	bluewaterhealth.ca	@julia.oosterman
Julie Bernard	julieheatherphotography.com	@julieheather12
Julie Drapeau	puritylife.com	@jd_girlpower
Julie Kim	juliekim.ca	@kooliejim
Julie Samant	Facebook: Chiffon Boutique By Julie Samant	

Karen Angelucci	birthrightinvestment.com	
Karen Cliche	@karencliche	
Karen Kristjanson	beyondlimitscoaching.com	
Karen Lee	glou.co	@gloubeauty
Karen Reid Sidhu		@kreidsidhu
Katayoon Webb	katayoonwebb.com	@katayoonwebb
Katherina Taylor	Enquire with Book Publisher	
Katherine Dines		@KatherineDines
Katherine McEachnie	Katherinethegrape.com BCWineworld.com	@katthegrape
Kathy Swift	kathyswift.com	@kathy_swift_artist

Katie Allan	katie.allan@kiewit.com	linkedin.com/in/katie-allan-a10063b0/
Katie Fuller	thefoxandhound.ca	@foxandhoundcanineretreat
Kelly Arsenault	Enquire with Book Publisher	
Kelly Mallinson	kellymallinson.com	@kelly_mallinson
Kelly Trerise	glossboudoir.com	@kellytrerise
Khadija Jiwani	simplyoffice.ca	@simplyofficevan
Kim Appelt	stylebykimxo.com	@stylebykimxo
Kim Chhay	doesthisbaby.blogspot.com	@doesthisbaby
Kim Drury		@kimdrury15
Kim Page Gluckie	truthandtonic.com	
Kim Vopni	vaginacoach.com	@vaginacoach
Kimberley Payne	fb: kimberley.payne.798	@kimberpayne
Kimberly Dolan		@kimberlydolanmusic
Kristal Barrett Stuart		@kristalbarrett
Kristin Hazzard	lawrenceandco.com	fb: LawrenceAndCo1
Kristina Matisic	kmcreative.ca	@kristinamatisiccreative
Kristy Powers	kristypowersphotography.com	@kristypowersphotograpy
Krystal Gabriel	krystalgabriel.com	
Krystal Lunardo	dauphine.ca	@dauphinemagazine
Kym Klopp	ecoexistence.ca	@ecoexistence
Kyra Wong	magicalunicornproject.com	@magicalunicornproject

L

Laura Branson	laurabranson.com	@laurabranson
Laura Burns	flexiblelifecoach.com	@withlauraburns
Laura Lee Lofgren	turningpointz.ca	@yourturningpointz
Lauren Labas	vancouverwinefestivals.com	@vancouverwinefestivals
Leanne Myles	tteamclinton.ca	@halifaxmortgage
LeiLani Kopp	sweetleilani.com	@sweetleilanicosmetics
Leslie Diamond	womenmovingmillions.org	
Lia Murrain	buggysnuggle.com	@liamurrain
Lily Ling	lilydoesmakeup.com	@lilydoesmakeup
Lily Yuan	lilyyuanartstudio.com	@lilyyuanartstudio
Lily Zhao		@lilyzhaoxx
Linda Bickerton-Ross	bickerton-rossphotography.com	@bickertonrossphotography
Linda Mackie	lindamackie.ca	@lindamackiecreative
Lisa Blake	Enquire with Book Publisher	
Lisa Chan	trufelle.com	
Lisa Holly	lisaholly.ca	
Lori Burke	fickledesignsartstudio.com	@loriburke3667

Lori Joyce	betterwith.com	@betterwith
Lorna Vanderhaughe	lornahealth.com	@lornavanderhaeghe
Lorraine Zander	faze.ca	@fazemagazine
Lynda Honing	theurbanoasis.info	@theurbanoasisblooms
Lynda Manson	lyndamanson.com	
Lynda Moffat	lyndamoffatt.com	@artist.lynda.moffatt
Lynda Turner	zengarry.com	@zengarryveg
Lynne Roy	elleroy.ca	@elleroyconsulting

M

Madeleine Marentette	grailsprings.com	@madeleine_marentette
Mandi Sellers	icldgroup.com	
Marcela Bahar	whitesquirrelgolfclub.com	@whitesquirrelgolfclub_
Margarita Romano	leapzonestrategies.com	@leapzone.strategies
Maria DeCotiis	mariadecotiis.com	@maria.decotiis
Maria Kritikos	ladieswholunchnetwork.com	@lunchwithmaria
Maria Velve	greenbeautyexpert.ca	@greenbeautycurator
Mariah Owen	gteproductionsinc.com	@mariahowen
Mariana Carneiro	@kajucreations.com	@kajucreations
Marika Houston	Enquire with Book Publisher	
Marilyn Wilson	marilynrwilson.com	@marilynrwilson
Marisa Pothier	honestcleaningandservices.com	@onestcleaningandservices
Mary Daniel	Enquire with Book Publisher	
Mary Lynn Fluter	fluterfineart.com	@marylynnfluter
Mary Painter	Enquire with Book Publisher	
Mary Zilba		@maryzilba
Marzena Skowronski	greenenvycosmetics.com	@greenenvycosmetics
Marzia Bellotti Molatore	mammamarzia.ca	@bellacibo
Maxine Cunningham	pickmybrain.world	@pickmybrain_ceo
Mélanie Bernard	minitipi.ca	@mini.tipi
Melanie Phillips	madhurimethod.com	
Melissa Deally	yourguidedhealthjourney.com	@guidedhealthjourney
Melissa Rosas		@violetdaecommunications
Melissa Wormington	Enquire with Book Publisher	
Mellisa Mills	spreademkitchen.com	@spreadem_kitchen
Mercedes Blanc		@sadie_ashley
Michaelee Lazore	sequoiasoaps.com	@sequoiasoaps
Michaella Shannon	michaellashannon.com	@michaella.shannon

Michele Partridge	yourconfidencecoach.ca	@mpartridgeconfidencecoach
Michelle Abraham	amplifyou.ca	
Michelle Chapin	campyhome.com	@campyhome
Michelle Epstein	elleondemand.com	@ellefitnessto @ellefitmichelle
Michelle Fedosoff	Enquire with Book Publisher	
Michelle Kam	michelle-kam.com	
Mishel Schwartz	mishelschwartzart.com	@mishelart2
Missy Mackintosh	missymackintosh.com	@missymackintosh
Monika Tupholme	monikatupholme.com	@monika_tupholme

N

Nahla Hopfe		@nahlahopfe
Natali Harea	natsbreadcompany.com	@natsbreadco
Natasha Reay	bloomelix.com	@nraey
Nazanin Afshin-Jam	nazanin.ca	
Nicola Arndt	Enquire with Book Publisher	
Nicole O'Keefe	otwgraphix@gmail.com	
Nina Bains	Enquire with Book Publisher	
Nisha Khare	nishakhare.com	@nishakhare
Nova Stevens		@thenovastevens

Olivia Repnicki	crystalobsessions.com	@crystalobsessionsbyolivia
Oresta Korbutiak	oresta.ca	@orestaorganics
Oyeta Kokoroko	okokocosmetiques.com	

Paddy Meade	paddymeade.com	@meade52
Patricia Heart Clum	evolutionoftheheart.com	@evolutionheart
Patricia Lapena	patricialapena.com	
Patricia Wilson		@fearflying
Paula Castellon	hipaula.ca	@hipaula.ca
Paula Lyons	gustochocolates.ca	@lifewith_gusto
Paula Skaper	kinetixdigital.ca	@paula.sk_official

Randa Derkson	randaderkson.com	@randanutrition
Randi Winter	paradise2perfection.com	@live_thep2plife
Rebekkah Stainton	westcoastvitality.com	@westcoast_vitality
Renée Chan	truenosh.com	@truenosh
Robin Farr	robinfarr.neora.com	@fitnessfarr22
Robyn Marshall	mementomoristudios.ca	@robynmarshalltattoo
Roseanne Parke	beyouthfulco.com	@beyouthfulco
Rosie Abigail Smith		@rosieabigailsmith
Roz McLean		twitter: rozzyrozmclean
Rycarda Smith	Enquire with Book Publisher	

S

Sam van Born	samvanborn.myalovea.com	@samvanborn
Samantha Brazeau-Wilson	birchjewellery.com	@birch.jewellery
Sandra Pike	thepikegroup.ca	@dealsinheels.halifax
Sara Nishi	illoleather.com	@illoleather
Sarah Jansel	sarahjansel.com	@sarahjansel
Sarah Khan	linchpin.virtual	@linchpin.virtual
Sarah Zoschke		@_sarahlouz
Senator Mobina Jaffer	mobinajaffer.ca	
Shana Recker	shanarecker.com	@quantumleapqueen
Shantel Taylor		@innershantiheals
Sharon Sloane	Enquire with Book Publisher	
Sharon Storoschuk	cranialsacralvancouver.com	@sharonstoros
Sheila Neufeld	sheilaneufeld.com	@sheilaneufeld
Shelby Kargl	weedance.com	@weedance2
Shelley Essery	revivedinteriors.com	@revivedinteriors
Shelly Smee	oakwyn.com	@residentgenius007
Sherice Langedahl-Kirby	sherrice.ca	@studiosherrice
Sherry Downes Sobey	generationgreenwpg.com	@sherry_sobey
Sherry Kallergis	atfortyfive.com	@atfortyfivemag
Sherry Klassen	roamgallery.com	@sheklas
Shirley Weir	best-of-menopause-chicks-2020.square.site	@menopausechicks
Simona Gozner	being49onthe49thparallel.blog	
Siobhan Coates	@siobhans_sparkup	fb: sparkupyourlifewithlaughter

Spencer O'Brien	@arthritisresearch	@spencerobrien
Stacey Wells	artistwells.net	@artistwells
Stephanie Barnes	stephaniebarnesdesign.com	
Stephanie Gust	benessehealth.com	@benessehealth
Stephanie Lehr	stephanielehr.ca	@stephanielehrofficial
Styawat Leigh Joseph	skwalwen.com	leighjoseph.com
Sue Clement	sueclement.com	@velocityinbusiness
Summer Dhillon	slapcommunications.com	@slapcommunications
Susan Greig	susanlgreigfineart.com	@susanlgreigart
Susan McCart	suzeinteriors.ca	@suzeinteriors
Susie Doré	joyridebranding.com	@joyridebranding
Suzanne Aujla	Valkofinancial.ca	@suzanne_fleurdelysaujla
Suzanne Carter	myocosmeticcases.com	@ecomyocase @myocosmeticcases
Suzanne Sendel	theoriginalftg.com	@theoriginalftg

T

Talia Beckett Davis	fempreneur.com	@taliadavispr
Tamara Barker Watson	whitestonedevelopments.ca	@xwhitestonebuilders
Tamara Spence	tamaraspencefineart.com	@tamaraspenceart
Tammy Bailey	roamgallery	@the_art_of_tammy_bailey
Tammy McNabb	tammylynnmcnabb.com	@tammylynnmcnabb
Tanya Farlinger	exhalo.ca	@exhalospa
Tanya Horne	tanyahorne.com	@sitdownstandupcomedian
Tanya Slingsby	tanyaslingsby.com	@tanyaslingsby
Tara Lavoie	taralavoie.com	@taralavoiedesign
Tawnya Ritco	tawnyaritco.com	@tawnyaritco
Teresa Phillips	paintontario.com	@paintontario
Teresa Simmonds	teresasimmonds.com	
Theresa Lambert	theresalambertcoaching.com	@theresalambertcoaching
Tiffany Reid	tiffanyreidart.com	@tiffanyreidart
Tina Llewellyn	imaginetruehealth.com	@imaginetruehealth
Tina Marie Springham		@tinamariespringham
Tina Richardson	Enquire with Book Publisher	
Toni Desrosiers	abeego.com	@abeego
Tonia LaRiviere	Enquire with Book Publisher	
Tori Dolmans	mortgagebytori.com	@mortgagebytori
Tosca Reno	toscareno.com	@toscareno
Tracy Donald	tracydonald.ca	
Tracy Valko	tracyvalko.ca	@thevalkoteam
Trisha Pitura	minitipi.ca	@mini.tipi

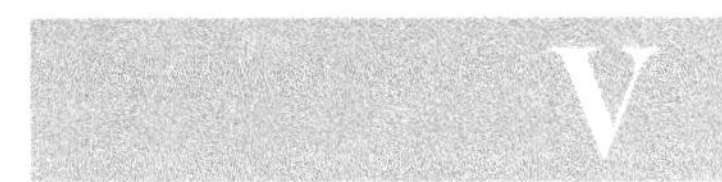

Name	Website	Social
Valerie Blackstock	valerieblackstock.com	@blackstinova
Verna Bohn	curvesisfashion.com	@curvesisfashion
Vicki Saunders	sheeo.world	
Victoria Kirsten Theriault	facebook.com/VictoriaDISC	

Z

Name	Website	Social
Zahra Efan	zahraefan.com	@zahraefan

Pursuit 365

Ann Kaplan	@annkaplan_ownit
Andreia McLean	@andreiavanessaa
Shelly Lynn Hughes	@shellylynn.hughes
pursuit:365	@pursuit_365

www.ingramcontent.com/pod-product-compliance
Lightning Source LLC
Chambersburg PA
CBHW080912190726
48294CB00009B/2065
9781777612412